Thoracic Surgery

Surgical Procedures on the Chest and Thoracic Cavity

Edited by
H. Pichlmaier and F.W. Schildberg

Foreword by
David B. Skinner

Translated by T.C. Telger

Contributors
U. Demmel, R. Grundmann, H. Hamelmann, H. Hofmann
Th. Junginger, E. Kiffner, J.M. Müller, H. Pichlmaier
F.W. Schildberg, M.H. Schoenberg, M. Thermann, R. Thoma
M.M. Wanke, K. Zilles

With 343 Figures in 763 Separate Illustrations
and 15 Anatomic Color Plates (Inside Back Cover)

Springer-Verlag Berlin Heidelberg NewYork
London Paris Tokyo Hong Kong

Professor Dr. Dr. H. PICHLMAIER
Chirurgische Universitätsklinik
Köln-Lindenthal
Joseph-Stelzmann-Str. 9
D-5000 Köln 41

Professor Dr. F.W. SCHILDBERG
Chirurgische Universitätsklinik
Klinikum Großhadern
Marchioninistr. 15
D-8000 München 70

Title of the German Edition: Thoraxchirurgie
(Volume VI, Part 1 of Kirschnersche allgemeine und spezielle Operationslehre,
edited by H. PICHLMAIER and F.W. SCHILDBERG)

Softcover reprint of the hadrcover 1st edition 1989

Library of Congress Cataloging-in-Publication Data. Thoraxchirurgie. English. Thoracic surgery: surgical procedures on the chest and thoracic cavity/edited by H. Pichlmaier and F.W. Schildberg; foreword by David B. Skinner; translated by Terry C. Telger; contributing authors, U. Demmel ... [et al.]. p. cm. "Translated form Kirschnersche allgemeine und spezielle Operationslehre, Band VI, dritte, völlig neubearbeitete Auflage, Teil 1: Thoraxchirurgie" – T.p.verso. Includes bibliographies and index. ISBN (invalid) 0–540–18464–3 (US). 1. Chest–Surgery. I. Pichlmaier, H. (Heinz) II. Schildberg, F.W. (Friedrich W.) III. Demmel, U. IV. Title. [DNLM: 1. Thoracic Surgery. WF 980 T48725] RD536.T4913 1989 617'.54059–dc19 DNLM/DLC for Library of Congress 89–4208 CIP

Illustrations: Jörg Kühn and Rüdiger Himmelhan, Heidelberg; Julius S. Pupp, Arnstein, Irene Schreiber, Köln

ISBN 978-3-642-48989-1 ISBN 978-3-642-83256-7 (eBook)
DOI 10.1007/978-3-642-83256-7

List of Contributors

U. DEMMEL, Dr., Anatomisches Institut der Universität Köln, Joseph-Stelzmann-Straße 9, D-5000 Köln 41

R. GRUNDMANN, Prof. Dr., Chirurgische Universitätsklinik Köln-Lindenthal, Joseph-Stelzmann-Straße 9, D-5000 Köln 41

H. HAMELMANN, Prof. Dr., Chirurgische Universitätsklinik, Abteilung Allgemeine Chirurgie, Arnold-Heller-Straße 7, D-2300 Kiel 1

H. HOFMANN, Ltd. Krankengymnastin, Chirurgische Universitätsklinik Köln, Joseph-Stelzmann-Straße 9, D-5000 Köln 41

Th. JUNGINGER, Prof. Dr., Chirurgische Klinik und Poliklinik der Johannes-Gutenberg-Universität, Postfach 3960, Langenbeckstraße 1, D-6500 Mainz

E. KIFFNER, Priv.-Doz. Dr., Medizinische Universitätsklinik, Klinik für Chirurgie, Ratzeburger Allee 160, D-2400 Lübeck 1

J.M. MÜLLER, Prof. Dr., Chirurgische Universitätsklinik Köln-Lindenthal, Joseph-Stelzmann-Straße 9, D-5000 Köln 41

H. PICHLMAIER, Prof. Dr. Dr., Chirurgische Universitätsklinik Köln-Lindenthal, Joseph-Stelzmann-Straße 9, D-5000 Köln 41

F.W. SCHILDBERG, Prof. Dr., Chirurgische Universitätsklinik, Klinikum Großhadern, Marchioninistr. 15, D-8000 München 70

M.H. SCHOENBERG, Dr., Chirurgie I, Universität Ulm, Steinhövelstraße 9, D-7900 Ulm

M. THERMANN, Prof. Dr., Klinik für Allgemein- und Thoraxchirurgie der Städtischen Krankenanstalten Bielefeld-Mitte, Akademisches Lehrkrankenhaus, Oelmühlenstraße 26, D-4800 Bielefeld 1

R. THOMA, Prof. Dr., Krankenhaus der Augustinerinnen, Innere Abteilung, Jakobstraße 27–31, D-5000 Köln 1

M.M.WANKE, Chirurgische Universitätsklinik, Operationsabteilung, Joseph-Stelzmann-Straße 9, D-5000 Köln 41

K. ZILLES, Prof. Dr., Anatomisches Institut der Universität Köln, Joseph-Stelzmann-Straße 9, D-5000 Köln 41

Foreword

It is a great pleasure and honor to be asked to participate in the translation of this important and historical volume on thoracic surgery and to provide this foreword. Martin Kirschner of Mannheim/Heidelberg was an early pioneer in thoracic and esophageal surgery. His operation for bypass of the esophagus using the entire stomach remains a standard of the surgical armamentarium to this date. The original Kirschner Textbook of Surgery was a standard in its day. We are fortunate that Professors H. Pichlmaier and F.W. Schildberg and other colleagues have provided us with this important modern successor of a classic textbook.

The reader is rewarded by an extensive treatise which includes not only the most up to date techniques in pulmonary, esophageal, mediastinal, and chest wall (including breast) surgery but also provides an excellent perspective on the techniques used by pioneers in the field. Although some of these early techniques are not commonly used today, knowledge of their use and application broadens the capability of the thoracic surgeon. Changing times bring renewed problems with infectious diseases. Knowledge of the management of the pleural space and pulmonary infectious problems is a critical part of the education of the thoracic surgeon.

The illustrations in this book are detailed and helpful. They provide a broad spectrum of useful technical information for a thoracic surgeon. The text is extensive and describes procedures, indications, complications and their management in great detail. This volume is a major contribution to the world literature on thoracic surgery and marks the revitalization of an important school of non-cardiac thoracic surgery in Germany which has provided us with so many pioneers in the specialty.

New York

DAVID B. SKINNER

Preface

The last thoracic volume of the surgical text series begun by M. Kirschner and continued by R. Zenker was published in 1967. That year marked the end of a lengthy postwar period during which German surgery was again able to attain the international standard. Many questions of surgical methodology were resolved, and new procedures were developed and applied clinically. The editors of the last volume sought to detail those procedures and make them accessible to the surgical community.

In the past two decades, noncardiac thoracic surgery has been concerned less with the development of fundamentally new operative methods than with the refinement and standardization of existing procedures. This has shifted the emphasis away from spectacular innovation toward safety and the anticipated postoperative status of the patients undergoing chest surgery. Risk assessment and limitation, prognostic assessment, and an individualized approach to patient selection have become matters of increasing concern for surgeons and have led to a dramatic reduction in operative risk. Significant improvements have also been seen in late functional results.

Surgery of the esophagus has been expanded by the development of techniques for the transfer or free grafting of bowel, and it has been enriched by the rediscovery and perfection of esophagectomy without thoracotomy. Advances in long-term parenteral alimentation have been a major factor in these developments.

Operations on the lung and especially on the tracheobronchial tree have been refined and individualized by the perfection of special ventilation and intubation techniques as well as suturing techniques using absorbable materials

Systematic mediastinal lymph node dissections have become an indispensable part of carcinoma surgery.

In operations for malignant breast disease, new insights into tumor biology and the introduction of effective adjunctive treatment modalities have shifted the emphasis away from ultraradical surgery toward less mutilating operations that conserve greater amounts of breast tissue.

This development and its results prompted the editors and publisher to create an up-to-date version of the thoracic volume. It was our intention not only to cover the points mentioned above but also to present a range of surgical treatment options and then weight those options on the basis of personal experience. True innovations relating, for example, to microsurgical techniques or advances in anesthesiology and perioperative management are described in detail. It was our special wish to advance the systematization of standard procedures while touching on organizational aspects (instrument layouts, etc.) that facilitate the conduct of surgical operations. Finally, we considered a thorough knowledge of anatomy to be an essential prerequisite for every surgeon. The publisher has made every effort to accommodate the authors' wishes in the production of this book.

We are grateful to all those who have made it possible for this book to be published in such a relatively short time. We convey special thanks to Springer Verlag and especially to Mr. Bergstedt for his always obliging and helpful support and advise. We acknowledge the great skill, insight, and patience of our illustrators, Misters Kuhn, Himmelhan and Pupp and Mrs. Schreiber. Special thanks go to the translator, Mr. Terry C. Telger, for providing a fluent and concise version of the German text.

Köln
München

H. Pichlmaier
F.W. Schildberg

Contents

A. Functional Operability in Thoracic Surgical Procedures

R. THOMA

CONTENTS

1 Physiologic and Pathophysiologic Considerations

The bronchopulmonary system, like most other organ systems in the body, possesses a significant functional reserve. This is most apparent during exercise, when the pulmonary tidal volume and oxygen consumption can increase by a factor of 10–20 over basal values. Under normal conditions exercise tolerance is limited not by the bronchopulmonary system, but by the cardiovascular system. Respiratory limitation generally is seen only in advanced diseases involving the bronchial system, the lung parenchyma, or the pulmonary vascular system. Exercise limitation due to problems of respiratory mechanics may be presumed to exist when the absolute value of the one-second forced expiratory volume (FEV_1) is less than 800 ml [8]. This lower limit must be considered, therefore, when predicting residual postoperative function after pulmonary resection. A vital capacity of approximately 15 ml/kg body weight represents another critical value, with lower values implying, at the least, pulmonary exercise limitation [13].

Critical values for pulmonary gas exchange are more difficult to define due to the importance of adaptive mechanisms in this component of lung function. Studies in patients with pulmonary sarcoidosis have shown that if the diffusion capacity of the lung for CO falls to 40% of normal or less, exercise intolerance with pulmonary hypertension will exist in the majority of cases [12]. With regard to arterial blood gases, a PCO_2 exceeding 50 mm HG and a PO_2 less than 50 mm Hg are usually indicative of exercise intolerance. Generally these values are seen only when there is a severe impairment of respiratory mechanics which by itself is sufficient to limit exercise tolerance.

It is even more difficult to establish a critical value for pulmonary hemodynamics that would imply exercise limitation. The reserve capacity of the pulmonary vascular bed is exhausted when a mean perfusion pressure of about 30 mm Hg is reached [10]. If this value is reached under resting conditions, it is certain that exercise limitation exists. A loss of hemodynamic reserve is assumed when the exercise pulmonary artery pressure rises to 40 mm Hg at a mild level of exertion (1/2–1 W/kg body weight).

Questions of exercise tolerance are of crucial importance in potential candidates for pulmonary resection, because an inaccurate assessment of the patient's functional reserves can leave him a respiratory cripple after the surgery. Preoperative tests of pulmonary function center on the parameters that correlate most closely with performance. The foremost of these in terms of respiratory mechanics are the vital capacity and the FEV_1, whose determination requires a high level of patient cooperation. The alternative in less cooperative patients is to assess the pulmonary compliance and airway resistance. These values do not represent capacities, however, and so the prognosis is less certain.

The functional reserve for gas exchange can be assessed by determining the diffusion capacity for CO. Determination of the arterial oxygen pressure can be misleading in terms of predicting postoperative function, because shunts created by tumors can sustain a hypoxemic state.

In summary, the vital capacity, FEV_1, and exercise pulmonary artery pressure may be considered the most reliable indicators of pulmonary function in potential surgical candidates.

2 Function Studies for Assessing Operability

2.1 Thoracic Procedures without Pulmonary Resection

Even in thoracic surgical procedures that do not involve the removal of lung parenchyma, the function of the respiratory organs will be compromised at least temporarily during and after the operation. Generally this functional impairment persists for no more than 3–6 months after the thoracic surgery [7]. Pulmonary dysfunction is of minor significance in cardiac operations, for often it reflects only the extent of the hemodynamic compromise. As hemodynamics improve after the cardiac procedure, generally there will be full recovery of the patient's preoperative respiratory function.

Operability considerations for thoracic surgery without pulmonary resection follow the same general guidelines that apply to other surgical procedures, especially abdominal. The pulmonary parameters of greatest interest are also the simplest: the vital capacity and the FEV_1. The absolute value of FEV_1 is especially useful, for it represents a summation of airway obstruction, airway instability, restriction, and the level of patient cooperation. If both of these functional parameters are found to be normal, it is unnecessary to perform additional tests of respiratory mechanics. This does not apply to the parameters of gas exchange, however. One should at least obtain a blood gas analysis under resting conditions to get a baseline for predicting postoperative defects of gaseous exchange. If the vital capacity and FEV_1 deviate from normal by more than 20%, further differential pulmonary function tests should be conducted.

If evidence of airway obstruction is found, the airway resistance should be determined if possible using body plethysmography. The airway resistance measured by this technique provides a sensitive and objective basis for planning bronchospasmolytic therapy. This method is excellent for predicting functional improvement and estimating the time of optimum response. The oscillometric measurement of airway resistance is also useful in directing bronchospasmolytic therapy and enables respiratory mechanics to be quantitated even in less cooperative individuals. If there is evidence of pulmonary restriction (low vital capacity with a normal relative FEV_1) or airway obstruction, the effect of the impaired respiratory mechanics on gas exchange should be determined by analyzing the glood gases at rest and during ergometric exercise. The ergometric study yields information on the gas exchange reserves and also gives an impression of the patient's circulatory and metabolic work capacity. If the blood gas analysis during ergometry shows significant deviation from normal values ($PACO_2 > 45$, $PAO_2 < 60$ mmHg), the hemodynamic effect should be evaluated by measuring pulmonary circulatory parameters, and appropriate treatment should be instituted.

The following guidelines may be applied when utilizing the FEV_1 as an index of operative risk:[1]

1. $FEV_1 < 0.8$ l: High anesthetic and operative risk. Indication for operation must be urgent. Resting arterial blood gas analysis is performed for further risk assessment; generally exercise cannot be tolerated.
2. $FEV_1 > 0.8$ l, < 2.0 l: Increased risk. Arterial blood gases should be measured at rest and during exercise (work rate increased by 25 W/2 min to about 50% of maximal capacity) for further risk assessment. If the $PACO_2$ rises above 45 mmHg and the PAO_2 falls below 60 mmHg, surgery is justified only if the indication is urgent. Supplementary measurement of pulmonary circulatory hemodynamics is advised.

In cases 1 and 2, airway obstruction should be excluded or, if present, optimally treated.

3. $FEV_1 > 2.0$ l: The operative risk is not increased, but in patients with a history of asthma or dyspnea attacks, hyperreactive airways should be excluded by provocative testing with acetylcholine, carbachol, or histamine.

[1] Based on the recommendations for preoperative pulmonary function testing of the German Society for Pneumology and Tuberculosis [6].

2.2 Thoracic Procedures Involving Pulmonary Resection

Not only must the global function impairment be known in this type of operation, but the location of the functional defect within the bronchopulmonary system must be ascertained. It must be determined whether the defect is ipsilateral, i.e. involving the lung that is to be operated, or contralateral (e.g., in patients with a complicating condition like emphysema, pleural thickening, tuberculosis, or embolism). Preoperative risk assessment, therefore, must rely on regional function testing-generally by perfusion scanning of the lungs with a quantitative comparison of both sides. Besides the pulmonary functional status, special attention must be given to the cardiac status in lung resections, as the loss of parenchyma will diminish the reserve capacity of the pulmonary capillary bed. Because of this loss of reserve capillaries, a postoperative expansion of the intrapulmonary blood volume will be more likely to precipitate an interstitial or alveolar pulmonary edema. It is imperative, then, that a cardiologic evaluation be done to exclude left heart failure. Besides special physical and radiologic studies of the cardiovascular system, including a resting and stress ECG, the pulmonary capillary pressure should be measured in patients who report dyspnea on exertion and angina pectoris. A previous myocardial infarction (within the last year) constitutes a relative contraindication to pulmonary resection. A history of myocardial infarction within six months before the contemplated surgery is considered to be an absolute contraindication.

Pulmonary resections should leave the patient with a postoperative vital capacity of 1500 ml and a FEV_1 of about 1000 ml, since lower values would imply cardiorespiratory insufficiency at mild levels of exercise. The immediate postoperative vital capacity should be no less than 15 ml/kg body weight, since lower values generally signify a need for prolonged ventilatory support [13]. The collective statistical data of several authors indicate that vital capacity is reduced by about 60% in the first weeks following pneumonectomy and by 20%–60% following lobectomy. In contrast to pneumonectomy, the functional deficit after lobectomy usually shows marked improvement (to less than half the initial deficit) within the first six months after surgery [7].

2.2.1 *Assessing Candidates for Pneumonectomy*

By following a prognostic scheme based on the FEV_1, the perfusion scan, and the exercise pulmonary artery pressure, it is possible to keep the postoperative mortality rate well below 10% following pneumonectomy or extended pneumonectomy [6].

A knowledge of additional pulmonary functional parameters such as residual volume, arterial oxygen tension, and airway resistance is less important for determining operability than for selecting appropriate pre- and postoperative therapeutic measures (broncholytics, O_2 therapy, respiratory training).

The significance of preoperative hypoxemia should not be overestimated in candidates for pneumonectomy, because deficient oxygen saturation can result from venous admixture through tumor-created shunts that will be eliminated by surgery. The prognostic scheme based on FEV_1, the perfusion scan, and the exercise pulmonary artery pressure satisfies the demand for a definitive postoperative FEV_1 of approximately 1 liter and for an acceptable rise in the pulmonary artery pressure during exercise. It should be noted that the absolute values cited in the prognostic scheme are only guidelines, and that individual values may deviate somewhat in either direction. This applies both to the FEV_1, which may be as low as 800 ml postoperatively without causing a prohibitive rise in mortality, and to the exercise pulmonary artery pressure, which may rise less after surgery than predicted.

A safety factor in this regard is the slight rise in the cardiac output during exercise and concomitant rise in the Hb level that are consistently observed after surgery [9].

While there is general agreement on the safe lower range for FEV_1 in pneumonectomized patients (800–1000 ml), reports vary regarding the behavior of the pulmonary artery pressure after lung resections. While Konietzko and his group claim that a rise of the pulmonary artery pressure above 45 mmHg during exercise contraindicates surgery, the follow-up data of a group of Swiss surgeons suggest that functional inoperability exists when the pressure reaches the range of 35–40 mmHg at an exercise rate of 40 W [3].

Because pneumonectomy offers the only hope of cure for most patients, the goal of preoperative evaluation should be to maximize the number of patients referred for resective surgery. The withholding of curative surgery on grounds of functional inoperability must be based on highly persuasive data. Thus, operability considerations in patients with airway obstruction should always take into account the FEV_1 after maximal broncholytic therapy, since the greater preexpansion of the remaining lung makes it likely that the airway obstruction will regress after the pneumonectomy. When assessing the hemodynamic risk, it also may be assumed that the reserve capacity of the pulmonary capillaries not open at rest will be sufficient to absorb a portion of the expected postoperative pressure rise in the pulmonary vascular system. Thus, in patients who have borderline exercise pressures in the pulmonary circuit (around 40 mmHg), it is advisable to simulate the postoperative status before surgery by occluding the main pulmonary artery branch supplying the lung that is to be removed. This makes it possible to investigate selectively the circulatory and gas-exchange reserves of the remaining lung [11]. This knowledge gives the surgeon a high degree of confidence that the success of the operation will not be jeopardized by the development of cardiopulmonary insufficiency. Daum et al. [1] advise testing the pulmonary circulation at rest and after exercise, with and without occlusion of the main pulmonary artery branch to the operative side, before every pneumonectomy, for it is common during occlusion to see a rise of pulmonary capillary pressure that correlates with an accompanying arterial hypoxemia. These authors believe that exercise testing with occlusion of the affected main pulmonary arterial branch should be routinely done before every proposed pneumonectomy to safeguard the patient against left heart failure developing postoperatively. We are unable to recommend pulmonary artery occlusion as a routine measure, because it is not without risk for the patient, and because severe postoperative exercise hypoxemia is a relatively uncommon occurrence. We believe that the test should be restricted to patients whose exercise pulmonary artery pressure reaches the upper tolerance limit of about 40 mmHg.

It has been found that pneumonectomy patients selected by the indices discribed above are well able to tolerate mild levels of exercise following their surgery. Moreover, they are not at increased risk for the accelerated development of a cor pulmonale.

2.2.2 *Assessing Candidates for Lobectomy*

In contrast to pneumonectomy, where functional recovery is slight during the months following the operation, lobectomy (or bilobectomy) may be followed by a disproportionately severe ("early") function loss occurring immediately after the surgery, or by a much less severe ("late") function loss seen after a period of about six months [7]. Thus, it is necessary to consider both an immediate and a late effect when assessing candidates for lobectomy or bilobectomy. Understandably, the postoperative function loss cannot be predicted as accurately as it can for pneumonectomy.

When patients are selected according to the prognostic scheme and given suitable postoperative management, the postoperative mortality rate is lower than 2%.

2.3 Thoracic Procedures to Improve Respiratory Function

2.3.1 *Decortication*

Pleural decortication is done to improve respiratory dysfunction caused by a residual empyema cavity, bronchopleural fistula, or scoliosis of the thoracic spine. An indication for this procedure exists when:

1) the vital capacity is 30% or more below the desired value,
2) perfusion of the affected lung half is decreased by more than 50% according to the perfusion scan, and
3) the "trapped" lung below the pleural peel is still intact and able to expand (bronchography!) [6].

2.3.2 *Bullectomy*

Patient selection for bullectomy demands careful preoperative function testing due to the very high rate of postoperative complications that is associated with generalized pulmonary emphysema, the leading cause of bulla formation. The procedure is appropriate only when:

1) there is little or no demonstrable airway obstruction during quiet respiration (as measured by body plethysmography),

2) perfusion scanning shows that the bulla occupies more than 50% of the affected hemithorax and is compressing "healthy lung", and
3) the contralateral lung shows no significant perfusion defects.

A single-stage bilateral thoracotomy for bilateral involvement should be contemplated only if it will provide a decompressive effect that will improve function [6].

2.3.3 Tracheal Stenosis, Tracheal Dyskinesia

Pulmonary function tests in tracheal stenosis are able to localize the site of the stenosis (intra/extrathoracic), establish its severity, and monitor any changes. The clinical or bronchoscopic diagnosis of tracheobronchial dyskinesia or tracheomalacia must be confirmed by careful pressure, flow, and volume measurements during quiet and forced respiration before "operative stabilization" of the major airways is justified.

The best technique for establishing the site of a tracheal stenosis is body plethysmography. An S-shaped resistance loop in this study is characteristic of extrathoracic stenosis, a club-shaped loop signifies an intrathoracic stenosis, and an egg-shaped loop signifies stenosis of a main bronchus. Simultaneous measurement of the residual volume with body plethysmography makes it possible to differentiate stenoses of the major airways (residual volume not increased) from generalized respiratory tract diseases (residual volume increased).

Body plethysmography can also quantitate the severity of the stenosis, especially with extrathoracic lesions. Increased airway resistance is measurable when the lumen of the trachea decreases to about 8 mm or less, and a massive resistance increase is apparent when the tracheal lumen is smaller than 5 mm [2, 5]. Stenosis to less than 4 mm increases the airway resistance by more than a factor of 15 and poses an acute risk of asphyxiation. Since a rise in airway resistance is measurable when the diameter of the tracheal lumen is 8 mm, surgical correction of the stenosis generally should be contemplated only when the lumen is substantially smaller. Conversely, a normal tracheal lumen is not an essential goal of tracheal reconstructive surgery [5].

3 Appendix

3.1 Calculation of Postoperative Pulmonary Function

Flowchart for identifying patients at risk[1]

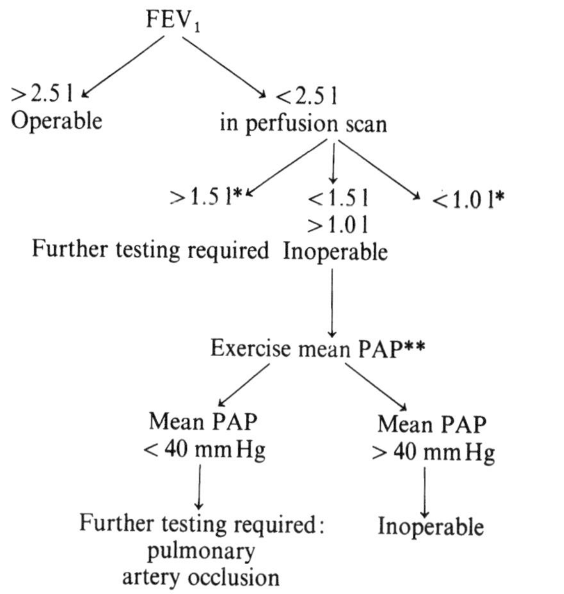

[1] Modified from Recommendations on Preoperative Pulmonary Function Testing. Prax Klin Pneumol 37:1199 (1983).

* Calculated postoperative FEV_1 (a semiquantitative assessment based on the evaluation of perfusion scans in four projections by an experienced examiner or an exact calculation of the fractional loss over areas of interest yield comparable results).

** Mean PAP = mean pulmonary artery pressure at a mild to moderate level of exercise (50–70 W).

Calculation of Postoperative Pulmonary Function [6]

$$FEV_1\ \text{postop} = FEV_1\ \text{preop}\ \frac{100 - A - k \times B}{100} \quad \text{(I)}$$

FEV_1 postop = forced expiratory volume calculated for the early postoperative period

FEV_1 preop = FEV_1 measured preoperatively

A = perfusion of the resected specimen as % of total lung

B = perfusion of the rest of the operative side as % of total lung

k = 0.37, a constant for the early postoperative period

The preoperative FEV_1 is determined by spirometry. A and B are calculated by scanning over areas of interest.

Example
A 56-year-old man has a malignant coin lesion in the right upper lobe. His preoperative FEV_1 is 1.4 l. Perfusion scans show an absence of perfusion in the right upper lobe that is to be resected, and the remaining perfusion of the right lung is 40% of the total lung perfusion. For an upper lobectomy, we calculate

$$FEV_1 \text{ postop} = 1.4\,\frac{100-0-0.37\times 40}{100} = 1.19\ \text{l}$$

The calculation for a pneumonectomy would be:

$$FEV_1 \text{ postop} = 1.4\,\frac{100-40-0.37\times 0}{100} = 0.84\ \text{l}$$

The calculations indicate that lobectomy would pose an increased but acceptable risk in this patient, while the risk of pneumonectomy would be prohibitively high.

References

1. Daum S, Goerg R, Mack D, Horbacher A (1979) Hämodynamische Untersuchungen bei einseitiger temporärer Okklusion der Pulmonalarterie. Herz 1:47
2. Dragojevic B, Buess G, Thoma R, Klaschik E, Pichlmaier H (1980) Probleme der Indikation und Beatmung bei Segmentresektion der Trachae. Langenbecks Arch Chir 351:99
3. Keller R, Kopp C, Zutter W, Mlczoch J, Herzog H (1976) Der Lungenkreislauf als leistungsbegrenzender Faktor bei Patienten. Verhandlungen der Gesellschaft für Lungen- und Atmungsforschung. Ulmer WT (Hrsg). Springer, Berlin Heidelberg New York
4. Konietzko N (1981) Lungenfunktionsprüfung. In: Hamelmann H, Troidl H (Hrsg) Behandlung des Bronchialkarzinoms, Symposium Kiel 1970, Thieme, Stuttgart New York
5. Konietzko N, Petro W (1980) Lungenfunktionsdiagnostik bei Stenosen im Bereich der großen Atemwege. Langenbecks Arch Chir 352:277
6. Konietzko N, Ferlinz R, Loddenkemper K, Magnussen H, Schlimmer P, Toomes H, v Wichert P (1983) Empfehlungen zur präoperativen Lungenfunktionsdiagnostik. Prax Klin Pneumol 37:1199
7. Schäfer P, Meyer Erkelenz JD, Effert S (1978) Lungenfunktion und Operabilität. Dtsch Med Wochenschr 102:123
8. Segall JJ, Butterworth BA (1966) Ventilatory capacity in chronic bronchitis in relation to carbodioxide retention. Scand J Resp Dis 47:215
9. Taube K, Konietzko N (1980) Prediction of postoperative cardiopulmonary function in patients undergoing pneumonectomy. Thorac Cardiovasc Surg 28:348
10. Thoma R, Pöhler E, Siemon G (1982) Pathophysiologie der Wechselbeziehungen zwischen kardiovaskulären und respiratorischen Funktionsstörungen. Med Welt 33:1330
11. Thoma R, Voigtmann R, Magnussen H (1980) Präoperative Diagnostik beim Bronchialkarzinom. Therapiewoche 30:6737
12. Widimysky J (1982) Pulmonale Hypertonie. Thieme, Stuttgart New York
13. Wolff G (1977) Die künstliche Beatmung auf Intensivstation. Springer, Berlin Heidelberg New York

B. Surgical Instruments, Materials, and Approaches

H. PICHLMAIER

CONTENTS

Surgical operations on the chest and chest wall and in the thoracic cavity require knowledge of many general and specialized techniques. The relatively poor accessibility of the thoracic cavity through the bony thorax requires the use of special positions to ensure optimum exposure with minimal trauma. To aid the operating team in organizing and preparing for thoracic procedures, we present the basic surgical techniques (of the approaches, etc.) along with the necessary materials and instrumentation. Besides possessing a knowledge of general surgical techniques, the operator must be experienced in vascular surgery, bone surgery, plastic surgery, and perhaps even microsurgery as well as in the use of modern stapling instruments. The list of necessary surgical instruments makes this clear.

1 Instruments for Thoracic Surgery

A thoracic operation can be made more efficient and less costly, and the work of the OR staff simplified, by making up basic instrument sets and extra sets that are selected according to the requirements of the procedure. With modern container systems it is possible to set up an exact program that will simplify handling, cleaning, sterilization, and sterile storage of the instrument sets. When implementing a container system of this kind, careful consideration must be given to the physical layout of the OR suite and the hospital practices that are followed (e.g., centralized or decentralized sterilization, large or small stock of sterile supplies, centralized or decentralized surgery department, separation of septic and aseptic areas, demands on sterilization service, etc.).

1.1 Basic Set

The *basic set* contains the instruments needed for every operation on and in the thorax. The components of the set are listed in the Appendix at the end of this chapter.

1.2 Extra Sets

The following *extra sets* have proven useful:

(1) Extra thoracic set
(2) Rib resection set
(3) Set for funnel chest and ribs
(4) Extra vascular set
(5) Pediatric set
(6) Thoracic vascular set
(7) ASIF small-fragment instrument set

In addition to these items, other special instruments, instrument sets, and supplies are kept in separate, sterile packages. They are listed at the end of the Appendix.

2. Materials

2.1 Materials for Asepsis

The materials needed for aseptic preparation of the operative field and for maintaining a sterile field during the operation include proper antiseptic solutions for the skin prep as well as towels, clamps, basins, and sterile gloves.

Conventional draping material consists of sterile towel drapes held in place with clamps, but it is preferable to use disposable drapes with an adhesive border, which come in various sizes. Incise drapes with full adhesive backing also may be used.

2.2 Special Materials Needed for Thoracic Surgery

See Appendix.

3 Positioning of Patient and Disposition of Operating Team

3.1 General

Positioning for intrathoracic surgery must make allowance for the frequent use of large incisions, the fact that the operative field is often distant from the chest tubes used to drain the pleural space, and that a combined approach (thoracocervical, thoracoabdominal, or even thoracoabdominocervical) may be required. Accordingly, the side of the chest to be operated must be freely accessible and unobstructed by pads or rests. The shave prep is performed on the unit and should include the axilla; if necessary the abdomen is shaved as far down as the symphysis. Care is taken during positioning that body parts, especially the arms, are insulated from metal parts of the operating table when diathermy instruments are used. Antiseptic solutions can create skin-metal contact, so a layer of absorbent cellulose should be placed

Fig. 1. Diagram of a patient in the full lateral position for a standard thoracotomy. The positions of the operating team are indicated

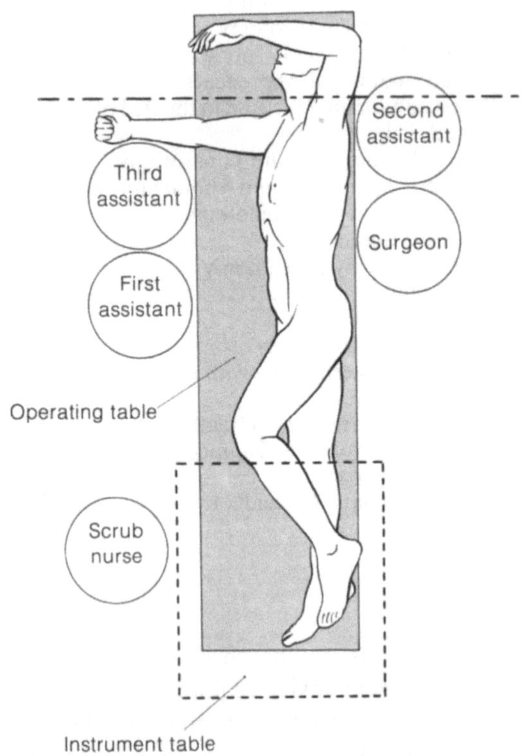

between the patient and the table when these solutions are applied. If the patient is on his side, it is customary for the surgeon to stand at the patient's back, with the first assistent standing opposite the surgeon, the second assistent next to the surgeon, and the third assistant opposite the second (Fig. 1). The patient's back should be even with the table edge so that the operative field is close to the surgeon.

3.2 Supine Position

The patient is secured in the supine position for anterior approaches, including the various types of sternotomy, and for blunt dissections involved in abdominocervical esophagectomy or subcutaneous and retrosternal esophageal reconstruction.

Fig. 2. The supine position for procedures on the cervical esophagus. The neck is slightly hyperextended, and the head is turned toward either side to give right- or left-sided access to the cervical esophagus. This may be combined with exposure of the abdominal esophagus or with retrosternal transposition of the colon. For the cervical exposure, the surgeon stands on the side that the patient is facing

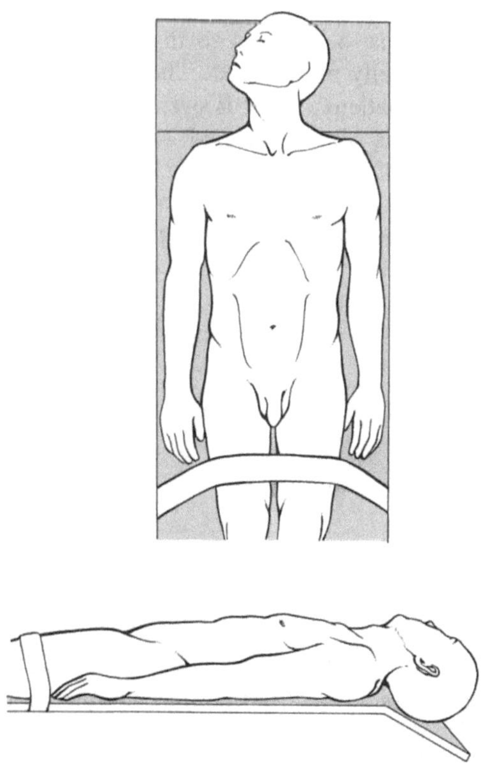

For exposure of the cervical esophagus, the head is hyperextended and turned away from the surgeon (Fig. 2). It is very useful in thoracic procedures, especially those extending up to the neck, to lengthen the infusion lines and place the patient's arms at his sides, since an abducted arm can be a hindrance when working on the neck. Suitable padding is provided. After the neutral electrode has been applied (usually a disposable adhesive electrode applied to shaved skin), a safety belt is placed above the knees, the arms are held to the table with braces, and the operative field is packed off in preparation for the final skin prep. This position does not differ from the standard supine position for abdominal operations.

3.3 Semilateral Position for the Anterolateral Approach

The anterolateral approach can be made from the right or left side, with the operative side elevated. The semilateral position can be effected in either of two ways:

3.3.1 On a Horizontal Table

For limited anterolateral exposures it is sufficient to elevate the thorax by placing a sandbag beneath the operative side. The pad can be secured by winding a gauze bandage around it, passing the bandage under the patient and securing it to the other side of the table (Fig. 3). The pelvis and lower extremities lie in the supine position. The arm on the operative side may be flexed over an arm rest or suspended over the patient's head on an anesthesia screen. Alternatively, the arm may be supported on a second arm rest introduced from the opposite side.

The pelvis is stabilized by placing a strap over the thighs, as it may be necessary to tilt the table laterally to obtain the best visualization of intrathoracic structures.

3.3.2 On a Tilted Table

The patient can be placed in a more lateral position by tilting the operating table toward the unaffected side and placing a brace behind the iliac crest to support the pelvis. The shoulder girdle is fixed by taping the arm to the anesthesia screen

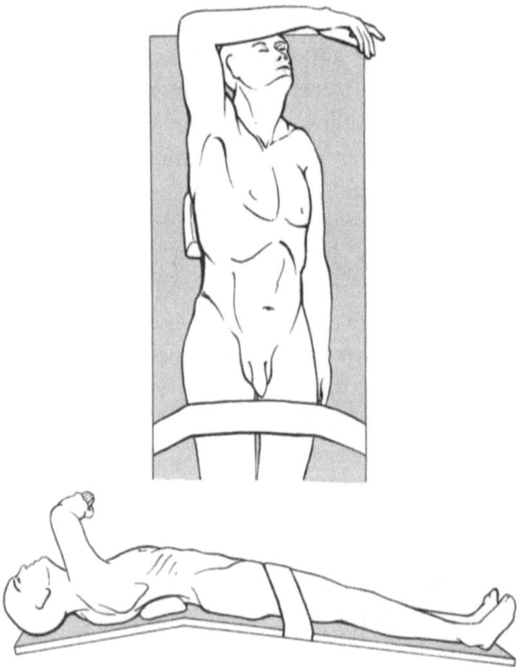

Fig. 3. Semilateral position for anterolateral thoracotomy. The patient is supine with the chest slightly elevated by a pad or sandbag on the operative side

(taking care to maintain insulation) or by supporting it on an arm rest as described above (Fig. 4).

While the pelvis is positioned approximately at right angles to the table surface, the upper body can be turned slightly away from the table by adjusting the position of the arm on the operative side. Special care is taken to avoid brachial plexus injury when this type of position is used. For both positions, the table is broken at the mid-thorax to hyperextend the upper part of the thorax and widen the intercostal spaces to facilitate surgical access. The operative field is moved to a comfortable position for the surgeon by tilting the table laterally toward either side.

3.4 Full Lateral Position

This position is used for the standard thoracotomy. The pelvis, thorax, and shoulder girdle are in a full lateral position. The pelvis is stabilized with a rest placed in front of the anterior iliac spine, and the arm is secured to the ether screen or a separate rest. Again, it is essential to break the table below the thorax. In all these positions the patient must be secured so that the table can be tilted laterally as required. The surgeon must see that the patient's back is even with the table edge, as this is often neglected and can increase the difficulty of the operation (Fig. 5). In all lateral and semilateral positions the lower leg is extended while the upper leg is flexed slightly at the hip and knee. A foam wedge is placed between the legs to protect pressure points.

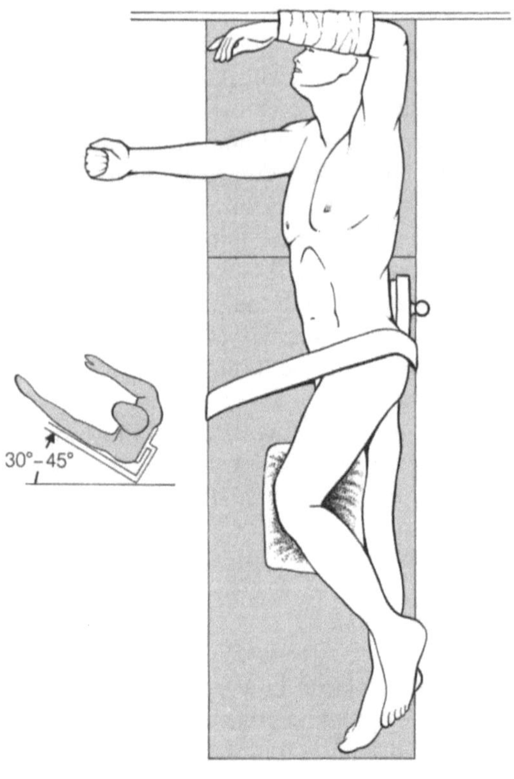

Fig. 4. Semilateral position for anterolateral thoracotomy. As an alternative to Fig. 3, the patient may be positioned on his side and supported so that he can be placed in an anterolateral position by rotating the table. The arm on the uppermost side is supported on a rest or taped to the anesthesia screen

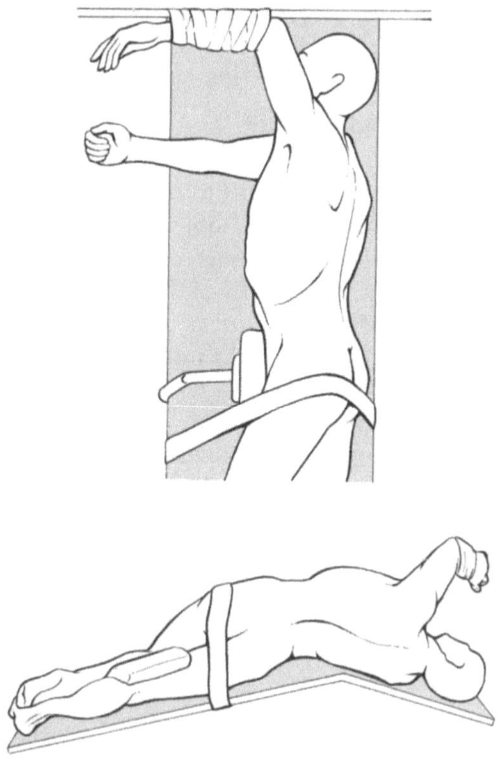

Fig. 5. Full lateral position with the table broken about 25° at the thorax

3.5 Positioning for the Posterolateral Approach

This position is similar to the full lateral position, except that the patient's upper body is turned toward the table to give a better view of the posterior aspect of the thorax. This is done by keeping the pelvis and legs in the full lateral position while rotating the abdomen and shoulder girdle slightly forward and securing the shoulders in that position. Access can be further improved by tilting the table to one side.

3.6 Prone Position

This position is used only exceptionally, as for exposing a lesion at the costal angle or between the costal angle and the spine at the level of the scapulae. A tumor arising from the ribs in this region or a neurogenic hourglass-shaped tumor requiring laminectomy and neurosurgical assistance could likewise be an indication for this unusual position. The prone position has been largely abandoned for exposures of the lungs. Today intratracheobronchial measures are used to prevent purulent secretions from entering the unaffected lung; special positioning is no longer necessary.

The prone position is effected by placing the patient on a table with an upper and central break (Fig. 6). We prefer to support the head on a special laminectomy pillow. The arms hug the head section of the table and are supported on rests. The head is appropriately fixed to avoid lordotic curvature of the neck. The patient is intubated while still supine and is then carefully turned onto the abdomen. The legs are slightly flexed at the hip and knee, and the table is adjusted to that position.

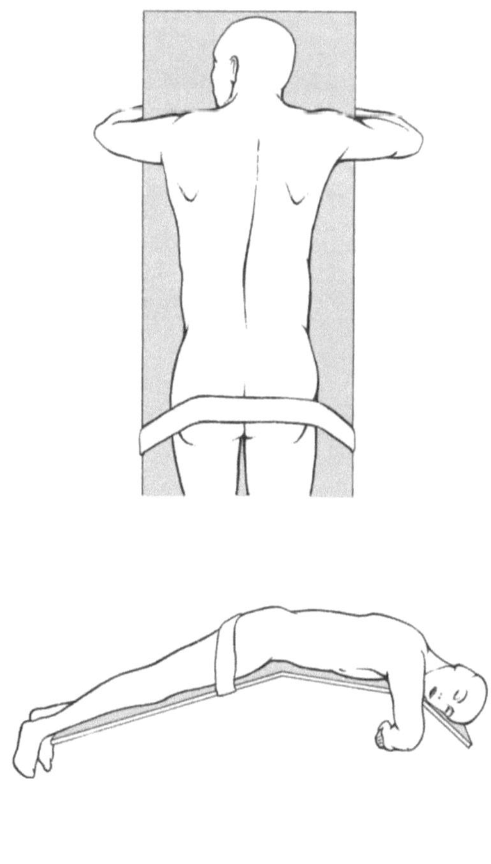

Fig. 6. The prone position. The table is broken at the neck and abdomen; the patient's arms are flexed about the table and supported. A laminectomy pillow is recommended to support the head

4 Standard Approaches to the Thoracic Organs

4.1 Standard Thoracotomy

This may be performed on the right or left side and opens the hemithorax from the costal angle to the sternal end of the intercostal space. The skin incision consists basically of three curved incisions (Fig. 7). Major landmarks are the angle of the scapula, the axilla, and the nipple; it is helpful to mark the tip of the scapula. The incision starts behind and above the angle of the scapula and passes down around the scapular border at a distance of about 2 cm from it. The incision swings fairly high up into the axilla and curves down along the lateral border of the pectoralis major muscle before turning back up to a point about 5 cm below the nipple in men. In women the inframammary fold is marked preoperatively with the patient erect, and the incision is carried along the inframammary fold to the sternal border. Next an electrocautery is used to divide the subcutaneous fat and secure hemostasis. In women it is usually necessary to mobilize the breast between the superficial thoracic fascia and subcutaneous fat so that the costal incision can be placed higher than the submammary incision. After division of the superficial thoracic fascia, the latissimus dorsi muscle is incised with the cautery in line with the cutaneous incision (Fig. 8). The entire serratus lateralis muscle is divided in similar fashion. At that point the angle of the scapula is freed from its distal soft-tissue attachments, and for a right-sided thoracotomy the surgeon can pass his left hand (or his right hand for a left-sided thoracotomy) beneath the scapula and identify the uppermost palp-

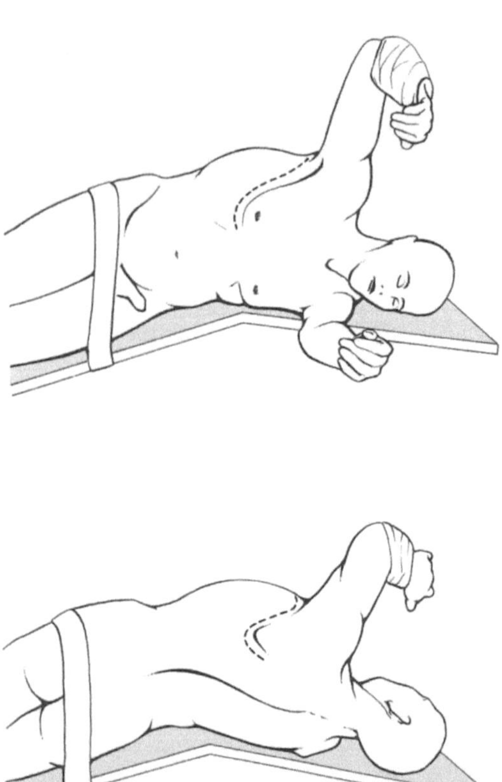

Fig. 7. The standard thoracotomy incision

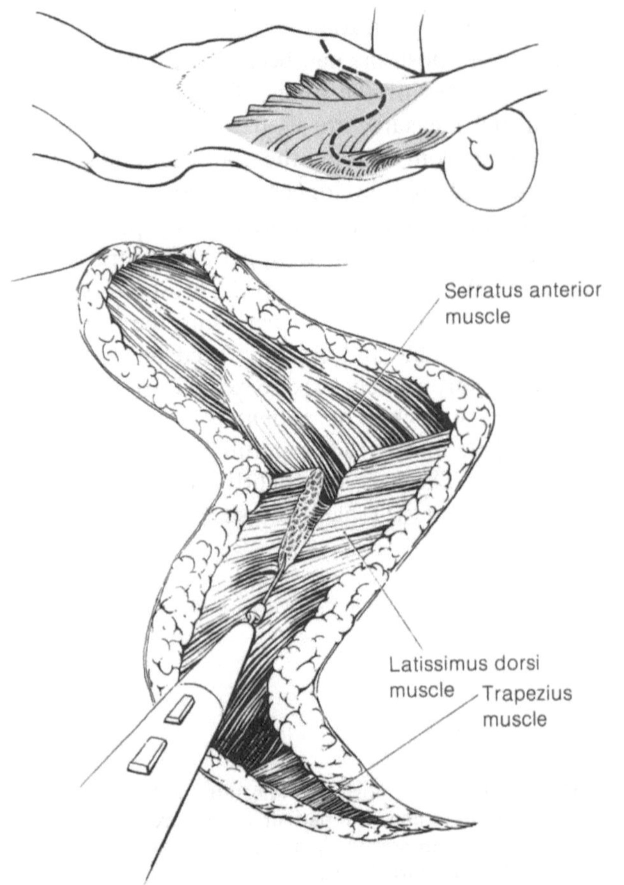

Fig. 8. Standard thoracotomy: The skin, subcutaneous tissue, and superficial thoracic fascia are divided. The latissimus dorsi muscle is divided to expose the serratus lateralis muscle, which also is transected

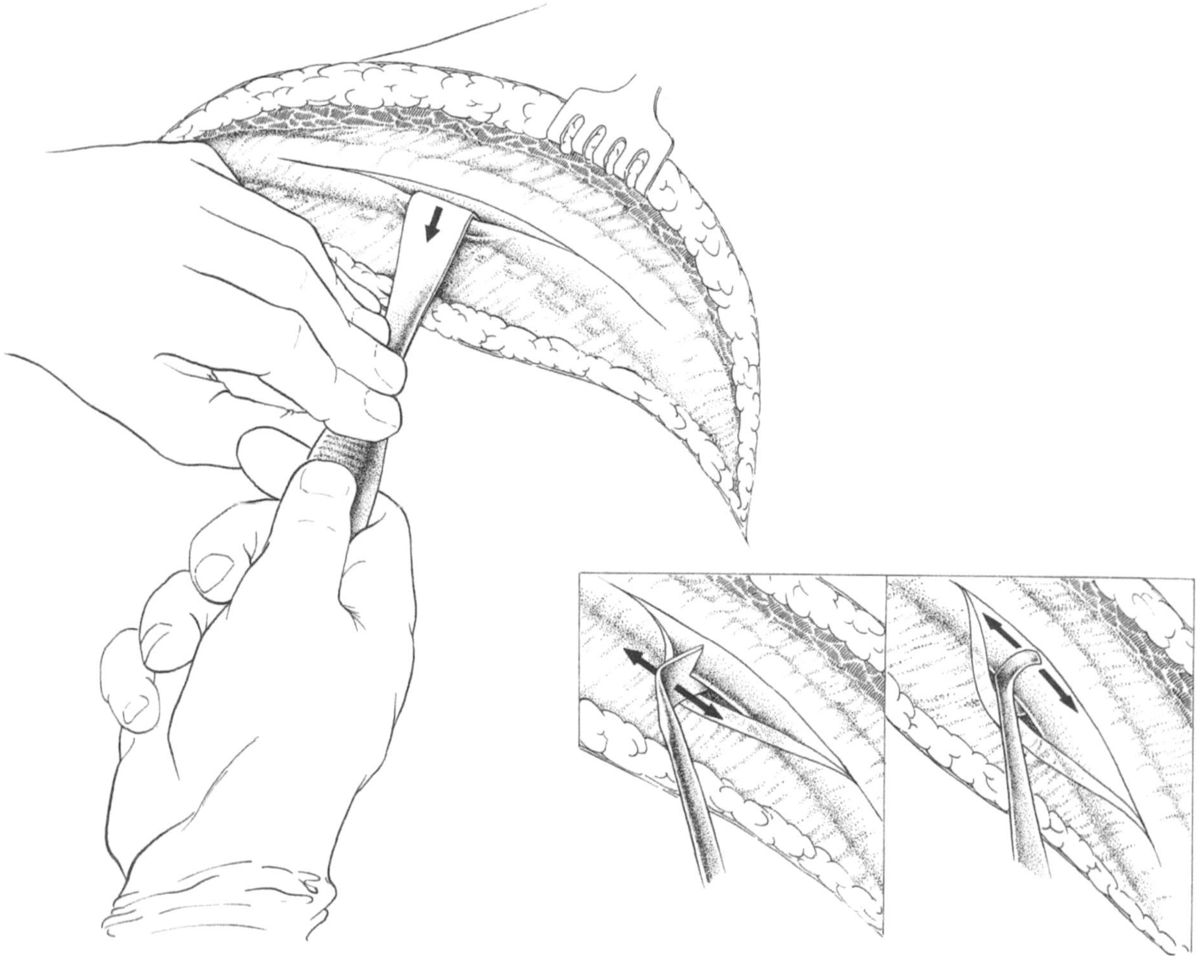

Fig. 9. Standard thoracotomy: The periosteum or perichondrium is stripped from the rib, sparing the intercostal vessels

able rib as the second rib. Depending on the type of disease anticipated, the scapula is now elevated, and the chest is opened in the bed of the fourth, fifth, or six rib. The upper rib bordering the incision is identified first. The overlying periosteum is incised with the cautery down the middle of the rib, and a raspatory is used to strip the periosteum from the bone; anteriorly the same technique is used to push the perichondrium back from the cartilage (Fig. 9), avoiding injury to the intercostal vessels. A Semb 1 raspatory is used to initiate stripping of the lower edge of the rib, and this is completed with a Semb 2. A Gaubatz rib spreader is inserted between the ribs adjacent to the proposed incision and slowly opened to place the intercostal tissues on stretch; the handle of the retractor points toward the surgeon (Fig. 10). Next the periosteum and parietal pleura are carefully incised with the scalpel at about the center of the rib bed. After about a 1-cm incision has been made, the anesthetist, who is ventilating the patient manually at this point, allows the lung to collapse once air has entered the pleural space. A sponge stick introduced into the chest protects the lung while the nonadherent parietal pleura and the periosteum of the rib bed are incised for the full length of the intercostal space. At this point the Gaubatz retractor is opened further, a plastic ring drape is laid down, and a Hegemann rib spreader is introduced. The Gaubatz retractor is now removed, taking care not to tear the plastic film, and the Hegemann spreader is opened until the desired exposure is obtained.

After completion of the intrathoracic procedure, the pleural space should be drained. One or two drainage tubes will be needed, depending on the nature of the operation. A single tube is

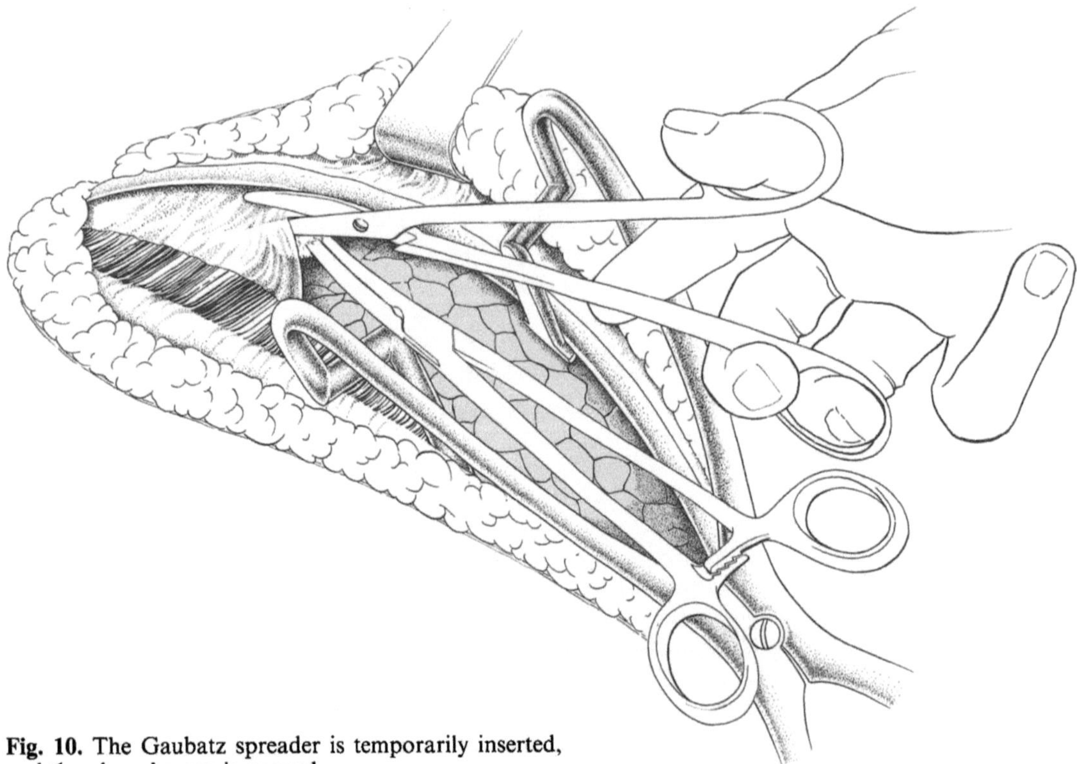

Fig. 10. The Gaubatz spreader is temporarily inserted, and the pleural space is opened

Fig. 11. a One or two pleural drains are placed before the thoracotomy is closed. **b** The upper drain is fixed in the apex of the chest

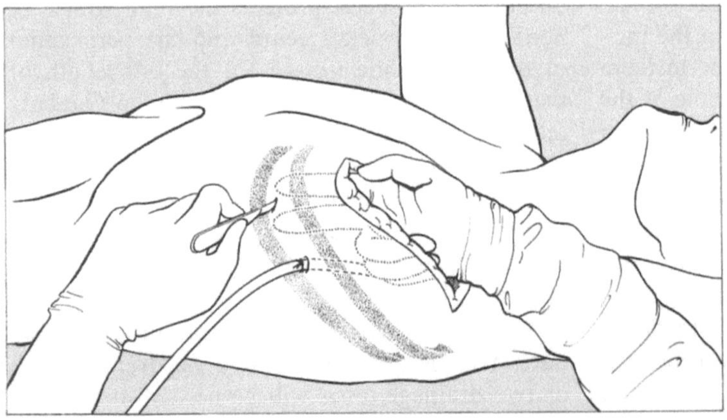
a

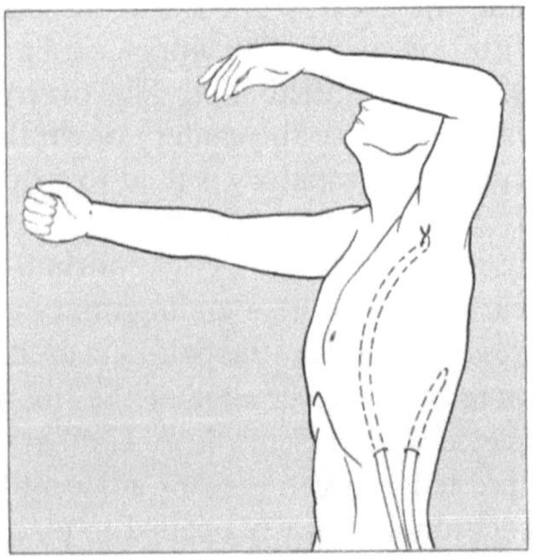
b

placed on the midaxillary line, or two tubes are placed on the anterior and posterior axillary lines and brought out through stab incisions spaced about 4 cm apart. The surgeon passes the hand that is closer to the patient's head into the deepest part of the phrenicocostal sinus and marks that point with the index and middle fingers; with the other hand he makes a 1 $^1/_2$-cm-long incision, following the skin lines, several centimeters below the sinus. A scissors is used to tunnel obliquely upward from the incision and open the pleural space over the palpating hand of the surgeon (Fig. 11a, b). Next a hemostat is introduced and is used to pull the rubber tubing out through the skin incision. This procedure is repeated if two drains are used. A single tube should drain the posteroinferior floor of the pleural cavity, for that is where fluid collects in the recumbent patient. When two drains are used, the anterior tube is placed as the procedure requires; after an upper lobectomy, for example, the tube is loosely fixed at the apex of the thorax with fine surgical gut so that it passes anteriorly over the hilus. Immediately afterward, skin sutures are placed to seal the tube sites. A purse-string suture is placed through the skin around the site so that when the tube is removed, the suture can be promptly tied to prevent air from entering the chest.

Fig. 12. Internal blockade of the intercostal nerve directly affected by the thoracotomy and of the adjacent nerves with a long-acting local anesthetic

After placement of the drains, the thoracotomy is closed in layers. First the intercostal nerve of the interspace is resected for a length of several centimeters at the level of the costal angle to prevent entrapment of the nerve by scar tissue and minimize scar pain. We additionally inject the intercostal nerves adjacent to the thoracotomy with a local anesthetic, as this will give several hours of postoperative analgesia (Fig. 12).

Next a suture of No. 2 absorbable material on a large round needle is passed down through the full thickness of the intercostal tissue at the lower edge of the incision. It is then passed into and out of the intercostal tissue above the upper adjacent rib and brought back out through the divided intercostal tissue (Fig. 13). A series of 8–12 of these sutures are placed, whereupon a Hegemann rib approximator is inserted and carefully tightened to close the intercostal space. A scissors is inserted temporarily to displace the rib above the incision beneath the inferior adjacent rib. This maneuver is made easier by partially eliminating the table break and suspending the "thoracic position." Then the sutures are individually tied to close the pleural space. The muscles that were divided during entry to the chest are reapproximated with 2-0 sutures in reverse sequence: first the pectoralis major and serratus lateralis, then the inferior part of the rhomboideus major, and lastly the latissimus muscle, the posterior fascia, and the border of the trapezius. The subcutaneous tissue and superficial fascia are reapproximated with 2-0

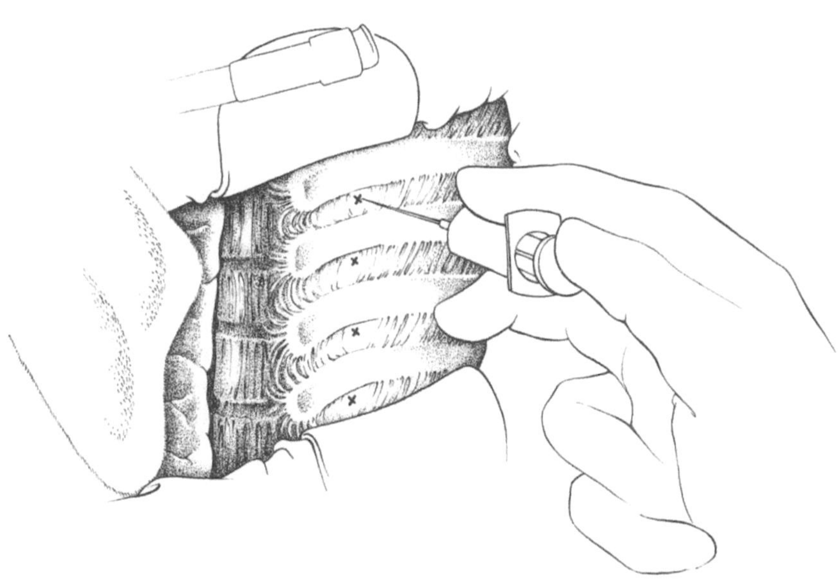

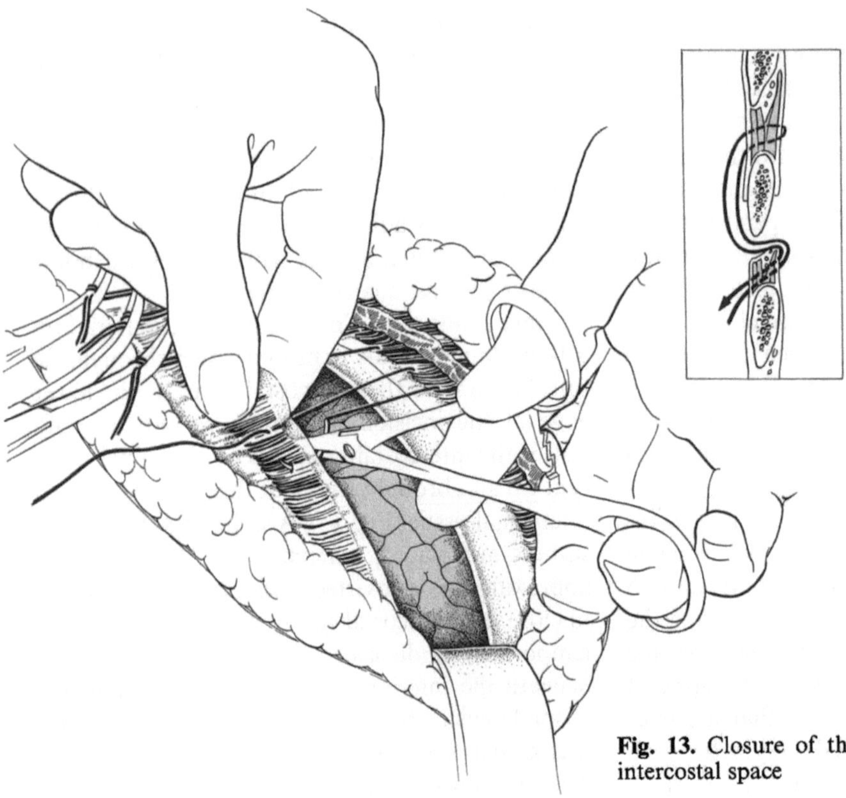

Fig. 13. Closure of the bony thorax by suture of the intercostal space

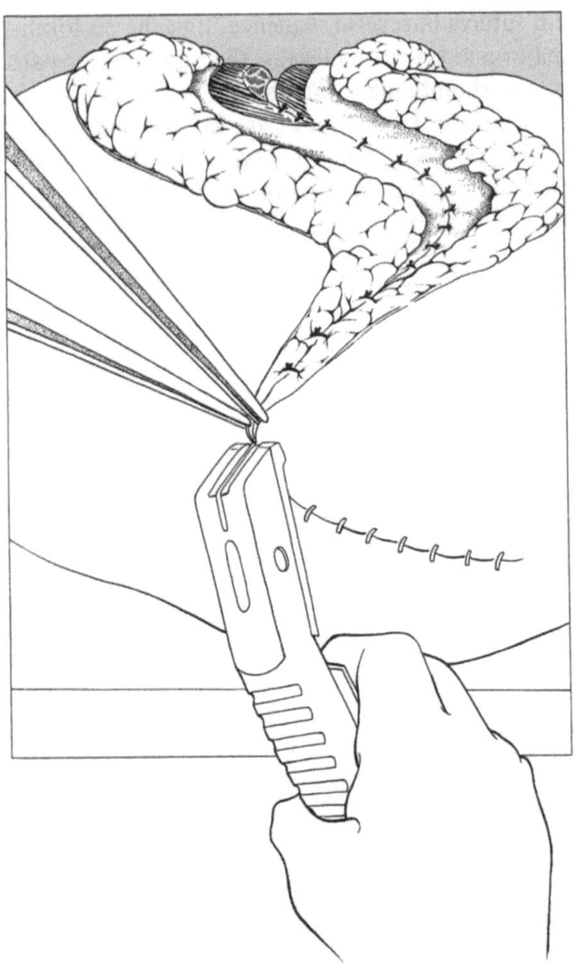

threads (Fig. 14), and finally the skin is closed with a running suture (over-and-over or vertical mattress) of No. 1 nonabsorbable monofilament. We can also recommend the use of skin staples, which save time and produce a cosmetically appealing scar, but are somewhat more costly than sutures.

4.2 Anterolateral Thoracotomy

This approach is very favorable functionally, as it requires only that the fibers of the pectoralis major be separated; it does not involve division of any chest wall muscles. It is suitable for all lung procedures and for most procedures on the bronchial system and pulmonary artery (Fig. 15).

The skin incision follows the line of the standard thoracotomy from the axilla to the anterior sternal margin. The tissues also are divided as they are in the standard thoracotomy. But in the anterolateral thoracotomy, it is possible to spare the

Fig. 14. Reapproximation of the muscles, superficial fascia, subcutaneous fat, and skin. Here a stapling instrument is being used to close the skin

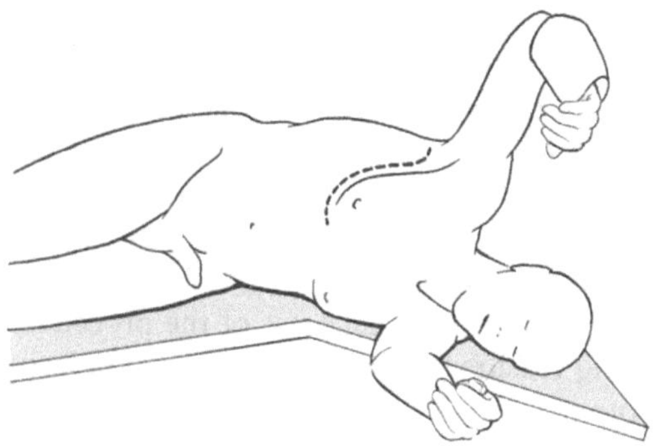

Fig. 15. The anterolateral thoracotomy incision

neurovascular bundle of the long thoracic nerve, a major advantage of this type of incision.

If the exposure is inadequate, additional spacc is gained by resecting about a 1-cm segment of costal cartilage from the rib above the incision in the subperichondrial plane. In this case the involved intercostal vessels must be divided and ligated. Closure of the incision is accomplished as for a standard thoracotomy following placement of the drain(s) and resection of the involved intercostal nerves. A small thoracotomy extending only 3–4 cm along the submammary part of the skin incision should suffice for a lingula biopsy. Aside from the shorter length of the incision in all layers, the technique is the same.

4.3 Posterolateral Thoracotomy

Like the anterolateral thoracotomy, the posterolateral thoracotomy is relatively nontraumatizing and has become the preferred approach for many operations. The posterior part of the incision is generally like that for a standard thoracotomy, i.e., it curves around the angle of the scapula, passes up into the axilla, then turns forward and downward (Fig. 16a, b). The axillary part of the incision is basically the same for the anterolateral and posterolateral approaches. Both approaches spare the neurovascular structures of the long thoracic nerve (see Sect. 4.2). The posterolateral thoracotomy requires that a larger portion of the latissimus dorsi be divided, but generally it is possible to spare at least part of the serratus anterior. By mobilizing the posterior border of this muscle, enough space usually is gained to enter the pleural cavity posterolaterally through the desired intercostal space. The details of the procedure correspond to the standard thoracotomy, and the closure technique is the same after the placement of one or two drains and resection of the involved intercostal nerves. The posterolateral thoracotomy is used mainly for operations on the trachea and bifurcation and certain pleural procedures; a modified form is used to expose the esophagus (see Sect. 4.4).

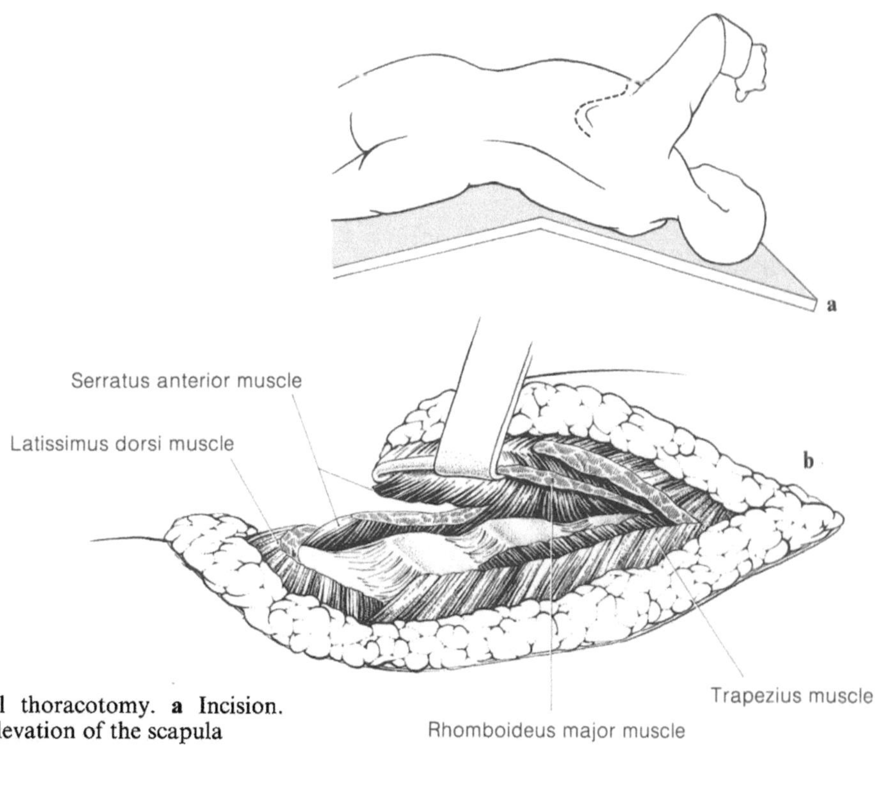

Fig. 16a, b. Posterolateral thoracotomy. **a** Incision. **b** Division of the muscles, elevation of the scapula

4.4 Oblique Posterolateral Thoracotomy

This is a modification of the posterolateral thoracotomy in which the incision, rather than sweeping up toward the axilla after rounding the scapula, passes downward and forward from the tip of the scapula in a gentle S-shaped fashion (Fig. 17a). The line of the incision roughly follows the costal axis. This approach is used mainly for exposures of the esophagus, posterior mediastinum, and diaphragm. When extended, it may be used for a double thoracotomy: Here the soft tissues over the chest wall are divided, and the chest is entered through two intercostal spaces separated by one or two intact intercostal spaces, affording access to the thoracic apex and to the diaphragm through a single skin incision. This approach is excellent for exposing the full length of the esophagus. It is also suitable for pleuropneumonectomy. After division of the skin, subcutaneous tissue, and superficial fascia, it is necessary to divide a small portion of the trapezius and latissimus dorsi muscles (Fig. 17). Then the connective tissue that binds the scapula between the rhomboideus major and serratus anterior muscles can be incised. The latter muscle is released along its posterior border, whereupon the scapula and serratus anterior are mobilized anteriorly so that the desired intercostal space can be identified. Peripheral fibers and tendinous insertions of the erector trunci muscle may have to be divided. The periosteum is incised over the selected rib, which is stripped and retracted as described in Sect. 4.1. The rest of the procedure, including closure, corresponds to the standard thoracotomy.

4.5 Thoracoabdominal Approaches

Thoracoabdominal incisions are required for extensive procedures on structures occupying portions of both body cavities. Indications would include procedures on the whole descending aorta, diaphragm, esophagus, or stomach, certain types of hepatic surgery (e.g., tumor or parasitic involvement of the pleural or pericardial space), procedures on the vena cava in the portocaval region, etc. Two types of situation may exist: On the one hand, a combined approach may be needed to gain exposure of a borderline thoracoabdominal lesion; on the other, it may be necessary to expose a lengthy portion of, say, the stomach, cardia, and esophagus. Cases of the first type are exposed directly through a single field; cases of the second

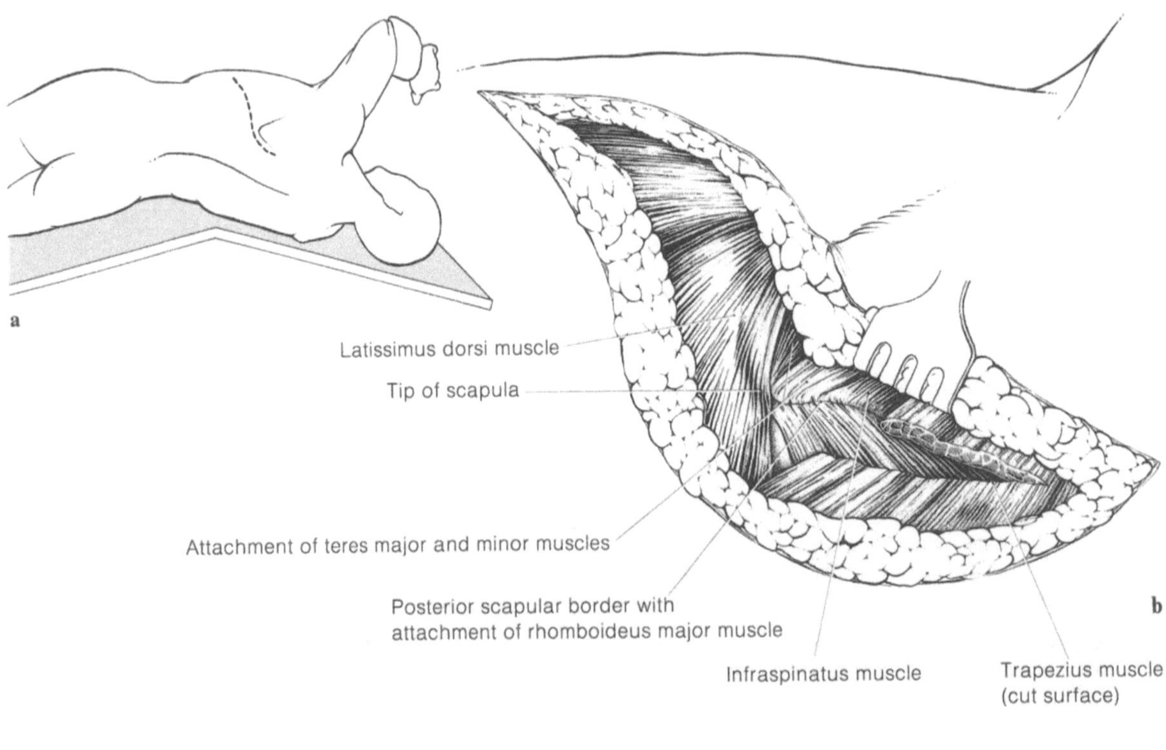

Fig. 17a, b. Oblique posterolateral thoracotomy. **a** Incision. **b** Division of the superficial layers and musculature

type may be approached through multiple incisions providing separate access to the abdominal and thoracic cavities. The type of incision will vary accordingly.

4.5.1 Thoracoabdominal Incision in the Bed of the Seventh Rib

This is used to expose organs that traverse the diaphragm, such as the entire descending aorta or the cardioesophageal junction. A left-sided thoracotomy is generally required, although special approaches to the liver may require a mirror-image thoracotomy on the right side.

The technique of the left-sided thoracotomy is described below:

The patient is placed in the semilateral position with a pad beneath the left thorax (see Sect. 3.3.1) and the thoracoabdominal region hyperextended. The left arm is elevated. The surgeon stands on the patient's left side.

The incision is first marked on the skin. It consists of an upper midline laparotomy (or right subcostal incision) combined with a low anterolateral thoracotomy, which join above the xiphoid (Fig. 18). The incisions having been made, the subcutaneous tissue is divided to expose the superficial thoracic fascia and the linea alba of the abdominal cavity. The linea alba is divided on the midline. If necessary, the incision may be extended downward to curve around the left side of the umbilicus. The peritoneal cavity is opened (for exposure of the aorta, it is best to leave the peritoneal sac closed and mobilize it toward the opposite side). Now the seventh rib is identified (the sixth rib may be chosen if the lesion is situated higher). The fibers of the pectoralis muscle are separated along the course of the selected rib, and the underlying periosteum or perichondrium is incised longitudinally with cutting current over the middle of the rib. The rib is stripped using a periosteal elevator and the Semb 1 and 2 raspatories. Then the pleural space is opened with a scalpel. After the lung has fallen away from the pleura, the pleural space is opened for the desired distance along the rib bed. At this point the abdominal and thoracic incisions are separated only by the cartilaginous costal arch, which is divided after incision of the perichondrium (Fig. 19). To apply the correct force, we

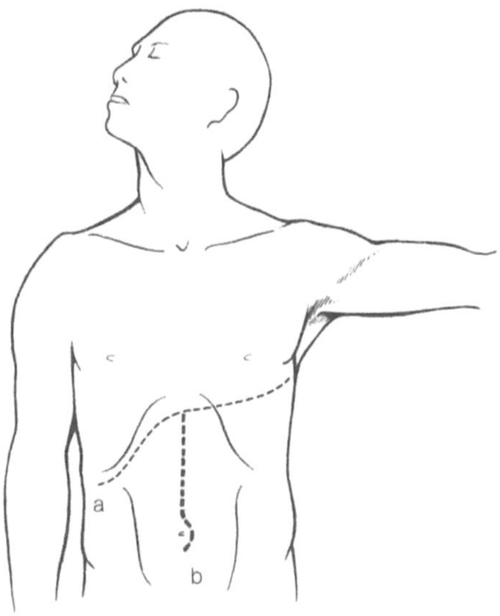

Fig. 18. Thoracoabdominal incision, combining a thoracotomy in the bed of the seventh left rib with *a* a right upper transverse laparotomy and *b* an upper midline laparotomy

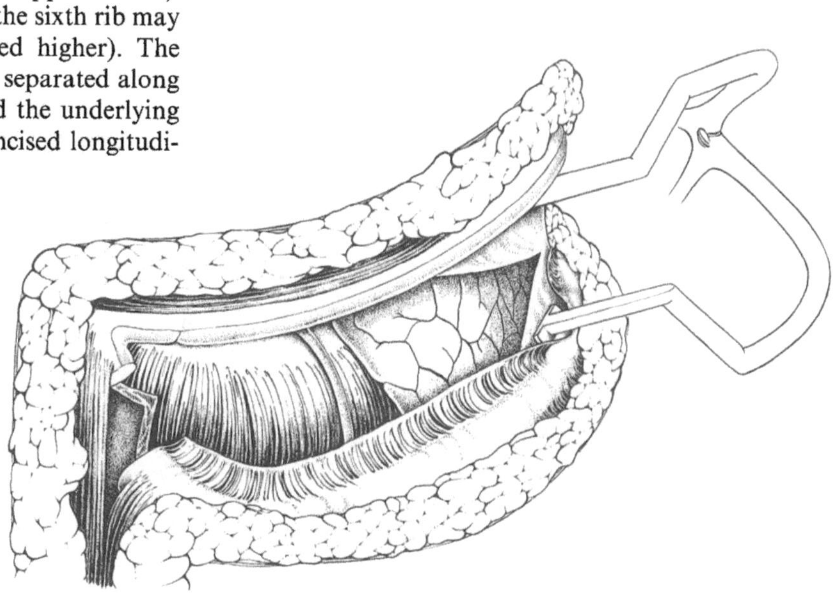

Fig. 19. Division of the costal arch with thoracoabdominal incision in the bed of the seventh rib

find it helpful to place the left thumb directly on the back of the blade and carefully press the scalpel through the cartilage. Further exposure is resisted by tension from the diaphragm. It should be noted that a radial incision of the diaphragm always severs part or all of the phrenic nerve, with consequent paralysis of the diaphragm. Whenever possible, therefore, the diaphragm should be incised in a circular fashion near its costal attachment so that the esophageal hiatus or aortic hiatus are approached from the posterior aspect. This is the only way of perserving diaphragmatic function. The diaphragm itself is incised in stepwise fashion with the electrocautery, using ligating sutures to control the often heavy bleeding from the diaphragmatic vessels (Fig. 20a). These sutures are excellent for elevating and retracting the cut diaphragm out of the surgeon's field of vision (Fig. 20b). This must be done cautiously to avoid injury to the spleen, which is in contact with the diaphragm in the left lower posterior part of the field.

After the necessary procedure has been carried out, the diaphragm (if still intact) is reapproximated to its narrow costal attachment with strong (No. 1) interrupted sutures of an absorbable material. Horizontal mattress technique may be employed. An abdominal drain is placed if necessary, and the mandatory pleural drain is inserted. The costal arch is repaired with two or three heavy (No. 2) atraumatic absorbable sutures placed through the cartilage (Fig. 21). Next the thoracic incision is closed in layers as in the standard thoracotomy. Finally the abdominal cavity is closed using continuous sutures in the peritoneum (1-0) and interrupted sutures in the fascia (No. 1) and subcutaneous space. Time can be saved and the cosmetic result improved by using a stapling instrument to close the extensive thoracoabdominal skin incision. Otherwise the wound may be closed with a continuous vertical mattress suture.

4.5.2 Median Sternotomy with Laparotomy

This approach, which is used for cardiac procedures and to expose lesions of the anterior and inferior pericardium, consists of a median sternotomy that is extended down into the abdominal cavity. The xiphoid may be included in the sternotomy, but it is best to remove it subperiosteally with a rongeur. Division of the various tissue layers and their reapproximation during closure are described in 4.5.1 and 4.6.1.

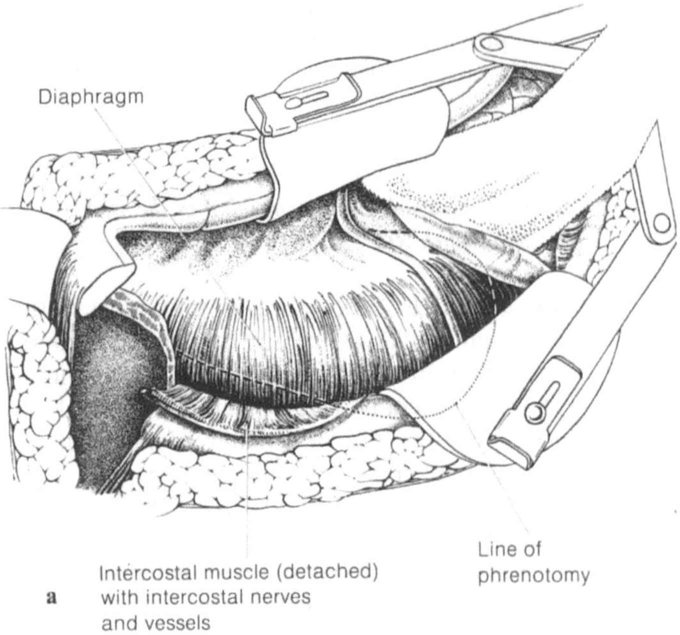

a

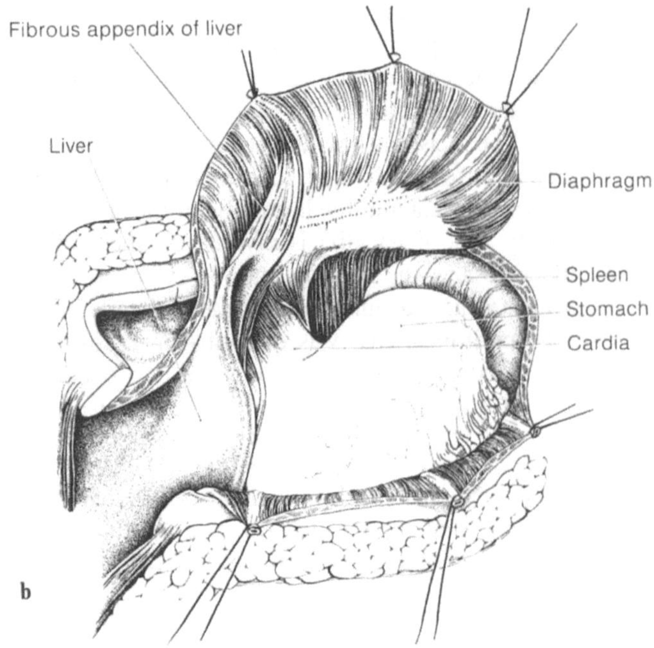

b

Fig. 20a, b. Thoracoabdominal incision. **a** Operative field, with broken line indicating the line of the phrenotomy. **b** The diaphragm has been incised circumferentially and raised to expose the stomach, spleen, and esophagus

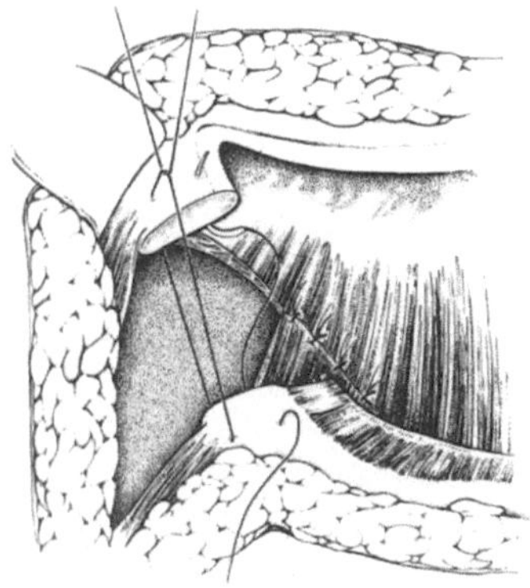

Fig. 21. Repair of the costal arch

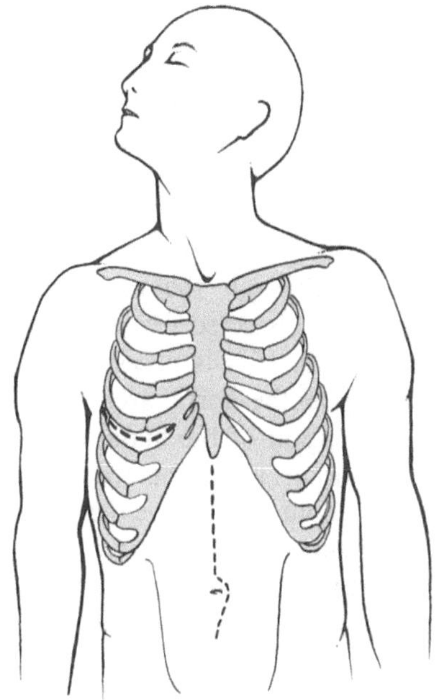

Fig. 22. Incisions for separate laparotomy and thoracotomy

4.5.3 *Separate Laparotomy and Thoracotomy*

This approach is recommended for procedures on the esophagus, stomach, and gastric cardia (Fig. 22). The individual situation and the surgeon's preference will determine the type of approach used. Options include a combined thoracoabdominal approach (see 4.5.1); an anterolateral thoracotomy in the bed of the sixth and seventh rib, without division of the costal arch, combined with a separate laparotomy (usually a midline laparotomy); or an upper abdominal incision and a thoracotomy, usually a right-sided posterolateral thoracotomy in the bed of the fifth rib or a double thoracotomy, performed in separate stages. The thoracotomy may be performed first, followed by the laparotomy, or the laparotomy may be done first and the abdominal cavity reopened at a later time if required. These questions are addressed during preoperative planning. The technique depends on the thoracic and abdominal incisions that are used. The laparotomy may be a midline, right subcostal, or left subcostal type, while the chest may be entered anterolaterally or posterolaterally through the selected rib bed.

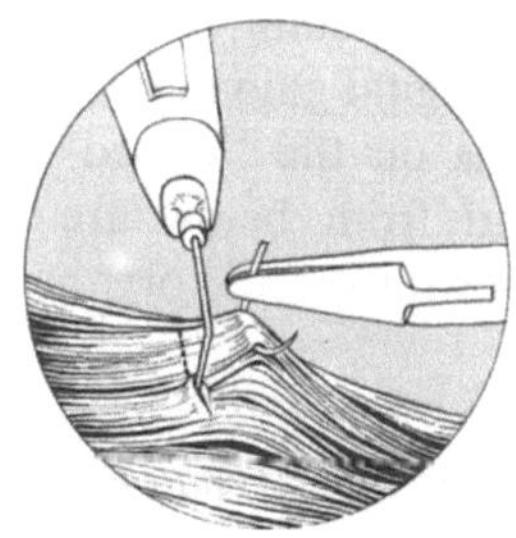

Fig. 23. Opening the diaphragm from the thoracic aspect is safer for the underlying organs (spleen!) if the diaphragm is first picked up on a sutureless needle before it is incised

4.5.4 *Thoracotomy with Phrenotomy*

This approach is occasionally used for a small carcinoma of the gastric cardia. The diaphragm is opened through a left-sided thoracotomy in the bed of the sixth or seventh rib, and the cardia is exposed in its entirety. The stomach is easily mobilized through this approach, so it is possible to perform a high subtotal gastrectomy and distal esophagectomy and then reconstruct with a gastric tube fashioned from the greater curvature. The procedure is like that described in Sect. 4.5.3, with the laparotomy omitted. Again, the diaphragm is incised in semicircular fashion 1–2 cm from its costal attachment to give posterior access to the esophageal hiatus. Since the abdominal cavity remains closed anteriorly, special care must be exercised in the area where the spleen is subjacent to the diaphragm and is palpable. An effective technique is to catch part of the diaphragm with a threadless needle in a needle holder and elevate it before incising it with an electrocautery a safe distance from the underlying viscera (transverse colon, spleen) (Fig. 23). All remaining steps are described in 4.5.1.

4.5.5 "Closed Thoracotomy"

This term applies to measures that give access to the mediastinum without opening the chest from the outside. Examples include mediastinoscopy from above and blunt mobilization of the esophagus from below or from above. Access from below can be gained through the esophageal hiatus, which is carefully dissected free and identified by its muscular crura. If it is necessary to pass the hand as far up as the aortic arch, access can be increased by incision of the hiatal crura. Profuse bleeding can occur from the left phrenic vein, which courses about 1 cm above the muscular arch in the diaphragm, so it is wise to identify, clamp, and ligate that vessel. Entry into the pleural space should be avoided if at all possible. If the pleural space is opened, the anesthetist should raise the end-expiratory pressure to 2–5 cm H_2O to keep the lung inflated and prevent air and fluid from entering the pleural cavity. If this nevertheless occurs, a pleural drain must be introduced before the laparotomy is closed. The drain is inserted through the pleural opening from the outside, preferably aided by digital guidance within the thorax (Fig. 24). Details on the "closed thoracotomy" from above and from below are given in the chapters dealing with specific organs.

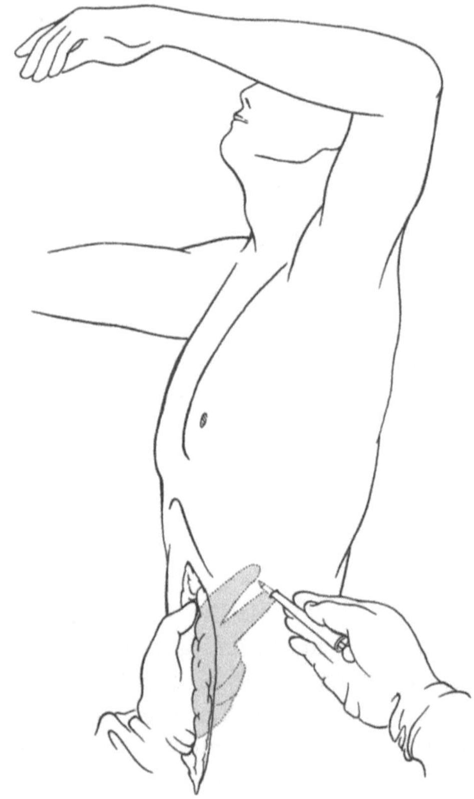

Fig. 24. In the "closed thoracotomy" the tube insertion is guided by the surgeon's fingers within the pleural space

4.5.6 Thoracotomy by Phrenotomy

Occasionally it is necessary to trace a pathologic process (tumor, parasitism) surgically from the abdominal cavity into the thorax to ensure the removal of all disease. It then becomes necessary to open the diaphragm from the abdominal aspect and, in some circumstances, to resect portions of it. As this is not a standard thoracotomy technique, its details will be described in the appropriate chapters.

4.6 Sternotomies

4.6.1 Median Sternotomy

This incision is used in noncardiac surgery for exposures of the anterior mediastinum (Fig. 25). With the patient supine, we use a ruler to draw a straight line from the jugular fossa to the tip of the xiphoid process. The skin is incised along this line, followed by electrocautery division of the

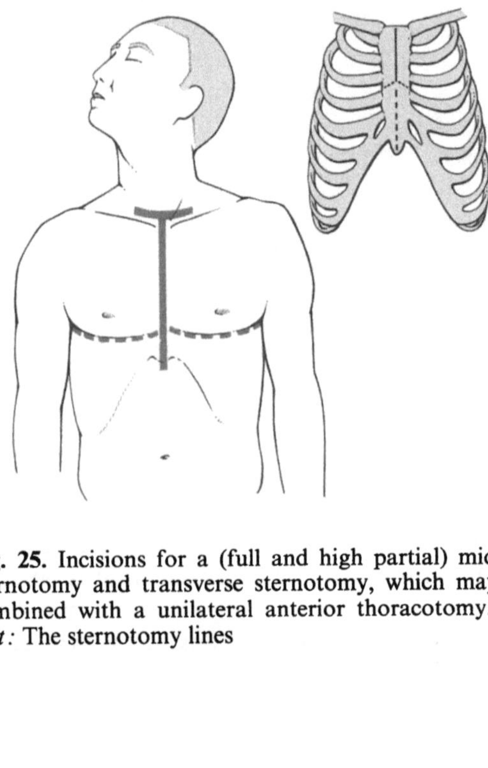

Fig. 25. Incisions for a (full and high partial) midline sternotomy and transverse sternotomy, which may be combined with a unilateral anterior thoracotomy. *Insert:* The sternotomy lines

subcutaneous tissue and sternal periosteum. Hemostasis at this stage must be meticulous. Next the sternum is osteotomized along the periosteal incision with the oscillating saw. Special care is taken in the area of the manubrium and jugular fossa to avoid injury to the closely subjacent brachiocephalic vein. A strong retrosternal ligamentous attachment also must be divided with scissors in this area. At that point the transected sternum is separated with two sharp hooks, and a sternal retractor is introduced (Fig. 26). Bleeding from the marrow spaces of the sternum is usually light and can be controlled by compression or cautery. Heavier bleeding is usually from the retrosternal periosteum and is controllable with the cautery. We have not had good results with bone wax on the sternal margins, and we abandoned its use some time ago.

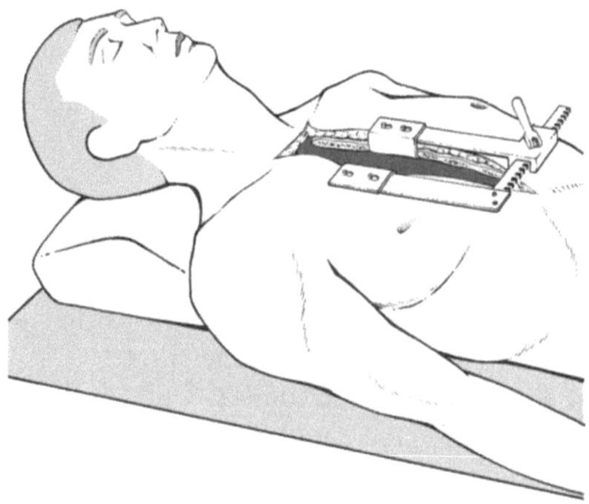

Fig. 26. Chest opened by a standard midline sternotomy

The intrathoracic procedure having been completed, closure of the sternotomy wound begins by reapproximating the sternal halves. While most surgeons use steel wire for that purpose, we prefer No. 2 absorbable suture material. Before placing the sutures, we perforate the sternum in five or six places with an awl and thread the suture in through a channel in the awl. The awl is similarly drilled through the sternum on the opposite side, and the mediastinal end of each suture is brought out through it. When all sutures have been placed, an assistant progressively tightens the threads and approximates the sternum, crossing some of the threads before tying them. Knot slippage can be prevented by grasping the thread with a hemostat after the first loop and placing the second loop over it so that the thread cannot slip between the first and second loops, and the bone edges are apposed under tension. Next the periosteum is closed with 2-0 absorbable sutures, followed by the subcutaneous tissue. The skin is closed with a stapling instrument.

4.6.2 High Partial Sternotomy

Median division of the upper half of the sternum may be used to expose the upper anterior mediastinum, e.g., for removing a small thymus tumor. The skin incision combines a small Kocher incision with a two-thirds sternotomy skin incision (Fig. 25). Again, the line of the incision is first marked on the skin with the aid of a ruler. The upper half of the sternum is exposed as for a full sternotomy, but at the level of the third or fourth intercostal space the periosteum is incised transversely on each side with the electrocautery, directing each cut toward the adjacent interspace. Similar cuts are made through the sternum with the oscillating saw, producing an inverted T-shaped osteotomy. Care is taken that the saw cuts are not carried past the bony margin into the intercostal space, where injury to the internal mammary vessels can cause brisk bleeding that is difficult to control. Finally a sternal retractor is inserted to expose the upper mediastinum.

Closure is the same as for a complete sternotomy, except that the divided segments are reapproximated with three absorbable interrupted sutures, and a fourth suture is used to join the upper sternal halves to the undivided lower part of the sternum. The rest of the closure is performed as described in 4.6.1.

4.6.3 Unilateral Partial Sternotomy with Anterolateral Thoracotomy

This seldom-used approach opens the apex of the thorax and can be useful for exposing tumors that have grown laterally from the sternum into the lung or mediastinum or for exposing the brachial vessels leading into the chest. It consists of a high unilateral sternotomy incision that is extended laterally into the intercostal space (usually the third). The mammary vessels are ligated. This technique represents a combination of the high partial sternotomy and anterolateral thoracotomy. The clavicle can pose an obstacle, but it may be divided if necessary to gain better access to the thoracic apex. In this case the clavicle is repaired with a nail or small plate during closure.

4.6.4 Transverse Sternotomy (Usually with Bilateral Anterolateral Thoracotomy)

This incision is occasionally used in cardiac surgery; its role in general thoracic surgery is in the treatment of metastatic tumors. Curved incisions are made below and about 3 cm from the nipples, turning upward at the sternum so as to create a pair of shallow U-shaped incisons. In women the lateral incisions follow the inframammary fold and leave cosmetically favorable scars. The sternum itself is transversely osteotomized with the oscillating saw through a periosteal electrocautery incision. The mammary vessels on both sides are ligated, and anterolateral thoracotomies are performed to open the pleural spaces.

The sternum is reapproximated with two or three sutures. The rest of the closure is like that for a median sternotomy combined with anterolateral thoracotomy.

4.7 Axillary Approach

This approach is used almost exclusively for thoracic sympathectomies. The skin incision is made transversely through the axilla on the axillary folds and is carried several centimeters forward along the lateral border of the pectoralis major muscle. The total length of the incision is about 8–10 cm. The long thoracic nerve, exposed by division of the fatty tissue, is retracted posteriorly, and the selected intercostal space, usually the third, is reached by blunt dissection. That space is opened subperiosteally as in other thoracotomies. Care is taken not to injure the pleura, which is bluntly mobilized away from the thoracic apex by patty dissection. This extrapleural thoracotomy gives relatively atraumatic access to the sympathetic thoracic ganglia. Meticulous attention is given to hemostasis, as it is not unusual for a torn intercostal vessel to be overlooked at operation and then bleed heavily after the chest is closed.

The incision is closed as in other minor thoracotomies. One suction drain is brought out of the wound; since the pleural space was not entered, an intrapleural chest tube is not required.

5 Appendix. Monika Meike Wanke

Suture Materials

Organ – tissue	Raw material	Absorbable	Non-absorbable	Needle code	Suture length (cm)	Suture size: Ph. Eur. metric size[a] (mm)	Suture size: USP[a]
Vascular snare	Silicone rubber		×		75	1.3, 2.0	
Vascular snare	Polyester green		×		75	4	
Vascular suture:							
Vena cava	Polypropylene		×	RB1–RB1	75	1–1.5	5/0–4/0
Pulmonary artery	Polypropylene		×	RB1–RB1	75	1.5	4/0
Aorta	Polypropylene		×	V7–V7	75	2	3/0
Trunk	Polypropylene		×	C1–C1	75	1	5/0
Subclavian artery	Polypropylene		×	C1–C1	75	1	5/0
Carotid artery	Polypropylene		×	BV1–BV1	75	0.7	6/0
Gastrointestinal anastomoses:	Polyglycolic acid	×		HR 22	75	2–3	3/0–2/0
	Polcglycolic acid	×		HR 26	75	2–3.5	3/0–2/0
	Polyglyconate	×		HR 22	75	1.5–2	4/0–3/0
	Polyglyconate	×		HR 26	75	2	3/0
Vessel ligation in stomach wall	Polyglyconate	×		HR 22	75	1–1.5	5/0–4/0
Purse-string suture for EEA	Polypropylene		×	SH	75	3.5	0
Purse-string suture for feeding gastrostomy	Polyglycolic acid	×		HR 26	75	3.5	0
Fixation of feeding tube	Polyester thread		×	HR 37s	4	1	
Suture ligation in EEA after exclusion of leak	Polyglyconate	×		HR 22	75	1.5	4/0
Cervical esophagostomy	Polycycolic acid	×		HR 26	75	3	2/0
	Polyglyconate	×		HR 26	75	2	3/0
Suture ligations	Polyglycolic acid	×		HR 26	75	3–3.5–4	3/0–0–1
Suture ligations	Polyglycolic acid	×		HR 37 s	75	3–3.5–5	2/0–0–1
Suture ligations	Polyglyconate	×		HR 22	75	1.5–2	4/0–3/0
Suture ligations	Polyglyconate	×		HR 26	75	2–3–3.5	3/0–2/0–0
Suture ligations	Polÿgluconate	×		HR 37	75	3.5–4	0–1
Suture ligation of afferent and efferent pulmonary vessels	Polyglycolic acid	×		HR 26	75	3.5–4	0–1
Pulmonary suture	Polyclycolic acid	×		HR 26	75	2–3	3/0–2/0
				HR 37	75	3–3.5	2/0–0
Pulmonary suture	Polyglyconate	×		HR 22	75	1.5–2	4/0–3/0
				HR 26	75	2–3	3/0–2/0
				HR 37	75	3.5	0
Sutures for bronchial closure:							
Segmental resection	Polyglyconate	×		HR 22	75	3	2/0
Lobectomy	Polyglycolic acid	×		HR 22	75	3–3.5	2/0–0
	Polyglyconate	×		HR 22	75	3–3.5	2/0–0
Pneumonectomy	Polyglycolic acid	×		HR 26	75	3.5–4	0–1
Pneumonectomy	Polyglyconate	×		HR 26	75	3.5–4	0–1
Trachea	Polyglycolic acid	×		HR 22/26	75	3–3.5	2/0–0
Trachea	Polyglyconate	×		HR 22/26	75	3–3.5	2/0–0

Suture Materials (continued)

Organ – tissue	Raw material	Absorbable	Nonabsorbable	Needle code	Suture length (cm)	Suture size: Ph. Eur. metric size[a] (mm)	Suture size: USP[a]
Skin: abdomen, thorax, sternum	Polyamide		×	DS-30	75	3–3.5	2/0–0
	Stainless steel		×				
Tube sites in skin	Polyamide		×	DS-30	75	3–3.5	2/0–0
Ligatures	Polyglycolic acid	×			45	3.3, 5–4	2/0, 0.1
Ligatures	Polyglycolic acid	×			75	3.5–4	0.1
Subcutaneous suture	Polyglycolic acid	×			45	3	2/0
Muscle	Polyglycolic acid	×		HR 37s	75	3.5–4	0–1
Fascia	Polyglycolic acid	×		HR 37s	75	3.5–4–5	0–1–2
Peritoneum	Polyglycolic acid	×		HR 37s	75	4–5	1–2
Pleura, mediastinum	Polyglycolic acid	×		HR 26, 37s	75	3–3.5	2/0–0
Diaphragm	Polyglycolic acid	×		HR 37s	75	4	1
	Polyester		×	HR 37s	75	4	1
Intercostal suture	Polyglycolic acid	×		HR 43	45	5	2
Sternal closure	Polyglycolic acid	×		HR 43	75	5	2
Sternal closure	Stainless steel monofilament		×	LS–1	60	5	2
Coverage of xiphoid process	Polyglycolic acid	×		HR 37s	75	4	1
Pediatric surgery:							
Intercostal sutures	Polyglycolic acid	×			45	3.5	0
Muscular layer	Polyglycolic acid	×			45	3	2/0
Fascial layer	Polyglycolic acid	×			45	3.5	0
Subcutaneous	Polyglycolic acid	×			45	2	3/0
Skin suture or staples	Polyamide		×	DS-24	75	3.5	0
	Stainless steel		×	35 W			
Vascular ligatures	Polyglycolic acid	×			75	3	2/0
	Polyglycolic acid	×			45	2	3/0
Suture ligation of vessels	Polypropylene		×	RB1		1.5	4/0
	Polypropylene		×	RB1		1	5/0
	Polydioxanone	×		C1		1	5/0
Bronchial anastomoses	Polyglycolic acid	×		HR 22 or TA 30		3	2/0
	Polyglycolic acid	×		HR 22 or TA 30		2	3/0
	Polyglycolic acid	×		HR 22 or TA 30		2	3/0

[a] Size designation for suture materials
Old: USP = United States Pharmacopeia. New: Ph. Eur. = European Pharmacopeia

The Europeanon Pharmacopeia (Ph. Eur.) is the standard currently followed by all European manufacturers and users of suture materials. In the present monograph we adhere to the USP system. Suture sizes in the Ph. Eur. system are given in metric units, with thread diameters stated in $^1/_{10}$ mm. For example, a No. 1 suture has a diameter of at least 0.1 mm and no more than 0.14 mm.

Suture Materials

Designation	Raw material	Manufacturer	Absorbable
Dexon	Polyglycolic acid	B. Braun-Dexon	yes
Vicryl	Polyglactin 910	Ethicon	yes
Maxon	Polyglyconate	B. Braun-Dexon	yes
PDS	Polydioxanone	Ethicon	yes
Synthofil	Polyester fiber, braided	B. Braun-Dexon	no
Ethibond	Polyester fiber, braided	Ethicon	no
Miralene	Polyester fiber monofilament	B. Braun-Dexon	no
Prolene	Polypropylene monofilament	Ethicon	no
Supramid	Polyamide pseudomonofilament	B. Braun-Dexon	no
Suturamid	Polyamide 6 pseudomonofilament	Ethicon	no

Instrument Sets for Thoracic Surgery

I. Basic Set

1 Surgical scissors, straight, sharp/blunt, 14.5 cm, matte
1 Surgical scissors, curved, sharp/blunt, 14.5 cm, matte
2 Lexer dissecting scissors, curved, 16.5 cm, matte
2 Metzenbaum dissecting scissors, straight, 14.5 cm, matte
1 Nelson-Metzenbaum dissecting scissors, 23 cm, curved, matte
1 Nelson-Metzenbaum dissecting scissors, 25 cm, curved, matte
1 Nelson-Metzenbaum dissecting scissors, 28 cm, curved, matte
1 Nelson-Metzenbaum dissecting scissors, 30.5 cm, matte
1 Toennis-Adson dissecting scissors, curved, 17.5 cm, matte
2 Dissecting forceps, narrow, 14.5 cm, matte
3 Tissue forceps, 1 × 2 teeth, 16.0 cm, matte
2 Tissue forceps, 1 × 2 teeth, 20.0 cm, matte
1 Maier polyp forceps, with lock, straight, matte
1 Maier polyp forceps, with lock, curved, matte
10 Backhaus towel clamps, 11 cm, matte
6 Halsted hemostatic forceps, curved, 12.5 cm, matte
15 Rochester-Pean hemostatic forceps, 16 cm, matte
2 Kocher hemostatic forceps, curved, 16 cm, matte
2 Collin hemostatic forceps, oval, 15.5 cm, matte
6 Overholt-Geissendoerfer dissecting forceps, matte
4 Zenker dissecting and ligature forceps, 29.5 cm, curved, matte
6 Mikulicz peritoneal forceps, 20 cm, matte
1 Needle case, 150 × 90 × 10 mm, perforated, 7 comp., matte
2 DeBakey Durogrip needle holders, 18 cm, matte
2 DeBakey Durogrip needle holders, 23 cm, matte
2 Hegar Durogrip needle holders, heavy, 20 cm, matte
2 Hegar Durogrip needle holders, heavy, 24 cm, matte
2 Wangensteen needle holders, 265 mm, matte
1 Hollow sound, plastic, 185 mm
2 Roux retractors, large, matte
1 Caspar explor. and coagul. hook, 5 mm, matte
2 Volkmann retractors, sharp, 6 prong, matte
2 Ollier retractors, blunt, 4 prong, matte
2 Mikulicz abdominal retractors, 120 × 50 mm, matte
1 Mikulicz abdominal retractor, 155 × 50 mm, matte
1 Fritsch abdominal retractor, 45 × 75 mm, matte
1 Kader intestinal spatula, 40 mm wide, matte
2 Allis intestinal forceps, 5 × 6 teeth, 190 mm, matte
2 Babcock intestinal forceps, 170 mm, matte
2 Kocher intestinal clamps, curved, 230 mm, matte
1 Luer hemorrhoidal forceps, 26 cm, matte
1 Guyon kidney clamp, 230 mm, matte
2 Martin vaginal speculum, 105 × 27 mm, matte
1 Mayo uterine sound, straight, flexible, 5 mm, matte
1 Museux tenaculum forceps, medium, 2 × 2 teeth, 240 mm, matte
2 Atr. forceps, straight, jaw 2.0 mm, 150 mm, matte
2 Atr. forceps, straight, jaw 3.5 mm, 200 mm, matte
2 Atr. forceps, straight, jaw 3.5 mm, 240 mm, matte
2 Atr. forceps, straight, jaw 2.8 mm, 300 mm, matte
1 Electrode handle with 2 pushbuttons
1 Surgical lancet-cutting electrode, angled
3 Kidney basins, 250 ml
8 Retractors, 250 mm
2 Langenbeck retractors, blade 48x15 mm, matte
1 Kader spatula, matte
2 Vein hooks, matte
2 Basins 100 ml
2 Basins 200 ml
1 Suction drain tip No. 8
1 Suction drain tip No. 10
1 Suction drain tip No. 12
1 Suction drain tip No. 18

II. Extra Thoracic Set

1 Needle holder, Aesculap model, 200 mm, matte
2 Volkmann retractors, sharp, 1 prong, matte
1 Allison lung retractor, pediatric, matte
1 Allison lung retractor, 32 cm, blade 53 mm, matte
1 Organ spatula, 26 cm, matte
1 Hammer with lead core, matte
1 General operating scissors, one blade serrated, matte
1 Collin intestinal forceps, fenestrated, 200 mm, matte
1 Finochietto rib spreader, light model, matte
1 Bailey-Gibbon rib contractor, 200 mm, matte
1 Lebsche sternum chisel, matte
1 Duval lung forceps, 23 cm, matte
3 Semb raspatories, 225 mm, matte
1 Championniere bone drill, 17 cm
1 Flat-nosed pliers, grooved jaws, 170 mm, matte
1 Flat-nosed pliers, 19 cm, matte
1 Gaubatz spreader, Ulrich CT 2015

III. Set for Rib Resection

1 Volkmann retractor, sharp, 1 prong, matte
1 Sauerbruch-Frey rib shears, 370 mm, matte
1 Brunner rib shears, 340 mm, matte
4 Semb raspatories, 225 mm, matte
1 Doyen rib rasp/elevator, adult, left, matte
1 Doyen rib rasp/elevator, adult, right, matte
1 Volkmann bone curet, size 0, matte
1 Volkmann bone curet, size 2, matte
1 Volkmann bone curet, size 5, matte
1 Hammer, 250 mm, head diam. 50 mm, plastic
1 Lexer chisel, 22 cm long, 10 mm wide, matte
1 Lexer chisel, 22 cm long, 15 mm wide, matte
1 Lexer chisel, 22 cm long, 20 mm wide, matte
1 Langenbeck bone holding forceps, matte
1 Semb bone or rib holding forceps, 20 cm, matte
1 Zaufal-Jansen ronguer, 18.5 cm, matte
1 Stille ronguer, curved on the side, 23 cm, matte
1 Luer-Stille ronguer, curved, 270 mm, matte
1 Ruskin-Liston bone splinter forceps, rounded, matte
1 Liston bone splinter forceps, curved, 275 mm, matte
1 Rib raspatory for the 1st rib, Ulrich CT 3003

IV. Set for Funnel Chest and Ribs

1 Raspatory, 8 mm wide, 170 mm long, matte
1 Volkmann bone curet, size 0, matte
1 Volkmann bone curet, size 2, matte
1 Volkmann bone curet, size 5, matte
1 Flat-nosed parallel pliers, wire cutter on side, 18 cm, matte
1 Sewall raspatory, 20 cm, matte
1 Hammer
1 Sternum pin 140 mm
1 Sternum pin 160 mm
1 Sternum pin 180 mm
1 Sternum pin 200 mm
1 Rib stripper, straight
1 Rib stripper, curved

V. Extra Vascular Set

1 Steel rule, millimeters and inches, 30 cm
1 Reynolds scissors, 180 mm, matte
1 Metzenbaum dissecting scissors, curved, 22.5 cm, matte
1 Toennis-Adson dissecting scissors, 17.5 cm, matte
1 Toennis dissecting scissors, straight, 18 cm, delicate, matte
1 Thorek scissors, full curve, 19 cm, matte
1 Potts-DeMartel scissors, curved 45° on the side, matte
1 Potts-DeMartel scissors, curved 60° on the side, matte
1 Durogrip forceps anat., 14.5 cm, matte
1 Durogrip forceps anat., 18.5 cm, matte
1 Kelly polyp forceps, matte
6 Halsted hemostatic forceps, curved, 12.5 cm, matte
1 Rumel dissecting forceps, 23 cm, size 3
1 Rumel dissecting forceps, 23 cm, size 5
2 Durogrip vascular needle holder, delicate, 20 cm, matte
2 Hegar-Mayo durogrip needle holders, 20 cm, matte
1 Costroviejo needle holder, 140 mm, matte
4 Mayo-Adams self-retaining retractors, 2 blade, matte
2 Atr. forceps, straight, jaw 2.0 mm, 200 mm, matte
2 Atr. forceps, straight, jaw 2.4 mm, 240 mm, matte
2 Bulldog clamps, straight, jaw 30 mm, 85 mm, matte
1 Atr. bulldog clamp, curved, jaw 30 mm, 85 mm, matte
6 DeBakey coarctation clamps, straight, 240 mm, matte
8 DeBakey atr. peripheral vascular clamps, 180 mm, matte
3 DeBakey atr. aortic aneurysm clamps, 250 mm, matte
1 DeBakey atr. aortic aneurysm clamp, 255 mm, matte
1 DeBakey atr. aortic aneurysm clamp, 265 mm, matte
2 DeBakey atr. vascular clamps, jaw 30 mm, 19.5 cm, matte
1 DeBakey atr. vascular clamp, jaw 40 mm, 26.0 cm, matte
1 DeBakey atr. vascular clamp, jaw 50 mm, 26.5 cm, matte
1 Rummel-Belmont tourniquet, 6.4 mm diam.
2 Basins
1 Abdominal retractor
1 Abdominal retractor
1 Vollmar ring stripper, 2 mm diam., Ulrich CV 1300
1 Vollmar ring stripper, 4 mm diam., Ulrich CV 1300
1 Vollmar ring stripper, 6 mm diam., Ulrich CV 1300
1 Vollmar ring stripper, 7 mm diam., Ulrich CV 1300
1 Vollmar ring stripper, 8 mm diam., Ulrich CV 1300
1 Vollmar ring stripper, 10 mm diam., Ulrich CV 1300
1 Vollmar ring stripper, 12 mm diam., Ulrich CV 1300
1 Vollmar ring stripper, 14 mm diam., Ulrich CV 1300
1 Dissecting spatula
1 Vascular clamp

VI. Pediatric Set

1 Haight rib spreader
1 Gaubatz rib spreader, pediatric model
1 Bailey rib spreader, 150 mm
1 Artmann rib raspatory
1 Doyen-O'Brien rib rasp/elevator
2 Allison retractors, 225 mm
2 Allison retractors, 320 mm
2 Tuffier abdominal spatulas, 200 mm
4 Overholt-Geissendorfer ligature forceps, 200 mm
4 Bulldog clamps, straight, 45 mm
4 Bulldog clamps, curved, 45 mm
2 Duval-Collin tissue grasping forceps, 200 mm
1 Rumel B ligature forceps
2 Derra vascular clamps, 165 mm
2 Derra vascular clamps, 175 mm
1 Clip applying forceps, 150 mm
2 Durogrip forceps (Gold forceps)
1 Potts-DeMartel vascular scissors, 190 mm (angled)
2 Derra atr. infant anast. clamp, large model, 17.5 cm, matte
2 Satinsky anastomotic clamps, 150 mm, matte
2 Wylie vascular clamps

VII. Thoracic Vascular Set

2 DeBakey atr. aortic aneurysm clamps, 315 mm, matte
1 DeBakey atr. vascular clamp, jaw 40 mm, 26.0 cm, matte
1 DeBakey atr. vascular clamp, jaw 50 mm, 26.5 cm, matte
1 DeBakey atr. vascular clamp, jaw 40 mm, 26.0 cm, matte
1 DeBakey atr. vascular clamp, jaw 60 mm, 27.5 cm, matte
1 DeBakey atr. vascular clamp, jaw 70 mm, 28.0 cm, matte

VIII. Special Instruments and Instrument Sets

ASIF Small-Fragment Instrument Set
Small air drill with snap-in chuck
Double hose
Oscillating bone saw
Saw blades with double hose attachment

Implants:
Grob sternum pins
Judet rib staples
Vecsei rip plates
Strut splints
Rehbein splints for pectus excavatum
Vascular prostheses, woven
Lyophilized dura
Marlex mesh
Neville tracheal-bronchial prosthesis

Stapling instruments and accessories:
EEA, straight, diam. 25, 28, 31 mm
EEA curved, diam. 21, 25, 28, 31 mm
TA 30-V stapler (for vessels)
Clip-A-Matic
Surgiclip
Skin stapler

Endoesophageal tubes and dilators:
Haering esophageal endoprosthesis
Atkinson endoesophageal tube
Celestine endoesophageal tube
Ruschelit esophageal dilators Ch 7–40
Soft rubber dilators, diam. 14–18 mm
ESKA-Buess multistage dilator

Special materials:
Trachea/bronchus
Spiral endotracheal tube with 15-mm connector, Ch 24–34
Connecting hose for endotracheal tube and ventilator, transparent, 1 m long, with connector for tube and ventilator hose
Ruesch balloon-tipped catheter, silicone latex, double-lumen, Ch 16, 18, 20
Chest tubes, Ch 16, 20, 24, 28, 32
Chest tube set 1081, connective tubing
Chest tube collecting bottle
1 l gas bottle, graduated
Trocar chest catheter, Ch 12, 32
Easy-flow AN, 6 mm and 12 mm
Vastrip (vein stripper), 15 mm diam., for esophageal dissection
Dennis probe
Unoplast stomach tube with stylet, Ch 14, 16, 18
Ruesch gastrostomy catheter, Ch 24, 26
Long-term feeding catheter for parenteral nutrition
Fibrin glue
Tabotamp
Indigo carmine
Carbosthesin 0.25%
Antiseptic solution for use on skin and in body cavities

Esophagoscope
Mediastinoscope
Bronchoscope
Thoracoscope

C. Perioperative Management

1 Parenteral Nutrition

J. M. Müller

CONTENTS

1.1 Definition

Parenteral nutrition, known also as total parenteral nutrition (TPN) or normocaloric parenteral nutrition (NPN), denotes the intravenous administration of nutrients in a composition and quantity which satisfy the patient's nutritional requirement. This is determined by the patient's basal metabolic rate, his level of activity, the nature of his illness, the extent of surgical trauma, and any preexisting deficiency syndrome that may be present. The limiting factor in nutritional support is the ability of the patient to metabolize the parenterally administered substrates [24].

Parenteral hyperalimentation [11] is not generally advised, because the administered substrates are either excreted or stored as fat. Both impose an added stress on the body and should be avoided, especially in the perioperative period.

Hypocaloric parenteral nutrition is based on the concept that in patients who are in normal nutritional status preoperatively and undergo moderately extensive surgery, an infusion of amino acids corresponding to normocaloric parenteral nutrition (1–1.5 g/kg b.w./d) combined with a low carbohydrate intake (2 g/kg b.w./d) is sufficient to preserve the protein resources of the body [22, 23]. Energy needs are met by mobilization of the body's own fat stores. Biochemical studies have demonstrated the validity of this concept, although comparative clinical studies have been unable to show that hypocaloric parenteral nutrition is superior to water-electrolyte solutions in terms of reducing postoperative morbidity. However, the ability to use peripheral veins for the infusion and the commercial availability of compounded solutions have simplified the routine use of "parenteral nutrition."

1.2 Indications

Parenteral nutrition is indicated in patients undergoing thoracic surgery who cannot be adequately nourished by the enteral route for three or more days postoperatively. Prime candidates for parenteral nutrition are patients who have had resective and reconstructive procedures on the esophagus and gastric cardia, as well as patients who require prolonged ventilatory support.

The indication for preoperative parenteral nutrition depends on the patient's nutritional status and the extent of the proposed surgery. A number of anthropometric, biochemical, immunologic, and radiologic techniques have been devised for assessing nutritional status. It does not matter what parameters are selected, as long as they are sensitive and specific enough in a given population to enable risk groups to be identified with reasonable certainty. Currently the most effective techniques of nutritional assessment rely on multifactorial indices covering various factors that are weighted differently [7, 27].

Preoperative parenteral nutrition should be maintained for at least seven days to achieve significant amelioration of nutritional status. Comparative prospective studies have shown that preoperative parenteral nutrition can significantly lower the complication rate following the resection of esophageal or cardial carcinoma [26].

1.3 Routes for Parenteral Nutrition

Hypocaloric parenteral nutrition can be administered by peripheral vein. Because the clinical efficacy of this nutrition has not yet been established, protection of the veins should be the primary concern when selecting a parenteral solution. It is safe to assume that solutions with an osmolarity of less than 900 mosmol and a pH greater than 5 will be well tolerated by the peripheral veins.

Because of the osmolarity of the highly concentrated amino-acid and carbohydrate solutions, parenteral nutrition requires access to the central venous system. It is widely agreed that a central venous catheter introduced via the basilic vein is associated with the lowest incidence of clinically significant complications. This is the preferred route in patients receiving short-term perioperative support. However, this route is far less acceptable if solutions must be administered for several days, because it is associated with a 100 times higher rate of phlebitis and 20 times higher rate of thrombosis than alimentation via the internal jugular vein or subclavian vein. Although, for anatomic reasons, use of the subclavian vein for the insertion of a central venous catheter carries a higher risk than use of the internal jugular vein, we nevertheless prefer subclavian vein catheterization for parenteral nutrition. In our own series of 182 consecutive subclavian catheter insertions, we encountered only one complication, a pneumothorax, that required treatment. We feel that this constitutes an acceptable risk. Because the subclavian catheter emerges from a site on the relatively rigid chest wall, its fixation and care are much easier than with an internal jugular vein catheter placed on the mobile neck close to the hairline. It is reasonable to expect that the risk of infection would be less with a subclavian catheter, although this has not yet been proven by clinical studies.

Table 1. Complication rates associated with the placement of central venous catheters, for various routes of insertion

Author	Burri			Müller
Route of insertion	Basilic vein	Internal jugular vein	Sub-clavian vein	Sub-clavian vain
Patients	7027	10 013	20 451	182
Complications (%)				
Pneumothorax	–	0.05	1.1	0.6
Arterial puncture	–	0.51	1.4	1.6
Faulty placement	9.5	0.9	6.0	6.6
Insertion not possible	4.1	1.8	6.2	2.8

The insertion of a central venous catheter for preoperative parenteral nutrition or for elective surgery is not an emergency procedure and should always be performed under aseptic conditions. A meticulous skin prep is done about the puncture site, sterile drapes are applied, and sterile clothing is worn. Although catheter sets are available that permit the catheter to be inserted without touching it, "semi-sterile" conditions (as in anesthesia induction) should never be tolerated when placing a central venous catheter. Moreover, because a radiologic check of the catheter placement is routinely performed and is necessary to exclude pneumothorax, it may be best to insert the catheter under optimum conditions on the day before the operation.

Long-term parenteral nutrition and home parenteral nutrition require the use of special catheter systems. They are described fully in the section on esophageal procedures.

Besides the complications that can occur during catheter insertion, other complications can result from the presence of the catheter in the venous system. The most important of these are catheter-related sepsis and the thrombosis of major veins. The incidence of catheter-related sepsis depends on a variety of factors, including the nature of the patient population and the length of time the catheter is left indwelling. Thus, figures reported in the literature are not always comparable and do not tell us which techniques are superior. A statistical review by Allen [1] showed that gram-positive cocci were the most frequent organisms detected (53% of cases). The only sure way to minimize the risk of catheter-related sepsis is the strict maintenance of a catheter care protocol. At most centers the provision of continual nursing care for patients on parenteral nutrition has dramatically reduced the incidence of catheter-related sepsis. However, as few centers will be able to provide this level of care for patients with central venous catheters, it is responsibility of the physician to see that specific guidelines are adhered to. These include changing the dressing over the catheter site daily and also changing the administration tubing under sterile conditions. In addition, the catheter should not be used for the bolus injection of medi-

Table 2. Incidence of catheter-related sepsis in parenteral nutrition

Author (year)	Patients	Sepsis rate (%)
Ryan (1974)	200	11
Filler (1976)	264	16
Dudrick (1977)	406	7
Müller (1982)	215	4

cation or for the drawing of blood for routine laboratory studies. Some of these "rules" of catheter care are controversial. Comparative prospective studies have shown no evidence that the incidence of sepsis is increased by the careful drawing of blood via the catheter or by limiting dressing changes to twice weekly [28]. The extent to which the formation of a subcutaneous tunnel or the addition of heparin to the infusion solution lowers the sepsis rate is unclear, because several comparative prospective studies have yielded different results [15, 34]. The treatment of catheter-related sepsis consists in removal of the catheter; it is unnecessary to administer antibiotics. Bozetti and Terno [5] and Newsome et al. [29] recommend changing the catheter over a stylet when sepsis is recognized. According to their studies, this does not significantly increase the reinfection rate compared with the placement of a new central venous catheter, and it avoids the risks associated with a second venipuncture.

The incidence of clinically overt thrombosis of the superior vena cava or its tributary veins in patients on parenteral nutrition ranges from 0.5% to 5% in prospective series. The coexistence of venous thrombosis with catheter-related sepsis is quite frequent. It is unclear whether the hypercoagulability in sepsis promotes thrombus formation, or whether the thrombus provides a favorable medium for bacterial growth. The incidence of asymptomatic thrombosis as a complication of central venous parenteral nutrition cannot be stated with certainty. Using phlebography, Burt et al. [9] found thrombotic changes in the superior vena cava or its tributaries in 33% of patients whose catheters had been in place an average of 7 days. The treatment of subclavian or internal jugular vein thrombosis is conservative. With thrombosis of the superior vena cava, the treatment of choice is thrombectomy.

1.4 Planning of Parenteral Nutrition

The planning of parenteral nutrition is guided by the patient's energy needs. The basal metabolic rate (BMR) can be determined before and after surgery by indirect calorimetry. If this is not possible, the BMR can be calculated from the Harris-Benedict formula [4] with an error of 10%–30% depending on the disease and type of surgical procedure. According to our own investigations, the BMR measured in patients with esophageal carcinoma is 15% higher on average than the calculated BMR. Assuming that the physical activity of hospitalized patients accounts for 20%–30% of the BMR, we obtain a caloric requirement of 22–27 kcal/kg b.w./d, depending on the patient's age, sex, and constitution. To correct a preexisting deficit, the energy intake may be increased to a maximum of 40 kcal/kg b.w./d.

Studies by Kinney [21] and his group have shown that the measured energy requirement of surgical patients can be 10%–40% higher than the calculated BMR, depending on the type of procedure. Sepsis can increase the energy requirement by as much as 70%.

The energy requirement can be satisfied by carbohydrate solutions alone or by a mixture of carbohydrates and fat emulsion.

It matters little whether the carbohydrate source is glucose or a mixture of glucose and sugar substitutes. We prefer glucose because its blood level and excretion are easily determined. The upper limit for postoperative glucose intake is 5 mg/kg b.w./min. If this volume is exceeded, the exogenous glucose is no longer oxidized and leads to increased lipogenesis and CO_2 production. The associated stress on the liver and lungs can have adverse effects in patients with marginal hepatic and pulmonary function.

Fat emulsions provide a satisfactory caloric source by the second or third postoperative day. They should contribute no more than 30% of the total energy intake. A higher proportion can ad-

Table 3. Optimum contributions of individual nutrients to total energy intake

Nutrient	Energy contribution (%)
Protein	15
Carbohydrate	55
Fat	30

Table 4. Planning of parenteral nutrition

Energy requirement
Basal metabolic rate (BMR) in kcal
For males: 66+(13.7 W)+(5 H)-(6.8 A)
For females: 655+(9.6 W)+ (1.7 H)-(4.7 A)
Preoperative
Normal activity: BMR 1.3
Malnutrition: BMR 1.5–1.7
Postoperative
Depending on type of procedure: BMR 1.4–1.7
Protein requirement
Nitrogen (g) $\frac{\text{Energy requirement (kcal)}}{\text{100–150 (kcal)}}$

W = weight in kg, H = height in cm, A = age in years

Table 5. Recommended daily intake of electrolytes

Electrolyte	Daily requirement (mmol/kg body weight)
Sodium	2–3
Potassium	1–2
Chloride	2–3
Calcium	0.1–0.2
Phosphate	0.2–0.5

versely affect the immune system, e.g., by compromising the phagocytic and bactericidal activity of granulocytes or macrophages. We never supply more than 15% of the total energy requirement with fat emulsion perioperatively.

Protein intake in the form of l-crystalline amino acid solutions is related to caloric intake by the ratio of 1 g nitrogen per 100–150 calories [20, 32]. This ratio leads to maximum utilization of the administered amino acids for protein synthesis. The specific composition of the amino acid solutions is of minor importance. None of the solutions currently on the market is clearly superior to any other for pre- or postoperative use.

The electrolyte requirement varies with the postoperative course and with the patient's energy and fluid intake. The basic daily requirement is added to the solutions. Repeated measurements of serum levels are necessary in order to adjust the electrolyte balance, especially after surgery. The actual vitamin and trace element requirements in the postoperative period are largely unknown, and recommendations (Table 7) are based on requirements during long-term parenteral nutrition.

When parenteral feeding is maintained for no more than seven days after uncomplicated thoracic surgery, a deficit should not arise if these guidelines are followed. The requirements in sepsis are less clearly defined.

Table 6. Recommended daily vitamin intake during parenteral nutrition

	AMA/NAG	Guthy[a]
Vitamin B_1 (mg)	3.0	25–50
Vitamin B_2 (mg)	3.6	5–10
Niacin (mg)	40	50–100
Vitamin B_6 (mg)	4	7.5–15
Vitamin B_{12} (mg)	5	10–30
Folic acid (mg)	0.4	0.5–15
Panthothenic acid (mg)	15	12.5–25
Biotin (mg)	0.06	
Vitamin C (mg)	100	250–1000
Vitamin A (IU)	3300	5000–10,000
Vitamin D (IU)	200	500–1000
Vitamin K_1(mg)	10	5–10
Vitamin E (IU)	10	2.5–5

[a] Postoperative period

Table 7. Recommended daily intake of trace elements during parenteral nutrition (in mg)

	AMA/NAG	Wretlind	Brennan
Zinc	2.5–4	1.4	5
Cooper	0.5–1.5	0.3	1.4
Manganese	0.15–0.8	2.3	0.5
Iron	–	3.9	10
Iodine	–	0.075	0.06
Chromium	0.001–0.015	–	0.02
Fluorine	–	0.9	–
Selenium	–	–	–

1.5 Conduct of Parenteral Nutrition

The individual components of the parenteral nutrition may be administered separately or combined in a nutrient solution. We prefer nutrient solution mixtures, because it is easier to guarantee the proper component ratios during the infusion. The individual components of mixed solutions must be compatible with one another (check manufacturer's recommendations), and the mixtures must be prepared under sterile conditions. At our center the nursing staff prepare the nutrient solutions in 3-liter bags. Regular tests for bacterial contamination have shown that, even without special mixing facilities, the rate of contamination does not exceed 2% when proper guidelines are followed. This is comparable to the contamination rate associated with the use of glass or plastic bottles. The mixed solutions differ from one another only in the concentration of the individual components.

In the ICU population we prefer highly concentrated solutions that permit low fluid volumes to be infused on a continuous basis. The water and electrolyte balance tend to be unstable after trauma and infection, and rapid adjustments can be made via a separate i.v. line without disturbing the alimentation. The nutrient solutions for ICU patients are essentially the same as for other patients, except that lower concentrations are infused. By adjusting the rate of the infusion, it is possible to meet the nutritional and fluid requirements of 95% of patients with a single mixed solution. This greatly facilitates the conduct of the nutritional support for ICU personnel and helps to avoid complications associated with the too rapid infusion of certain components.

1.6 Metabolic Complications of Parenteral Nutrition

Each of the components contained in parenteral solutions has the potential of causing or exacerbating a metabolic abnormality. If we disregard complications that have occurred during the development of certain types of solution (e.g., hypochloremic metabolic acidosis from amino acid solutions or erythropoietic disturbances from cottonseed oil) and reject the use of sugar substitutes, we may attribute the metabolic complications of parenteral nutrition to underdosing and overdosing, i.e., to factors that are user-related rather than method-related. Usually these complications can be avoided by the use of solution mixtures and infusion pumps. However, it is still possible for the physician to assess incorrectly the daily requirements of a patient whose metabolic status is not clearly recognized. We therefore favor a staged approach to parenteral support which takes into account the clinical presentation and various metabolic parameters. When glucose is administered as the main energy source, it is common to observe hyperglycemia and glucosuria in the early postoperative period. This results from a disturbance of peripheral glucose utilization caused by metabolic alterations in the stressed patient. Treatment consists of reducing the glucose intake or administering insulin directly or with the nutrient solution. With both measures it is almost always possible to keep the blood glucose level and urinary glucose excretion within limits not exceeding 200–250 mg/dl and 2 g/24 h, respectively. A rise of transaminases is another common finding during parenteral nutrition. Potential causes are:

- tryptophan breakdown products resulting from the addition of sodium bisulfite to the amino acid solution [17],
- permanent blood glucose levels exceeding 200 mg/dl or a glucose intake exceeding 600 g/d [30],
- a deficiency of amino acids necessary for the formation of bile salts [36],
- overloading of the Krebs cycle by an excessive amino acid intake [16],
- lack of stimulation of bile secretion due to absence of oral food intake [31],
- folic acid deficiency [18],
- uneconomical nitrogen-caloric ratio [12],
- copper deficiency [12, 13],
- deficiency of essential fatty acids [16].

Most of these factors do not become active during short-term parenteral nutrition in the postoperative period. The major factor would appear to be a glucose intake that markedly exceeds the patient's requirement. It should be pointed out, however, that a moderate transaminase elevation after surgery is not necessarily referrable to the parenteral nutrition. Upper abdominal procedures are consistently followed by a rise of transaminases caused by manipulations of the liver.

Table 8. Metabolic complications of parenteral nutrition and their causes (modified from Dudrick [12, 13] and Thomas [35])

Potential complications	Causes
I. Carbohydrate metabolism	
A. Hyperglycemia, glucosuria, osmotic diuresis, nonketotic hyperosmolar dehydration and coma	Too rapid infusion of excessive glucose doses; inadequate endogenous insulin production; glucocorticoid medication; infectious process; latent or overt diabetes
B. Ketoacidosis in diabetes	Inadequate endogenous insulin production; inadequate exogenous insulin administration
C. Postinfusion hypoglycemia	Persistence of high insulin level after prolonged stimulation of islet cells by high-dosage glucose infusions
D. Lactic acidosis	Infusion of large amounts of fructose, especially in the presence of hypoxia or acidosis
E. Hyperuricemia	Fructose or xylite infusion, dep. on administered dose
F. Oxalosis	High doses of xylite
II. Amino acid metabolism	
A. Hyperchloremic metabolic acidosis	Too much chloride and monohydrochloride in crystalline amino acid solutions
B. Serum amino acid imbalance	Unphysiologic amino acid profile in parenteral solutions; poor amino acid utilization secondary to disease (genetic metabolic disturances, hepatic cirrhosis)
C. Hyperamonemia	Too much free NH_3 in protein hydrolysates; absence of arginine, ornithine, or glutaminic acid in crystalline amino acids; hepatic disease
D. Prerenal azotemia	Excessive doses of amino acids; deficient intake of calorie sources
III. Fat metabolism	
A. Hyperlipidemia, colloid syndrome	Excessive fat emulsion; insuffi cient adaptation time; cottonseed oil
B. Depletion of essential fatty acids;	Inadequate intake of essential fatty acids, vitamin E
IV. Calcium and phosphorus metabolism	
A. Hypophosphatemia	Inadequate phosphate intake; deposition of phosphate in cells and bone; intracellular phosphate shift with high carbohydrate intake
1. Decreased erythrocytes 2,3-diphosphoglycerate	
2. Increased O_2 affinity of hemoglobin	
3. Malutilization of metabolites of erythrocyte metabolism	
B. Hypocalcemia	Inadequate Ca^{++} intake; reciprocal relationship of phosphorus intake without concurrent Ca^{++} replacement; hypoalbuminemia
C. Hypercalcemia	Excessive calcium intake; vitamin D overdose
V. Miscellaneous	
A. Hypo- or hypernatremia	Inadequate Na^{+} intake in relation to H_2O, especially in patients with abnormal losses (fever, ileus, diuresis)
B. Hypokalemia	Inadequate potassium intake combined with increased protein turnover; diuresis
C. Hyperkalemia	High K^{+} intake, especially in metabolic acidosis; renal failure
D. Hypomagnesemia	Inadequate magnesium intake coupled with high demand due to increased protein synthesis
E. Anemia	Inadequate intake of iron, folic acid, B_{12}
F. Hemorrhage	Inadequate vitamin K intake
G. RHS blockage	Fat infusion

1.7 Supervision of Parenteral Nutrition

The supervision of parenteral nutrition in the pre- and postoperative period requires obtaining a daily blood glucose profile and determining electrolytes (sodium, potassium, calcium) and transaminases daily for the first three days. As these studies are performed routinely after major surgery, they do not impose an additional burden on the patient. When findings have stabilized, it is sufficient to perform these studies every three days, barring the development of postoperative complications that require closer supervision.

References

1. Allen JR (1978) The incidence of nosocomial infection in patients receiving total parenteral nutrition. In: Johnston IDA (ed) Advances in parenteral nutrition. MTP
2. American Medial Association; Department of Foods and Nutrition (1979) Multivitamin preparations for parenteral use. A statement by the Nutrition Advisory Group. JPEN 3:258
3. American Medical Association; Department of Foods and Nutrition (1979) Guidelines for essential trace elements preparations for parenteral use. Expert Panel for Nutrition Advisory Group. JAMA 241:2051
4. Benedict FG (1915) A study of prolonged fasting. Carnegie Inst. of Washington, Publication no. 203
5. Bozzetti F, Terno G (1982) Prevention and treatment of central venous catheter sepsis by exchange via a guidewice. A prospective controlled trial. 4th ESPEN-Congress (abstract), Wien
6. Brennan MF (in press) Trace metal deficiency and replacement during total partenteral nutrition. Surgical Metabolism Section, Surgery Branch, National Cancer Institute, Bethesda, Md, USA
7. Brenner U, Müller JM, Keller HW, Schmitz M, Horsch S (1983) Ein neuer Ernährungsindex zur präoperativen Beurteilung der Mangelernährung als Risikofaktor in der Chirurgie. Infusionstherapie 10:302
8. Burri CF, Ahnefeld FW (1977) Cava-Katheter. Springer, Berlin Heidelberg New York
9. Burt ME, Dunnick NR, Krudy AG et al. (1981) Prospective evaluation of subclavian vein thrombosis during total parenteral nutrition by contrast venography. Clinical Research 29:264 A
10. Dudrick SJ, Steiger E, Long JM, Ruberg RL et al. (1979) General prinziples and techniques of intravenous hyperalimentation. In: Cowan JR (ed) Intravenous Hyperalimentation. Lea and Febiger, Philadelphia
11. Dudrick SJ, Long JM, Steiger E, Roads JE (1970) Intravenous hyperalimentation. Med Clin North Amer 54:577
12. Dudrick SJ, McFadyen BV, van Buren CT (1972) Parenteral hyperalimentation. Metabolic problems and solutions. Am Surg 176:259
13. Dudrick SJ, Long JM (1977) Applications and hazards of intravenous hyperalimentation. Annu Rev Med 28:517
14. Filler RM, Coran AG (1976) Total parenteral nutrition in infants and children: Central and peripheral approaches. Surg Clin North Am 56:395
15. Garden OJ, Sim AJW (1982) Subclavian catheter infection. A prospective study of tunneling versus non-tunneling. 4th ESPEN-Congress (abstract), Wien
16. Ghadimi H, Abaci F, Kuma S (1971) Biochemical aspects of intravenous alimentation. Pediatrics 48:955
17. Grant JP, Cox CE, Kleinmann LM, Mahler MM, Pittmann MA, Tangrea JA, Brown JH, Gross E, Meacley RM, Jones S (1977) Serum hepatic enzyme and bilirubin elevations during parenteral nutrition. Surg Gynecol Obstet 145:573
18. Green PJ (1977) Folate deficiency and intravenous nutrition. Lancet 1:814
19. Guthy E (1980) Zur Frage des postoperativen Vitaminbedarfs. In: Heberer G, Schultis K, Günther B (Hrsg) Postaggressionsstoffwechsel II. Schattauer, Stuttgart New York, S 103–106
20. Hartig W, Czarnetzki H-D, Faust H, Fickweiler E (1976) Zur Verwertung von Aminosäure-Infusionslösungen beim Gesunden und bei Patienten im Stress, untersucht an 15N-Glyzin. Infusionsther u klin Ernährung Basel 3:268–273.
21. Kinney JM (1976) Energy requirements for parenteral nutrition. In: Fischer (ed) Total parenteral nutrition, Little, Brown and Comp, Boston, pp 135–142
22. Löhlein D (1979) Veränderungen des postoperativen Proteinstoffwechsels bei peripher-venöser Infusionstherapie. Habilitationsschrift. Hannover
23. Löhlein D (1981) Untersuchungen zum proteinsparenden Effekt verschiedener Konzepte der peripheren parenteralen Ernährung. Z Ernährungswiss 20:81–95
24. Molnar JA, Wolfe RR, Burke JF (in press) Metabolism and nutritional therapy in thermal injury. In: Nutritional support of medical practice, 2nd edn, Harper & Row, New York
25. Müller JM (1982) Der Einfluß der präoperativen parenteralen Ernährung auf den klinischen Verlauf und das Stoffwechselverhalten bei Karzinompatienten in der prä- und postoperativen Phase. Habilitationsschrift. Köln
26. Müller JM, Brenner U, Dienst C (1982) Preoperative parenteral feedings in patients with gastrointestinal carcinoma. Lancet 1:68
27. Mullen J, Buzby GP, Waldmann MT, Gertner MH (1979) Prediction of operative morbidity and mortality by preoperative nutritional assessment. Surg Forum 30
28. Murphy LM, Lipman TO (1983) Safety of twice per week central venous catheters dressing changes in total parenteral nutrition. 7th ASPEN-Congress (abstract), Washington DC

29. Newsome HH Jr, Armstrong CW, Mayhall GC (1983) Comparison of denovo percutaneous venipuncture to change of catheter over guidewire for insertion of subclavian venous feeding catheters. 7th ASPEN-Congress (abstract), Washington DC
30. Parsa MH, Habif DV, Ferrer JM, Lipton R, Yoshimura NN (1972) Intravenous hyperalimentation: Indications, technique and complications. Bull NY Acad Med 48:920
31. Rager R, Finegold (1975) Cholestasis in immature newborn infants: is parenteral alimentation responsible? J Pediatr 86:264
32. Rutten P, Blackburn GL, Flatt JP, Hallowell E, Cochran D (1975) Determination of optimal hyperalimentation infusion rate. J Surg Res 18:477
33. Ryan JA (1974) Catheter complications in total parenteral nutrition. N Engl J Med, 290:757
34. Tanner WA, Delaney PV, Hennessy TP (1980) The influence of heparin on intravenous infusions: A prospective study. Br J Surg, 67:311
35. Thomas DW (1977) Practical metabolic problems. Klin Anaesth Intensivmed 13:184
36. Touloukian RJ, Downing SE (1973) Cholestasis associated with longterm parenteral hyperalimentation. Arch Surg 106:58
37. Wretlind A (1972) Complete intravenous nutrition: Theoretical and experimental background. Nutr Metab 14 (Suppl):1

2 Perioperative Antibiotic Therapy

R. GRUNDMANN

CONTENTS

The perioperative use of antibiotics can have two goals: 1) therapeutic for treating an established infection or 2) prophylactic, where agents are given at the time of contamination to prevent a subsequent infection. The latter application is preferred, although fears of promoting the development of resistant organisms have, until recently, greatly curtailed the indications for prophylactic antibiotic therapy [8]. However, perioperative antibiotic prophylaxis on a strictly short-term basis has become widely accepted as a means of preventing infection following a variety of operations, including procedures on the esophagus and lung [17].

2.1 General

2.1.1 Timing of Antibiotic Therapy

The antibiotic can be fully effective only if it is present in high levels at the potential infection site at the time of bacterial contamination. Initial animals studies on the effective period of antibiotic action were performed by Burke [2], who showed that maximum efficacy is achieved when the antibiotic is administered at least 1 h before the organisms have entered the tissue.

These animal studies have been confirmed clinically [19], indicating that prophylactic antibiotics should be initiated during premedication so that optimum levels of activity are present when the surgical incision is made.

2.1.2 Duration of Therapy

In principle, the duration of the antibiotic therapy should be as brief as possible to discourage superinfection by resistant organisms and minimize the side effects of the drug. Evidence indicates that it is unwise to continue antibiotic prophylaxis for more than 24 h [5]. Today it is generally recommended that the antibiotic should be given maximally in three doses spaced 6 h apart, although other regimens have been successful. Hoffmann et al. [11], for example, achieved good prophylaxis with an antibiotic administered in three successive doses spaced 2 h apart. Other authors report good results with a single dose administered preoperatively [9, 21].

2.1.3 Selecting an Antibiotic

The choice of antibiotic depends on the proposed operation and thus on the types of bacteria that are to be encountered. Antibiotic choice is also guided by the nature of the resistant bacterial strains that exist in the hospital. Side effects and costs should also be considered.

Cephalosporins or broad-spectrum penicillins, such as mezlocillin, are recommended for procedures in which the gastrointestinal tract is opened (e.g., surgery of the cardioesophageal junction). The necessity of adding a drug active against anaerobes (metronidazole) is unclear. For procedures on the lung, suitable antibiotics besides cephalosporins and mezlocillin are penicillinase-resistant penicillins, penicillin G, and azlocillin (see below).

2.2 Indications

2.2.1 *Resections of the Esophagus and Cardia*

The rationale for perioperative antibiotic prophylaxis in resections of the esophagus and gastric cardia [12] derives from bacteriologic studies showing a link between the intragastric pH and the size of the bacterial population in the stomach [16]. When the intragastric pH was less than 4, the gastric juice was usually sterile, but when the pH was greater than 4, bacteria were almost always found. This led Muscroft and Deane [16] to conclude that perioperative antibiotic prophylaxis is appropriate for all gastroesophageal resections where the gastric juice is found to have a relatively high pH.

This does not mean that the gastric-juice pH and bacterial count need to be determined routinely for these operations. Because patients with a cardia or gastric carcinoma are normally achlorhydric, and the carcinomas are heavily colonized by bacteria, prophylactic antibiotics are indicated in carcinoma patients as a standard precaution.

Prospective studies have confirmed the prophylactic value of perioperative antibiotics in resections of gastric and cardia carcinoma [12]. Similar considerations apply to resections involving the esophagus: The bacteria found in this region are the same as those identified in the stomach of achlorhydric patients [16]. Finlay et al. [6], who found both aerobic and anaerobic organisms, noted a close relationship between the bacterial colonization of the esophagus and postoperative infections [16].

These studies demonstrate the value of administering a broad-spectrum antibiotic (cephalosporin or mezlocillin) combined with a drug active against anaerobes (metronidazole) perioperatively to patients scheduled for an esophageal resection.

2.2.2 *Pulmonary Procedures*

Perioperative antibiotics are considered appropriate for all procedures that involve division of the bronchial tree (segmental resections, lobectomies, pneumonectomies) [17], although it must be added that research in this area has not been as comprehensive or thorough as one would wish [10]. Thus, while Kvale et al. [15] showed in a prospective study that perioperative antibiotics were of value in pulmonary surgery, Truesdale et al. [22] concluded that this type of prophylaxis was ineffective. Nevertheless, we feel that perioperative antibiotic prophylaxis should be recommended for all pulmonary resections. It must be considered that the bacteria encountered in pulmonary procedures (e.g., Staphylococcus aureus [7]) can be quite different from those encountered in esophageal procedures, and that the selection of antibiotic must be adjusted accordingly (penicillin or cephalosporin; activity against anaerobes is not required; see above).

2.3 Local Antibiotic Prophylaxis in Patients on Ventilatory Support

It has been shown that the bacterial flora of the upper airways does not change appreciably until the patient has been on ventilatory support for about 48 h, at which time the respiratory tract becomes increasingly colonized by pathogenic organisms [1].

This colonization does not constitute infection, however, and indeed there is much evidence against a direct link between mechanical ventilation and the incidence of pneumonia [3, 4]. Cause-and-effect relationships between ventilation and respiratory tract infection become very difficult to establish in patients requiring prolonged ventilation.

But while a direct link between the postoperative pneumonia rate and mechanical ventilation cannot be proved, there is no question that the risk of pneumonia due to hospital organisms increases with the duration of ventilatory support [4]. Potential sources of infection include a tracheostoma or the effects of intratracheal suctioning. Storm [20], for example, showed that the routine suctioning of ventilated patients can cause bacteria present in the tracheobronchial tree to invade into the blood stream. The result is an initially asymptomatic bacteremia that can progress to a systemic infection. This transient bacteremia can be avoided by reducing the bacterial colonization of the upper airways. Klastersky et al. [13] and Vogel et al. [23] accomplished this by the intratracheal instillation of gentamycin. This *prophylaxis* was found to reduce significantly the incidence of respiratory tract infection [23], and it is additionally recommended for the *treatment* of bronchopneumonia in ventilated patients [14].

It should be added that the routine use of this technique in the intensive care unit requires frequent determinations of aminoglycoside serum levels, because gentamycin, even when applied locally, is absorbed and thus can accumulate in the serum. Systemic and potentially toxic side effects are a danger, especially in patients with renal failure [18].

References

1. Bryant LR, Trinkle JK, Mobin-Uddin K, Baker J, Griffen WO (1972) Bacterial colonization profile with tracheal intubation and mechanical ventilation. Arch Surg 104:647–651
2. Burke JF (1961) The effective period of preventive antibiotic action in experimental incisions and dermal lesions. Surgery 50:161–168
3. Comhaire A, Lamy M (1981) Contamination rate of sterilized ventilators in an ICU. Crit Care Med 9:546–548
4. Cross AS, Roup B (1981) Role of respiratory assistance devices in endemic nosocomial pneumonia. Am J Med 70:681–685
5. Daschner F (1981) Antibiotikaprophylaxe – sinnvoll oder sinnlos? Dtsch med Wochenschr 106:1150–1153
6. Finlay IG, Wright P, Mcardle CS (1980) Oesophageal bacterial flora in carcinoma of oesophagus. Brit J Surg 67:815–836
7. Frimodt-Møller N, Ostri P, Pedersen IK, Poulsen SR (1982) Antibiotic prophylaxis in pulmonary surgery. A double-blind study of penicillin versus placebo. Ann Surg 195:444–450
8. Grundmann R (1982) Die perioperative Antibiotikaprophylaxe. Krankenhausarzt 55:879–884
9. Hamelmann H, Erttmann M (1984) Antibioticapro phylaxe in der Chirurgie des Gastrointestinaltraktes. Chirurg 55:218–221
10. Hirschmann JV, Inui TS (1980) Antimicrobial prophylaxis: A critique of recent trials. Rev infect Dis 2:1–23
11. Hoffmann CEJ, McDonald PJ, Watts J McK (1981) Use of peroperative Cefoxitin® to prevent infection after colonic and rectal surgery. Ann Surg 193:353–356
12. Keighley MRB, Burdon DW, Gatehouse D (1982) Rate of wound sepsis with "selective" short-term antibiotic prophylaxis in gastric surgery. World J Surg 6:445–449
13. Klastersky J, Cappel R, Noterman J, Snoeck J, Geuning C, Mouawad E (1973) Endotracheal gentamincin for the prevention of bronchial infections in patients with tracheotomy. Int J Clin Pharmacol 74:279–286
14. Klastersky J, Carpentier-Meunier F, Kahan-Coppens L, Thys JP (1979) Endotracheally administered antibiotics for gram-negative bronchopneumonia. Chest 75:586–591
15. Kvale PA, Ranga V, Kopacz M, Cox F, Magilligan DJ, Davila JC (1977) Pulmonary resection. South Med J 70:64–68
16. Muscroft TJ, Deane SA (1982) Prevention of sepsis in gastroesophageal surgery. World J Surg 6:293–300
17. Sandusky WR (1977) Prophylaxis in surgery. J Am med Ass 237:1003–1008
18. Schulz E, Busse FW, Strasburger C, Herhahn J, Wood WG, Sack K (1983) Gentamicin-Serumspiegel nach intratrachealer Applikation bei Beatmungspatienten mit normaler und eingeschränkter Nierenfunktion. Dtsch med Wochenschr 108:1964–1967
19. Stone HH, Haney BB, Kolb LD, Geheber CE, Hooper CA (1979) Prophylactic and preventive antibiotic therapy. Timing, duration and economics. Ann Surg 189:691–699
20. Storm W (1981) Transitorische Bakteriämien nach endotrachealem Absaugen. Dtsch med Wochenschr 106:1496–1498
21. Strachan CJL, Black J, Powis SJA, Waterworth TA, Wise AR, Wilkinson AR, Burdon DW, Severn M, Mitra B, Norcott H (1977) Prophylactic use of cephazolin against wound sepsis after cholecystectomy. Br med J 1:1254–1256
22. Truesdale R, D'Alessandri R, Manuel V, Daicoff G, Kluge RM (1979) Antimicrobial vs placebo prophylaxis in noncardiac thoracic surgery. J Am med Ass 241:1254–1256
23. Vogel F, Werner H, Exner M, Marx M (1981) Prophylaxe und Therapie von Atemwegsinfektionen bei beatmeten Patienten durch intratracheale Aminoglykosidgabe. Dtsch med Wochenschr 106:898–903

C. Perioperative Management

3 Physiotherapy in Thoracic Surgical Patients

H. Hofmann, with Assistance from H. Ehrenberg

CONTENTS

3.1 Introduction

The goals of pre- and postoperative physiotherapy in thoracic surgical patients relate to the prevention of postoperative respiratory complications and gross postural defects. The causes of pulmonary complications in this population may be divided into two groups:

3.1.1 Causes Relating to the Surgical Procedure

- Effects of anesthesia, i.e., anesthetic gases paralyze the bronchial ciliary epithelium and stimulate mucus production, which can lead to retention of secretions.
- Wound and chest-tube pain, which can deter deep breathing and effective coughing.

3.1.2 Patient-Related Causes

- General condition, age, obesity.
- Cigarette smoking, preexisting pulmonary disease (especially obstructive bronchitis).
- Level of patient understanding and cooperation.

3.2 Goals, Principles, and Conduct of Physiotherapy

3.2.1 Therapeutic Goal: Prevention of Pneumonia

Pneumonia prophylaxis consists in eliminating the postoperative factors that promote infection by pneumonia-causing bacteria.

3.2.1.1 Correction of Alveolar Underventilation or Nonuniform Ventilation

Principles	*Techniques*
Increasing inspiratory excursions to the range of the inspiratory capacity (ventilatory stimulation)	Physiotherapeutic techniques: patient performs deep inhalations, holding the breath at the end of inspiration (inhalation exercises) [2].
Increased respiratory excursions with an increased respiratory effort (ventilatory increase)	Dead-space tubing [3]
Increasing respiratory excursions with a decreased respiratory effort	Intermittent positive pressure breathing (IPPB)

3.2.1.2 Management of Airway Secretions

Principles	*Techniques*
Gravitational effect	Physiotherapeutic techniques: position changes, i.e., change from supine position, decubitus, sitting; postural drainage as needed
Mechanical stimulation of the chest wall	Chest vibration or percussion
Respiratory fluctuations in bronchial calibers.	Sessions of deep inhalation and exhalation (deep breathing exercises) [2] Dead-space tubing, see 1.1

3.2.1.3 Raising Bronchial Secretions by Coughing

Principles	*Techniques*
Coughing assisted by pain relief	Physiotherapeutic techniques: patient coughs while the wound area is supported (anxious patients are taught to cough in short bursts).
Coughing with minimal rise of intrathoracic pressure (e.g., for procedures on the tracheobronchial tree)	Damp unproductive coughing with closed lips, coughs in short bursts or performs "throat clearing."

3.2.1.4 Prevention of Pulmonary Hypostasis

Principles	*Techniques*
Redistribution of pulmonary blood (gravitational effect	Physiotherapeutic techniques: frequent repositioning, see 2.1.2

3.2.2 Therapeutic Goal: Improvement of Ventilation-Perfusion Ratio

This is accomplished by correcting maldistribution of ventilation, following the principles and techniques for pneumonia prophylaxis.

3.2.3 Therapeutic Goal: Support of Lung Expansion

Indicated after segmentectomy, atypical resection, lobectomy, decortication, and in pneumothorax.

Principles	*Techniques*
Reinflation of all alveoli	Physiotherapeutic techniques: spontaneous deep breathing (see 2.1.1); mechanical aids (see 2.1.1); breathing against an expiratory resistance, e.g., exhalating against water pressure in a bottle or blowing up a prestretched balloon.

3.2.4 Therapeutic Goal: Prevention of Pleural Thickening

Effective prophylaxis depends on the rapid elimination of pleural effusion.

Principles	*Techniques*
Increase movement of pleural layers to inhibit pleural thickening	Physiotherapeutic techniques: deep breathing exercises with breath held at end-inspiration in various "stretch-positions" of the chest wall

3.2.5 *Therapeutic Goal: Correction of Postural Defects*

This involves the correction of upper body postural defects following a lateral thoracotomy incision (especially after lung resections and thoracoplasties and in growing patients; scoliosis prevention).

Principles	*Techniques*
Vertical realignment of the spinal column	Physiotherapeutic techniques: postural and motor exercises of the upper body

3.2.6 *Therapeutic Goal: Prevention of Contractures*

This involves the prevention of contractures about the shoulder joint on the operative side, especially after mastectomy.

Principles	*Techniques*
Repeated stretching of incipient fibrous tissue contraction (scar, muscle, joint capsule)	Physiotherapeutic techniques: arm movements and positioning

3.2.7 *Therapeutic Goal: Prevention of Thrombosis*

Principles	*Techniques*
Stimulation of venous return	Physiotherapeutic techniques: dynamic muscular contractions to activate the muscle pump, compression by stockings or bandages

3.3 Conduct of Physiotherapy

3.3.1 *Preoperative Period*

Experience has shown that the level of patient cooperation and motivation after surgery depends greatly on the quality of the preoperative management and the degree to which the patient has been prepared for postoperative care measures. The following preparatory steps are essential:

- The patient is told what to expect after surgery and is informed about potential complications to reduce his anxiety and improve his level of cooperation.
- The patient is taught to increase chest wall movements in the area of the proposed incision while maintaining a normal tidal volume to avoid hyperventilation. He is taught how to cough effectively while supporting the proposed wound area to alleviate pain.
- Practice in breathing through dead-space tubing to increase pulmonary ventilation [3] (see Postoperative Management).
- Practice with IPPB devices both for assisted ventilation and for inhalation therapy with secrolytic and bronchodilator agents (4 × daily) where an obstructive ventilatory defect is present (after pulmonary function testing).

3.3.2 *Postoperative Period*

In the initial days following thoracic surgery, patients manifest an altered breathing pattern characterized by frequent, shallow respirations. Movements of the wound area are reflexly diminished, with upper abdominal surgery leading to a predominance of costosternal respiratory movements, and lateral thoracotomy leading to a predominance of forward and lateral costoabdominal excursions toward the unaffected side. These patients, unlike patients with sternotomies, are at increased risk for developing respiratory problems.

There is reluctance to move the arm on the operated side, and movements of the entire upper body are diminished. Coughing is largely suppressed due to fear of pain.

In cooperative patients, deep breathing can be acccomplished through spontaneous respirations with manual assistance. If the depth of respiration is not increased in this way, due for example to pain, fear, chest tubes, or pleural effusion, we utilize dead-space tubing. It is our experience that this technique distracts the patient sufficiently to enable deeper respirations.

The dead-space tubing is made of plastic and can be lengthened in volume increments of 100 ml. The tubing causes the patient to rebreath expired air and therefore increases the inspired concentration of CO_2, effectively increasing the dead-space volume. This leads to a rise of CO_2 tension in the alveoli and secondarily in the arterial blood, while the oxygen tension falls slightly. Central respiratory centers respond to the elevated arterial PCO_2 by increasing the total ventilation in an effort to restore a normal PCO_2 – a process known as compensation. But this ventilatory increase requires a corresponding adjustment in respiratory mechanics that will enable the patient to match the depth of respiration to the respiratory rate, i.e., the patient must make an increased respiratory effort. If this is not possible due to pain or general postoperative debility, the respiratory rate during dead-space breathing will rise to levels above 24/min, which can result in hypoventilation with a falling PO_2 and rising PCO_2. The patient becomes dyspneic and is forced to terminate the dead-space breathing. The respiratory rate is counted before the tubing is used and 3 min afterward, as that is the time needed to compensate a dead-space volume of 300–500 ml. When the dead space is properly selected, the respiratory rate after 3 min should be less than 24/min, in which case a ventilatory increase can be maintained for a prolonged period without the detrimental effects of hyperventilation. The duration is determined with the following objectives in mind:

- Breathing with tubing volumes of 200–400 ml for 10–15 min 8–10 times per day is adequate for the prevention of microatelectases and for the clearing and raising of secretions.
- The tubing should be used for at least 10 min hourly to correct maldistribution of ventilation.
- Coughing can be induced by 5–10 breaths with 400–700 ml of tubing, without regard for the respiratory rate.

Contraindications to the use of dead-space tubing are:
- A rise in the respiratory rate above 24/min
- Severe emphysema
- Severe bronchial asthma
- Excessive hypoxic risk (e.g., in coronary patients).

It is our experience that most patients can compensate a dead-space volume of 200–300 ml in the initial days following surgery. But if the patient cannot make the necessary effort (e.g., if his respiratory rate becomes too high), assisted ventilation with IPPB devices is indicated. This will permit inspiration to the designated end-inspiratory pressure even in anxious patients and those with significant wound pain. In patients who have undergone lung resections or tracheobronchial anastomoses, the inspiratory pressure should not exceed 25 cm H_2O to avoid bronchopulmonary fistulae. In the presence of pneumothorax, treatment should be deferred until the second postoperative day, provided there is free chest tube drainage. Since failure to humidify the inspired air can damage the bronchial epithelium (viscous secretions are a culture medium for infection and can form crusts), water should always be used in the nebulizer. Exceptions are patients with obstructive bronchitis, who require special management. These patients with chronic obstructive ventilation defects should continue to receive bronchiolytic therapy. Sputum production varies a great deal, and it should be determined whether a persistent and possibly troublesome cough is productive, in which case the patient should be helped several times daily to raise secretions, or whether the cough is unproductive, in which case it should be suppressed until sputum can be raised.

The early repositioning of lateral thoracotomy patients into the unaffected side is performed in conjunction with breathing exercises, dead-space tubing, and IPPB treatments. This program is effective in increasing respiratory excursions and producing a stretching effect that inhibits pleural thickening. In patients who are expected to develop pleural thickening, stretching postures are employed in conjunction with deep breathing exercises and dead-space tubing. This is a long-term regimen that should be continued independently at home.

Starting on the first postoperative day, patients are encouraged to use the arm on the operative side as much as possible. As recovery progresses, the range of shoulder motion can be increased as scar tissues become stretched.

In mastectomized patients whose tissues are compromised by pre- or postoperative radiation or who have undergone axillary dissection, contractures are prevented by a gradual but persistent stretching of the soft tissues over a period of up to four months. With incipient lymphedema, the arm should be elevated and the muscular pump activated by dynamic exercises of the hand and forearm muscles, assisted by compression therapy.

Training in the maintenance of an upright posture is started right away in the sitting position and is combined with breathing exercises. Long-term therapy for scoliosis prevention is indicated after certain operative procedures (see 2.2.5) and is of major importance in children.

References

1. Brünger B, Stühmer B (1980) Krankengymnastik aktuell. Pflaum-Verlag, München
2. Ehrenberg H (1982) Krankengymnastik, Bd I, Grundlagen der Krankengymnastik (Krankengymnastische Techniken der Atemtherapie) Thieme, Stuttgart
3. Giebel O (1962) Der Einfluß künstlicher Totraumvergrößerung auf Ventilation und Blutgase. 79. Tagung d. Dtsch. Gesellschaft f. Chirurgie, Langenbecks Arch Chir und Dtsch. Z. f. Chirurgie 301:543–548

3a. Giebel O (1967) Über das Verhalten von Ventilation, Gasaustausch und Kreislauf bei Patienten mit normalem und gestörtem Gasaustausch unter künstlicher Totraumvergrößerung. Habilitationsschrift Springer Bd 41.

3b. Giebel O (1976) Totraumvergrößerer. Fortbildungskursus für Krankenschwestern- und Pfleger. 116. Tagung der Vereinigung Nordwestdeutscher Chirurgen: Inhalationstherapie und Atemgymnastik. Die Schwester/Der Pfleger 15:48–50

3c. Giebel O, Horatz K (1967) Die Anwendung künstlicher Totraumvergrößerung zur Behandlung von Atelektasen. Bruns-Beitr klin Chir 214:375–381

4. Siemon G (1976) Physikalische Atemtherapie im Rahmen operativer Eingriffe. Fortbildungseminar für Krankengymnasten „Prä- und postoperative Atemtherapie“ 93. Tagung der Deutschen Gesellschaft für Chirurgie

D. Surgical Treatment of Thoracic Trauma and Chest Wall Diseases

F. W. SCHILDBERG, E. KIFFNER, and M. H. SCHOENBERG

CONTENTS

1 Procedures for Thoracic Trauma

1.1 Management of Musculoskeletal Injuries

The spectrum of thoracic trauma ranges from simple contusions to fractures of the thoracic cage and acutely life-threatening injuries of intrathoracic viscera. Certain injuries that are visible on roentgenograms, such as fractures of the first rib or sternum, usually signify massive chest trauma and always raise the question of associated injuries within the chest. In other cases serious injuries may be masked by the presence of apparently trivial ones. Thoracic injuries, then, should always be evaluated in relation to the overall condition of the patient.

1.1.1 Management of Subcutaneous Emphysema

Isolated subcutaneous emphysema is a common finding. It indicates injury to aerated structures and is usually of little significance in itself. Treatment is directed toward the underlying cause, which may be a pneumothorax, tension pneumothorax, mediastinal emphysema, respiratory tract injury, or esophageal injury. The symptomatic treatment of subcutaneous emphysema by multiple skin incisions is rarely advised.

1.1.2 Treatment of Mediastinal Emphysema

Posttraumatic mediastinal emphysema can result from esophageal or tracheobronchial injuries and from pneumothorax with a tear in the mediastinal pleura. Occasionally it results from alveolar rupture in patients on prolonged ventilatory support. The condition is first manifested clinically by a subcutaneous emphysema about the neck and head. Treatment generally is not required. Increased mediastinal pressure with inflow stasis will necessitate surgical decompression by a collar mediastinotomy.

1.1.2.1 Collar Mediastinotomy (Fig. 1 a–c)

Indication: Impending rise of mediastinal pressure.

Surgical goal: Decompression of mediastinal emphysema.

Preoperative preparation: Local skin prep.

Incision: Transverse incision about 5 cm long over the jugular fossa.

Instruments: Basic set, drainage tube.

> *Steps in procedure:*
>
> (1) Transverse incision over the jugular fossa
> (2) Division of subcutaneous tissue and platysma
> (3) Blunt dissection on the trachea to the bifurcation
> (4) Insertion of drainage tube
> (5) Wound closure over tube

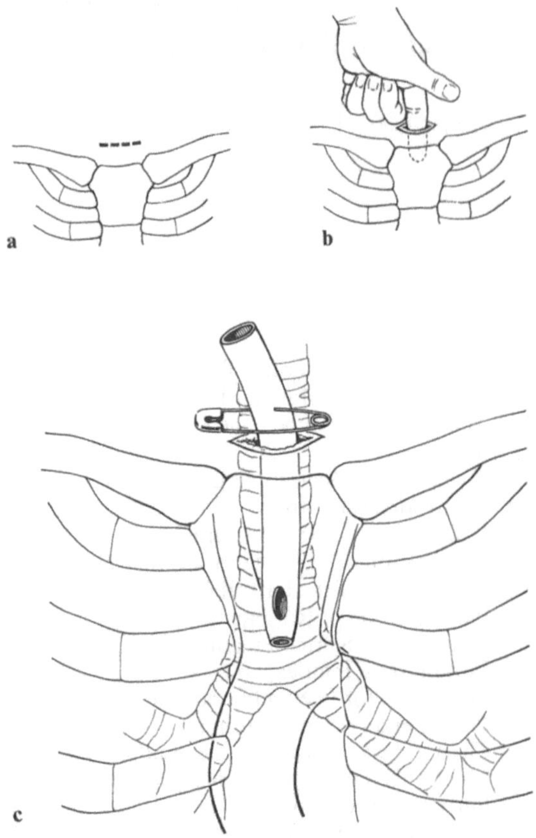

Fig. 1 a–c. Collar mediastinotomy: Transverse incision over the jugular fossa, pretracheal finger dissection, insertion of drainage tube

Following division of the skin and subcutaneous tissue, the platysma is sharply incised, and the straight neck muscles are bluntly separated to expose the trachea distal to the thyroid, sparing the lowest thyroid artery and vein. The finger is passed bluntly down along the trachea; air usually escapes from the mediastinal tissue at this time. The blunt dissection can be carried as far as the tracheal bifurcation, at which point a drainage tube is inserted and brought out through the wound or, preferably, through a separate incision. The tube does not need to be connected to a waterseal system as long as the pleural spaces have not been entered. If the mediastinal emphysema is the result of a tension pneumothorax, primary decompression of the pneumothorax will usually obviate the need for a mediastinotomy. The incision is approximated with sutures, and the tube is secured.

1.1.3 Management of Rib Fractures

Rib fractures and costochondral separations are the most common thoracic injuries. The goal of primary treatment, after the exclusion of associated injuries, is to relieve pain to enable adequate spontaneous respiration. In most patients this can be accomplished with oral analgesics, although unresponsive cases will require intercostal nerve block or peridural anesthesia. When respiratory insufficiency is caused exclusively by chest wall instability, or if a thoracic procedure is indicated for other reasons, operative stabilization of the thoracic skeleton should be considered. Several options exist in these cases, including traction on the sternum for anterior instability, fixation of the unstable fragments with steel splints, Kirschner wire fixation of the rib, and bone plating.

1.1.3.1 Stabilization of the Anterior Chest Wall (Figs. 2 and 3)

Indication: Chest wall instability secondary to serial segmental rib fractures.

Surgical goals: Stabilize the chest wall to avoid prolonged respiratory support, prevent posttraumatic chest deformities.

Preoperative preparation: Chest hair is removed, the rib fractures and flail portion of the chest wall are marked.

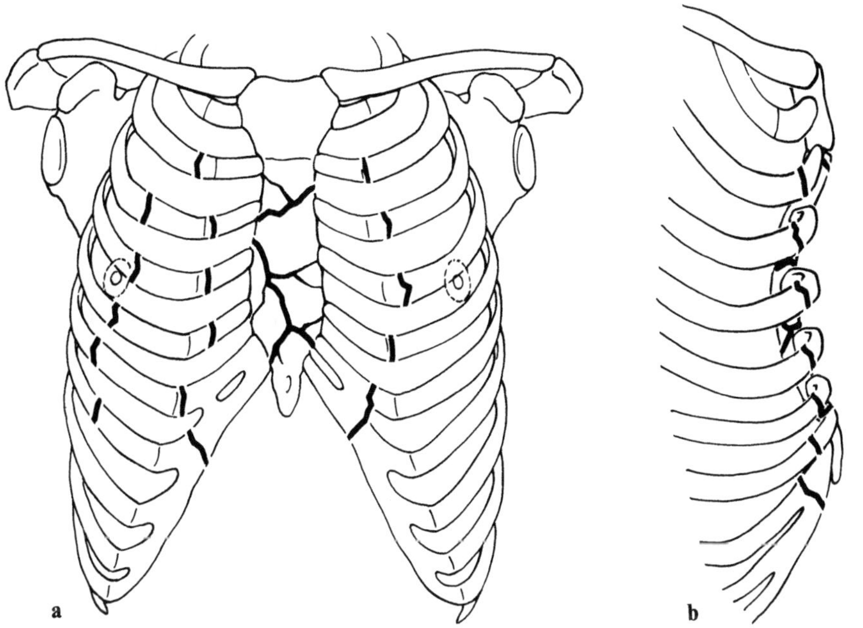

Fig. 2a, b. Anterior chest wall instability: Common fracture sites. a Anterior and b lateral view

Position: Supine.

Incisions: Three incisions are made, each 5 cm long: two over the ribs that will support the fixation material, and one auxiliary incision over the xiphoid process.

Instruments: Basic set, set for funnel chest and ribs, Sulamaa steel splint [20].

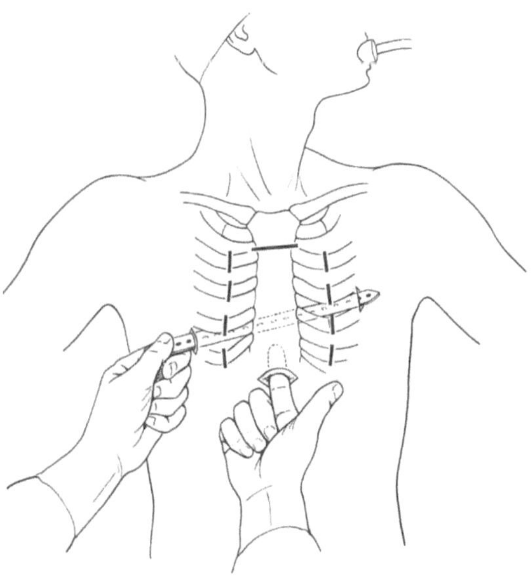

Fig. 3. Surgical treatment of anterior chest wall instability: The depressed chest wall is elevated by blunt dissection through an incision over the xyphoid. The sternum is supported on a steel splint inserted obliquely through separate incisions and anchored to the ribs

Steps in procedure:

(1) Incision over the rib sites that will support the splint
(2) Elevation of the sternum through an auxiliary incision over the xyphoid process
(3) Insertion of the steel splint
(4) Fixation of the splint
(5) Skin closure

With the patient in the supine position, intact areas of rib lateral to the fracture are identified, and the sites of support are designated. These should be selected such that the splint, when inserted, will be positioned at about the center of the flail segment. For better stability we insert the splint obliquely so that the sharpened end is one interspace higher than the blunt end. Each rib site that will support the splint is exposed through a 5-cm incision parallel to the rib. A third, longitudinal incision can be made over the xiphoid process as an auxiliary incision for elevating the sternum and assisting the dissection. Through the incision, a finger is passed bluntly beneath the sternum and elevates it outward. The chest wall is then stabilized with a narrow, pointed steel splint of the type used for funnel chest operations. It is inserted under digital guidance so that it lies deep to the sternum and external to the pleura, and it is fixed to the supporting rib sites with nonabsorbable polymer threads (Fig. 3).

1.1.3.2 Stabilization of the Lateral Chest Wall (Fig. 4a, b)

Indication: Operative treatment is very rarely indicated. Stabilization is usually performed for serial segmental rib fractures or in conjunction with the operative treatment of other chest injuries.

Surgical goals: Stabilize the chest wall, prevent paradoxical motion, shorten the duration of ventilatory support.

Preoperative preparation: Removal of chest hair.

Position: Lateral or oblique.

Incision: Depends on the site of the injury and the selected operative procedure.

Instruments: Basic set, rib resection set, special instruments and instrument sets. Kirschner wires, ASIF one-third tubular plate, special Vecsei plates [21] or steel splints.

Several procedures have been devised for operative stabilization of the lateral chest wall. The procedure requiring the least time involves the application of steel splints in a V-shaped configuration. For this purpose drill holes are made at the ends of the splints to permit their fixation to intact ribs and to the clavicle. An incision is made over the clavicle, and the steel splints are introduced subcutaneously such that they bridge the unstable fragment in an inverted V-shaped fashion. The splints are fixed to the clavicle, the lower supporting ribs, and to the flail fragment with nonabsorbable threads.

1.1.3.3 Plate Fixation of Rib Fractures (Figs. 5–7, 8a–c)

With the patient under general endotracheal anesthesia, the unstable area is exposed. After the rib fractures are identified and reduced, a sufficiently long ASIF one-third tubular plate is appropriately contoured and temporarily held in place with Lambott or Verbrugge forceps before it is definitively fixed with small-fragment cortex screws

Fig. 4a, b. Stabilization of an unstable lateral chest wall with steel struts: The splints are introduced through a small incision over the clavicle. Counterincisions are made over the supporting rib sites, and another incision is made in the area of the unstable fragment for attachment to the splints

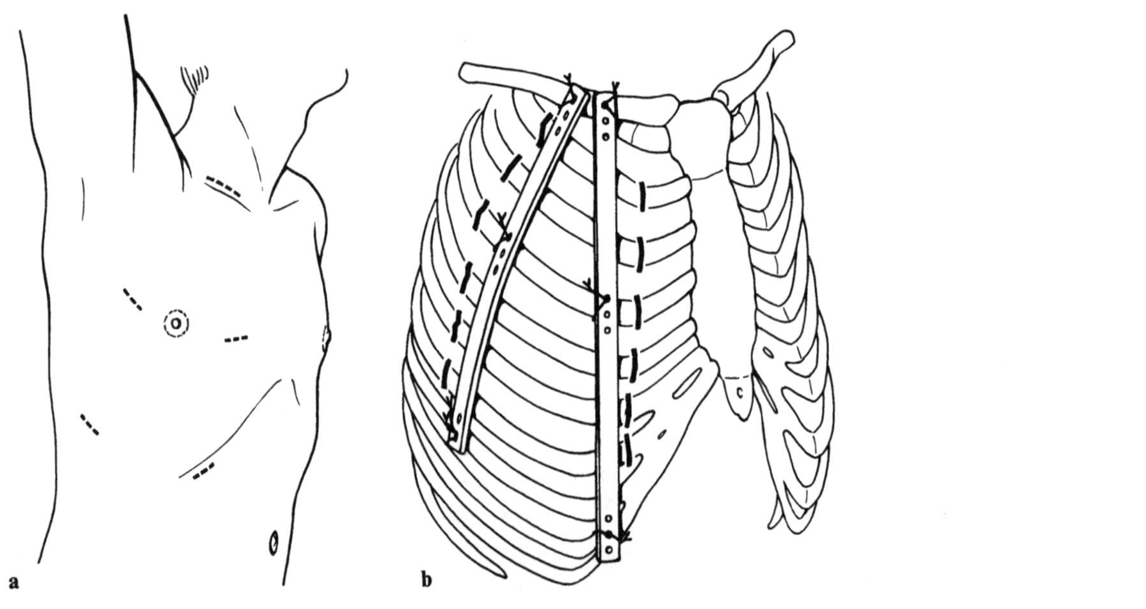

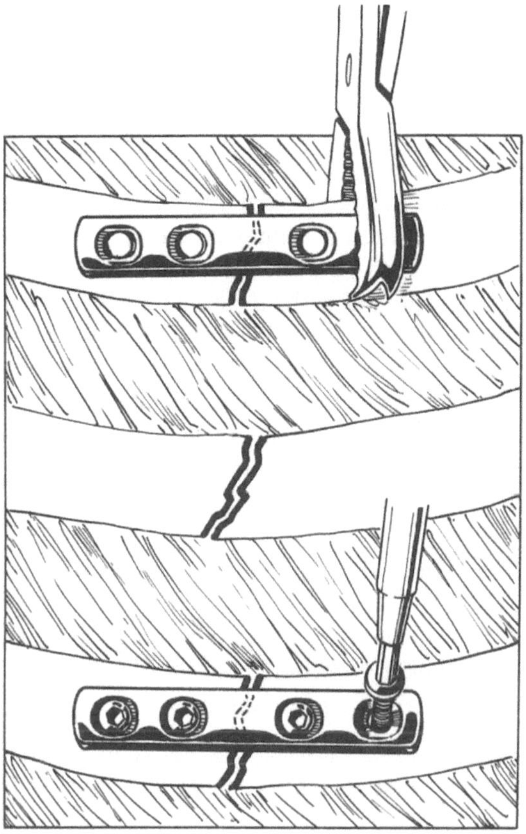

Fig. 5. Internal fixation of the lateral chest wall: When stabilizing the ribs with the ASIF one-third tubular plate, it is sufficient to stabilize the major pillars. The plate is contoured to the rib surface and temporarily held in place with a forceps (Verbrugge or Lambott) before it is definitively fixed with screws

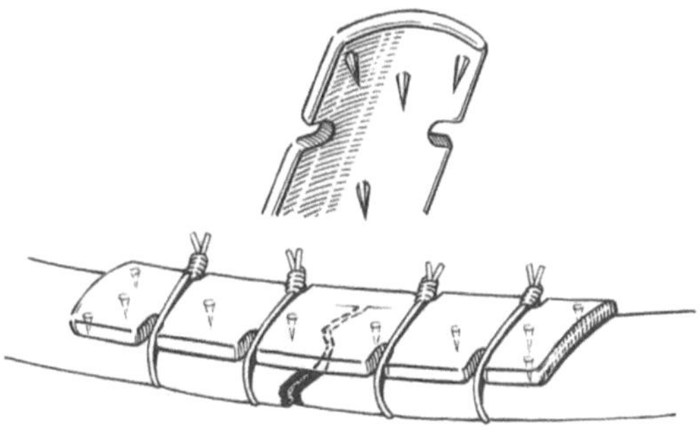

Fig. 6. The Vecsei plate is contoured to the rib surface and temporarily held in place with a forceps while the definitive wire loops are applied. Small teeth keep the plate from slipping

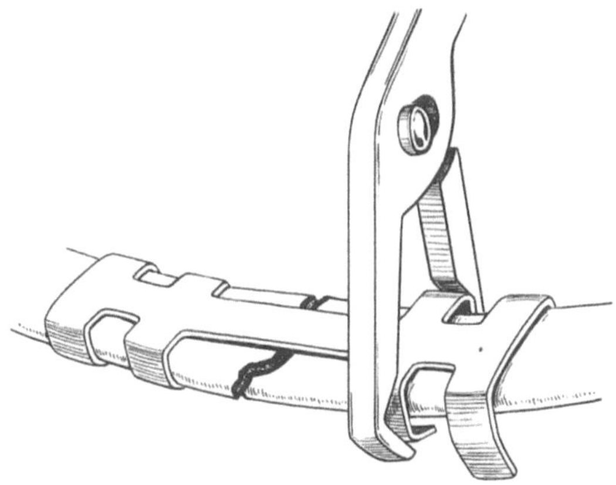

Fig. 7. The Judet plate is designed for quick application. The tabs are crimped around the rib with a special forceps

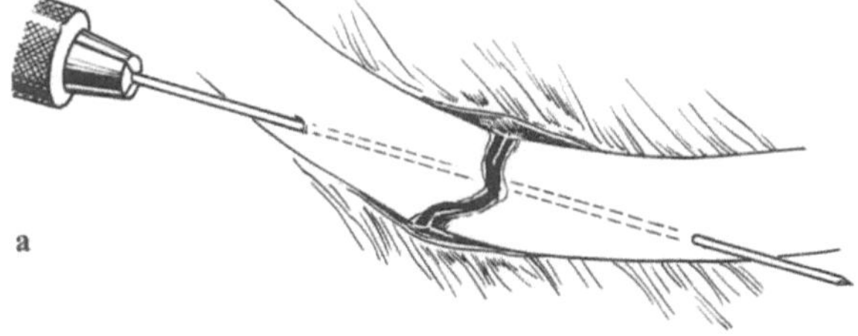

a

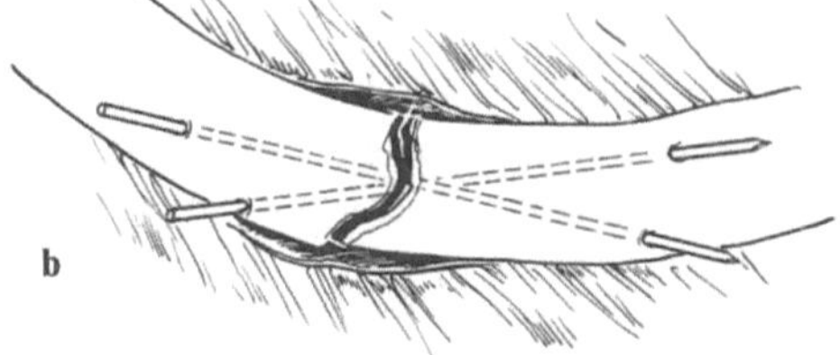

b

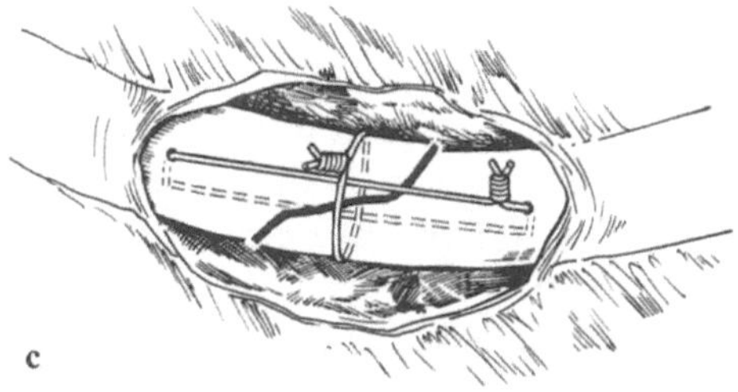

c

Fig. 8. a, b Fixation of a rib fracture with crossed Kirschner wires that transfix the fracture tangentially. **c** Fixation of a rib fracture with a wire suture and wire loop

(Fig. 5). All the fracture do not require operative fixation; it is sufficient to stabilize, say, every second rib in order to prevent paradoxical movement of the chest wall.

To make plating easier, Vecsei [21] has developed a plate that can be attached to the reduced fracture with cerclage wire. The small spikes on the plate ensure a solid seating (Fig. 6).

Another special plate developed by Judet has fixation tabs that can be crimped around the rib with the aid of special forceps (Fig. 7).

Kirschner wires are the oldest devices for the internal fixation of rib fractures, and currently they are the least used. After reduction of the fracture, a Kirschner wire is drilled across the center of the fracture site, utilizing the curvature of the rib for access. If enough space is available, two wires may be inserted in crossed fashion (Fig. 8a, b).

Cerclage wires and wire sutures provide yet another technique for the operative fixation of rib fractures (Fig. 8c).

1.1.4 Treatment of Sternal Fractures

Fracture of the sternum is frequently associated with other severe intrathoracic injuries, such as pulmonary or cardiac contusion. Tears of great vessels like the aorta, brachiocephalic trunk, and the supraaortic branches as well as lacerations of the tracheobronchial system are well-known coexisting injuries. The isolated fracture itself is characterized clinically by a protracted, painful course. In the absence of associated injuries, the reduction of a displaced sternal fracture may be attempted by lordotic positioning of the thoracic spine.

Operative fixation is usually performed only in conjunction with the treatment of other injuries. In these cases the fragments may be fixed with wire sutures or Kirschner wires.

1.2 Intrathoracic Injuries

1.2.1 Procedures for Pneumothorax, Hemothorax, and Hemopericardium

Traumatic pneumothorax can result from a rupture or perforation of the lung by a fractured rib and also from tears of the trachea, bronchi, or esophagus.

A mild pneumothorax without associated injuries requires no special treatment initially. However, a larger accumulation of air in the pleural cavity or a tension pneumothorax is an emergency situation necessitating chest tube insertion. For pure pneumothorax the tube may be inserted anteriorly through the second intercostal space, $2^1/_2$ fingerwidths from the sternal margin (avoiding injury to the internal thoracic artery). If effusion is also found to be present (hydropneumothorax) or if there is blood in the pleural space (hemopneumothorax), the tube is introduced through the fifth intercostal space anterior to the midaxillary line. A rule of thumb is that the chest tube should not be inserted distal to the nipple, but at the level of the fourth or fifth interspace (Fig. 9).

1.2.1.1 Chest Tube Drainage for Pneumothorax

Indications: Drainage of pneumothorax or tension pneumothorax, decompression of hemopneumothorax or hydropneumothorax.

Surgical goals: Remove accumulated air, reexpand the lung, remove tension, evacuate intrapleural fluid.

Preoperative preparation: Local skin prep, local anesthesia.

Incision: 2-cm incision over the selected intercostal space, parallel to the rib.

Instruments: Chest tube, wound care set.

Steps in procedure:

(1) Incision parallel to the rib in the 4th or 5th interspace anterior to the midaxillary line
(2) Blunt dissection to the pleural surface
(3) Incision of parietal pleura with a scissors
(4) Insertion of large-gauge chest tube
(5) Fixation of tube with suture
(6) Connection of tube to waterseal system
(7) Postoperative check roentgenograms

Local anesthetic is injected in the selected interspace to produce analgesia in the skin, subcutaneous tissue, and especially in the rib periosteum and pleural layers. A 2-cm stab incision is made, and the pleural surface is reached by blunt dissection with a scissors. Under digital guidance, the pleura is opened with the scissors, and the chest tube is

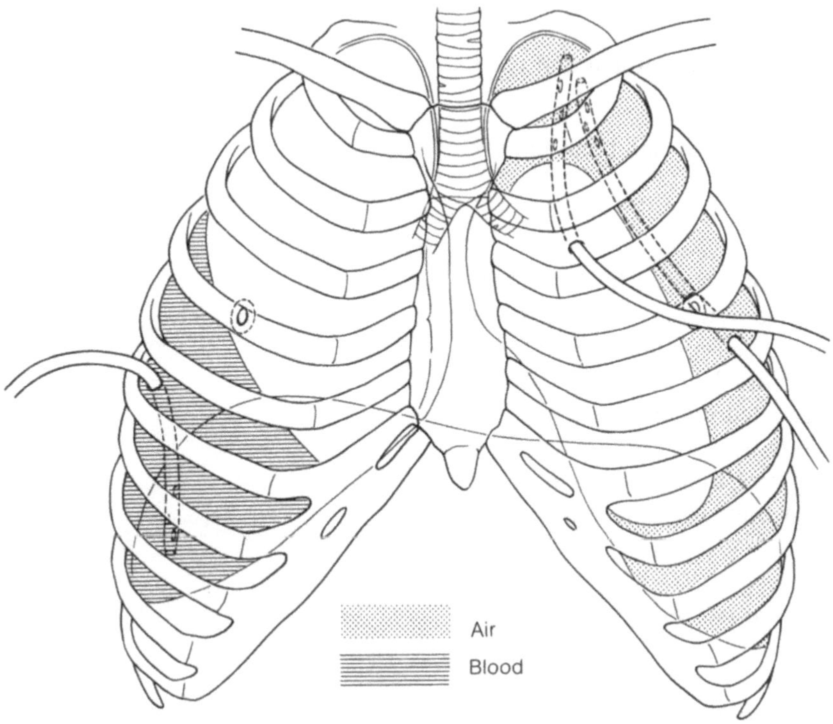

Fig. 9. Pleural drainage: The left half of the figure shows the tube placement for drainage of hemothorax, the right half for drainage of pneumothorax

inserted. Alternatively, a trocar chest tube may be used to penetrate the parietal pleura. In this case the left hand guides the tube while the right hand presses gently on the trocar to introduce it into the pleural space. The trocar method carries a greater risk of injury to parenchymatous organs (lung, liver, spleen). A large-gauge chest tube (No. 28) is preferred. After the tube has been inserted, it is sutured to the skin, and a horizontal mattress suture is placed that will be tied at the time of tube removal. The chest tube is connected to a waterseal apparatus.

In the ventilated patient, air loss through preexisting parenchymal fistulas can occasionally be so significant that multiple chest tubes are needed to handle the volume of air that accumulates.

1.2.1.2 Chest Tube Drainage for Hemothorax

Bleeding into the pleural space can result from injuries to the lung, intercostal vessels, internal thoracic artery, pericardial vessels, or great vessels. Coexistence with pneumothorax is common. Treatment is necessary to quantitate the blood loss, avoid lung compression, and prevent significant pleural thickening.

Hemothorax may be classified by volume as mild (less than 350 ml of collected blood)), moderate (350–1500 ml), or massive (more than 1500 ml). With a massive hemothorax or if bleeding persists after chest tube insertion, an emergency thoracotomy must be performed to eliminate the source of the hemorrhage. All other situations can be managed with a chest tube. The insertion technique is the same as for pneumothorax, except that the tube is placed against the lower chest wall to drain the dependent portions of the thoracic cavity.

1.2.1.3 Early Decortication

If a hematoma cannot be removed by a chest tube, and a significant accumulation of blood is present, early decortication is advised with evacuation of the hematoma through a small anterolateral thoracotomy.

Indication: Hemothorax

Surgical goals: Evacuate the hematoma and reexpand the lung.

Preoperative preparation: Local skin prep, removal of chest hair as required.

Position: Lateral.

An anterolateral thoracotomy is performed under general endotracheal anesthesia. The parietal pleura is opened, and a self-retaining retractor is inserted and slowly opened until the hematoma can be manually evacuated under vision. The entire pleural space and thoracic organs are carefully inspected for bleeding sites, a chest tube is inserted, and the thoracotomy wound is closed in layers.

1.2.1.4 Pericardiocentesis in Cardiac Tamponade (Figs. 10, 11)

Even a relatively small amount of blood collecting in the pericardial sac after trauma can cause compression of intrapericardial structures like the atrium and venae cavae and can impair diastolic filling of the heart. The fluid collection must be removed to prevent the deleterious effects associated with the fall in cardiac output.

Indication: Cardiac tamponade.

Surgical goal: Decompress the pericardium by aspirating the bloody effusion.

Preoperative preparation: Local skin prep.

Position: Supine.

Under local anesthesia, a large-gauge aspirating needle (No. 1) with syringe attached is inserted through Larrey's cleft at a 30° angle to the coronal plane, directed the point of the needle toward the center of the clavicle (Fig. 10). The needle is then advanced while the plunger is withdrawn. If the position of the needle tip is uncertain, inadvertent cardiac puncture can be avoided by attaching an ECG lead to the needle; contact with the myocardium will be signified by an injury potential (Fig. 11). A drainage tube may be inserted at the end of the procedure.

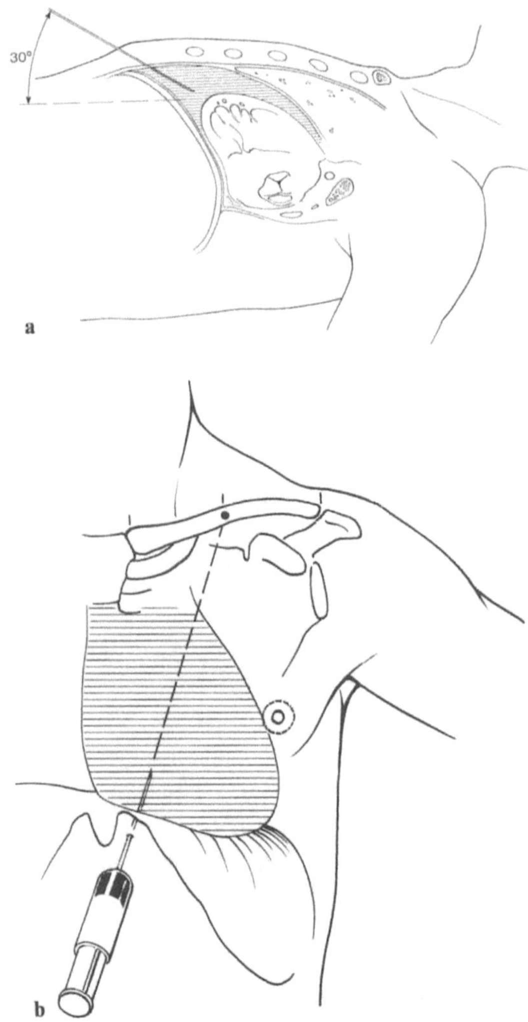

Fig. 10. a Pericardial aspiration. The aspirating needle is introduced at a 30° angle to the patient axis. **b** The angled needle is directed toward the middle of the clavicle

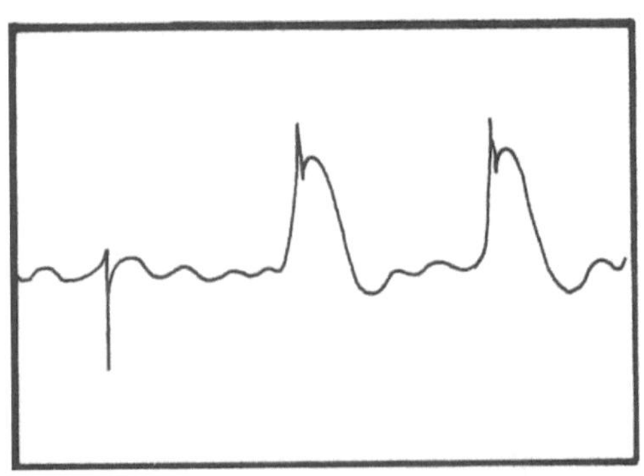

Fig. 11. ECG changes produced by myocardial injury

1.2.2 Treatment of Cardiac Herniation (Fig. 12a, b)

Most tears of the pericardium run longitudinally in front of or behind the phrenic nerve and are more common on the left side than on the right. With a large left-sided tear, part or all of the myocardium can herniate through the rent (Fig. 12 a,b). This condition, which may not develop until several days after the trauma, is marked by tachycardia, hypotension, and frequently by inflow stasis and can quickly become life-threatening. Differentiation is required from myocardial contusion and cardiac tamponade. The diagnosis can be difficult to establish but is aided by sonography, serial roentgenograms, and possibly by serial electrocargiograms showing displacement of the cardiac axis.

Indication: Cardiac herniation with impairment of cardiac function.

Surgical goals: Return the heart to the pericardium, repair the pericardial tear.

Patient advisement: Hemorrhage, nerve injury (phrenic nerve), pulmonary injury, chest tube.

Preoperative preparation: Removal of chest hair.

Position: Semilateral.

Incision: Anteromedial thoracotomy.

Steps in procedure:

(1) Left anteromedial thoracotomy in the fifth interspace
(2) Reduction of the herniation (may require extension of the pericardial tear)
(3) Closure of the pericardium, leaving an aperture for drainage
(4) Insertion of chest tube
(5) Wound closure in layers

A left-sided anteromedial thoracotomy having been performed in the bed of the fifth rib, the herniated portion of the myocardium is identified and returned to the pericardial sac. If this maneuver proves difficult, the tear in the pericardium should be extended. The pericardium is closed with absorbable No. 00 sutures, leaving (or creating) an aperture at the bottom of the suture line for the placement of a drain. Finally a chest tube is inserted, and the thoracotomy is closed.

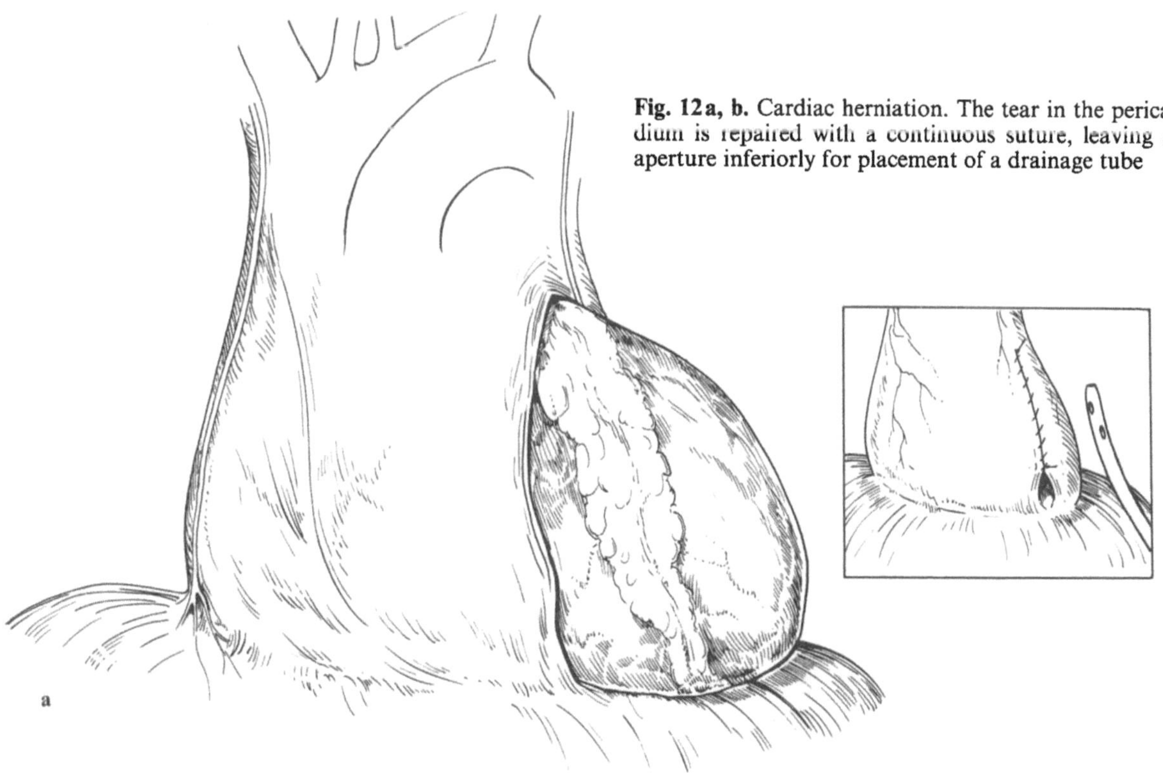

a b

Fig. 12a, b. Cardiac herniation. The tear in the pericardium is repaired with a continuous suture, leaving an aperture inferiorly for placement of a drainage tube

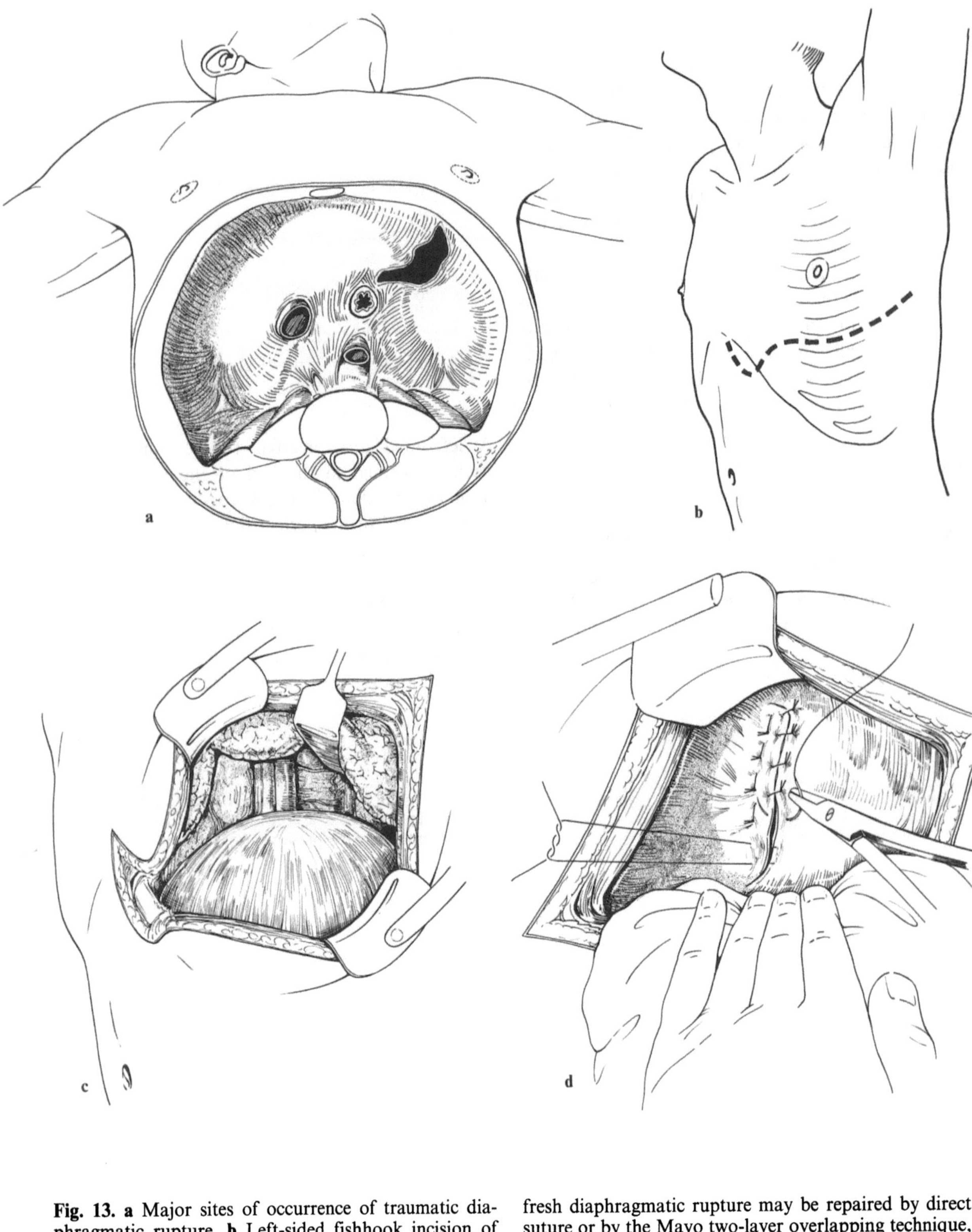

Fig. 13. a Major sites of occurrence of traumatic diaphragmatic rupture. **b** Left-sided fishhook incision of Kirschner. **c** The left thoracic cavity is exposed. **d** The fresh diaphragmatic rupture may be repaired by direct suture or by the Mayo two-layer overlapping technique, as shown

1.2.3 *Repair of Traumatic Diaphragmatic Rupture* (Fig. 13a–d)

Diaphragmatic rupture occurs predominantly on the left side and is most commonly diagnosed in patients with multiple injuries. A transabdominal approach is generally advised for left-sided ruptures, as this permits inspection of the abdominal viscera. If necessary the incision may be angled and extended to a thoracotomy.

Indication: Repair of diaphragmatic rupture and evaluation for associated injuries.

Surgical goal: Repair of diaphragmatic rupture and coexisting injuries.

Preoperative preparation: Epilation of the chest and abdomen.

Position: Supine, possibly with the left hemithorax slightly elevated. The left arm is flexed and suspended over the head.

Incision: Upper midline laparotomy with possible extension to a thoracotomy in the seventh interspace. Alternatives are the fishhook incision of Kirschner (Fig. 13b), upper transverse laparotomy (Drüner), or a left-sided subcostal incision.

Steps in procedure:

(1) Laparotomy and exploration of the abdomen
(2) Reduction of abdominal viscera
(3) Insertion of chest tube
(4) Direct repair of the ruptured diaphragm
(5) Abdominal drainage according to associated injuries
(6) Wound closure in layers

Following laparotomy, the abdomen is explored to exclude associated injuries of the spleen, liver, pancreas, or bowel. The pericardium is also inspected for injury and repaired as necessary. Then the herniated abdominal viscera are returned to the peritoneal cavity, and the diaphragm is repaired with interrupted sutures using the double-layer Mayo technique, carefully avoiding injury to the phrenic nerve branches (Fig. 13d). A coexisting pericardial tear is also repaired with sutures, leaving an aperture for a drainage tube.

If the diaphragm has been avulsed from the chest wall, it may not be possible to perform an anatomic repair, and the diaphragm will have to be reattached at a slightly higher level. Rarely, larger defects will have to be reconstructed using a suitable material such as lyophilized dura or Marlex mesh, but usually this is not necessary in the primary care of diaphragmatic ruptures. In all cases a chest tube should be inserted prior to the definitive diaphragmatic repair. An abdominal drain is placed according to the location of associated injuries.

1.2.4 *Repair of Chest Wall Hernias* (Fig. 14a, b)

Chest wall hernias are most common after blunt thoracic trauma with subcutaneous injury to muscle and fascia. Many are not true hernias, but involve a subcutaneous prolapse of lung through a tear in the pleura. The decision for surgery is made on the basis of subjective complaints (pain, pleural irritation, dyspnea). Repair may be carried out by the Sauerbruch-Doberer technique (Fig. 14), or the defect may be reconstructed using a graft or synthetic material.

Indication: Protrusion of lung through a defect in the chest wall.

Surgical goal: Closure of the chest wall defect.

Preoperative preparation: Epilation of the chest wall.

Incision: Parallel to the rib over the chest wall hernia, the length depending on the extent of the herniation.

Instruments: Basic set.

Steps in procedure:

(1) Skin incision over the hernia
(2) Exposure of chest wall defect
(3) Reduction of pleura and lung
(4) Closure of defect
(5) Insertion of chest tube and subcutaneous suction drain
(6) Skin closure

The skin is incised parallel to the ribs over the protrusion to expose the adjacent ribs and chest wall defect. With a true herniation the hernial sac is opened, its contents are reduced, and the sac is closed. The hernial opening itself is repaired by

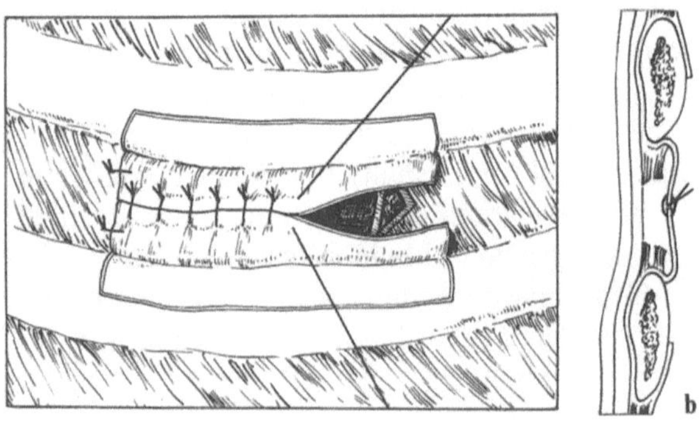
a b

Fig. 14a, b. Repair of chest wall hernia. The periosteum of the adjacent ribs is incised to create a pair of trapdoor flaps that are swung over the hernia and sutured together

mobilizing a pair of periosteal or osteoperiosteal flaps from the adjacent ribs, swinging them over the defect, and suturing their edges together (Fig. 14a, b). Meticulous hemostasis is established, and a suction drain is inserted. Temporary chest tube insertion is recommended if the pleural space has been entered.

Today it is more common to reconstruct the chest wall defect using autologous (skin flap), homologous (dura mater), or synthetic material (Marlex mesh, Vicryl mesh, etc.), still employing the same operative technique. This type of procedure is performed more quickly and easily than the classic repair, since there is no need to mobilize periosteal flaps. It is essential that the material used to reconstruct the defect be applied under tension.

2 Procedures for Chest Wall Diseases

2.1 Diseases of the Thoracic Skeleton

2.1.1 Rib Resections (Fig. 15a–e)

Rib resections are performed for the diagnosis and treatment of circumscribed rib lesions as well as for the harvesting of autologous bone or cartilage.

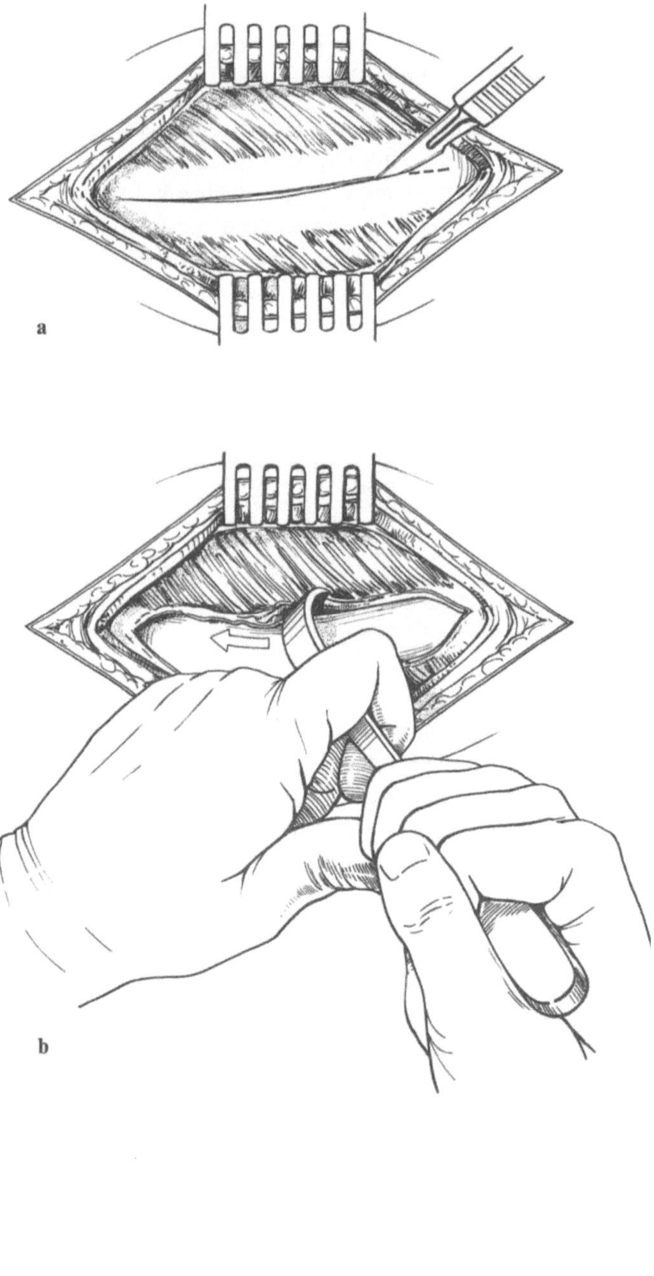
a b

Fig. 15a–e. Rib resection. a The periosteum is incised. b The periosteum is stripped from the rib with a raspatory. c Clearing of the rib surfaces is completed with Doyen elevators. d The rib is divided with a rib shear. e Rib tumors necessitate complete removal of the rib and periosteum. The rib is exarticulated at the costovertebral joint and divided parasternally

2.1.1.1 Rib Resection for Tumor, Necrosis, or for Grafting

Indications: Neoplastic changes, radionecrosis of bone, source for autologous graft material.

Surgical goal: Removal of the rib (extent of removal depends on indication).

Preoperative preparation: Removal of chest hair.

Position: Lateral.

Incision: Parallel to the rib.

Instruments: Basic set, extra thoracic set, rib resection set.

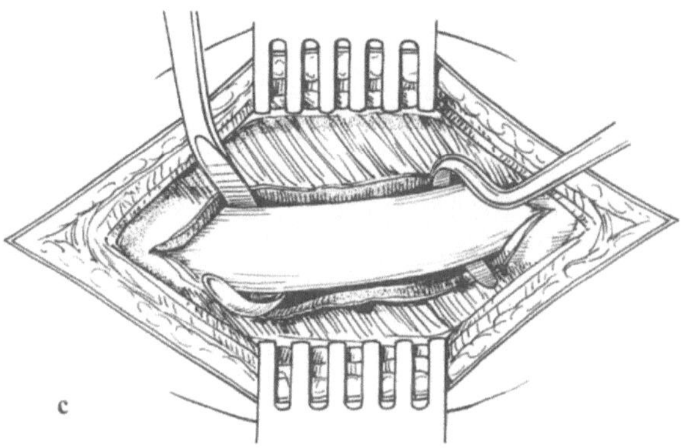

c

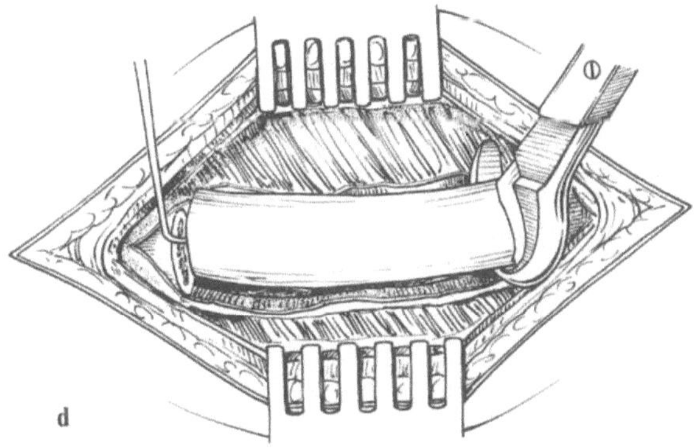

d

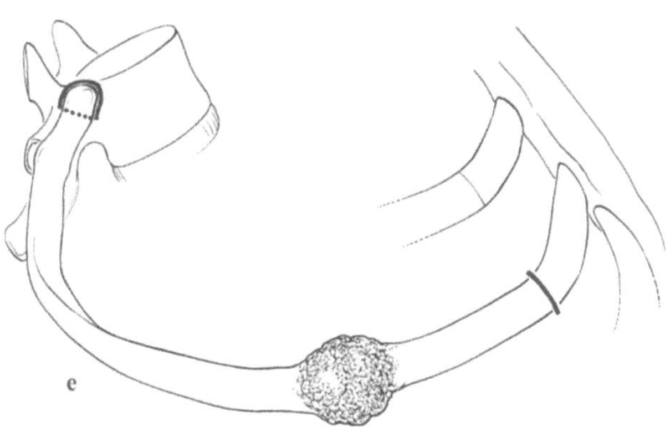

e

Steps in procedure:

(1) Incision parallel to the rib
(2) Sub- or extraperiosteal mobilization of the rib, depending on the indication
(3) Exarticulation of the whole rib for malignancy, otherwise division of the rib at the appropriate sites
(4) Hemostasis
(5) Skin closure

With the patient on his side, the incison is made along the rib, and the rib is exposed. The intercostal muscles are detached from it, sparing the intercostal vessels. With a primary rib malignancy, the periosteum and surrounding healthy tissue are included in the resection. The rib is divided in the region of the costochondral junction and is also disarticulated at the costovertebral joints. To harvest autologous graft material (e.g., for bridging a defect), the rib is dissected free subperiosteally and divided with the rib shears. Bleeding is carefully controlled, and the wound is closed.

With osteoradionecrosis of the ribs, histologic confirmation is needed even with unequivocal radiologic findings, since differentiation is required from metastatic tumor.

2.1.1.2 Rib Resection in Ostitis

Indication: Ostitis of the rib.

Surgical goal: Removal of the inflammatory focus.

Preoperative preparation: Removal of chest hair.

Position: Lateral.

Incision: Parallel to the rib.

Instruments: Basic set, extra thoracic set, rib resection set.

With a fistulous lesion secondary to osteomyelitis of the rib, the fistulous tract is excised, and the ostitic rib lesion sustaining the fistula is exposed. The focus is resected with a margin of normal rib. With a florid ostitis, secondary wound healing is the goal; with a more chronic infection in which antibiotic sensitivity has been ascertained, primary wound closure may be attempted.

2.1.2 *Chest Wall Resection* (Fig. 16a–c)

Resection is indicated for malignant diseases of the chest wall such as osteosarcoma, chondrosarcoma, soft-tissue sarcomas, and even metastatic tumors or bronchial carcinoma that have invaded the chest wall. With lymphomas, it is sufficient to establish the diagnosis and then treat the lesion by nonoperative means. Primary chest wall malignancies and some metastases have to be resected in accordance with the guidelines of tumor surgery. These procedures often result in large chest wall defects that must be reconstructed using a combination of measures.

Indication: Tumor resection.

Surgical goals: Radical tumor removal, closure of the chest wall defect, stabilization of the chest wall.

Preoperative preparation: Removal of chest hair.

Incision: Parallel to the involved ribs over the tumor mass; involved skin may also have to be excised.

Instruments: Basic set, extra thoracic set, rib resection set, set for funnel chest and ribs.

Steps in procedure:

(1) Exposure of the tumor (possibly with excision of skin)
(2) Excision of the tumor
(3) Closure of the chest wall defect
(4) Stabilization of the chest wall as required (with metal struts or ribs)
(5) Wound closure

The malignant tumor is resected with an adequate margin of healthy tissue; involved skin is also removed. Negative surgical margins are confirmed by frozen section. Further surgery depends on the extent of the chest wall defect. Smaller defects can be adequately reconstructed with lyophilized dura or other materials (Marlex, Vicryl or tantalum mesh, skin flaps, etc.) sutured into the defect under tension. A suction drain is then inserted, and the wound is closed primarily over the reconstruction site. Marlex mesh may also be suitable for the repair of extensive chest wall resections. However, additional stabilization is needed in these cases to prevent paradoxical motion. This can be accomplished with steel struts placed over the implant and fixed to the supporting ribs with nonabsorbable sutures (Fig. 16). Generally, two of these splints are sufficient. The remainder of the defect is covered with local tissue, assuming a primary closure can be obtained. Autologous ribs offer an alternative to steel splints. Either one entire rib may be used for this purpose, or a rib may be longitudinally split and grafted into the defect.

Fig. 16. a Resection of the chest wall. Smaller chest wall defects can be repaired primarily with lyophilized dura or Marlex mesh. **b** If additional soft-tissue coverage is needed, a pedicled flap of greater omentum can be mobilized through a laparotomy incision and transferred subcutaneously to the defect. **c** Larger chest wall resections can usually be repaired with Marlex mesh. If paradoxical motion develops, the repair can be stabilized by steel splints or autologous rib grafts. The steel splints are tied to supporting ribs with steel wire, or autologous ribs are pegged into the defect

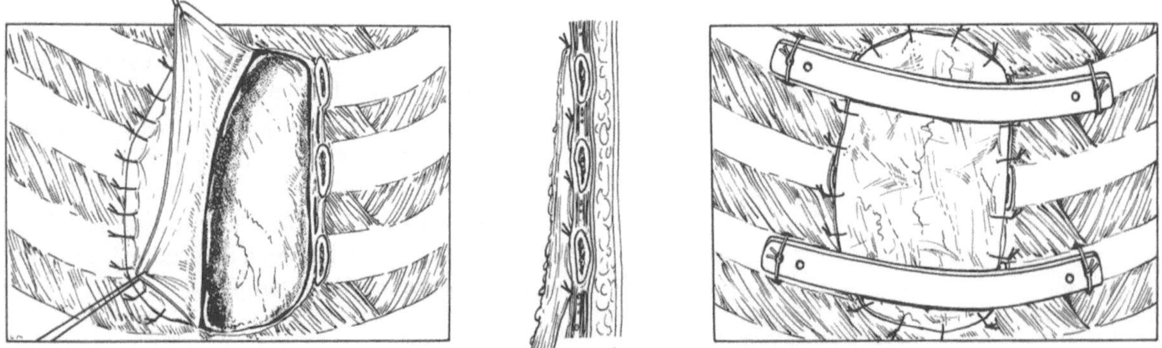

a b c

2.1.3 Resection of the Sternum
(Figs. 17a, b; 18a, b; 19; 20)

In cases of sternal malignancy, partial or complete resection of the sternum may be indicated. Complete sternal resection profoundly impairs respiratory mechanics.

Indication: Malignant tumors of the sternum.

Surgical goals: Removal of tumor with adequate margins, stabilization of the chest wall.

Preoperative preparation: Removal of chest hair.

Incision: Longitudinal incision over the sternum, possibly with excision of the skin.

Instruments: Basic set, extra thoracic set, rib resection set, set for funnel chest and ribs, possibly autologous rib.

Steps in procedure:

(1) Longitudinal incision over the sternum, possibly with local excision of skin
(2) Separation of costochondral attachments or osteotomy of the ribs
(3) Removal of sternum
(4) Coverage of defect with lyophophilized dura
(5) Insertion and fixation of steel splints or autologous ribs
(6) Drain insertion
(7) Skin closure

Following incision (or excision) of the skin overlying the sternum, the tumor and an adequate surrounding portion of the sternum are dissected free. The sternum is separated from the ribs at the costochondral junctions or if necessary by osteotomizing the ribs. It is always advantageous to leave the manubrium and sternoclavicular articulations intact if possible, as this will preserve some stability of the chest and shoulder girdle and will simplify reconstruction. If removal of the manubrium is necessary to achieve tumor free margins, the clavicles will need to be stabilized. Following the sternectomy, the defect is initially closed with prosthetic material (Marlex, Vicryl) sutured into place under moderate tension. The thoracic cage is then stabilized with two steel splints placed across the defect and fixed to the supporting ribs with nonabsorbable sutures. Autologous rib also may be used to bridge the defect.

Alternatively the chestwall can be reconstructed by closing the defect with Mesh (Marlex, Vicryl) placed under tension followed by a layer bonecement (Pallacos, Sulfix). This "sandwich" construction [8a] can be further improved by the addition of vascular tissue such as major omentum.

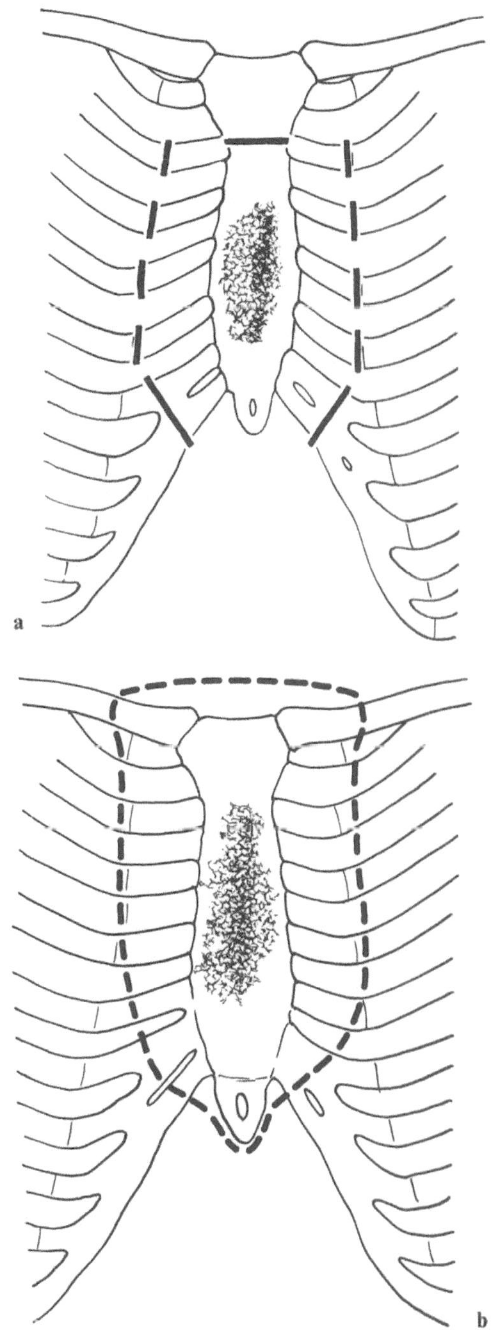

Fig. 17. a Partial sternectomy. The drawing illustrates the possible extent of the sternal resection, e.g., for a malignant chondroma. **b** Resection lines for a total sternectomy

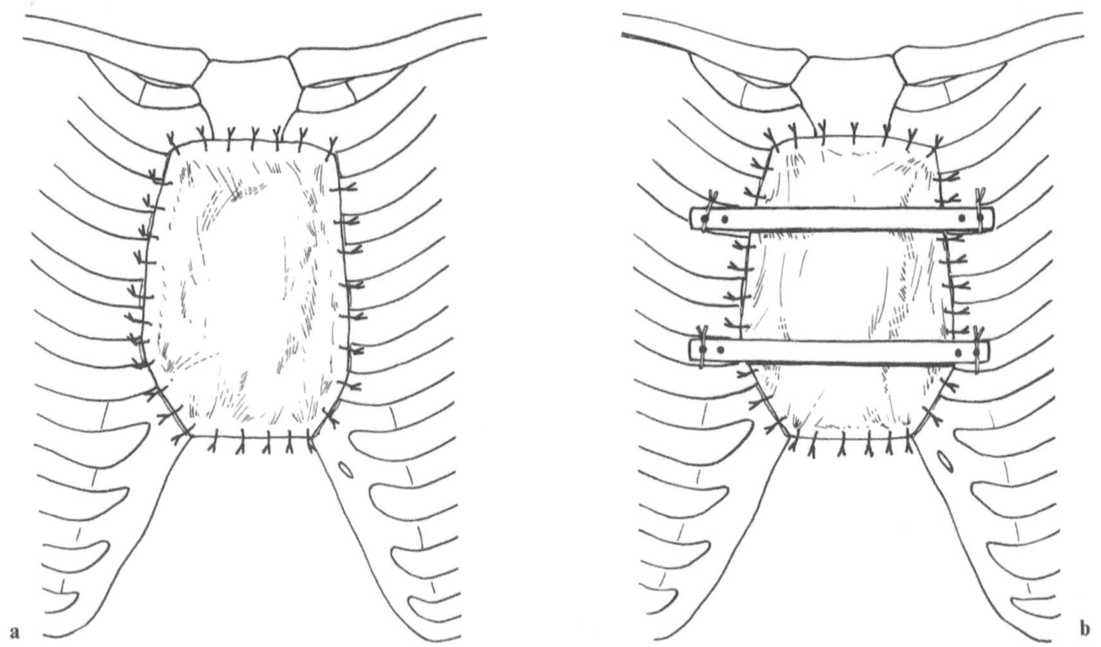

Fig. 18. a Reconstruction after sternectomy can be accomplished with lyophilized dura or Marlex mesh. **b** Steel struts may be placed to reinforce the anterior chest wall

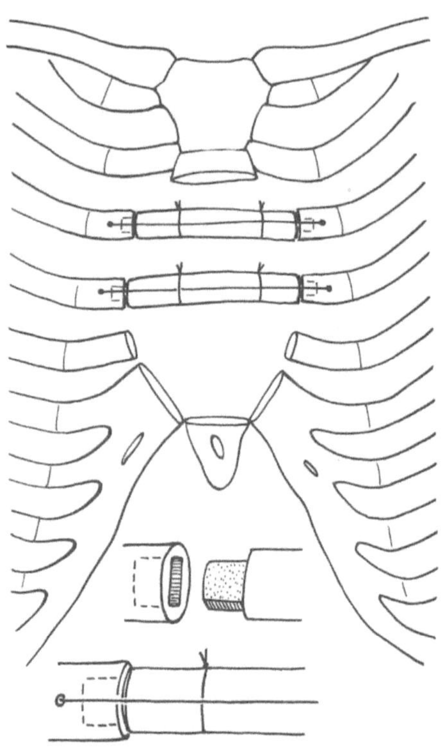

Fig. 19. As an alternative to steel struts, segments of autologous rib may be pegged into the defect to stabilize the thoracic skeleton

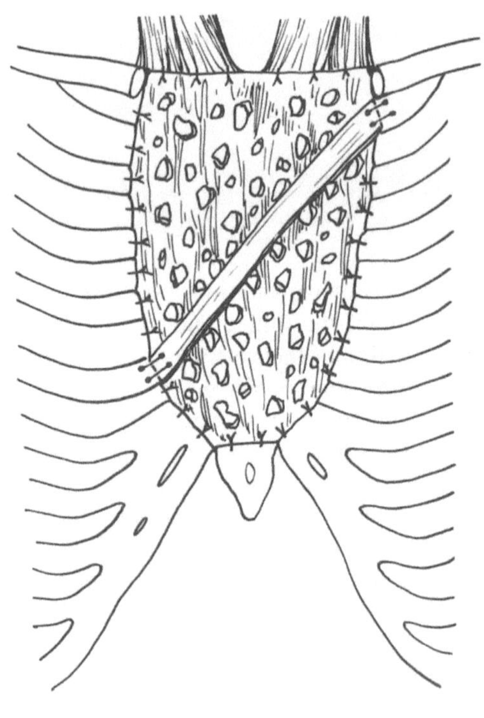

Fig. 20. The anterior chest wall can also be stabilized by cancellous bone grafts reinforced by a diagonally placed rib. The bone chips can regenerate to produce a solid bony surface

2.2 Surgical Treatment of Pleural Empyema (Fig. 21)

2.2.1 *Intercostal Tube Drainage of Empyema*

Indication: Pleural empyema.

Surgical goals: Remove collected pus, insert drainage tube.

Preoperative preparation: Epilation of the operative site.

Position: Sitting (or semilateral if the patient cannot sit up).

Incision: Stab incision for introducing the tube.

Instruments: Chest tube set.

Steps in procedure:

(1) Localization of the empyema
(2) Incision of an intercostal space on the anterior axillary line over the lowest point of the empyema
(3) Development of a soft-tissue tunnel and insertion of the drainage tube
(4) Fixation of the tube
(5) Connection of the tube to a waterseal or suction system

The empyema should be drained through an intercostal space above the lowest point of the fluid collection. The empyema may be localized by percussion and fluoroscopy. The drainage tube is inserted by the Buelau technique and can be used to irrigate the empyema cavity with antiseptic or enzyme-containing solutions.

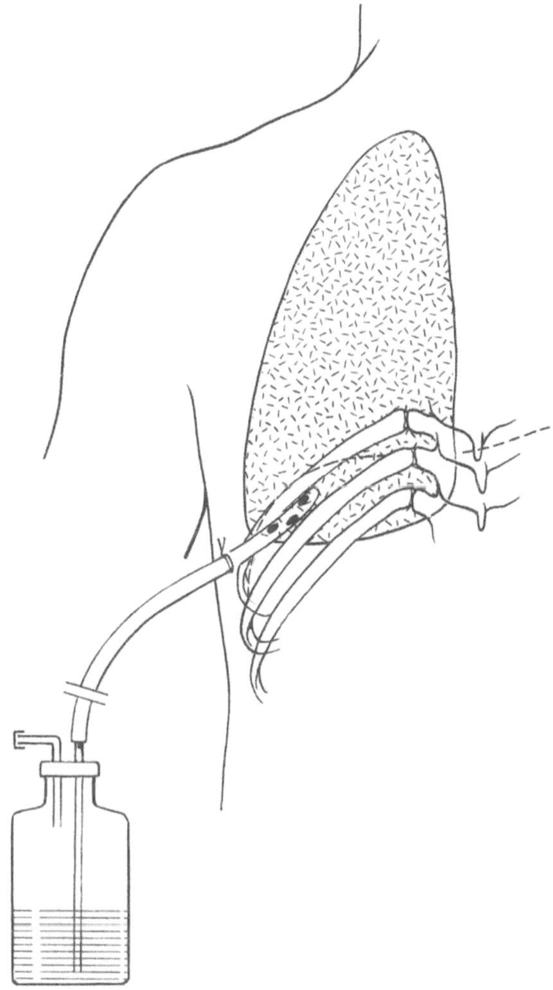

Fig. 21. Intercostal tube drainage of empyema. The fluid level is localized by radiography, and the drain is inserted through the interspace above the lowest part of the empyema

2.2.2 *Rib Resection Drainage of Empyema*
(Fig. 22a, b)

Rib resection drainage is indicated when more conservative methods have been unsuccessful (fibrinous debris or clotted blood, reinfection with a bronchopleural fistula).

Indication: Evacuation of pleural empyema refractory to intercostal tube drainage.

Contraindication: Tuberculosis.

Surgical goal: Evacuation of the empyema cavity.

Preoperative preparation: Epilation of the operative site.

Position: Semilateral.

Incision: Parallel to the rib at the lowest point of the empyema.

Instruments: Basic set, rib resection set.

Steps in procedure:

(1) Paravertebral incision starting at the medial scapular border, or incision parallel to the rib on the anterior or midaxillary line
(2) Exposure of the selected rib
(3) Incision of the periosteum
(4) Resection of about a 5-cm segment of rib
(5) Opening of empyema cavity and removal of purulent fluid
(6) Insertion of drainage tube
(7) Wound closure in layers
(8) Connection of the tube to a waterseal or suction system

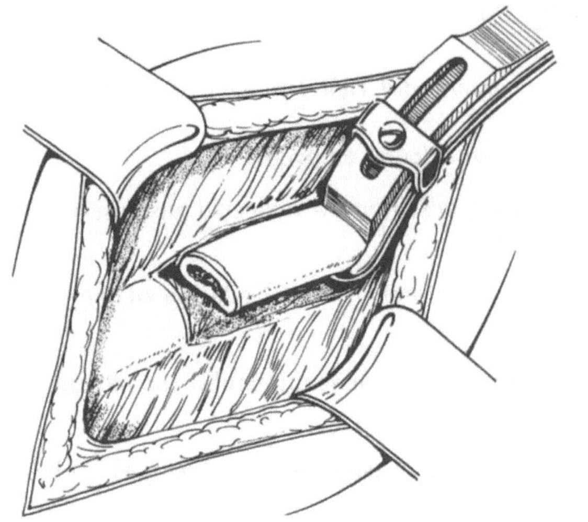
a

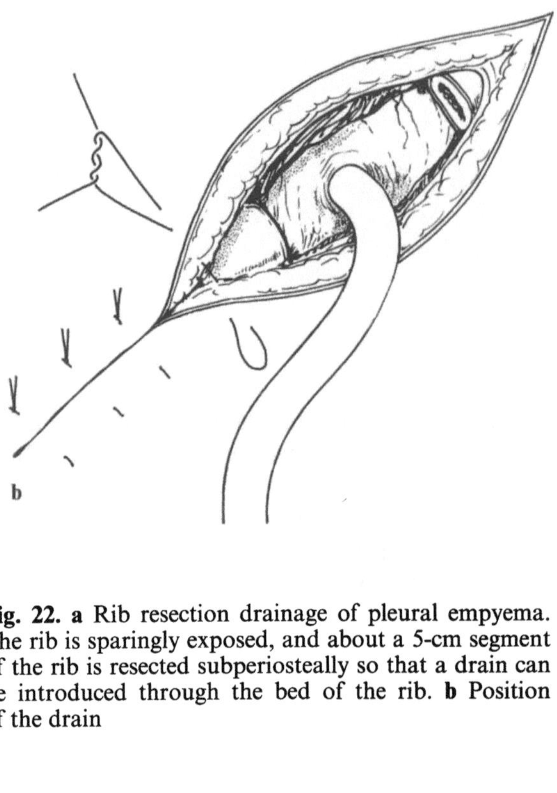
b

Fig. 22. a Rib resection drainage of pleural empyema. The rib is sparingly exposed, and about a 5-cm segment of the rib is resected subperiosteally so that a drain can be introduced through the bed of the rib. **b** Position of the drain

The advantage of this procedure over intercostal tube drainage is that it permits the empyema cavity to be visualized so that any cysts, membranes, blood clots, fibrinous debris, or other tissue residues can be identified and removed. A vertical incision about 5 cm long, extending down to the ribs, is made over the empyema. Alternatively, a parallel incision over the course of the seventh or eighth rib can be advantageous for postoperative care, as the patient is able to lie on his back. The selected rib is exposed, and the periosteum is incised with the cautery. The upper surface is stripped with a curved raspatory, a Doyen elevator is passed beneath the rib, and a rib shear is used to divide the rib and remove a segment about 5 cm long. The pleura is opened in the bed of the rib, sparing the neurovascular bundle if possible, and the empyema is drained. Special care is taken to remove all fibrinous debris and blood clots from the pleural surface. Then a silicone drainage tube of sufficient caliber is introduced into the empyema cavity and secured with sutures. The muscle and fascia may be coapted around the tube if necessary. The tube is connected to a waterseal or suction system.

2.2.3 Removal of a Residual Empyema Cavity (Fig. 23a–f)

Indication: Chronic empyema.

Surgical goal: Removal of pleural peel and residual empyema cavity.

Preoperative preparation: Epilation of the operative site, local skin prep.

Position: Lateral.

Incision: Lateral thoracotomy over the residual empyema cavity.

Instruments: Basic set, extra thoracic set, rib resection set.

Steps in procedure:

(1) Lateral thoracotomy
(2) Entry into pleural cavity, usually through the bed of the fifth rib
(3) Mobilization of outer peel from the chest wall
(4) Mobilization of peel from the mediastinum
(5) Mobilization of peel from the lung
(6) Hemostasis
(7) Insertion of drains
(8) Wound closure

The skin, subcutaneous tissue, and muscle are divided as in the standard lateral thoracotomy (q.v.), and the chest is entered through the bed of the fifth rib. A finger is passed extrapleurally between the thoracic fascia and the parietal pleura with the empyema sac, and the tissue is freed from the chest wall by a combination of blunt and sharp dissection. Considerable force may be needed to mobilize the pleura completely in this area. Special attention is given to freeing the peel about the apex of the thorax. This should be done under direct vision if possible to avoid injury to nerves and vessels. After the parietal peel has been freed from the chest wall, decortication is continued on the mediastinal side, avoiding injury to the subclavian artery, vena cava, azygous vein, and the vagus and phrenic nerves. Then the inner wall of the empyema sac is carefully separated from the lung using a combination of sharp and blunt dissection. Adhesions between the pulmonary lobes are divided along with other fibrous structures on the lung surface so that the lung will be free to expand. To conclude the operation, the anterior and posterior parts of the thoracic cavity are drained with two separate tubes brought out through the phrenicocostal sinus and connected to a waterseal or suction apparatus.

Fig. 23. a Basal standard thoracotomy for decortication. **b** The inflammatory exudate and peel are bluntly dissected off the lung. **c–f** see p. 66

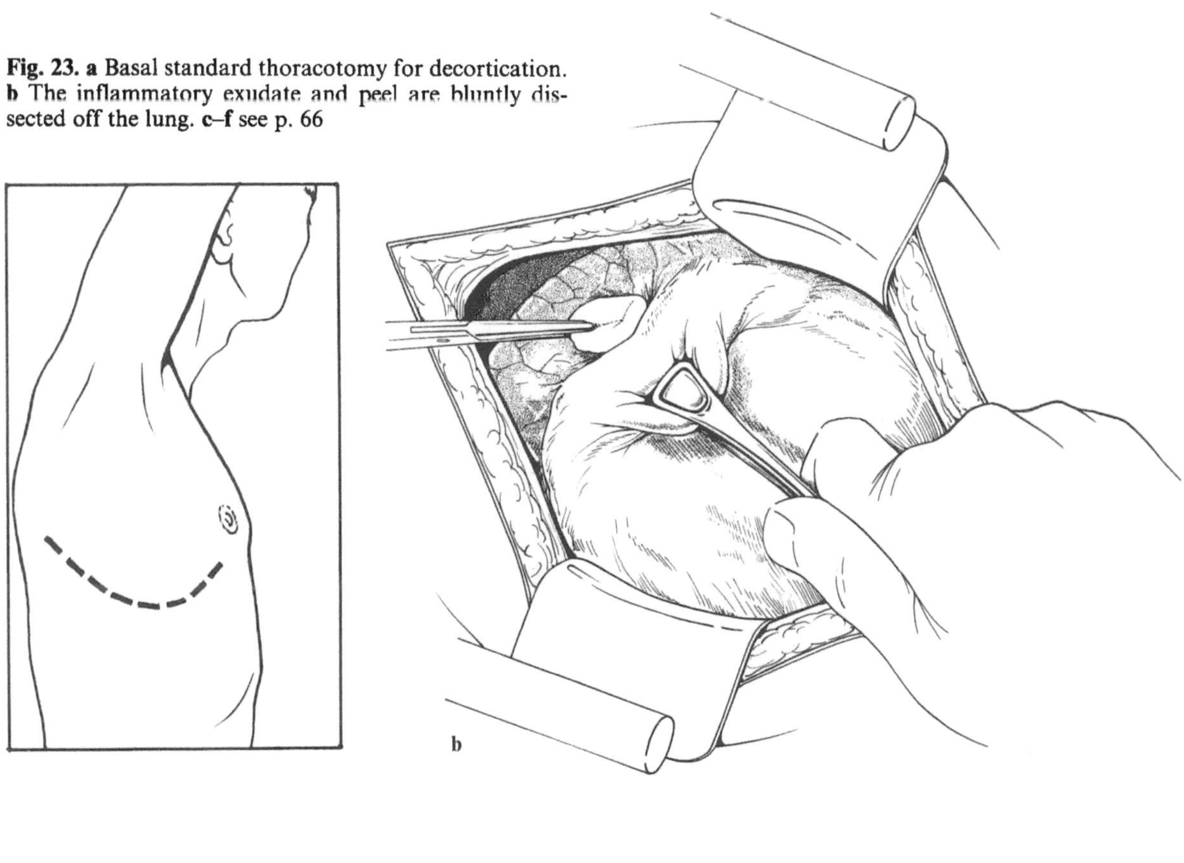

a b

Fig. 23.c The peel is separated from the hilus. d The decortication is nearly complete. e,f Schematic drawings of the decortication showing removal of the residual empyema cavity and the placement of the chest tubes

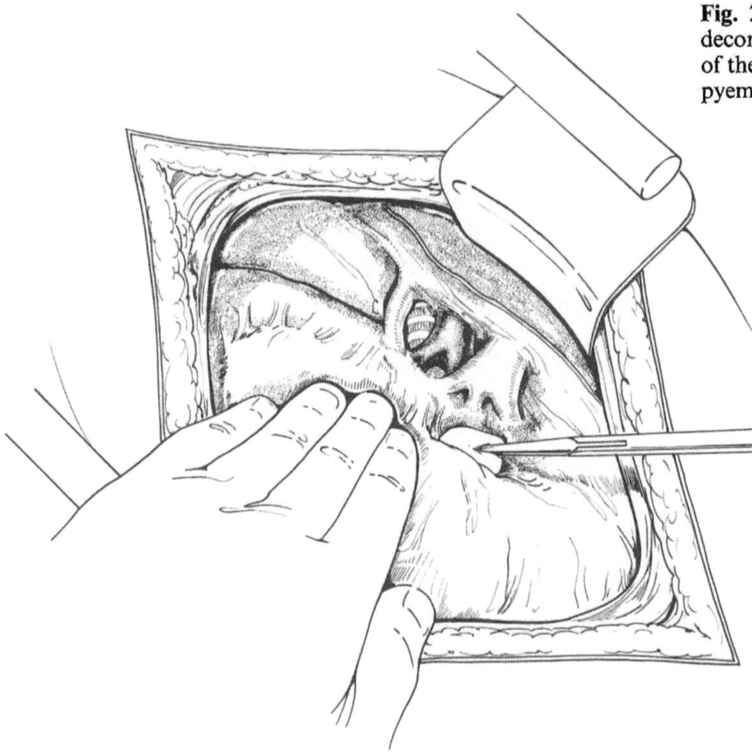

c

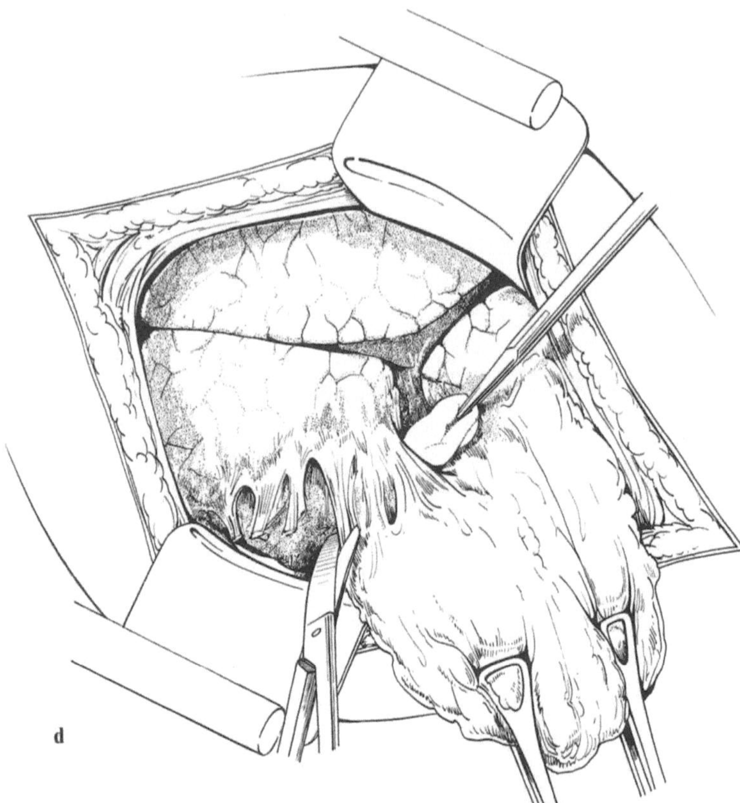

d

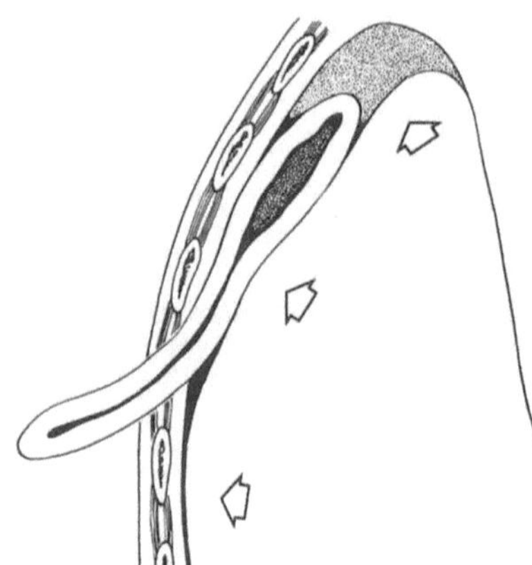

e

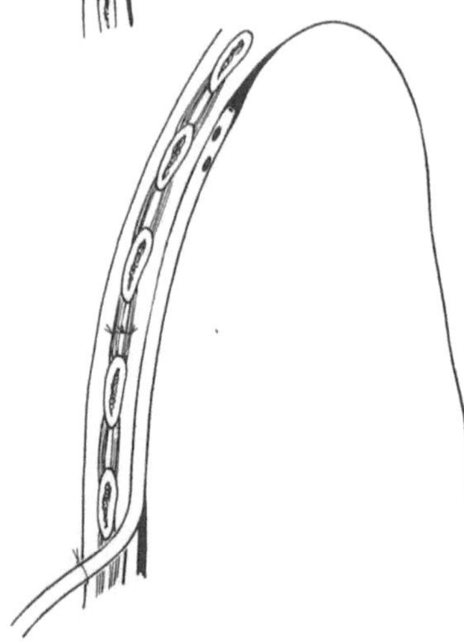

f

2.3 Congenital Deformities of the Chest Wall

2.3.1 Repair of Pectus Carinatum (Pigeon Breast) (Figs. 24, 25)

As a result of rickets prophylaxis, the clinical picture of pectus carinatum is rarely seen today. Operative treatment is indicated when there is significant chest deformity that interferes with respiration or is causing significant psychological anguish.

Surgical goals: Create a normal chest contour, improve respiratory function.

Preoperative preparation: Epilation of the anterior chest wall.

Position: Supine.

Incision: Transverse incision in the region of the submammary folds or medial sternotomy incision.

Instruments: Basic set, extra thoracic set, rib resection set, set for funnel chest and ribs, special instruments and instrument sets.

Fig. 24a, b. Pectus carinatum. Schematic drawings of the deformity and the extent of the resection, with the resulting alteration of chest contour. The sternotomy allows the sternum to retract, creating a more acceptable contour

Steps in procedure:

(1) Transverse incision on the submammary folds or vertical midline incision
(2) Mobilization of the skin, subcutaneous tissue, and muscles
(3) Exposure of the costochondral junctions
(4) Subperiosteal resection of the cartilaginous portions of the ribs
(5) Reefing of redundant perichondrium
(6) Approximation of the ribs and perichondrium to the sternum
(7) Reapproximation of the muscles
(8) Drain insertion
(9) Skin closure

A vertical midline incision is preferred in male patients and permits the skin, subcutaneous tissue, and chest muscles to be mobilized en bloc. The pectoral muscles and recti muscles are detached. A transverse submammary incision is preferred in females. It is more cosmetically appealing, although the muscles cannot be mobilized en bloc with the subcutaneous tissue. The skin of the chest wall is supplied by perforating branches from the internal mammary artery, so wide mobilization can endanger the vascular supply to the upper flap. After the sternum has been exposed, the muscular attachments are released from the sternum and costal cartilages with the electrocautery. Inferiorly the fascia of the rectus abdominis must be incised

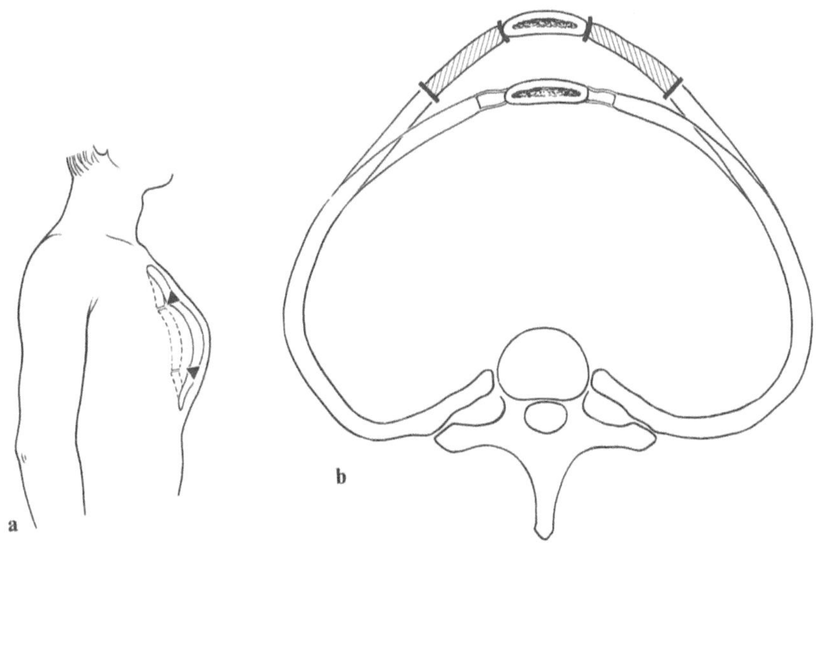

to expose the costal cartilage in that area. All costal cartilages involved in the deformity must be exposed. These portions of the cartilages are then removed subperichondrially; usually the resection must extend to the costochondral junctions (Fig. 25). A finger is passed behind the posterior surface of the sternum to mobilize it, and a transverse sternotomy is performed usually at the level of the second interspace so that the protrusion can recede. A second osteoteomy or partial sternectomy may have to be performed distally to achieve the desired result. The redundant periosteum is shortened with absorbable synthetic reefing sutures, and the rib stumps are approximated to the sternum and sutured in place. Usually these sutures will stabilize the detached portion of the sternum well enough to avoid the need for additional fixation. The pectoral muscles are reapproximated at the sternal midline, and the rectus abdominis is drawn up and sutured to the lower borders of the pectorals.

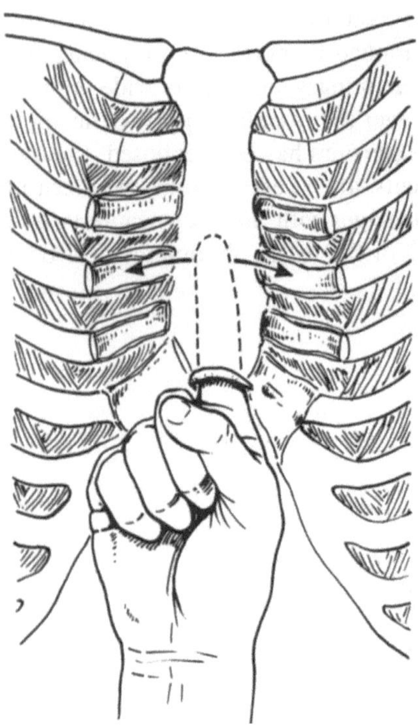

Fig. 25. The costal cartilages are resected subperichondrally, and the sternum is mobilized. Excess periosteum is reefed so that the sternum can be reapproximated to the ribs

2.3.2 Repair of Pectus Excavatum (Funnel Chest)

The massive form of funnel chest is usually associated with thoracic kyphosis and an asymmetric bulging of the ribs. Milder forms are common and do not require operation. The most severe forms with cardiopulmonary dysfunction are extremely rare and are the only absolute indication for operative treatment. Surgery on cosmetic grounds may be considered in less severe cases.

2.3.2.1 Operation of Sulamaa and Willital [20, 22] (Fig. 26a–c)

Surgical goal: Correct the excavatum deformity.

Preoperative preparation: Removal of chest hair. Biplane roentgenograms using a radiopaque strip to outline the depth of the deformity. Antibiotic prophylaxis.

Position: Supine.

Incision: Vertical midline incision over the sternum or transverse submammary incision in females (see Pectus Carinatum).

Instruments: Basic set, rib resection set, set for funnel chest and ribs.

Steps in procedure:

(1) Vertical incision over the sternum or transverse incision on the submammary folds
(2) Exposure of the costosternal junctions and the apical rim of the depression deformity
(3) Subperiosteal resection of cartilage para sternally, at the rim of the deformity, and if necessary at multiple sites on the lower costal arch
(4) Blunt mobilization of the sternum
(5) Transverse osteotomy in the second interspace; a second, more distal osteotomy may be required
(6) Transfixion of the sternum with the Sulamaa steel splint
(7) Fixation of the splint to the supporting ribs
(8) Closure of periosteal incisions
(9) Skin closure over subcutaneous suction drains

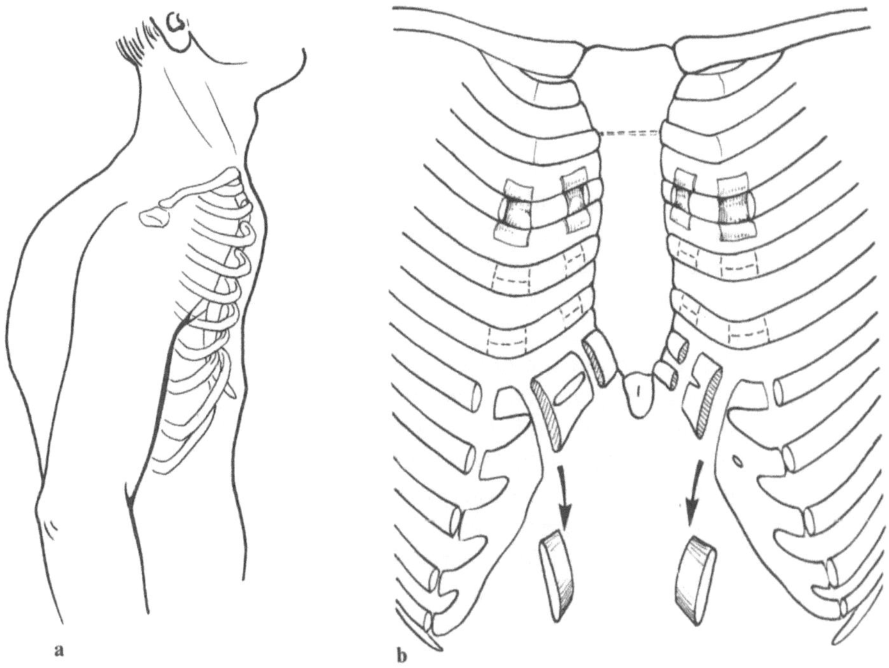

The skin and subcutaneous tissue are divided to expose the sternum and thoracic muscles. The latter are detached from the bony and cartilaginous portions of the chest wall with the electrocautery. The rectus abdominis muscle is divided distally so that the costal arches can be exposed for their full length. This is necessary to be able to bring the lower thoracic aperature level with the rest of the thorax through multiple incisions and excisions. Connections with the diaphragm in this area are also dissected free, and the sternum is bluntly mobilized in the region of the deformity (Fig. 25). The lateral extent of the presternal dissection depends on the extent of the depression. The entire deformity should be widely mobilized to a point beyond the rim of the depression. After all sternocostal attachments have been visualized, the perichondrium over the rib is incised in H-shaped fashion, and a 1-cm-wide segment of cartilage is resected. A second segment of comparable size is resected from the highest point on the rim of the deformity. Following the chondrotomy in children, the sternum is so mobile that it can be elevated without difficulty. In adults, this may additionally require a transverse sternotomy at the upper limit of the deformity, usually at the level of the second or perhaps the third interspace. The mobilized portion of the sternum that formed the floor of the depression is then transfixed with a

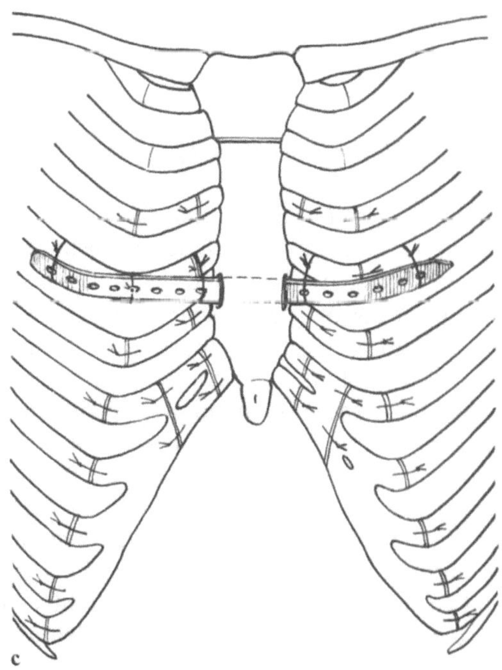

Fig. 26. a Pectus excavatum (lateral view). **b** Cartilage segments are removed parasternally and around the rim of the deformity, permitting elevation of the sternum. **c** The steel splint is temporarily fixed with sutures; it is removed after consolidation

flat, pointed steel bar. This splint is shaped (with bending irons) to fit the anatomic contour of the chest and is secured to the ribs. Alternatively, the splint may be attached to the sternum with screws and then fixed to the adjacent ribs with sutures. All the perichondrial incisions for the cartilage resections are closed with absorbable sutures (Fig. 26c). Care is taken to obtain an accurate apposition of all cut surfaces. Any projecting costal edges about the sternum that might tent the skin are sharply removed.

To maintain the correction and prevent shifting of the lower thoracic aperture, cartilage may be excised from additional sites, and the two costal arches can be joined together with Mersilene tape or a metal strip. Reattaching the posterior rectus abdominis fascia to the costal arch provides a similar effect. Even when the steel Sulamaa splint is passed through the sternum, it should be secured laterally to the ribs with nonabsorbable threads (see Fig. 26c). Meticulous hemostasis is established in the operative field before inserting two suction drains and closing the skin. Intraoperative pleural injury may necessitate the placement of a chest tube.

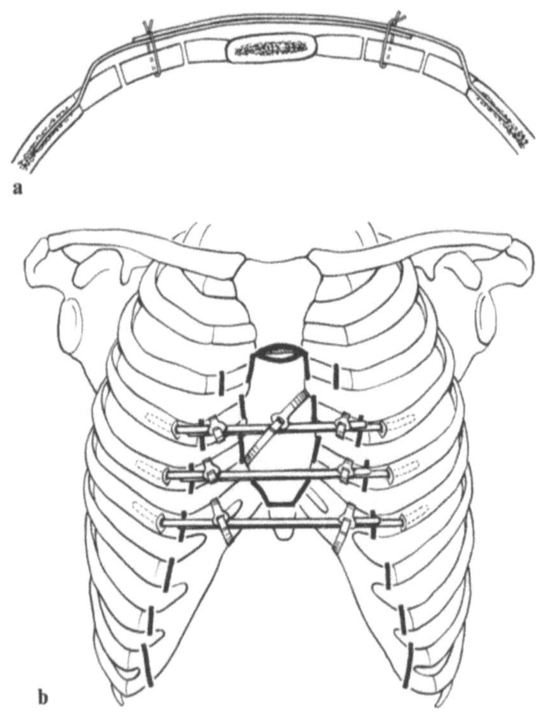

Fig. 27. a Pectus excavatum. In Rehbein's operation the sternum is mobilized, the depressed segment is elevated, and the recontoured chest is stabilized with special steel rods anchored in the medullary cavities of the ribs. **b** Appearance of the chest wall following application of Rehbein's splints

2.3.2.2 Rehbein's Operation (Fig. 27a, b)

In Rehbein's operation for pectus excavatum, the sternum is mobilized in standard fashion and transversely osteotomized, and the thorax is stabilized by means of special splints, which usually are anchored to the third, fourth, and fifth ribs. To apply the splints, the periosteum is incised 1–2 cm lateral to the costochondral junction, and the medullary cavity of the rib is opened. Each cavity is widened sufficiently to accommodate the splint, and the opening is beveled medially so that the splint can enter the cavity at a fairly direct angle. The sternum is fastened to the uppermost splints with two steel bands, securing it in a slightly overcorrected position, and looped steel bands are placed inferiorly to secure the costal arches to the lower pair of splints.

2.3.2.3 Operations of Ravitch and Brunner

In the operation of Ravitch, the sternum is completely mobilized by cartilage resection and blunt dissection of its dorsal wall (see operation of Willital and Sulamaa). A partial osteotomy is performed posteriorly through the upper part of the sternum, leaving an anterior bony lamella that enables the sternum to be greenstick fractured into the desired position. It is fixed in that position with modeling sutures placed in the sternum and costochondral junctions.

Brunner's operation utilizes a T-shaped sternotomy in which both bony lamellae are angled in roof-ridge fashion and secured in that position with "modeling" sutures.

2.3.2.4 Plastic Correction of Pectus Excavatum Using Prosthetic Material (Fig. 28)

In less severe forms of pectus excavatum where surgical treatment is desired for cosmetic reasons, the depression can be filled by implanting an appropriate silicone rubber prosthesis.

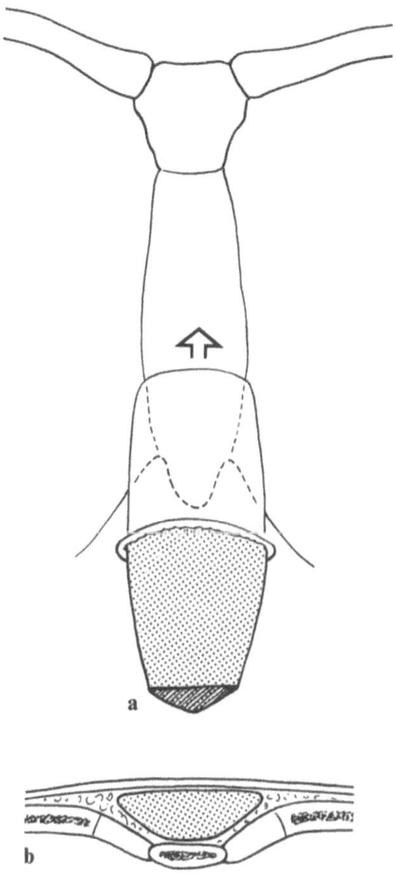

Fig. 28a, b. Smaller chest wall depressions can be filled with a synthetic material. A molded prosthesis is prepared, smoothed, sterilized, and implanted subcutaneously through an incision over the xyphoid

Indication: Cosmetically troublesome pectus excavatum.

Surgical goal: Eliminate depression deformity.

Preoperative preparation: Remove chest hair, prepare molded prosthesis; perioperative antibiotic prophylaxis.

Position: Supine.

Incision: Transverse incision over the distal xyphoid.

Steps in procedure:

(1) Preparation of molded prosthesis
(2) Silastic implant is smoothed and sterilized
(3) Blunt mobilization of the skin over the sternum
(4) Placement of the implant
(5) Insertion of drains
(6) Closure of subcutaneous tissue and skin

Prior to surgery the prosthesis is custom prepared by pouring a special plastic compound (RTV Silastic 382 Medical Grade Elastomer, Dow Corning) into the depressed area. It takes 5 min or less for the material to harden. We grease the skin beforehand so that the prosthesis is easier to remove. The polymerized mold is then mechanically worked, smoothed, and autoclaved. To insert the prosthesis, the skin is bluntly mobilized from the sternum through a 6-cm transverse incision below the xiphoid. All bleeding in the operative area is carefully controlled before introducing the implant. Two suction drains are inserted, and the subcutaneous tissue and skin are closed. It should be noted that seroma formation is common before fibrotic reactions definitively fix the implant.

2.4 Thoracoplasty

In thoracoplastic operations the chest wall over an intrapleural dead space or diseased portion of lung is mobilized by removing a portion of the rib cage.

Indications:

(1) To reduce the volume of intrapleural cavities by approximating thoracic soft tissues to the pulmonary or mediastinal wall, thus enabling spontaneous obliteration of the pleural cavity.
(2) To prevent mediastinal displacement due to contraction of lung and pleural tissues.
(3) To collapse tuberculous cavity-bearing portions of the lung without prior resective surgery.

The thoracoplasties of Semb and Björk are most commonly performed today.

2.4.1 Semb Thoracoplasty with Apicolysis (Figs. 29, 30a–c)

This procedure is chiefly indicated as a secondary operation to reduce the volume of intrapleural dead space following pulmonary resection. Its advantage is that it combines thoracoplasty with extrafascial mobilization of the chest wall and pleura in the region of the thoracic apex.

Surgical goals: Obliterate intrapleural cavities, collapse diseased portions of lung.

Contraindications: Septic processes involving the chest wall.

Preoperative preparation: Epilation, perioperative antibiotic prophylaxis.

Position: Lateral.

Incision: Posterolateral thoracotomy.

Instruments: Basic set, extra thoracic set, rib resection set.

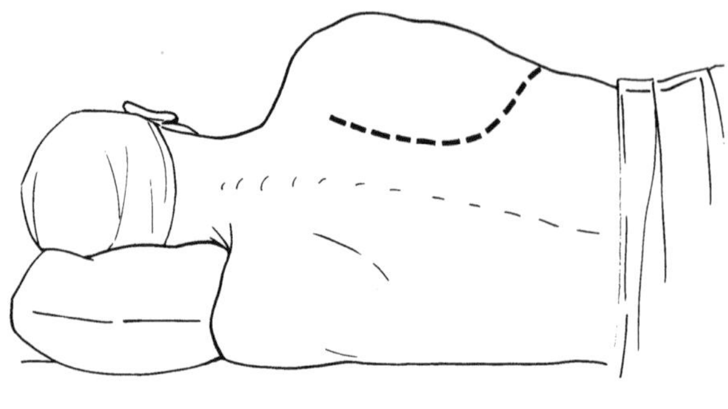

Fig. 29. The incision for the Semb thoracoplasty

Fig. 30. a The periosteum is incised over the ribs. **b** The second rib is removed. **c** The scalenus muscle is divided. **d** Appearance of the Semb thoracoplasty after the pleural apex has been freed

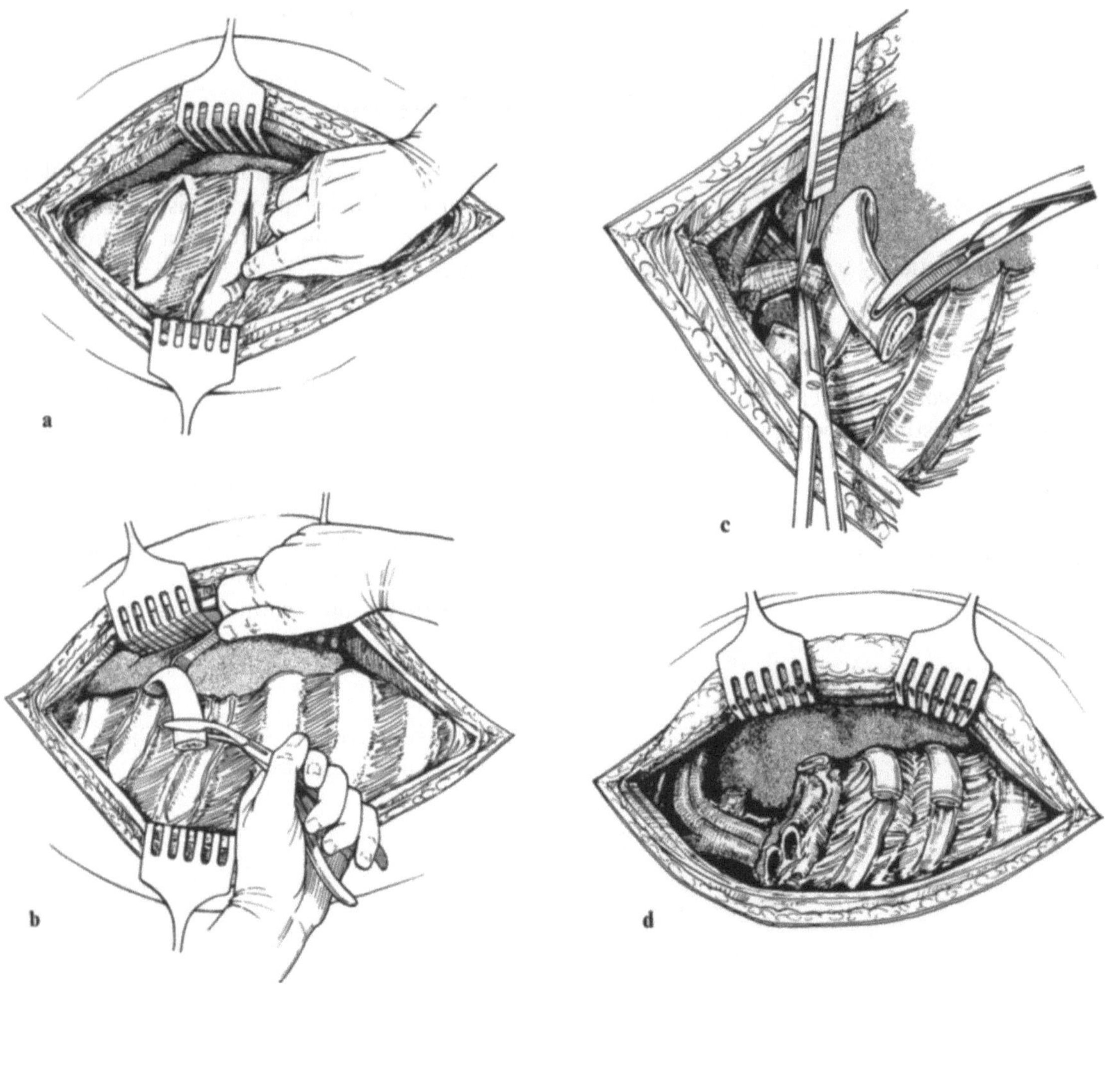

Steps in procedure:

(1) Posterolateral thoracotomy.
(2) Rib resections in increasing lengths from below upward, starting with the third rib
(3) Resection of the posterior portions of the ribs at the level of the costotransverse joint
(4) Paravertebral division of the periostea and intercostal bundles
(5) Division of scalenus attachments from the first rib
(6) Division of fibrous tissue attachments of the pleural apex
(7) Paramediastinal and paravertebral mobilization of the pleural apex
(8) Resection of the first rib
(9) Insertion of drains
(10) Skin closure

With the patient in the lateral position, a posterolateral thoracotomy is performed, and the posterior half of the third rib is resected (Fig. 30a). The second rib is resected anteriorly to its sternocostal attachment (Fig. 30b). As in the paravertebral thoracoplasty, the costotransverse joint is opened, and the posterior portions of the ribs are resected at that level. The periostea and intercostal bundles of the resected ribs are ligated and divided posteriorly. The scalenus attachments are dissected free and sharply divided (Fig. 30c). Below the first rib (not yet resected) the extrafascial layer is dissected free, and the pleural dome is freed from the apex of the chest by a combination of blunt and sharp dissection (Fig. 30d). The vertebropleural and costopleural ligaments are divided to free the pleural apex paramediastinally, whereupon the pleural dome can be mobilized downward and medially to the level of the lowermost resected rib. The first rib is resected only after the apicolysis has been completed. Hemostasis is secured, drains are inserted, and the wound is closed in layers.

2.4.2 *Osteoplastic Thoracoplasty of Björk* [3]

Indication: Equalize space after pulmonary resections and collapse cavity-bearing portions of the lung.

Surgical goal: Mobilize the chest wall to reduce the size of the pleural cavity (or collapse cavity-bearing lung).

Preoperative preparation: Epilation, perioperative antibiotic prophylaxis.

Position: Lateral.

Incision: Posterolateral thoracotomy.

Instruments: Basic set, extra thoracic set, rib resection set.

Steps in procedure:

(1) Posterolateral thoracotomy.
(2) Resection of the lowermost rib (fourth or fifth) from the costovertebral joint to the midaxillary line
(3) Resection of the uppermost ribs in increasing lengths from above downward
(4) Division of the second rib 2–3 cm from the vertebra
(5) Posterior resection of the ribs at the costovertebral joint
(6) Paravertebral division of the periostea and intercostal bundles of the resected ribs
(7) Blunt mobilization of the pleural apex (Semb apicolysis)
(8) Complete removal of the first rib (optional)
(9) The ends of the resected ribs are wired to the uppermost intact rib
(10) Drain insertion
(11) Skin closure

The fourth or fifth rib is exposed through a posterolateral incision and resected subperiosteally. In contrast to the previous technique, the lowermost rib is resected anteriorly as far as the midaxillary line, and progressively shorter portions of the higher ribs are resected, with only the posterior 2–3 cm of the second rib being removed. All the ribs are resected at the level of the costovertebral joint, and their periostea and intercostal bundles are divided paravertebrally. With the first rib left intact, the extrafascial layer is exposed, and apicolysis is performed. The pleural dome is bluntly mobilized down to the level of the lowermost resected rib. Herniation of the mobilized thoracic structures is prevented by fixing the pleural dome to the highest intact rib with several sutures. Then the scalenus musculature is cut from the first rib, and the first rib is completely resected. A new thoracic roof is constructed from the sternal ends of the resected ribs and from the periosteal-intercostal bundle. This is done by fixing the ends of the resected ribs to the first (uppermost) intact rib with stainless steel sutures. Finally drains are inserted, and the soft tissues are closed.

2.5 **Tumors of the Pleura** (Fig. 31)

The pleura may become involved by primary tumors or by secondary metastases. While the latter are more important clinically, they signify a generalized metastatic disease that precludes aggressive surgical therapy. The primary tumors include benign pleural neoplasms such as lipomas and hemangioendotheliomas as well as benign localized pleural mesothelioma. On the whole, however, these lesions are rare.

Malignant pleural mesothelioma becomes clinically manifest between the fifth and sixth decades of life, affecting males twice as often as females. Asbestos exposure is considered the prime etiologic factor.

Two pathoanatomic forms of malignant pleural mesothelioma are recognized:

(1) Solitary fibrous pleural mesothelioma, which arises from the visceral pleura and may be broad-based or pedunculated. The tumor produces clinical symptoms by its expansive growth and resulting displacement of intrathoracic structures. With early diagnosis, the lesion is amenable to surgical cure.
(2) Diffusely spreading pleural mesothelioma. This form invades the pulmonary lobes, infiltrates the diaphragm and the intercostal muscles, and can spread through the mediastinal pleura to involve the pericardium and great vessels.

The system of Butchart [4] is used to stage the extent of disease:

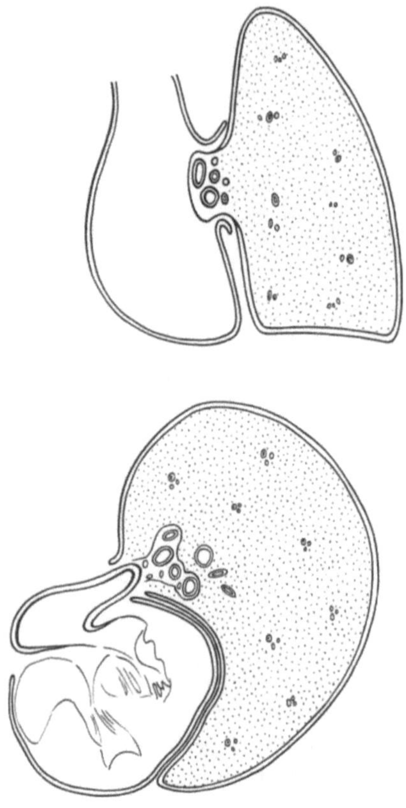

Fig. 31. Schematic diagram of the extent of the pleuropneumonectomy

Stage I. Tumor confined to the parietal pleura and involving only ipsilateral pleura, lung, pericardium, and diaphragm.

Stage II. Tumor invading the chest wall or involving mediastinal structures, e.g. esophagus, heart. Lymph node involvement inside the chest (N_2).

Stage III. Tumor penetrating the diaphragm to involve the peritoneum. Involvement of contralateral pleura and of lymph nodes outside the chest.

Stage IV. Distant blood-borne metastases. The longest postoperative survival times are still achieved in patients with stage I mesotheliomas that show an epithelial histology. This has led some authors to recommend that radical pleuropneumonectomy be reserved for these cases.

However, survival time aside, curative as well as palliative surgery has been shown to benefit patients and improve their response to cytostatic drugs and/or radiation. This underscores the importance of early detection by a systematic diagnostic procedure. Prompt surgical treatment may improve the prognosis and should not be withheld, especially in younger patients who are candidates for a radical and thus potentially curative operation.

Prognosis: With some exceptions, the survival times achieved in patients undergoing radical or palliative surgery for malignant pleural mesothelioma have been disappointing. Only a few patients are four-year survivors, and some reports indicate no difference between the results of palliative and curative surgery, although the studies were not controlled.

2.5.1 Palliative Parietal Pleurectomy

Indication: Malignant pleural mesothelioma, removal of the parietal pleura and part of the visceral pleura to prevent recurrent effusions.

Preoperative preparation: Removal of chest hair.

Incision: Posterolateral thoracotomy in the fifth or sixth interspace.

Instruments: Basic set, extra thoracic set.

Steps in procedure:

(1) Posterolateral thoracotomy in the sixth interspace
(2) Blunt, extrapleural mobilization of the parietal pleura and a portion of the visceral pleura
(3) Meticulous hemostasis (by coagulation or temporary packing)
(4) Insertion of chest tubes
(5) Closure of the thoracotomy

The parietal pleura is separated from the chest wall by a combination of blunt and sharp dissection. Bleeding at this stage may be profuse and is controlled by ligatures, coagulation, and temporary packing. Care is taken to spare the nerves and blood vessels in the region of the apex and mediastinum. Reducing the tumor bulk can be helpful when done as part of a combined oncologic therapy (radiation, chemotherapy).

2.5.2 Extended Pleuropneumonectomy

The objective of pleuropneumonectomy is the radical removal of all tumor-involved portions of the chest wall, diaphragm, mediastinum, and pericardium. Involvement of the lung and diaphragm by malignant pleural mesothelioma is common even in the early stage of the disease. Given the extent of the resection, the operative risk is high (approximately 10%).

Indication: Early-stage diffuse malignant pleural mesothelioma.

Contraindication: Significant cardiorespiratory dysfunction.

Surgical goal: Removal of all tumor-bearing thoracic organs.

Preoperative preparation: Removal of chest hair, perioperative antibiotic prophylaxis.

Position: Lateral.

Incision: Lateral thoracotomy.

Instruments: Basic set, extra thoracic set, rib resection set, extra vascular set.

Steps in procedure:

(1) Lateral thoracotomy in the sixth interspace
(2) Blunt, extrapleural mobilization of the parietal pleura
(3) Mobilization of the mediastinal pleura and adjacent pericardium
(4) Secondary thoracotomy in the eighth interspace
(5) Mobilization of the diaphragm at the level of the costophrenic angle and at the mediastinum
(6) Pneumonectomy by transecting the root of the lung after arterial, venous, and bronchial dissection
(7) Reconstruction of the diaphragm with prosthetic material (e.g., Marlex mesh).
(8) Pericardial reconstruction with dura
(9) Drainage of the pleura and abdomen
(10) Closure of the intercostal incisions
(11) Closure of the thoracotomy

A standard posterolateral thoracotomy having been performed in the sixth interspace, the tough, thickened parietal pleura is bluntly dissected off the chest wall. This often provokes heavy bleeding, which can be controlled by local packing. Then the mediastinal pleura is dissected free from the apex to the hilus of the lung, and the paratracheal lymph nodes are removed. Anteriorly, the internal mammary artery and vein are ligated at the level of the pulmonary apex, and the lymph nodes are removed with these vessels and with the pleura from the chest wall. Posteriorly, the paraesophageal lymph nodes and the lymph nodes at the bifurcation are removed. Then the pericardium is opened over the left atrium from the posterior aspect. At this point it is decided whether to deal with the hilus and vessels first or proceed with resection of the diaphragm. The sequence will depend on the location and extent of the tumor. The pulmonary hilus and vessels are transected and closed as in any intrapericardial (i.e., extended) pneumonectomy. Since the lower part of the pleura does not extend to the insertion of the diaphragm on the chest wall, it is possible to section the diaphragm outside the pleural fold after the pleura has been mobilized. A radical resection usually requires making a second, lower incision in the eighth to tenth interspace.

With the patient in the lateral position, there is a tendency for the liver to become displaced upward toward the mediastinum following removal of the diaphragm. This can compress the inferior vena cava, leading to disturbances of cardiac motion and blood flow. The resected diaphragm is reconstructed using Marlex mesh or dacron-silastic material. Some authors also use dura mater for this purpose. Whatever technique is used must provide a watertight seal between the thoracic and abdominal cavities to prevent leakage of blood or pleural fluid into the abdomen. The substitute diaphragm should be sutured tightly to the residual rim of the diaphragm with a continuous suture line to keep the abdominal organs from bulging into the thoracic cavity. Chest tubes are placed and connected to suction before the chest wall is closed.

References

1. Aigner PW, Klammer H-L, Blömer A (1975) Stabilisierung von Rippenserienfrakturen mit Hilfe von Lochplatten des Kleinfragment-Instrumentariums der AO – Erste klinische Erfahrungen. Hefte Unfallheilkunde 121:199–201
2. Aston ShJ, Pichrell KL (1977) Chest Wall Reconstruction. In: Converse JM (ed) Reconstructive Plastic Surgery, Vol 7, Chapt 88, 2nd ed. Saunders, Philadelphia London Torento, pp 3609–3660
3. Björk VO (1954) Thoracoplasty, a new osteoplastic technic. J Thorac Surg 28:194
4. Butchart EG, Ashcroft T, Barnsley WC, Hoden MP (1981) The role of surgery in diffuse maligment mesothelioma of the pleura. Semin Oncology 8 (3): 321–328
5. Cleland WP (1968) Decortication pleurectomy: excision of empyema. Operative Surgery, Butterworths, London, pp 47–51
6. Dalquen P, Dabbert AF, Hinz I (1969) Zur Epidemiologie des Pleuramesothelioms. Prax Pneumol 23 (8):547–558
7. Eiselsberg AV (1922) Im Protokoll der Gesellschaft für Ärzte Wiens. Klin Wochenschrift 1922, 509
8. Elmes PC (1973) Therapeutic openings in the treatment of mesothelioma. Biological effects of asbestos. International Agency for Research on Cancer, Lyon pp 277–280

8a. Eschapasse H, Gaillard J, Henry E, et al. (1981) Repair of large chest wall defects. Experience with 23 patients. Ann Thorac Surg 32:329–336

9. Gibson LD, Carter R, Himshaw DB (1962) Surgical significance of sternal fracture. Surg Gynec Obstet 1 (4):443–448
10. Grewe HE, Kremer K (1977) Thorakoplastik mit extrafaszialer Apikolyse nach Semb. Chirurgische Operationen. Ein Atlas für die Praxis, 2. Aufl, Bd I. Thieme Stuttgart 180–215
11. Antman KH (1980) Current concepts: Malignant mesothelioma. New Engl J Med 303 (4):200–202
12. Hegemann G (1967) Kosmetische und funktionelle Ergebnisse operativer Maßnahmen bei Trichterbrust. Langenbecks Arch Klin Chir 319:526
13. Hoyer J (1973) Rippen-Osteosynthese bei instabilem Thorax. Act Chir 8:87–94
14. Lemperle G, Exner K (1983) Die Behandlung der Trichterbrust mit RTV-Silikon Implantaten. Handchir 15:154–157
15. Löhr J, Klippe HJ, Kroeger C (1981) Chirurgische Behandlung des Pleuramesothelioms – gegenwärtige kurative und palliative Möglichkeiten. Prax Pneumol 35:394–399
16. Naclerio EA (1971) Chest injuries. Physiologic principles and emergency management. Grune and Stratton, New York London
17. v d Oelsnitz G (1983) Die Trichter- und Kielbrust. In: Daum R, Mildenberg Rehbein F (Hrsg) Bibliothek für Kinderchirurgie. Hippokrates, Stuttgart
18. Rothfeld A, Bromberg Ph (1983) Pneumothorax: Diagnose und Behandlung. Klin J 6:6–12
19. Salzer G (1951) Die diffusen Pleuratumoren als chirurgisches Problem. Thoraxchirurgie 7:377–382
20. Sulamaa M, Walgren J (1970) Trichterbrust. Z Kinderchir 8:22
21. Vecsei V (1982) Instabiler Thorax – chirurgische Therapie. Hefte zur Unfallheilkunde 158:353–371
22. Willital GH (1981) Operationsindikation, Operationstechnik bei Brustkorbdeformierungen. Z Kinderchir 33:244–252
23. Wolfart W, Schildge J (1963) Therapeutische Überlegungen zum Pleuramesotheliom aus chirurgischer Sicht. Atemwegs- und Lungenerkrankungen 11: 457–459

E. Operations on the Breast

F. W. SCHILDBERG and E. KIFFNER

CONTENTS

1 Diagnostic Procedures on the Breast

1.1 Indications

Lesions of uncertain nature that are detected by palpation, mammography, or sonography are an indication for incisional biopsy. Despite advances in aspiration cytology, the open excision and subsequent histologic examination of breast tissue, though more costly, offers the most dependable proof of the nature of breast disease. In all open biopsies an effort should be made to excise the lesion completely with adequate margins, even if this involves an appreciable sacrifice of breast tissue.

The operative technique does not depend on the extent of the resection. The goal is always the removal of the entire suspicious area. With palpable masses, then, the extent of the resection will correspond roughly to the size of the mass (tumorectomy). Nonpalpable lesions often necessitate a wider excision (e.g., a segmental resection) due to difficulties in localizing the tumor.

1.2 Preoperative Methods of Tumor Localization

Physical examination of the breast is preceded by accurate history taking that includes the age at menarche, the length of menstrual cycles, the use of oral contraceptives or other hormonal or nonhormonal medications, the family history for breast cancer, and the nature of the patient's symptoms. The physical examination should follow a standardized procedure. We start by inspecting the breasts with the patient erect, first with her arms at her sides and then with her arms raised or supported on the hips (Fig. 1). This position change makes it easier to recognize subtle skin changes, retractions, and protrusions. Changes also can be accentuated by having the patient lean forward. Inspection is followed by palpation, which is done with the patient erect and then su-

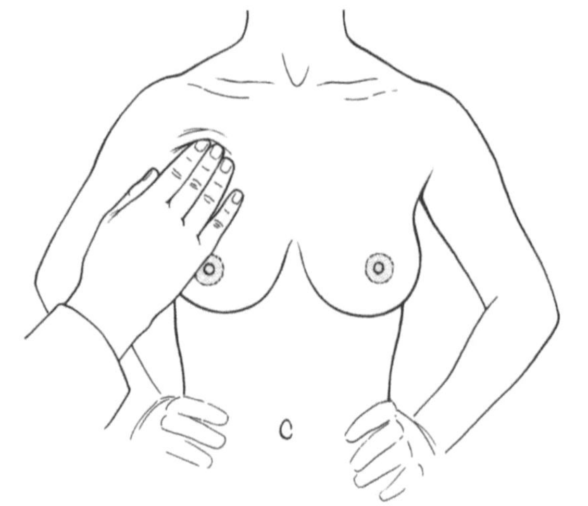

Fig. 1. Inspection and palpation of the breasts in the erect patient with the arms slightly abducted

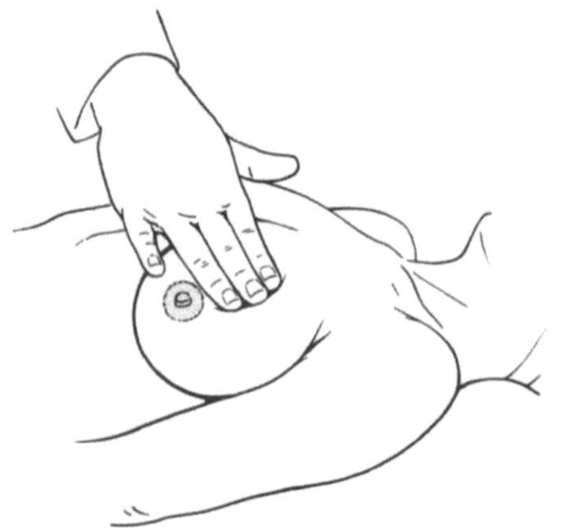

Fig. 4. Breast palpation in the supine patient. The contents of the breast are pressed against the chest wall

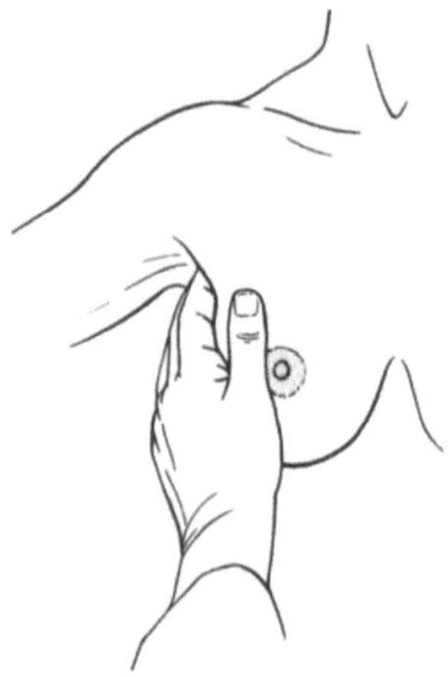

Fig. 2. Palpation of the axillary tail of the breast and axillary lymph nodes

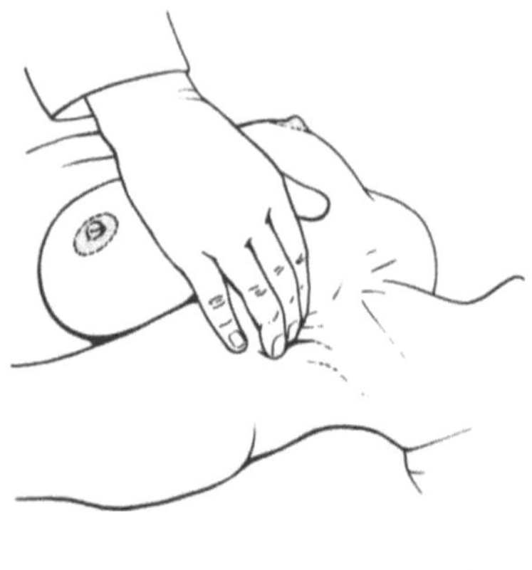

Fig. 3. Palpation of the supraclavicular lymph nodes

pine. All quadrants of the breast, including the axillary tail, are systematically examined (Fig. 2) as are the supra- and infraclavicular areas (Fig. 3). The contents of the breast are pressed gently against the rib cage with the tips of the fingers (Fig. 4) and are also examined bimanually for the presence of deep-lying masses. Lesions detected in this way are marked to facilitate operation.

Palpable masses lying inside or outside the breast tissue do not require further preoperative localizing measures. However, accurate preoperative localization is necessary for the excision of a mammographically suspicious lesion that is impalpable – a situation occurring in many women whose mammograms show suspicious microcalcifications. Any of several localizing techniques may be employed in these patients.

1.2.1 Geometric Localization (Fig. 5)

The geometric localization of a breast lesion utilizes mammograms taken on two planes; it is the technique that we prefer. Making allowance for magnification factors, the mammographic abnormality is localized in its relationship to the skin and nipple. The distance measured on the mammogram is transposed onto the patient's breast, ideally while reproducing the compression that was applied when the mammograms were taken. The coordinates are marked on the breast so that the surgeon can locate the lesion accurately from

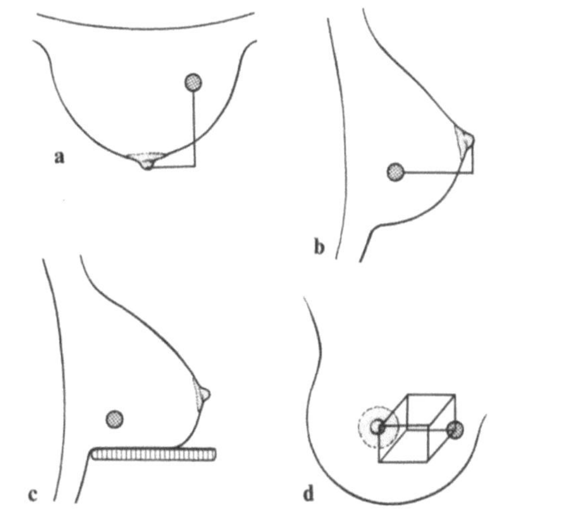

Fig. 5a–d. Geometric localization of a suspected breast lesion. The mammographic coordinates of the lesion are transferred to the breast

the geometric data. It should be noted with this method that the relative positions of the glandular tissue and skin can change when the patient changes position.

1.2.2 Radiologic Localization

To minimize the extent of the excision, several radiologic methods have been devised for the localization of mammographic abnormalities. In one method a mixture of visible dye and radiographic contrast medium is injected under mammographic control immediately before surgery both to guide the surgeon in his biopsy and to permit the suspicious area to be identified on specimen radiographs, faciliting the pathologic workup.

Another method involves the introduction of radiopaque particles, such as tiny metal beads, which likewise can be injected through a needle under mammographic control. Needle localization is another possibility, employing either conventional hypodermic needles or special needles with a barbed end (Fig. 6).

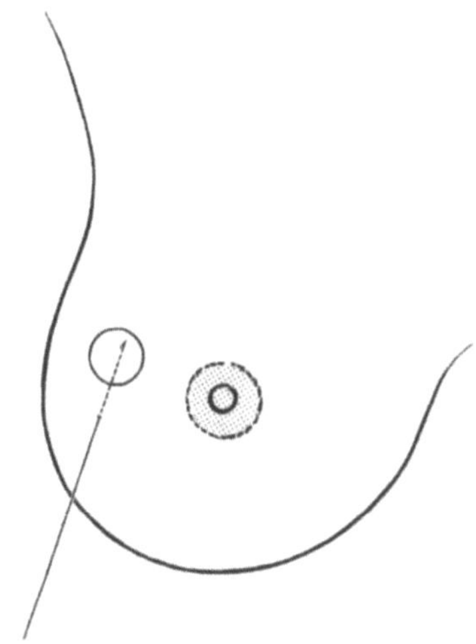

Fig. 6. Localization of a mammographically suspicious lesion by marking the area with a needle

1.2.3 Cyst Localization (Fig. 7)

Cysts can be sonographically visualized and diagnosed. Inserting a needle into the cyst and instilling air before taking another roentgenogram (pneumocystography) has both diagnostic and therapeutic value.

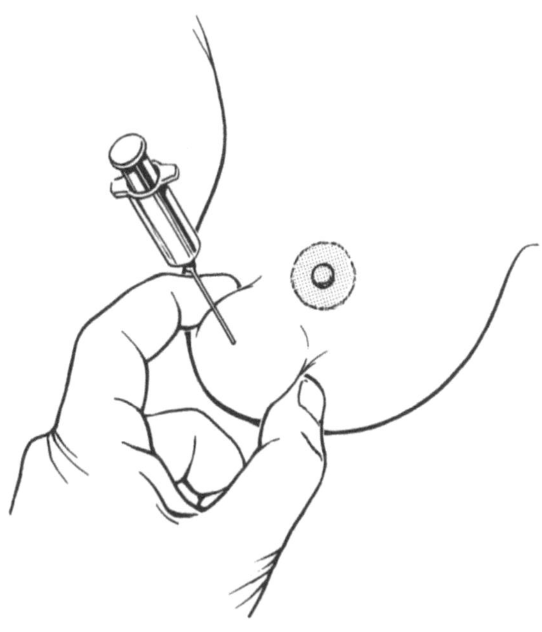

Fig. 7. Percutaneous aspiration of a cyst localized by palpation. Evacuation of the cyst should be followed by pneumocystography to detect changes located in the radiographic shadow of the cyst or papillary changes within the cyst wall

1.3 Breast Biopsy

Indication: Palpable mass, suspicious mammographic finding.

Surgical goal: Removal and histologic evaluation of the mass.

Preoperative preparation: Complete removal of axillary hair.

Position: Supine; the involved side may be elevated slightly with a thin cushion or a 3- to 5-cm thickness of towels. The arm on the involved side is abducted almost to 90°, avoiding hyperextension that might stretch the plexus or cause pressure injury to the radial and ulnar nerves. The arm need not be free to move, but it should be draped such that the surgeon and assistant can stand below and above the arm, respectively (Fig. 8).

Instruments: Basic set.

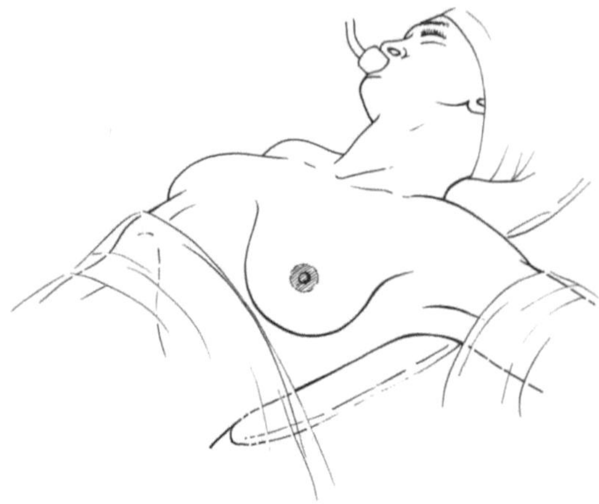

Fig. 8. Position of the patient for all diagnostic and therapeutic procedures on the breast. The arm on the involved side is extended, and the corresponding hemithorax is slightly elevated on a pad

Steps in procedure:

(1) Periareolar incision
(2) Division of subcutaneous tissue
(3) Mobilization of skin flap to expose the tumor
(4) Tumor excision, frozen section
(5) Reapproximation of breast tissue
(6) Drain insertion
(7) Skin closure

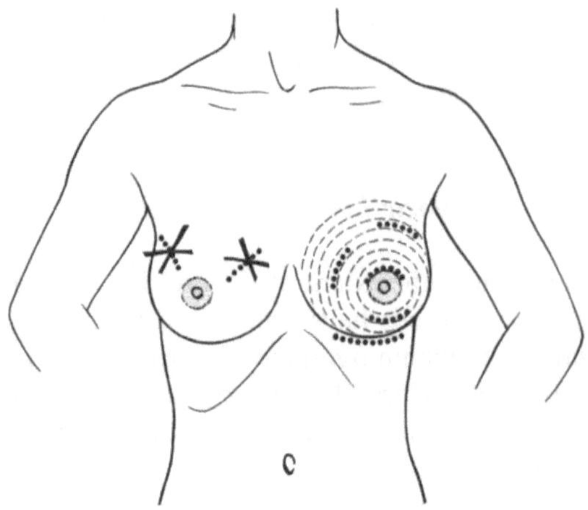

Fig. 9. Radial incisions should not be used on the breast. If a periareolar incision is not suitable, incisions should be made along skin cleavage lines

1.3.1 ***Incision*** (Fig. 9)

Of the many breast incisions that are available, the periareolar incision has established itself as the most cosmetically appealing. Other incisions (Fig.9) are used mainly when the location of the tumor would require prohibitive dissection of the soft tissues if a periareolar incision were used. Thus, with a peripheral tumor or in very large breasts, the cosmetic advantage of the periareolar incision is offset by the greater traumatization of breast tissue and perhaps by extensive scar formation that would hinder future clinical and mammographic evaluation. Generally this is the case when the area to be excised lies more than 5 cm from the areola. In these situations, incisions made in the skin lines or Bardenheuer's incision are safer and less traumatic.

Radial incisions should not be used for questionable or putatively benign lesions. However, a radial incision or scar is the inevitable result of the techniques used in "breast-conserving" operations (see Tylectomy). The radial scar in these cases does not become hypertrophic during subsequent irradiation.

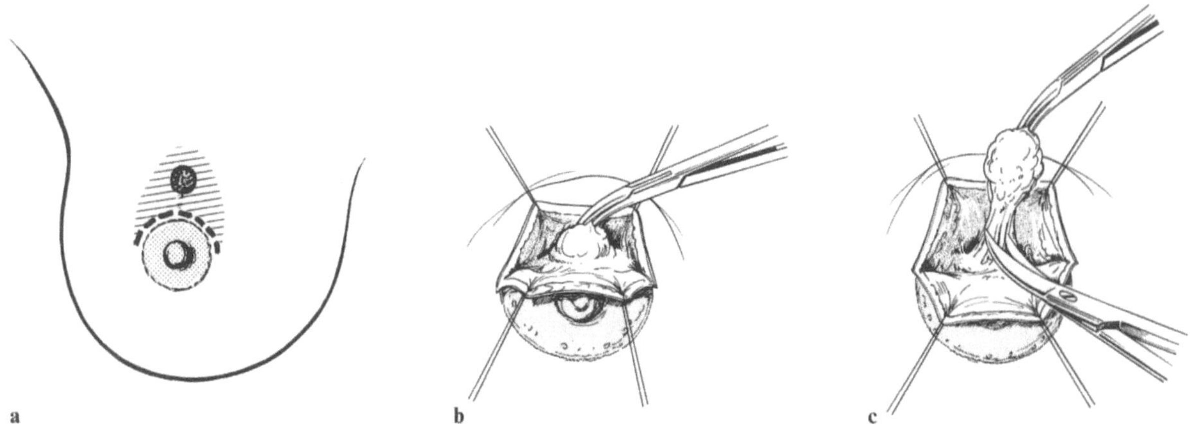

Fig. 10. **a** Incision and necessary extent of mobilization for the local excision of a benign lesion. **b** Stay sutures are placed in the skin, and the skin and subcutaneous tissue are dissected from the breast. **c** The tumor is dissected free, grasped with a small sharp forceps, and excised at its base with a scissors or electrocautery

1.3.2 Tumor Excision

Excisional biopsy is indicated in patients with a palpable breast mass or abnormal discharge or with an impalpable mammographic abnormality to exclude malignancy or to document the proliferative tendency of the breast tissue.

The exact placement of the periareolar incision is guided by the site of the lesion (Fig. 10a). The skin is incised with a small scalpel (No. 15), and the subcutaneous blood vessels are electrocoagulated. The edges of the incision are retracted with small hooks or, preferably, with intracutaneous stay sutures (Fig. 10b). The subcutaneous tissue is divided down to the breast parenchyma, and the flap is separated from the breast tissue using predominantly sharp dissection (Fig. 10b). Care is taken to maintain an adequate thickness of the skin flap to avoid scar plaque formation that would compromise the esthetic result and hinder postoperative evaluation. After the tumor has been identified, it is isolated with small Langenbeck retractors and grasped with a traction suture or a forceps (Allis, Museux) (Fig. 10c). While gentle traction is applied to the specimen, it is dissected free on all sides with the electrocautery or scissors, separating it as needed from the pectoral fascia. We recommend insulating the standard diathermy knife with a silicone rubber tube so that only 1–2 mm of the tip is exposed, as this lessens the danger of skin burns. If clinical and mammographic findings are suggestive of fibroadenoma, the dissection can be carried close to the tumor, although a wedge excision of the base of the tumor is recommended to prevent recurrence. All other tumors are excised with a margin of healthy tissue and sent for frozen section. If the biopsy was performed for microcalcification clusters on mammograms or if the lesion was radiologically marked before surgery, specimen radiography is indicated to confirm that the designated area has been removed and that a complete excision has been accomplished. After a correct and adequate excision has been confirmed, the operative field is checked for hemostasis, and bleeding points are coagulated. A suction drain is placed into the wound and brought out through a cosmetically acceptable site, either on the submammary fold or in the region of the axillary line. With larger defects the cosmetic result can be improved by approximating the breast tissue with 3-0 synthetic absorbable sutures.

1.4 Procedures for Abnormal Nipple Discharge

Indication: The indication for surgery is based on the presence of an abnormal nipple discharge and on preoperative mammographic and ductographic findings.

Surgical goals: Removal of the secreting area of the breast, histologic evaluation.

Preoperative preparation: See above.

Position: See above.

Instruments: Basic set.

Steps in procedure:

(1) Intubation of secreting duct
(2) Staining of duct with methylene blue
(3) Periareolar incision, nipple dissected free
(4) Secreting duct is identified and grasped with a forceps
(5) Excision of stained tissue
(6) Hemostasis
(7) Reapproximation of breast tissue (as required)
(8) Drain insertion
(9) Skin closure

At the start of the operation the nipple is squeezed to produce some discharge and identify the affected duct. Then the duct is intubated with either a No. 14 disposable beveled cannula or a special plastic catheter and stained with methylene blue (Fig. 11a). Next a periareolar incision is made in the appropriate quadrant, and intracutaneous stay sutures are applied. The nipple is dissected free on a plane immediately deep to the subcutaneous veins, which are electrocoagulated or ligated. Dissection on this plane spares the subdermal vascular plexus, preserving the blood supply to the nipple. The nipple is mobilized and elevated with stay sutures until the stained duct can be visualized. The duct is grasped with a small forceps, divided, and ligated (Fig. 11 b). Then the nipple is everted over the index finger of the left hand (Fig. 11c), and residual duct tissue is resected with the scissors. Finally, while gentle traction is applied, all of the stained duct system is dissected free with the electrocautery and excised (Fig. 11c). A frozen section is done right away to exclude malignancy, although the specimen will be processed later into serial sections for a more detailed evaluation. All bleeding points are carefully controlled. If the defect is large enough, the breast tissue may be mobilized and the resected edges approximated. The skin is closed over a suction drain with simple interrupted sutures.

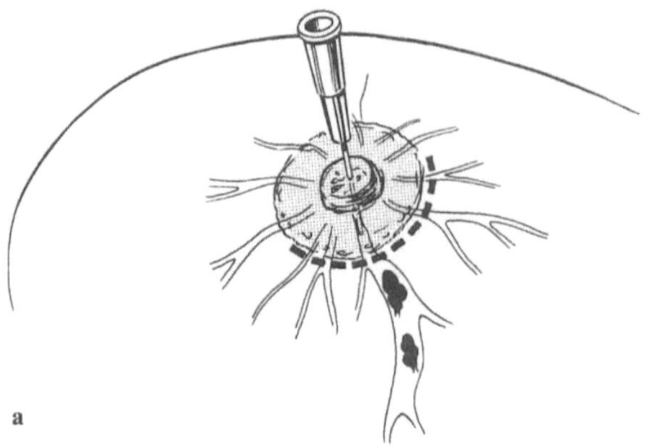

a

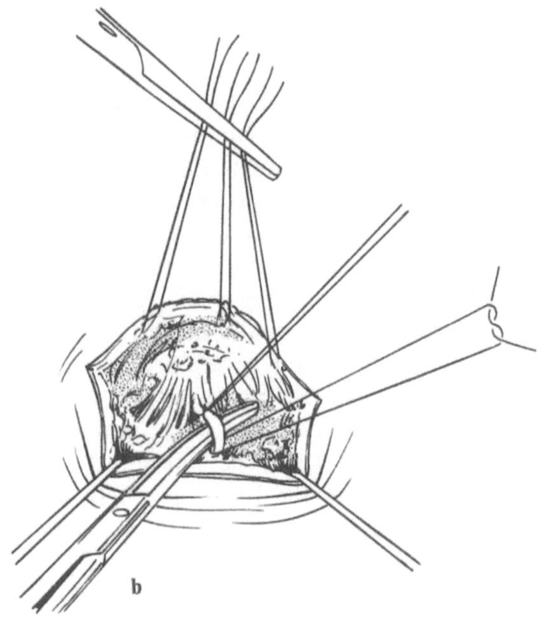

b

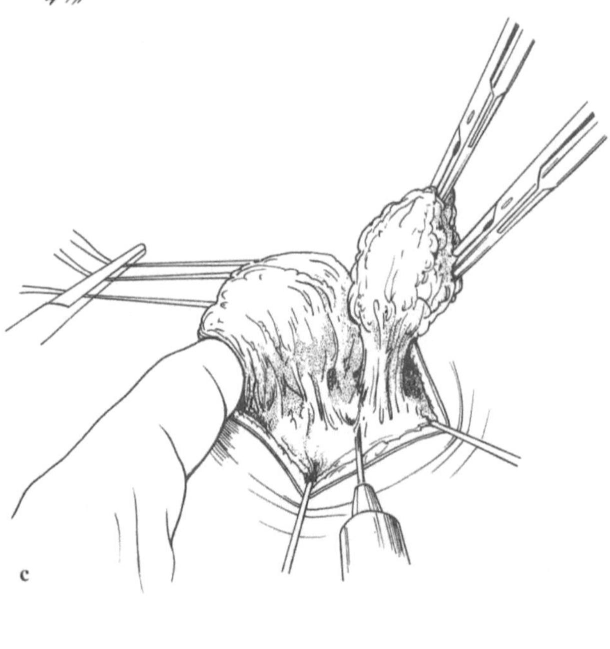

c

Fig. 11. a Intubation of a secreting milk duct containing intraductal papilloma. **b** A periareolar incision is made, the areola is dissected free, and the nipple is retracted with stay sutures. The stained duct is identified, grasped with a small forceps, and ligated. **c** The index finger of the left hand is passed beneath the retracted nipple to assist the removal of residual stained tissue. The entire stained area is excised with the electrocautery

1.5 Segmental Resection (Quadrantectomy)

Indication: Radiologically localized microcalcification clusters.

Surgical goal: Removal of affected breast quadrant, histologic evaluation.

Preoperative preparation: See above.

Position: See above.

Instruments: Basic set.

Incision: Periareolar; radial in exceptional cases.

Steps in procedure:

(1) Periareolar incision
(2) Dissection of skin and subcutaneous tissue
(3) Excision of breast segment with the electrocautery
(4) Reapproximation of the breast tissue
(5) Drain insertion
(6) Skin closure

The soft-tissue flap comprised of skin and subcutaneous tissue is dissected free over the affected quadrant while Cooper's ligaments are divided (Fig. 12a). The dissection is carried a short distance into the adjacent quadrants. When the edge of the breast is reached, it is grasped with small forceps, and a wedge-shaped segment corresponding in size to the mammographically localized area is resected with the electrocautery, trying to keep the width of the excised segment as small as possible. The resection is limited from below by the pectoral fascia (Fig. 12b). To further localize the changes, it is helpful to mark the area about the nipple with a clip or wire suture so that, following specimen mammography, it will be easier for the pathologist to locate, mark, and selectively examine the suspicious area. After meticulous hemostasis by electrocautery, the remaining breast tissue is mobilized (Fig. 12c) and reapproximated (Fig. 12d) with 3-0 synthetic absorbable sutures before placing a suction drain and closing the skin.

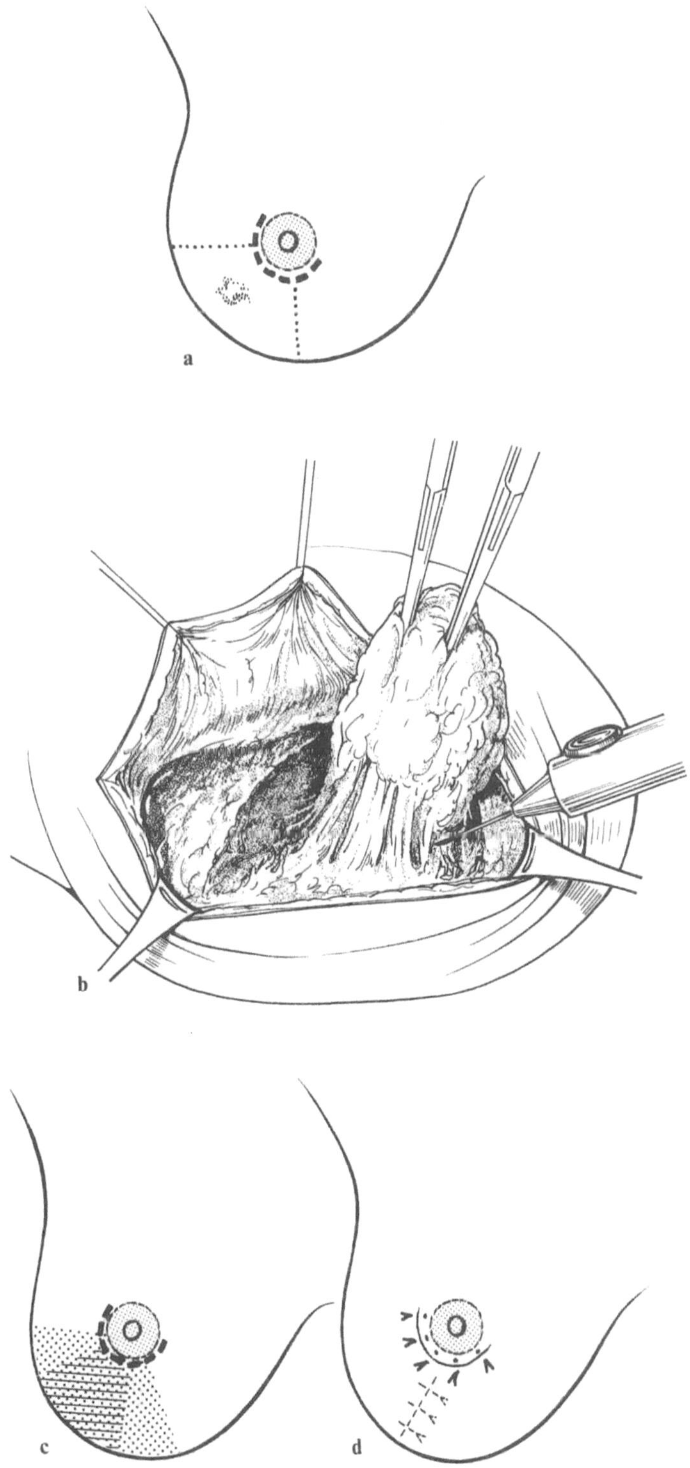

Fig. 12. a Segmental resection. The radiographically suspicious area is identified and marked, and the segment is dissected free through a periareolar incision. **b** First the nipple is dissected free, preserving the subareolar venous plexus. Then the skin and subcutaneous fat are mobilized, with division of Cooper's ligaments. Then, proceeding from the periphery of the quadrant toward the center, the specimen is divided from the pectoral fascia. **c** After the suspicious segment has been resected, the adjacent portions of the breast tissue are mobilized. **d** The remaining breast tissue is approximated to avoid troublesome defects, and the skin is closed

1.6 Subcutaneous Mastectomy

Indications: Premalignant disease, breast tissue difficult to evaluate by palpation and mammography due to prior surgery. Cystosarcoma, siliconoma, giant fibroadenoma.

Surgicial goal: Removal of all breast tissue from the cutaneous envelope.

Preoperative preparation: See above.

Position: Semisitting with the arm on the involved side extended.

Instruments: Basic set, silicone prosthesis.

Incision: Lateral Bardenheuer incision about 10 cm long.

Steps in procedure:

(1) Bardenheuer incision
(2) Dissection of the breast tissue on the pectoralis major muscle
(3) Sharp dissection of the overlying soft tissues
(4) Meticulous hemostasis and inspection for residual breast tissue
(5) Placement of suitable implant after insertion of a trial prosthesis
(6) Insertion of drains
(7) Skin closure

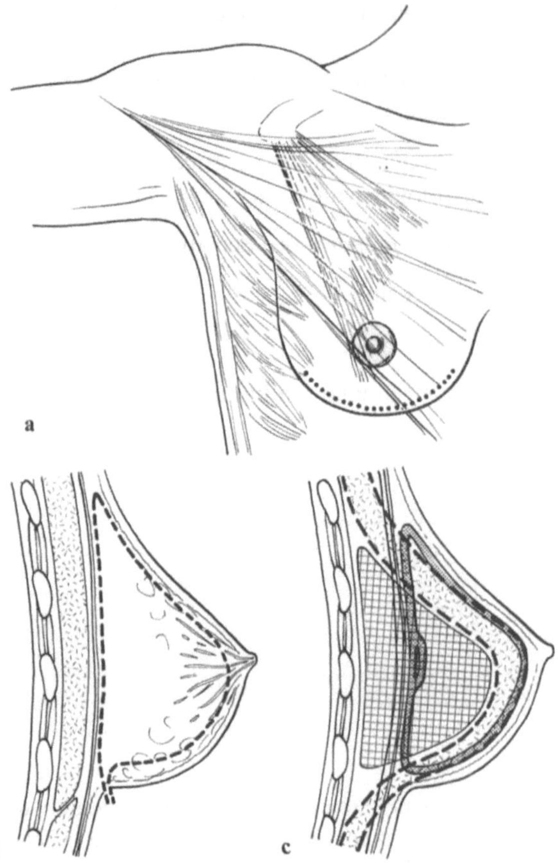

Fig. 13. a Incision for subcutaneous mastectomy. **b** Extent of dissection on the subcutaneous plane. **c** The silastic prosthesis may be implanted either subcutaneously or submuscularly (deep to the pectoralis major)

After incision of the skin (Fig. 13a), the breast tissue is first separated from the pectoral fascia. Some perforating vessels will have to be electrocoagulated at this time. Next the surgeon locates the plane of dissection between the skin flap and breast. Care is taken to cut the flap sufficiently thick, while also making certain that all mammary tissue is removed. Cooper's ligaments, which unite the breast to the subcutaneous tissue, are divided with a scissors. Dissection around the nipple must be performed with particular care. The plane of dissection should be deep to the subcutaneous veins to preserve the blood supply to the nipple, yet the excision of breast tissue must be as radical as possible (Fig. 13b). After the region behind the nipple has been mobilized, dissection of the breast tissue proceeds along the chest wall. The dissection is continued along the axillary tail, which must be completely removed. Small clamps and ligatures are used to control bleeding in the lateral part of the wound. A meticulous hemostasis is sought on all remaining wound surfaces to avoid hematoma and seroma formation. With painstaking technique, approximately 95% of the breast tissue can be removed by this operation. The remaining 5%–10% consists of tissue residues along Cooper's ligaments. Reconstruction of the breast may be performed in one or two stages. For a two-stage reconstruction, it is recommended that a temporary prosthesis[1] be inserted to prevent undesired shrinkage and scarring of the skin. Selection of the definitive prosthesis is guided by anatomic considerations; lately a preference has emerged in favor of silicone prostheses with an outer saline-filled lumen. In large breasts, the skin flaps should be adapted to the implant, creating in effect a reduction mammoplasty. If the skin

[1] Inlay or subcutaneous tissue expander, Heyer Schulte

flaps are too thin, a submuscular implantation can be performed by mobilizing the pectoralis major over the prosthesis (Fig. 13c). The muscle is incised along its margin, and a combination of finger and diathermy dissection is used to create an adequate pocket.

1.7 Mastectomy

Indication: Premalignant disease. Recurrent benign cystosarcoma phylloides.

Surgical goal: Removal of the breast tissue, overlying skin, and nipple.

Preoperative preparation: See above.

Position: Supine with the upper body slightly elevated on the involved side. The arm is extended and the field draped so that the surgeon can stand below the arm while an assistant stands above it.

Instruments: Basic set.

Incision: Transverse elliptical incision of Stewart. The medial limit of the incision should not cross the sternal midline; the lateral limit should not extend past the anterior axillary line.

Steps in procedure:

(1) Elliptical incision
(2) Development of skin flaps
(3) Medial-to-lateral dissection of the breast
(4) Removal of the axillary tail
(5) Hemostasis
(6) Insertion of suction drain
(7) Skin closure

If the mastectomy is being done for a putatively benign disease, the extent of skin removal can be minimized, i.e., the incision may be made close to the nipple without maintaining the 3-cm margin customary for malignant disease (Fig. 14a). This results in larger skin flaps that will facilitate a later reconstruction. In all cases the incision is first out-

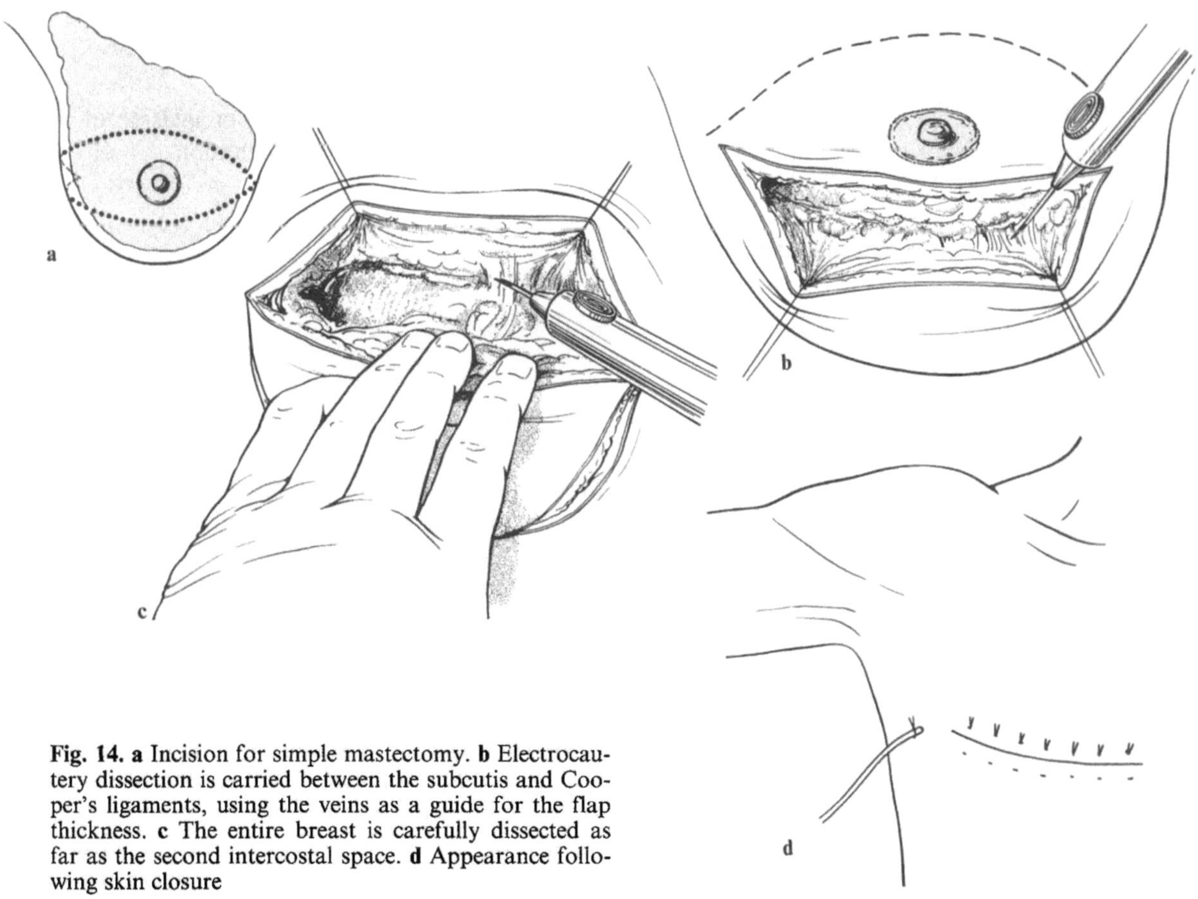

Fig. 14. a Incision for simple mastectomy. **b** Electrocautery dissection is carried between the subcutis and Cooper's ligaments, using the veins as a guide for the flap thickness. **c** The entire breast is carefully dissected as far as the second intercostal space. **d** Appearance following skin closure

lined with a marker. The skin and subcutaneous tissue are divided with a scalpel, and the skin is retracted with stay sutures. The plane of dissection is guided by the course of the superficial veins, resulting in a flap thickness of about 0.5 cm (Fig. 14b). The flaps are dissected upward to the level of the second intercostal space and downward to a point just below the submammary fold. After the flaps have been mobilized, the mammary tissue is dissected off the fascia, proceeding in a medial-to-lateral direction (Fig. 14c). For anatomic reasons it is best to begin the dissection somewhat lateral of center, as the plane of dissection is easier to locate in that area. Even with a simple mastectomy, the axillary tail of the breast (tail of Spence) must be included in the resection. For this purpose the mobilized breast is retracted laterally under slight tension, and the breast tissue is dissected on the pectoral fascia. Blood vessels entering the lateral part of the field are divided and ligated between Overholt clamps. Further hemostasis is effected by cautery or ligation of the vascular stumps. A suction drain is brought out in the area of the midaxillary line, and the skin is closed with 4-0 monofilament sutures (Fig. 14d).

1.7.1 Simultaneous Reconstruction of the Breast with Subcutaneous Tissue Expander

Indication: Small breast carcinoma T1/T2 N0 M0, premalignant disease.

Surgical goal: Restore the external appearance of the breast.

Preoperative preparation: See above.

Position: See above.

Instruments: Basic set, subcutaneous tissue expander (Heyer Schulte).

Steps in procedure:

(1) Modified radical mastectomy (q.v.)
(2) Placement of inflatable silastic prosthesis
(3) Placement of reservoir
(4) Filling of prosthesis with 50–100 ml NaCl
(5) Insertion of drains
(6) Skin closure

Concurrent reconstruction of the breast after a modified radical mastectomy may be possible by the (submuscular) insertion of a suitable, inflatable implant such as the subcutaneous tissue expander. The operative field must be painstakingly checked for bleeding sites. After the prosthesis is inserted beneath the muscle and the filler valve is installed in the axilla, drains are inserted and the skin is closed. A period of three to nine months is recommended for inflation of the implant, whose final volume should be about 1 $^1/_2$ times that of the definitive prosthesis. The implant is then exchanged for a silastic prosthesis of appropriate size.

1.8 Procedures for Inflammatory Breast Disease

Indication: Inflammation with abscess formation (usually in the puerperium).

Surgical goal: Open and evacuate abscess, histologic and microbiologic examination.

Preoperative preparation: Removal of axillary hair.

Position: See above.

Instruments: Basic set.

Incision: Bardenheuer incision, or incision at the lowest point of the area of fluctuation.

Steps in procedure:

(1) Incision
(2) Evacuation of necrotic tissues; histology and microbiology
(3) Drain insertion

Most inflammatory breast diseases occur in the initial days and weeks after childbirth, and most involve the lower outer quadrant of the breast. The recommended approach is either through a sufficiently long incision made on the skin lines at the lowest point of the fluctuation or, for disease of the lower outer quadrant (Fig. 15a), Bardenheuer's incision. The abscess cavity is opened and cleared of necrotic material (Fig. 15b), dividing any septa that are found. In all cases a histologic examination is done to exclude or confirm an inflammatory breast tumor. The material is cultured to identify the organisms present. Depending on the extent of the abscess formation, the wound cavity may either be drained with a silicone catheter (Fig. 15c) or packed loosely with iodoform gauze. Further treatment follows the guidelines for septic surgery.

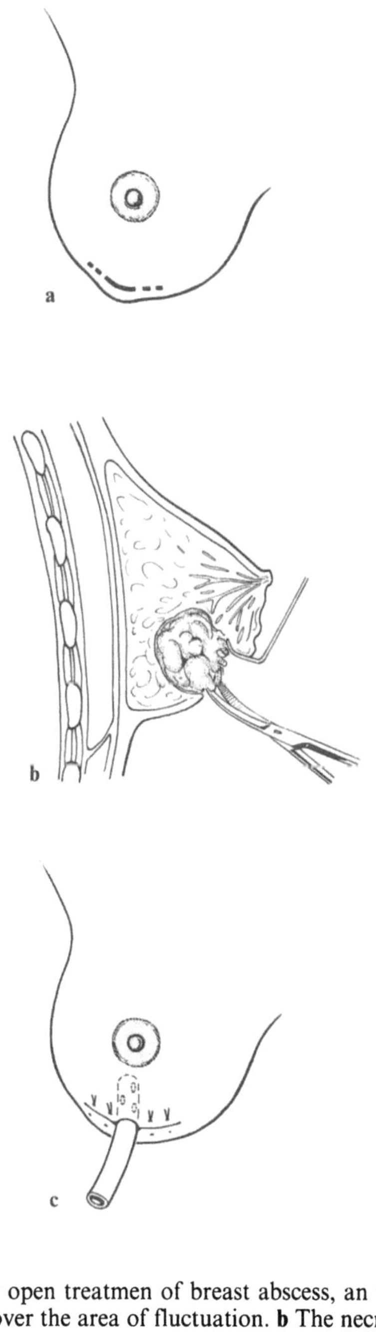

Fig. 15. a For open treatmen of breast abscess, an incision is made over the area of fluctuation. **b** The necrotic material is removed, and any septa are divided to permit mechanical cleansing of the abscess cavity; the material is sent for histologic study. **c** A silicone drainage tube is inserted, and retention sutures are placed

1.9 Gynecomastia

Preoperative measures: Symmetrical gynecomastia or unilateral hypertrophy of the male breast may be caused by an endocrine abnormality or testicular tumor. Differential diagnosis should additionally include hepatic disease and adverse drug effects. Preoperative mammography is helpful in establishing the nature of the lesion.

Indication for surgery: Palpable nodes (usually retroareolar), cancerphobia, unilateral occurrence.

Surgical goal: Removal of tumor, histologic diagnosis.

Preoperative preparation: Removal of chest and axillary hair.

Position: See above.

Instruments: See above.

Approach: Periareolar incision in the lower quadrants.

Steps in procedure:

(1) Skin incision
(2) Mobilization and elevation of the nipple
(3) Tumor excision
(4) Hemostasis
(5) Drain insertion
(6) Skin closure

The periareolar incision is made inferiorly to spare the blood supply to the nipple, dividing the skin with a small scalpel (No. 14). Stay sutures are placed, and the nipple is sharply dissected from the breast. The tumor is grasped with a stay suture or Museux forceps, and the node is excised with a rim of healthy tissue using the electrocautery. The node is sent for frozen section and for receptor analysis if malignancy is determined. Bleeding points are coagulated, a suction drain is inserted, and the skin is closed.

2 Therapeutic Procedures on the Breast

2.1 Malignant Breast Diseases

Malignant tumors can develop from any and all components of the breast tissue. Sarcomatous lesions such as fibrosarcoma, angiosarcoma, and carcinosarcoma are rarely encountered in the breast. Types deverving particular mention are lymphangiosarcoma (Kaposi's sarcoma), which can occur in the area of a previous mastectomy or in the arms of patients who have severe arm edema following mastectomy, and malignant cystosarcoma phylloides, which shows a peak incidence during periods of hormonal change (puberty, pregnancy, menopause). This tumor metastasizes chiefly by hematogenous spread; axillary lymph node metastases are rare, so local surgical treatment may be directed by clinical findings.

Carcinoma of the breast is the commonest form of cancer in women, affecting between 6% and 9% of the female population in Europe and the United States. In recent decades the incidence of the disease has been increasing steadily in western industrialized nations. Ethnic and genetic factors play a role in the etiology of breast carcinoma, and a familial occurrence is well documented.

Other known risk factors are an early menarche and a late first pregnancy. The age distribution for breast carcinoma shows two peaks: one around age 45 and another around age 60. At present it is believed that breast carcinoma is a hormone-dependent neoplasm that cannot develop before puberty. The tumors usually take 10 to 20 years to produce clinical signs, since the average doubling time is about 200 days, and many such doublings are needed for the tumor to attain a clinically palpable size of 1 cm, or a volume of 10^6–10^9 cells. An earlier manifestation is commonly seen in women with a positive family history, and bilateral occurrence is not unusual. Breast carcinomas can occur in males, but only with about 1/100 the incidence in the female population. The prognosis in men and women appears to relate closely to the TNM stage of the lesion.

Breast carcinoma is already considered to be a potentially generalized disease at the time of diagnosis, because a large percentage of patients go on to develop distant metastases regardless of the type of local treatment administered. The extent of surgical resection, then, is presumably not the only determinant of patient outcome. This is not inconsistent with Halsted's earlier claim that breast carcinoma is primarily a locoregional disease and that wide surgical excision is an important factor in determining the chance for a cure. Portions of this concept have been retained and provide the rationale for delivering postoperative radiation to the breast and lymph nodes to eradicate locoregional disease following a limited breast resection. Overall, there has been a definite trend in recent decades toward more conservative operations, which have been shown to yield favorable results in suitably selected patients.

Prognosis: The major prognostic factor in breast carcinoma, besides the tumor size, is the lymph node status. The tables show the 5- and 10-year survival rates in large collective series as a function of locoregional lymph node involvement.

Prognosis of female breast carcinoma
(after Henderson and Canellos [60, 61])

Histologic stage NSABP	Survival rate in %	
	5 years	10 years
All patients	63.5	45.9
Negative lymph nodes	78.1	64.9
Positive lymph nodes (all patients)	46.5	24.9
1–3 lymph nodes positive	62.2	37.5
4 or more lymph nodes positive	32.0	13.0

Prognosis of male breast carcinoma
(after Robinson and Montague [89])

Histologic stage NSABP	Survival rate in %
	10 years
All patients	50
Negative lymph nodes	70
Positive lymph nodes (all patients)	34

2.2 Classifications

Breast carcinomas are classified according to histologic criteria (WHO classification). A second, morphologic subclassification is based on the presence of estrogen and progesterone receptors in the tumor and provides additional useful information on prognosis and type of treatment. Besides the histologic type of carcinoma, which is useful prognostically, lesions may be further classified according to the TNM system.

TNM Classification of Female Breast Cancer (ICD-0 174)

The TNM classification takes into account the anatomic location of the primary tumor as well as the possible occurrence of lymph node involvement and distant metastases. The minimum requirement for TNM classification is a clinical examination that includes mammograms and a mammographic determination of the tumor extent. Lymph node involvement is assessed by clinical examination.

TN Classification by Clinical Examination before Treatment

T = Primary tumor
TIS = Preinvasive carcinoma (carcinoma in situ), noninfiltrating intraductal carcinoma or Paget's disease of the nipple with no demonstrable tumor [if Paget's disease is associated with a tumor (70%–80%), the disease is classified by tumor size]
T0 = No clinically apparent primary tumor

Note: A plateau phenomenon of the skin, nipple retration, or other skin changes except for those characterizing stage T4 may be seen in T1, T2, or T3 lesions without affecting the classification.

T1 = Tumor of 2 cm or less in its greatest dimension
T1a = No attachment to the pectoral fascia or muscle
T1b = With attachment to the pectoral fascia
T2 = Tumor between 2 cm and 5 cm in its greatest dimension
T2a = No attachment to the pectoral fascia or muscle
T2b = With attachment to the pectoral fascia or muscle
T3 = Tumor larger than 5 cm
T3a = No attachment to the pectoral fascia
T3b = With attachment to the pectoral fascia
T4 = Tumor of any size with direct attachment to the skin or chest wall

Note: The chest wall includes the ribs, intercostal musculature, and the seratus anterior muscle, but not the pectoralis.

T4a = With attachment to the chest wall
T4b = With edematous infiltration and ulceration of the skin, including peau d'orange, or lenticular skin metastases on the ipsilateral breast
T4c = Combination of a and b

Note: Inflammatory breast carcinomas constitute a separate group.

N – Regional lymph nodes
N0 = No palpable homolateral axillary lymph nodes
N1 = Homolateral axillary lymph nodes that are not fixed
N1a = Metastasis not suspected
N1b = Metastasis suspected
N2 = Homolateral axillary lymph nodes that are fused together
N3 = Homolateral supraclavicular or infraclavicular lymph nodes showing metastatic change

Note: Edema of the arm can be caused by lymphatic obstruction, in which case the lymph nodes themselves may not be palpable.

RT = Local recurrences also can be classified by the TNM system by placing the prefix R before the appropriate TNM category.

Stage grouping of TNM subsets

Stage I:	T1a	N0	or	N1a	M0
	T1b	N0	or	N1a	M0
Stage II:	T0	N1b			M0
	T1a	N1b			M0
	T1b	N1b			M0
	T2a	N0	or	N1a	M0
	T2b	N0	or	N1a	M0
	T2a	N1b			M0
	T2b	N1b			M0
Stage III:	Any T3 with any N				M0
	Any T4 with any N				M0
	Any T with N2				M0
	Any T with N3				M0
Stage IV:	Any T	Any N with			M1

2.3 Surgical Treatment of Malignant Breast Diseases

2.3.1 Biopsy Excision

Steps in procedure:

(1) Periareolar incision
(2) Division of subcutaneous tissue
(3) Mobilization of skin flap to expose the tumor
(4) Tumor excision, frozen section
(5) Change of instruments
(6) Hemostasis
(7) Drain insertion
(8) Skin closure

The excision of suspected breast malignancies is performed as described previously for benign disease (see Breast Biopsy p. 80), with special care taken to remove all of the gross lesion. To assist the pathologist, crushing of the specimen is avoided. All carcinomas should undergo a receptor analysis if possible, as this will furnish useful therapeutic and prognostic information. For this purpose the specimen must be cooled while still in the operating room. After pathomorphologic processing, the specimen is divided up for further biochemical processing, and if necessary it may be frozen at a temperature of −20° or lower. Gloves and instruments used for the excision are discarded at once so that tumor cells will not be seeded back into the wound.

Surgical treatment options

Procedure	*Extent of resection*	*Indication*
Extended radical mastectomy	Mammary gland Pectoralis major and minor muscles, axillary lymph nodes, mammary lymph nodes, supra- and infraclavicular lymph nodes	Operable breast carcinoma
Radical mastectomy	Mammary gland Pectoralis major and minor muscles, axillary lymph nodes	
Patey's operation	Mammary gland Pectoralis minor muscle, axillary lymph nodes	
Modified radical mastectomy	Mammary gland and axillary lymph nodes	
Mastectomy and lower axillary dissection	Mammary gland and lower axillary lymph nodes	
Subcutaneous mastectomy	Breast tissue within cutaneous envelope	Small, operable breast carcinoma
Segmental resection (tylectomy)	Breast segment + axilla (may include local excision of skin)	
Tumorectomy	Tumor with margin of healthy tissue	

2.4 Breast-Conserving Operations

2.4.1 Tumorectomy

Indication: Small operable breast carcinoma of stage T0 to T1 N0.

Surgical goal: Remove the tumor with a rim of normal tissue.

Preoperative preparation: Removal of axillary hair.

Position: See Breast Biopsy.

Instruments: Basic set.

Tumorectomy is appropriate only for small tumors of stages T0 to T1 (2 cm or less in size). It is acceptable when combined with postoperative irradiation of the breast and lymph nodes. The operative technique is the same as that for a diagnostic breast biopsy (q.v.), except that greater attention is given to removing a margin of grossly normal breast. Four marking sutures should be placed on the specimen to facilitate additional resection if positive margins are found. Axillary dissection is imperative as a staging procedure.

2.4.2 *Segmental Resection*

Indication: Small breast carcinoma T0 to T1 N0 M0.

Surgical goal: Removal of tumor along with overlying skin and muscle fascia.

Preoperative preparation: See above.

Position: See above.

Instruments: Basic set.

Steps in procedure:

(1) Elliptical excision of the skin over the palpable tumor (Fig. 16 a,b)
(2) Excision of the affected quadrant with the electrocautery, removing the pectoralis major fascia
(3) Meticulous hemostasis in the operative field
(4) Axillary dissection, either en bloc or through a separate incision
(5) Final hemostasis
(6) Insertion of drains
(7) Skin closure

Besides tumorectomy, the segmental resection with axillary dissection is the most widely used of the breast-conserving operations. The incision is made in an elliptical fashion around the skin overlying the palpable breast mass. With a laterally situated tumor, the axillary dissection can be performed through the same incision. With a medial tumor, a separate axillary incision is required. After the elliptical incision has been made with a scalpel, stay sutures are placed, and the affected breast segment is dissected down to the pectoral fascia with the electrocautery and is excised along with the fascia. With a lateral tumor, the axillary tail of the breast and the axillary fat and lymphatic tissue can be removed in continuity with the specimen. Negative margins should be confirmed histologically.

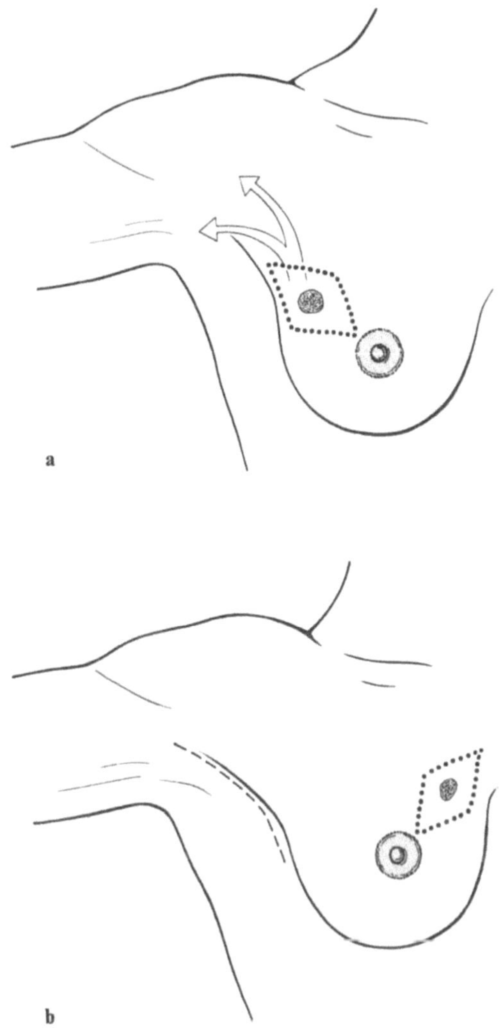

a

b

Fig. 16. a Elliptical excision of skin and breast tissue for a tumor of the upper outer quadrant. This incision also gives access for the axillary dissection and does not require significant extension. **b** If the tumor is in an inner quadrant, the axillary dissection is performed through a separate incision

2.4.3 Axillary Dissection

Indication: Tumor staging or debulking (Fig. 17).

Surgical goal: Remove the axillary lymph nodes within designated limits.

Preoperative preparation: Removal of axillary hair.

Position: See above.

Instruments: Basic set.

Steps in procedure:

(1) Incision along the border of the pectoralis major muscle or along the axillary hairline
(2) Exposure of pectoralis minor muscle and axillary vein
(3) Dissection of fat and lymphatic tissue
(4) Exposure of long thoracic nerve and thoracodorsal neurovascular bundle
(5) Hemostasis
(6) Insertion of drains
(7) Skin closure

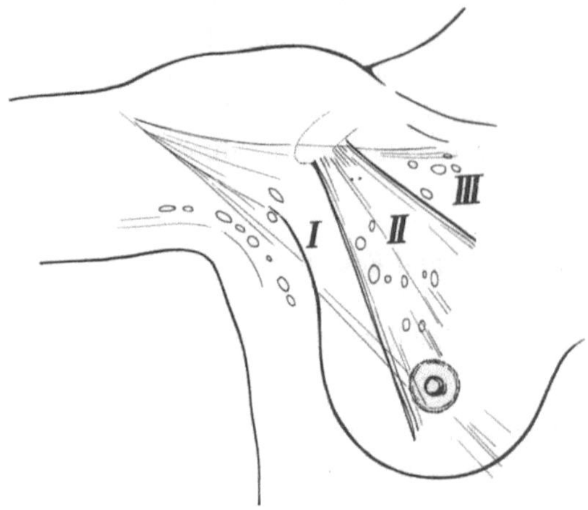

Fig. 17. The three major groups of axillary lymph nodes (after Leis). Group I lymph nodes are lateral to the pectoralis minor, group II lymph nodes are projected below the pectoralis minor, and group III nodes are medial to the pectoralis minor

A limited axillary dissection is most commonly performed, avoiding dissection of the infraclavicular lymph nodes. The limits of the dissection are formed by the lateral chest wall, the inferior border of the axillary vein, and the axillary skin. The muscles are left intact, as are the longitudinally coursing nerves and blood vessels of the axilla. This approach has proven adequate to define the stage of the disease, and there is no evidence that a more extensive dissection would be of therapeutic benefit in these patients. However, this does not diminish the importance of a radical local excision to prevent axillary recurrence or limit radiation to the breast. The axilla may be approached through a curved incision along the inferior edge of the axillary hairline or through a straight incision along the anterior border of the pectoralis major (Fig. 18a). With both incisions, the pectoral muscles can be exposed after division of the subcutaneous fat (Fig. 18b). Rotter's (interpectoral) lymph nodes are dissected free in the interval between the two muscles and sent for separate histologic evaluation. Further dissection is carried along the pectoralis minor to the inferior border of the axillary vein. The fatty and lymphatic tissue along the lower border of this vessel can then be divided between Overholt forceps (Fig. 18c). We use a synthetic absorbable suture for this purpose to avoid postoperative suture granulomas that could later mimic a positive lymph node. The pectoralis minor is retracted medially to expose the apical axillary lymph nodes (Fig. 18d). Dissection in this area can be facilitated by notching the muscle (Fig. 18e) or dividing it. Sharp division of the tissue without ligating it below the vein is apt to result in persistent exudation of lymph and should be discouraged. The thoracodorsal neurovascular bundle and the long thoracic nerve are identified and carefully dissected free. Besides having functional value, preservation of the thoracodorsal bundle is helpful in terms of a later flap procedure involving the latissimus dorsi muscle. The axillary fat and lymphatic tissue are dissected free from above downward while gentle manual traction is applied. The nerve fibers that cross the field transversely (intercostobrachial nerve) give sensory innervation to a skin area on the dorsal surface of the forearm. Because considerable dissection would be needed to spare these fibers, and since most patients are not bothered by the sensory loss that results from their division, these transverse neural structures generally are not preserved. At this stage the resected tissue is marked at its apex to facilitate the histologic workup. A suction drain is placed into the surgical cavity and brought out distally through a separate stab incision in the area of the midaxillary line. The skin is closed with 4-0 monofilament sutures.

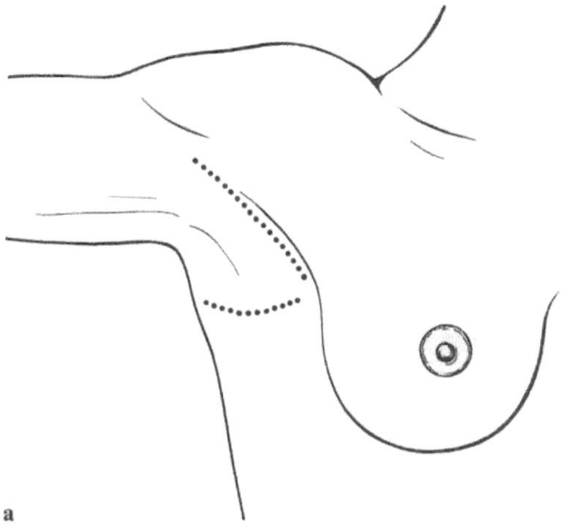
a

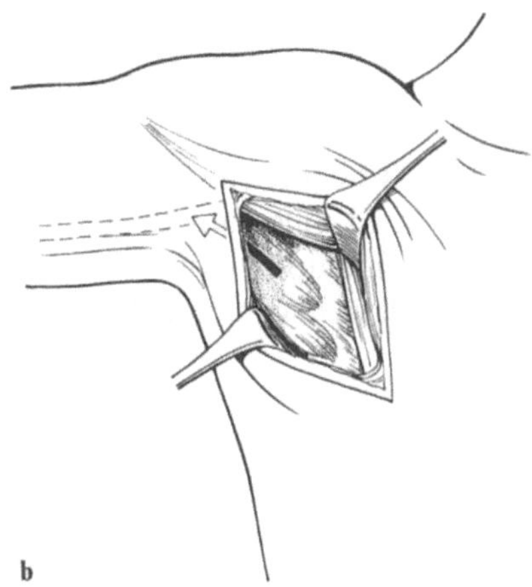
b

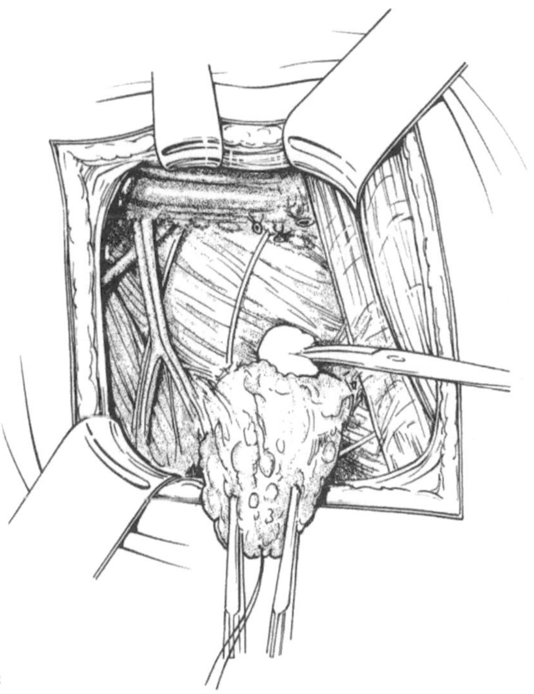
c

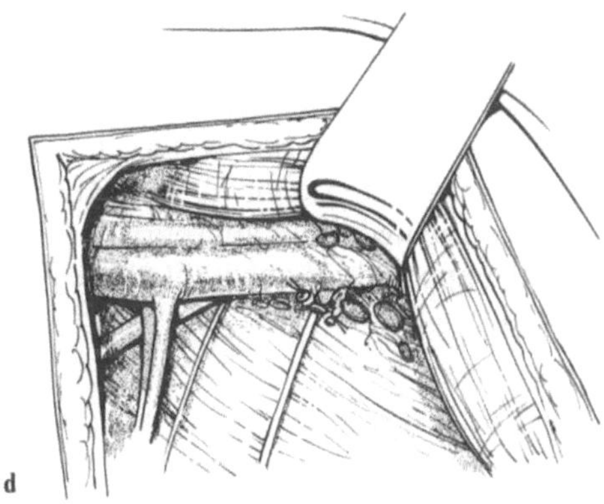
d

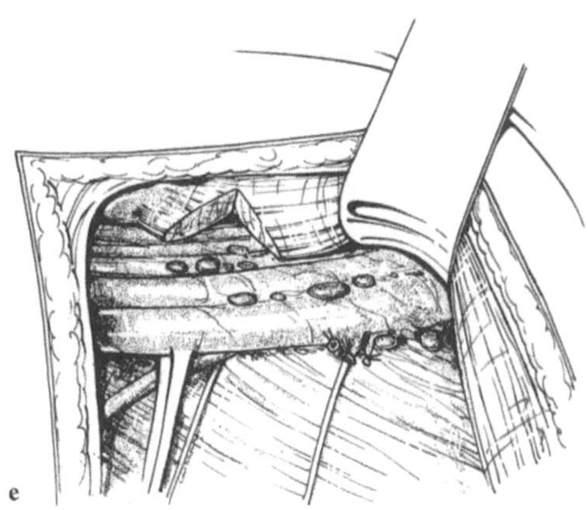
e

Fig. 18. a Possible incisions for axillary dissection. **b** The pectoralis minor muscle is exposed and serves as a guide for further dissection to the inferior margin of the axillary vein. **c** The axillary vein has been dissected free, exposing the long thoracic nerve and thoracodorsal neurovascular bundle. **d** The pectoralis minor muscle is retracted laterally upward for dissection of the axillary apex. **e** Here the pectoralis minor has been notched to facilitate dissection of the apical lymph nodes

2.5 Mastectomy

Mastectomy is performed for all malignant neoplasms that contraindicate a breast-conserving operation. Radical mastectomy, for decades the mainstay of breast cancer surgery, is rarely indicated today, e.g., for a T3 cancer invading the chest-wall musculature. In all other situations a limited surgical procedure combined with appropriate adjunctive therapies will yield comparable results.

2.5.1 *Skin Incisions*

Of the many skin incisions that have been devised, the transverse elliptical incision of Stewart has become the most widely used for the common operation of modified radical mastectomy. The vertical elliptical incision of Deaver or Halsted may be considered as an alternative for cases requiring a more radical excision (Fig. 19).

The basic Stewart incision extends from the sternal midline to the anterior axillary line, staying at least 3 cm from the tumor. A vertical elliptical incision is considered more appropriate for carcinomas in the upper outer quadrant at the junction with the axillary tail.

2.5.2 *Modified Radical Mastectomy*

Indication: Operable breast carcinoma (T1 to T3a).

Surgical goal: Remove breast tissue, lymph nodes, and skin.

Preoperative preparation: See above.

Position: See above.

Instruments: Basic set.

Steps in procedure:

(1) Transverse elliptical incision
(2) Placement of stay sutures
(3) Development of skin flaps
(4) Removal of breast in medial-to-lateral direction
(5) Removal of Rotter's lymph nodes in interval between pectoralis major and minor muscles
(6) Axillary dissection
(7) Hemostasis
(8) Insertion of drains
(9) Skin closure
(10) Correction of incongruities as required.

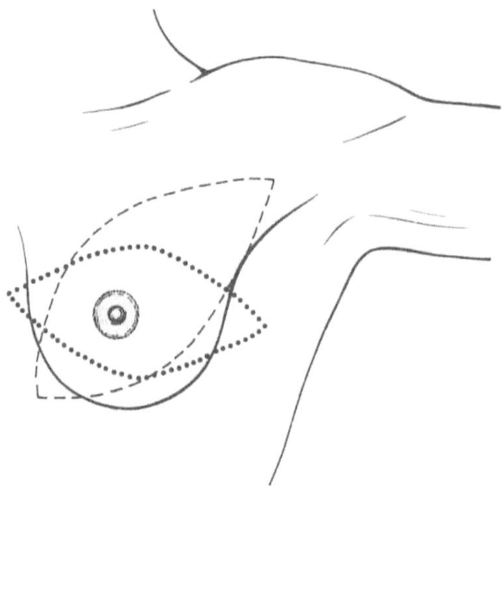

Fig. 19. Transverse elliptical mastectomy incision of Stewart, and the oblique Deaver modification

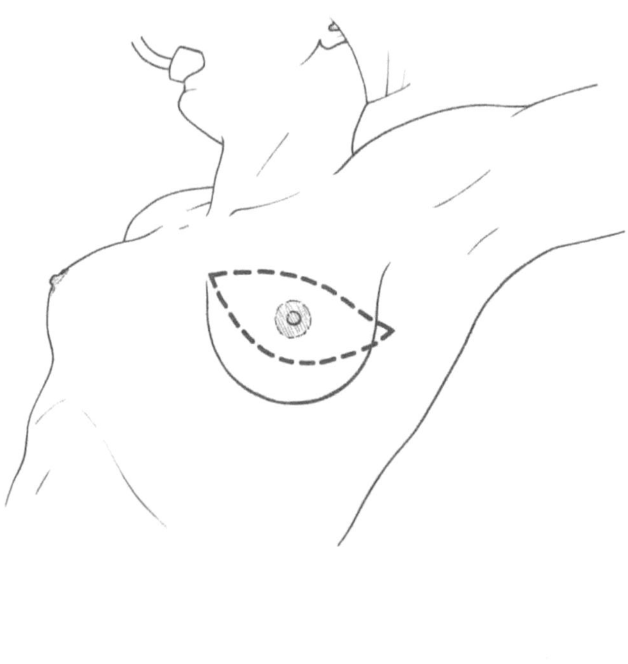

Fig. 20. Transverse elliptical incision for modified radical mastectomy

The modified radical mastectomy is usually a unilateral procedure, i.e., it is performed in the same session in which biopsy and frozen section confirmed malignancy. The instruments used to excise the tumor are discarded, and the surgeon's gloves are changed to avoid disseminating the cancer. The incision line is drawn with a marker, keeping a safety margin of at least 3 cm from the nipple and tumor to ensure a radical excision (Fig. 20). The skin flaps are developed outside the superficial veins, which provide a useful landmark for keeping to the desired plane of dissection. As in Stewart's incision, the dissection is first carried upward to the level of the first or second intercostal space (Fig. 21). Distally the dissection is carried only slightly past the submammary fold. The dissected skin flaps are retracted with sutures. The correct plane of dissection is most difficult to locate laterally, and special care is taken not to make the skin flap too thin in that region. Dissection of the breast tissue proceeds in a medial-to-lateral direction. The pectoralis major fascia may be removed at this time if the location of the tumor requires it. Some of the vessels perforating the chest wall can be coagulated; larger vessels may be grasped with small forceps and ligated. After the breast has been dissected from the chest wall,

Fig. 21. A skin flap about 0.5 cm thick is developed up to the level of the second intercostal space. The breast is dissected free in a medial-to-lateral direction, and the axilla is cleared as described. The dissection for a modified radical mastectomy may be performed en bloc

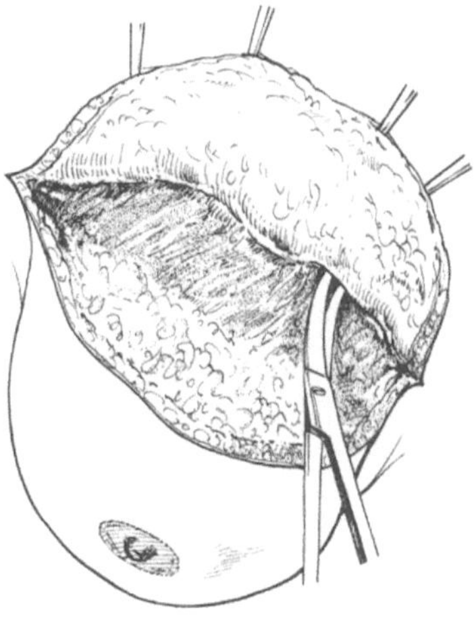

it remains in continuity with the axillary tail and with the axillary fat and lymphatic tissue. The borders of the pectoralis major and minor muscles are identified, and the interval between them is opened up to gain access to the interpectoral lymph nodes (of Rotter), which are dissected free. Several smaller blood vessels traversing this area are ligated. Care is taken to spare the nerve supplying the pectoralis major, which passes downward to the muscle accompanied by the pectoral branch of the thoracoacromial artery. The fatty and lymphatic tissue that was dissected free between the pectoral muscles is sent for separate histologic evaluation. Involvement of Rotter's lymph node group is seen in 1%–2% of all breast carcinomas. When axillary lymph node involvement is present, this incidence rises to 20%. Next the lateral border of the pectoralis minor is followed into the axilla until the inferior border of the axillary vein is visualized. Dissection is continued laterally along the lower border of this vessels. We recommend dividing the lymphatic tissue between ligatures to minimize postoperative lymph flow. Close attention is given to the axillary vein during the dissection, making sure that small branches are not avulsed from it. The vessels of the thoracodorsal neurovascular bundle must be clearly identified. The thoracic vein, which usually courses longitudinally through the axilla, passing anterior to the neurovascular bundle, is divided and ligated between Overholt forceps. The nerves crossing the axilla transversely–typically the intercostobrachial nerve from the second intercostal space–may be divided, as the resulting sensory deficit on the dorsal side of the forearm is minor. The thoracodorsal neurovascular bundle and the long thoracic nerve that emerge from below the vein are identified. Next the axillary fat and lymphatic tissue are dissected from above downward. Gentle traction on the tissue is helpful for this part of the dissection. Generally the tissues will separate from the nerves and vessels without difficulty; only one or two small side branches will need to be divided between Overholt forceps. After this step, the entire specimen is still in contact with the axillary skin and can be cut free with a scissors while gentle traction is applied. At this stage the inferior border of the axillary vein lies exposed, along with the subscapular muscles, the thoracodorsal nerve bundle, and the long thoracic nerve on the lateral chest wall (Fig. 22). The wound bed is carefully inspected to make sure it is dry, and two subcutaneous suction drains are placed–one in the chest wound and

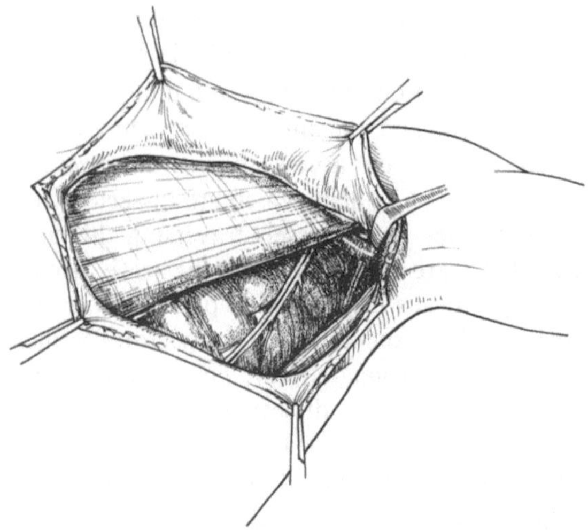

Fig. 22. The operative field after removal of the breast and axillary tissue, exposing the border of the pectoralis major, the inferior margin of the axillary vein, the long thoracic nerve, and the thoracodorsal neurovascular bundle

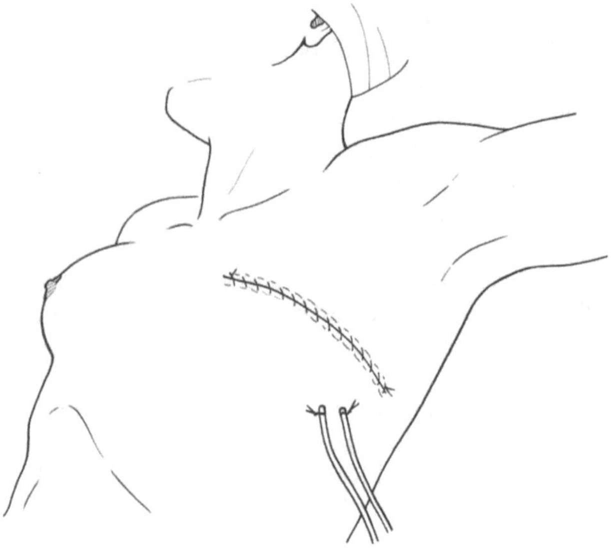

Fig. 23. Appearance on completion of the mastectomy

one in the axillary region against the lateral chest wall (Fig. 23). It is common for an incongruity to exist between the upper and lower edges of the incision in obese patients or patients with large breasts. In some cases this can be corrected by excising a "Burrow's triangle" in the region of the axillary tail. This creates an L-shaped surgical wound in the axilla or a T-shaped wound if the correction is done on both sides.

2.5.3 *Patey's Operation*

Patey's operation differs from the modified radical mastectomy by the additional removal or notching of the pectoralis minor muscle to facilitate apical axillary dissection. All the operative steps are the same up to exposure of the pectoralis minor (Fig. 24a), at which point the muscle is severed from its attachment on the coracoid and removed en bloc with Rotter's lymph nodes and the axillary fat and lymph tissue (Fig. 24b, d). The rest of the procedure follows the steps for the modified radical mastectomy.

Fig. 24. a Patey's operation. The breast dissection is carried upward while developing a skin flap 0.5 cm thick. **b** The breast is mobilized laterally, exposing the pectoralis minor which is severed from its attachment

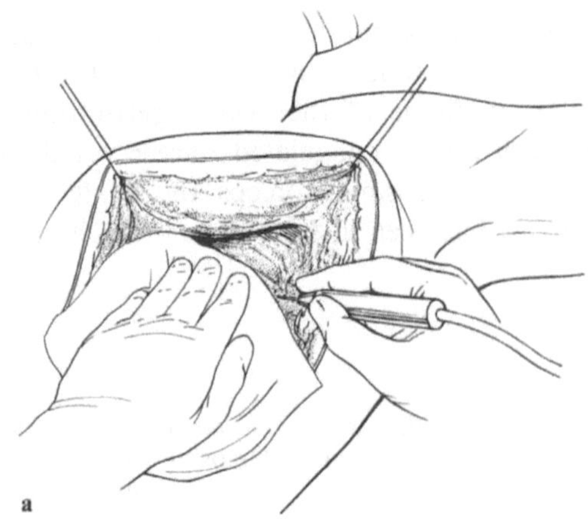

a

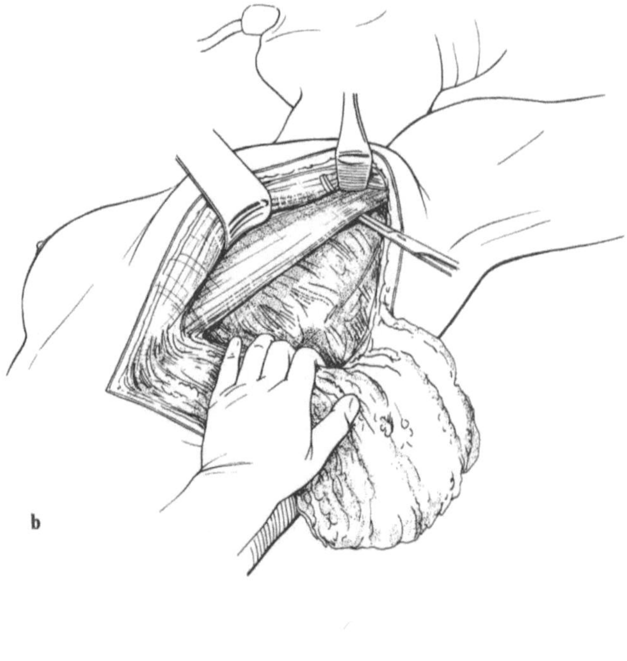

b

2.5.4 *Radical Mastectomy (Rotter-Halsted Modification)*

Indication: Operable breast carcinoma (T1–T3b).

Surgical goal: Remove the breast, skin, musculature, and axillary lymphatic tissue.

Preoperative preparation: See above.

Position: Supine with the involved side slightly elevated by a 5-cm thickness of towels or padding. The arm is extended at a right angle to the body.

Instruments: Basic set.

Steps in procedure:

(1) Incision
(2) Development of skin flaps
(3) Division of pectoralis major and minor muscles at their attachments
(4) Dissection of the deep fascia
(5) Axillary lymphadenectomy with division and ligation of the thoracodorsal neurovascular bundle
(6) Removal of the specimen from the chest wall
(7) Insertion of drains
(8) Skin closure or
(9) Coverage of the defect with a split-thickness skin graft

Fig. 24.c The pectoralis minor is removed from the chest wall. **d** Status following skin closure

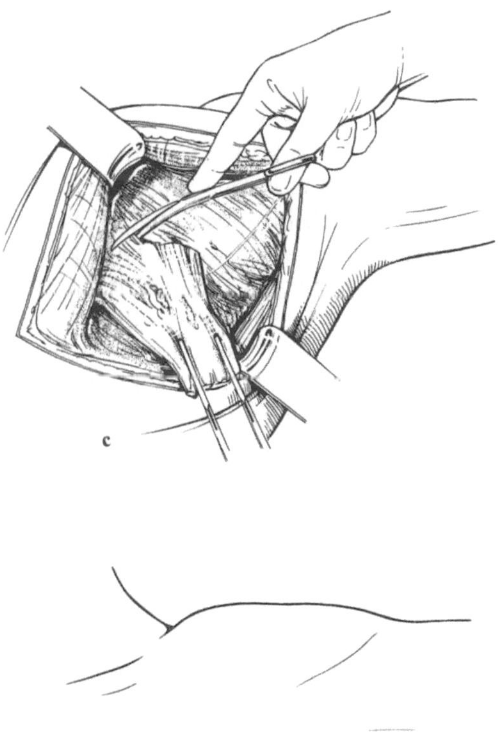

c

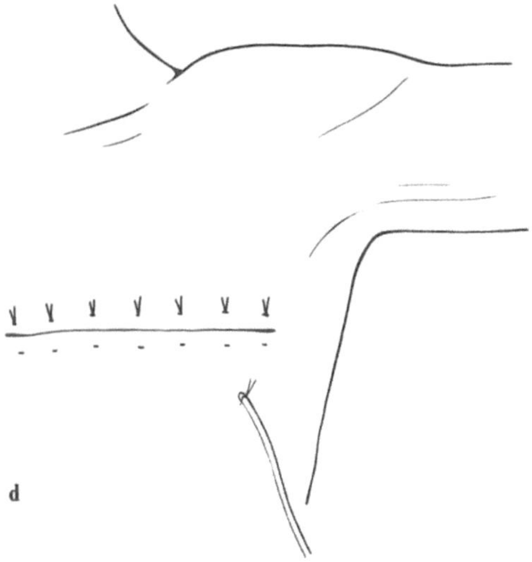

d

In the original method the incision extends from the midclavicle to the breast and widely encircles the breast in elliptical fashion, without regard for subsequent skin closure. The incision then runs in the ipsilateral hypochondrium in the region of the rectus sheath. Alternatively, Deaver's incision from the acromion to the hypochondrium may be used. Dissection of the skin flaps is done as in the modified radical mastectomy, maintaining a flap thickness of about 0.5 cm and following the plane of the superficial veins. The limits of the dissection are the sternal midline, the rectus sheath, and the skin of the axilla, which is dissected as far as the border of the latissimus dorsi. The next step in the dissection is exposure of the axillary vessels. The pectoralis major and minor are divided between clamps at their insertions (Fig. 25a). The perforating vessels from the internal mammary artery are divided between clamps. The entire specimen, including the breast, muscles, and the axillary fat and lymph tissue, is then mobilized from above downward. This step requires incising the deep pectoral fascia over the axillary vein and dissecting the fascia from above downward. The thoracodorsal vessels are ligated and divided. The thoracodorsal nerve is also resected, causing loss of latissimus dorsi function. Only the long thoracic nerve is spared in the original method (Fig. 25b). Meticulous hemostasis is secured, and the skin is closed over a suction drain. Because of the wide excision of skin, this operation often leaves a large central defect on the chest wall that must be covered primarily by a split-thickness skin graft.

Besides the cosmetic deformity, the classic radical mastectomy of Rotter-Halsted results in functional deficits occasioned by the absence of the

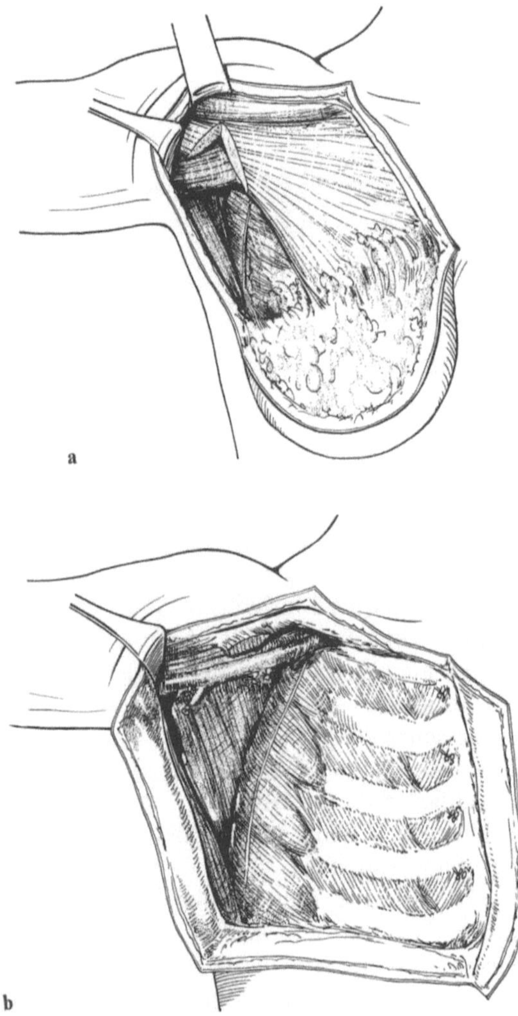

a

b

Fig. 25. a Radical mastectomy of Rotter-Halsted. The incision extends from the middle of the clavicle. After division of the skin and subcutaneous tissue, the pectoralis major and minor muscles are identified and divided. **b** Operative field after resection of the skin, subcutaneous tissue, breast, and pectoral muscles. In the original method only the long thoracic nerve is spared. The thoracodorsal neurovascular bundle is included in the resection

pectoral muscles and the sacrifice of latissimus dorsi function. The method gained wide acceptance initially because it lowered the incidence of locoregional recurrences by a factor of ten. But controlled studies have shown that less radical procedures can yield the same results, and the operation is rarely performed today for stage T3b cancers. Generally these tumors are managed by less radical surgery supplemented by an adjunctive therapy appropriate for the stage of the disease.

2.5.5 Extended Radical Mastectomy [103]

Indication: Operable breast carcinoma (T1–T3a).

Surgical goal: Removal of the breast, skin, musculature, and all regional lymph nodes.

Position: See above.

Instruments: Basic set, extra vascular set, chest tube set.

Urban extended the radical mastectomy to include an en bloc resection of the lymph nodes along the internal mammary artery. This extends the scope of the operation well beyond the mammary artery dissection practiced in Europe [30, 72]. Controlled studies have shown no differences in 10-year survival rates, although the status of these lymph nodes permits a more accurate prognostic assessment at the time of operation.

The skin incision and dissection are the same as for a radical mastectomy using the Deaver incision, except that the sternum, the entire infraclavicular fossa, and the rectus sheath are exposed. Following this step of the dissection, which is identical to that for radical mastectomy, the surgeon undertunnels the sternal attachment of the pectoralis major with his index finger (Fig. 26a). Next the sternum is divided with a Lebsche chisel or oscillating saw, placing the line of the osteotomy in the ipsilateral one-quarter of the sternum. The rips and intercostal tissue in the undertunneled area are divided with a scissors at the level of the costochondral junction. The blood vessels are ligated and sectioned. At this point the specimen can be retracted laterally en bloc (Fig. 26b). Next the mediastinal pleura is sutured into the medial edge of the wound. A Buelau drain is brought out through the fifth intercostal space (Fig. 26d). The chest-wall defect is partially closed with pericostal horizontal mattress sutures of monofilament nylon placed under high tension, and the residual defect is patched with lyophilized dura or other suitable material (Fig. 26c). The remaining steps in the procedure are identical to those in a radical mastectomy (Fig. 26d).

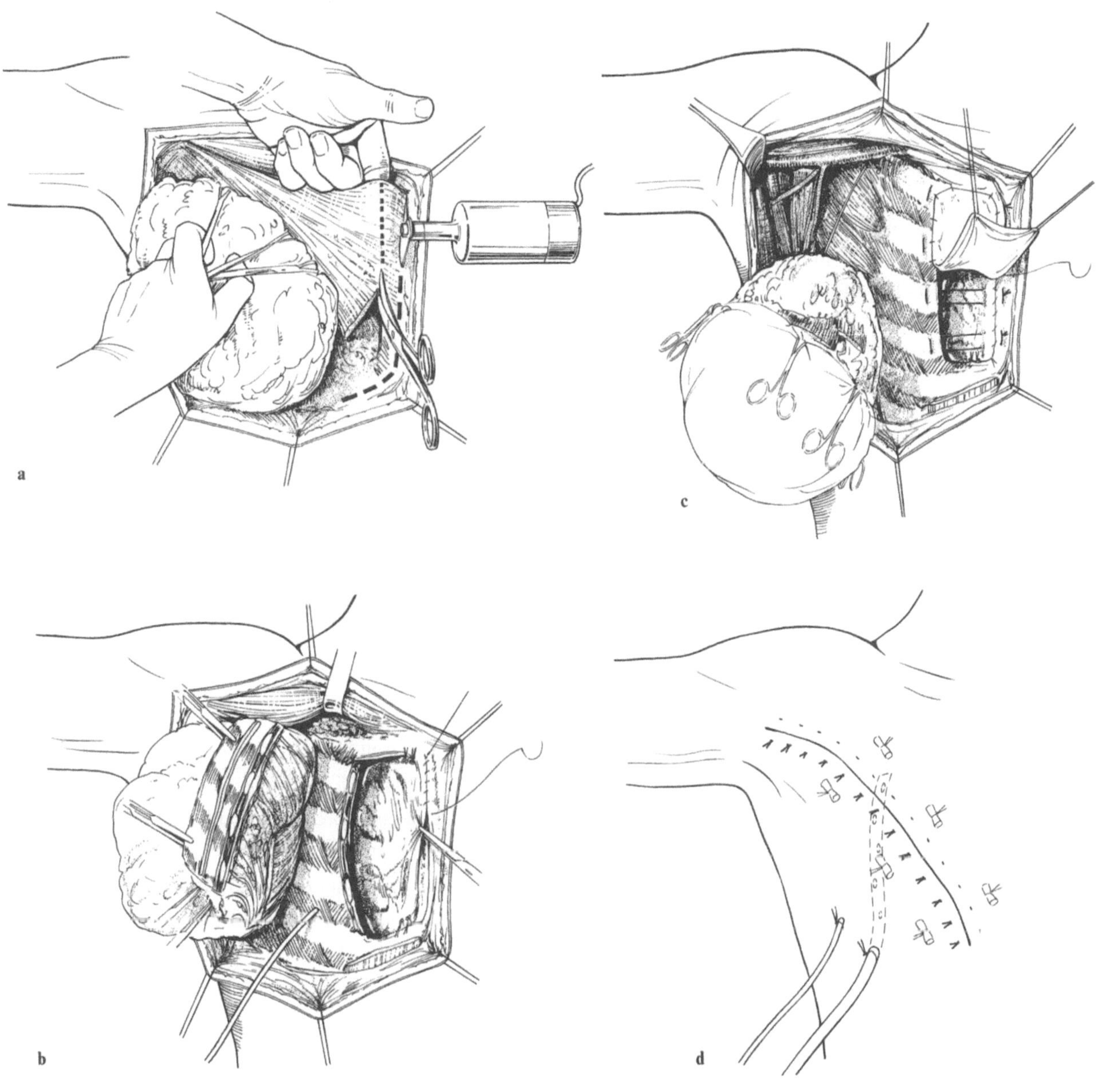

a b c d

Fig. 26. a Urban's modification of the extended radical mastectomy. A modified Deaver incision is made, and the breast, skin, and subcutaneous tissue are mobilized. The pectoralis major is undermined with the finger, and the sternum is osteotomized along the line of muscle attachment. **b** The mammary lymph nodes are removed en bloc with the breast and pectoral muscles. Mediastinal pleura is sutured into the defect. **c** Lyophilized dura or Marlex mesh is sewn under tension into the chest wall defect. The rest of the dissection is like that for a radical mastectomy, but the thoracodorsal neurovascular bundle is spared. **d** Tubes are placed to drain the wound and chest, and the skin is closed

2.6 Measures for Local Inoperability

Ulcerating breast carcinomas and stage T4-lesions are considered to be inoperable, because the disease is presumed to be generalized and cannot be influenced by a local surgical procedure. However, recent oncologic treatment concepts provide a rationale for surgery even in these cases, whether for the purpose of tissue removal, receptor analysis, or as part of an interdisciplinary treatment program in which a tumor-debulking mastectomy is performed as an intermediate measure between sessions of radiation or chemotherapy. Similar considerations apply to inflammatory breast carcinoma, which likewise is treated after biopsy confirmation by radiation or chemotherapy before a tumor-reducing mastectomy is carried out.

2.7 Measures for Difficult Skin Closure

Indication: Excessive tension on the wound margins.

Surgical goal: Tension-free wound closure.

Preoperative preparation: See Mastectomy.

Position: See above.

Instruments: Basic set.

Steps in procedure:

(1) Planning of flap procedure
(2) Cutting and elevation of flap
(3) Hemostasis
(4) Transposition of flap
(5) Mobilization of skin to cover donor defect
(6) Drain insertion
(7) Skin closure

In the classic radical mastectomy of Rotter-Halsted, great emphasis is placed upon a wide excision of the skin. A safety margin of 6 cm is advised, necessitating primary split-thickness skin grafting of the central defect. This contrasts with the less extensive skin excision of the standard modified radical mastectomy, which generally enables a primary wound closure to be obtained without difficulty. If this is not the case, tension in a transverse elliptical mastectomy incision can be relieved by mobilizing the skin into the hypochondrium from about the level of the umbilicus (Fig. 27a). Vessels entering the mobilized skin from the dorsal aspect are ligated between small clamps. Generally this technique will allow a tension-free wound closure without the need for more extensive plastic surgery.

Excessive tension in a vertical elliptical mastectomy incision (Deaver incision) can sometimes be relieved by additional mobilization of the flaps in the lateral and medial directions, taking care not to cause excessive displacement of the contralateral breast across the midline. If a tension-free closure is still not obtained, the defect can be covered in the same sitting with a thoracoepigastric flap. The length-to-width ratio of the flap should be approximately 2:1 to preserve its medial blood supply (Fig. 27b). Generally a flap length of 14 to 20 cm is sufficient. After the medially based flap has been carefully planned and outlined with a marker, the skin and subcutaneous tissue are divided down to the chest wall or rectus sheath, and the flap is elevated as atraumatically as possible. Even as the incision is made, care should be

Fig. 27. a If tension-free closure of the Stewart mastectomy incision cannot be obtained, the tension can be relieved by mobilizing the skin and subcutaneous tissue on the chest and abdominal wall. **b** If primary closure of Deaver's incision proves difficult, the defect can be covered by a thoracoepigastric flap. The flap is cut, the skin and subcutaneous tissue on the chest wall are mobilized, and the flap is slid into position. **c** The transposed flap is sutured in place, and the donor defect is primarily closed

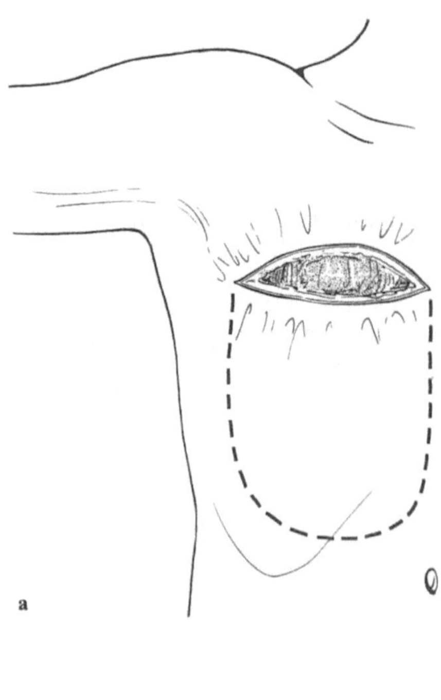

a

taken to preserve the flap's blood supply. Dissection past the midline might disrupt the nutrient vessels and should be avoided. The flap is advanced into the mastectomy defect and sutured in place without tension (Fig. 27c). The donor defect is closed by mobilizing the skin distally, yielding a roughly omega-shaped scar. The undermined area should be adequately drained to prevent serum accumulation. When the foregoing measures are applied, a primary wound closure can almost always be achieved following a radical or modified radical mastectomy. Split-thickness skin grafts are rarely necessary.

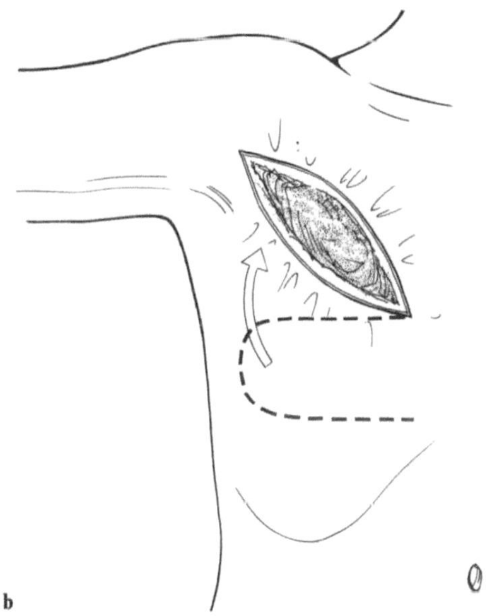

b

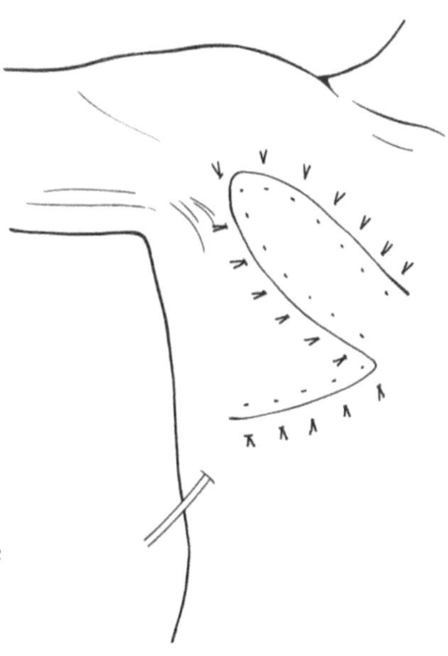

c

2.8 Carcinoma of the Male Breast

Indication: Male breast carcinoma.

Surgical goal: Locoregional excision of disease.

Surgical procedure: Modified radical mastectomy.

Preoperative preparation: Removal of chest hair and axillary hair.

Position: See above.

Instruments: Basic set.

Steps in procedure:

(1) Transverse elliptical incision (after marking) with a scalpel
(2) Removal of breast in medial-to-lateral direction
(3) Axillary dissection
(4) Hemostasis
(5) Drain insertion
(6) Skin closure

Breast carcinoma is about 100 times less frequent in men than in women. The surgical guidelines correspond to those for female breast cancer. The procedure of choice is a modified radical mastectomy followed by postoperative therapy appropriate for the stage of the disease. A receptor analysis of the tumor tissue is also advised, because the male carcinoma, too, is hormone-dependent and thus can be influenced by therapy.

2.9 Treatment of Local Recurrence

Indication: Local recurrence after mastectomy or modified radical mastectomy.

Surgical goal: Removal of the recurrence with adequate margins.

Preoperative preparation: Removal of axillary hair.

Position: See above.

Instruments: Basic set.

Steps in procedure:

(1) Excision of locoregional disease with adequate margins
(2) Frozen section and receptor analysis
(3) Hemostasis
(4) Drain insertion
(5) Primary closure

Eighty percent of all local recurrences of breast carcinoma occur in the first two years after primary treatment. Many are harbingers of generalized disease; few represent a strictly local problem. The therapeutic goal is excision of the local recurrence followed by receptor analysis. The extent of the resection is determined by local factors. Local surgery and diagnostic confirmation must be followed by systemic therapy and perhaps by local irradiation.

2.10 Treatment of Radiation Ulcers

Indication and surgical goals: Confirm benignancy of ulcer, remove ulcer, close defect.

Position: See above.

Radiation ulcers of the chest wall have become less common owing to changes in the type and quality of therapeutic radiation. They are most commonly seen in elderly women who underwent radiotherapy 10 to 15 years previously. Local excision of the ulcer followed by primary approximation of the wound edges is very rarely successful, and an attempt must be made to transpose viable tissue into the defect left by the ulcer excision. Various technique are available for this, depending on the size and location of the defect.

2.10.1 Thoracoepigastric Flap

See Measures for Difficult Skin Closure (Fig. 27).

After excision of the ulcer with a margin of healthy tissue, the proposed flap in the unirradiated skin is outlined with a scalpel and carefully elevated on the fascia. The flap is advanced into the defect, and the donor site is closed primarily. The flap is sewn into place with simple interrupted sutures or intracutaneous sutures. Suction drains are placed, and a sterile dressing is applied.

2.10.2 Latissimus Dorsi Flap

If the defect is located near the axilla, a latissimus dorsi flap can be used if the thoracodorsal neurovascular bundle has been preserved. A skin area corresponding to the size of the surgical defect is outlined with a scalpel and transposed on its muscular pedicle as an island flap into the defect (Fig. 28a–d).

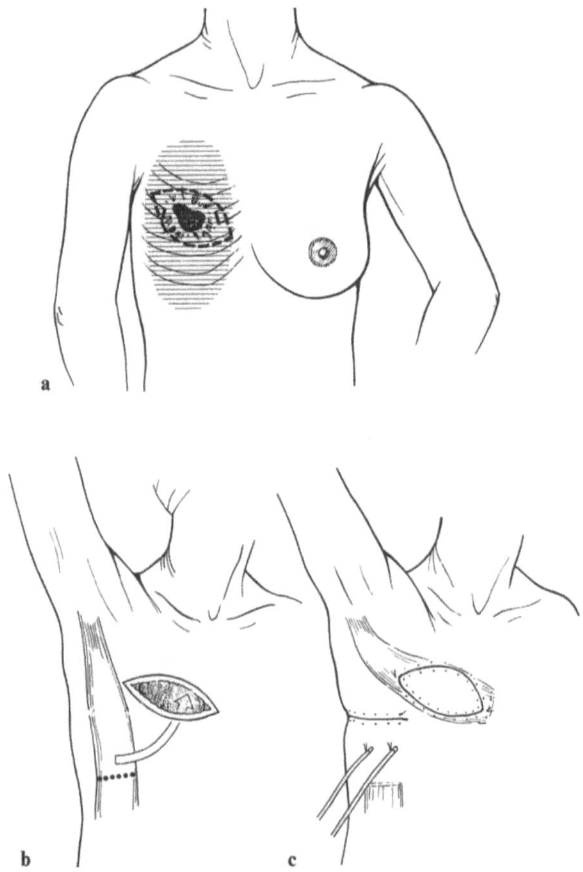

Fig. 28. **a** Closure of a radiation ulcer with a latissimus dorsi flap. First the ulcer is excised, preferably with a rim of healthy tissue. **b** Status after ulcer excision; the muscular pedicle is indicated. **c** An island flap is cut and mobilized on its latissimus dorsi pedicle. The skin and subcutaneous tissue are undermined, and the island flap is transposed into the defect. The donor site is primarily closed

2.10.3 Omentoplasty

Steps in procedure:

(1) Laparotomy and mobilization of the greater omentum on a vascular pedicle
(2) Excision of the ulcer
(3) Transfer of the omentum into the defect
(4) Closure of the laparotomy

Another method of closing an ulcer excision defect is omentoplasty. In this operation the greater omentum is exposed by laparotomy, mobilized on a nutrient pedicle, and passed from the laparoto-

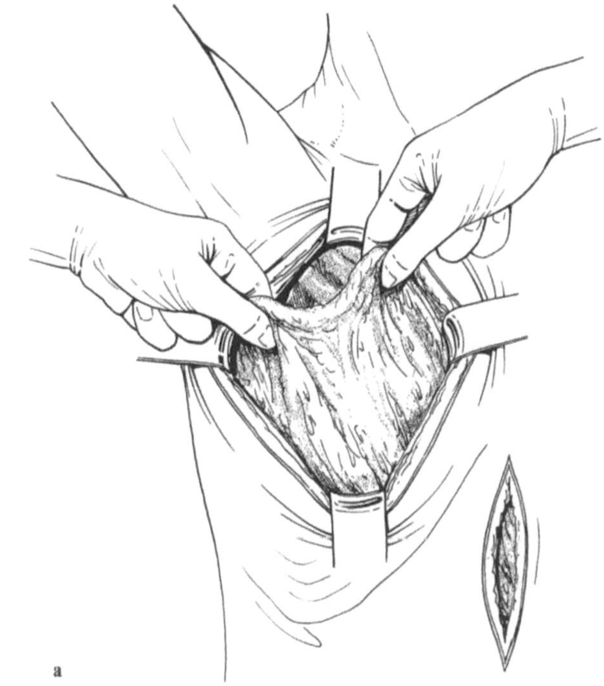

a

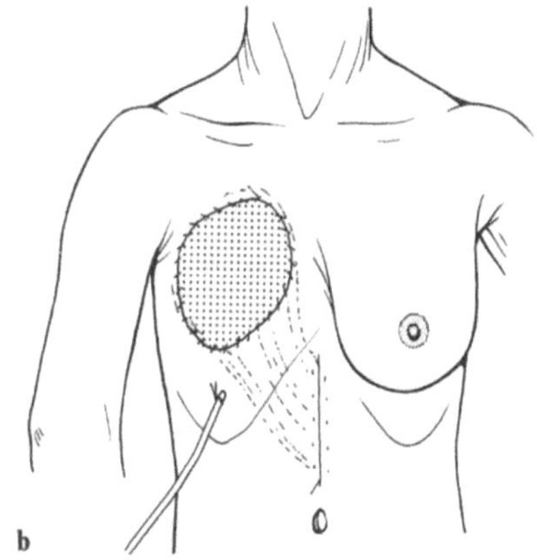

b

Fig. 29. **a** After excision of the radiation ulcer, a midline laparotomy is performed, and a pedicled flap of greater omentum is brought subcutaneously to the defect. **b** Following transfer of the omentum, the granulating wound surface can be covered with a split-thickness skin graft in a later sitting

my wound into the defect through a subcutaneous tunnel. There the viable tissue creates a granulating surface that can be covered secondarily by a split-thickness skin graft (Fig. 29a, b).

2.10.4 *Myocutaneous Rectus Flap* (Fig. 30a–c)

Indication: Radiation ulcer.

Surgical goal: Closure of the ulcer.

Preoperative preparation: Epilation.

Position: Supine.

Instruments: Basic Set.

Steps in procedure:

(1) Ulcer excision with rim of healthy tissue
(2) Cutting of adequate-sized island flap
(3) Incision of anterior rectus sheath
(4) Mobilization of muscle
(5) Creation of subcutaneous tunnel
(6) Transfer of flap into the defect
(7) Closure of rectus sheath

Fig. 30. **a** Radius for transfer of the myocutaneous rectus flap. **b** Resection of the radiation ulcer and outline of the rectus abdominis flap, showing its blood supply and the site of muscle division. **c** The donor defect is primarily closed, and the flap is sutured into the excisional defect

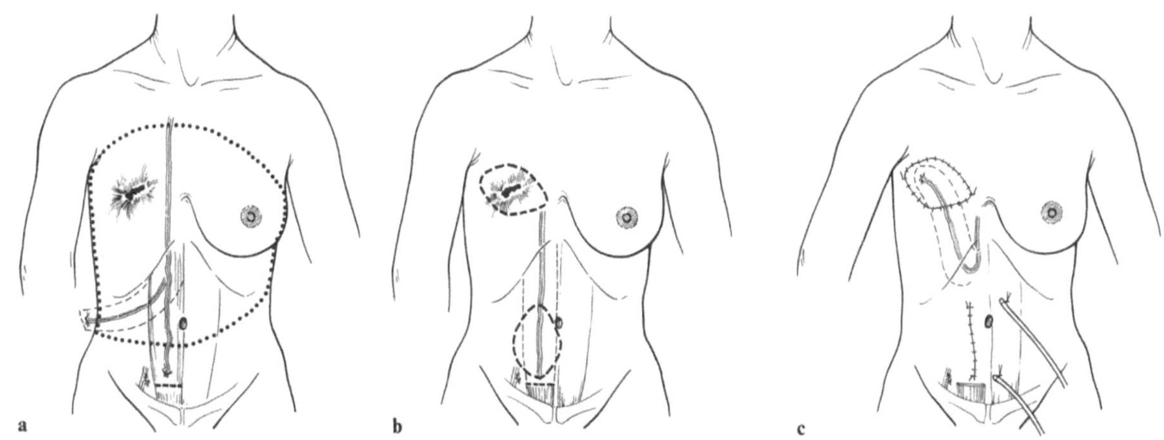

a b c

The radiation ulcer having been excised, an adequate area of skin is outlined with a scalpel over the middle third of the rectus muscle (Fig. 30a, b). The rectus fascia is incised 1–2 cm lateral to the linea alba, and a parallel incision is made 1–2 cm medial to the lateral border. This is followed by sharp dissection of the muscle; the dissection should not cross the semilunar line to avoid weakening the abdominal wall. The flap is mobilized, brought through a subcutaneous tunnel to the defect, and sutured in place (Fig. 30c). Care is taken that rotation of the flap does not compromise its venous drainage. The abdominal wall is repaired by direct suture, and the donor defect is directly closed.

References

1. Alpert S, Ghossein NA, Stacey P, Migliorelli FA, Efron G, Krishnaswamy V (1978) Primary management of operable breast cancer by minimal surgery and radiotherapy. Cancer 42:2054–2058
2. Amalric R, Santamaria F, Robert F, Seigle J, Altschuler C, Kurtz JM, Spitalier JM, Brandone H, Ayme Y, Pollet JF, Burmeister R, Abed R (1982) Radiation therapy with or without primary limited surgery for operable breast cancer. Cancer 49:30–34
3. Andersen PT, Pheils MT (1971) Primary carcinoma of the male breast: a report of 16 cases in Australian Ex-Servicemen. Aust NZ J Surg 41:148–152
4. Atkins SH, Hayward JL, Klugman DJ, Wayte AB (1972) Treatment of early breast cancer. A report after ten years of clinical trial. Brit Med J 2, 423–429
5. Baker RR, Montague ACW, Childs JN (1979) A Comparison of modified radical mastectomy to radical mastectomy in the treatment of operable breast cancer. Ann Surg 189:553–559
6. Barth V (1979) Brustdrüse. Thieme, Stuttgart New York
7. Bataini JP, Picco C, Martin M, Calle R (1978) Relation between time-dose and local control of operable breast cancer treated by tumorectomy and radiotherapy or by radical radiotherapy alone. Cancer 42:2059–2065
8. Baumeister RGH (1983) Mikrochirurgie des Lymphgefäßsystems. Chirurg 54:374–378
9. Bergholz M, Schauer A, Reck H, Gregl A (1979) Krebsrisiko bei papillären Proliferationen der Brustdrüse. Langenbecks Arch Chir 348:157–165
10. Bohmert H (1973) Die chirurgische Behandlung des Armlymphödems nach Mammaamputation. Fortschr Med 91:228–232
11. Bonadonna G, Rossi A, Valagussa P, Banfi A, Veronesi U (1977) The CMF program for operable breast cancer with positive axillary nodes. Cancer 39:2904–2915
12. Bonadonna G, Valagussa P, Rossi A, Tancini G, Brambilla C, Marchini S, Veronesi U (1982) Multimodal therapy with CMF in resectable breast cancer with positive axillary nodes: The Milan Institute Experience. In: Mathé G, Bonadonna G, Salomon S (eds) Recent Results in Cancer Research, Adjuvant Therapies of Cancer. Springer, Berlin Heidelberg New York
13. Bonadonna G (1982) Fortschritte bei der adjuvanten Chemotherapie des operablen Mammakarzinoms. In: Frischbier H-J (ed) Die Erkrankungen der weiblichen Brustdrüse. Thieme, Stuttgart New York
14. Bonk U (1983) Biopsie und Operationspräparat. Karger, Basel München Paris London New York Sydney
15. Boova RS, Bonanni R, Rosato FE (1982) Patterns of axillary nodal involvement in breast cancer. Predictability of level one dissection. Ann Surg 196:642–644
16. McBride ChM (1972) Extended simple mastectomy: anatomic. Definition and uses. South Med J 65:1427–1431
17. Brinkley D, Haybittle JL (1975) The Curability of Breast Cancer. Lancet I:95–97
18. Calle R, Pilleron JP, Schlienger P, Vilcoo JR (1978) Conservative management of operable breast cancer. Cancer 42:2045–2053
19. Calle R, Pilleron JP (1982) Nicht-verstümmelnde Behandlungsverfahren beim operablen Brustkrebs. In: Frischbier H-J (ed) Die Erkrankungen der weiblichen Brustdrüse. Thieme, Stuttgart New York
20. McCarty KS, Kesterson GHD, Wilkinson WE, Georgiade N (1978) Histopathologic study of subcutaneous mastectomy specimens from patients with carcinoma of the contralateral breast. Surg Gyn Obst 147:682–688
21. Charlson ME, Feinstein AR (1973) An analytic critique of existing systems of staging for breast cancer. Surgery 73:579–598
22. Cole Ph (1980) Major aspects of the epidemiology of breast cancer. Cancer 46:865–867
23. Crichlow RW (1972) Carcinoma of the male breast. Surg Gyn Obst 134:1011–1019
24. Crile G, Hoerr SO (1971) Results of treatment of carcinoma of the breast by local excision. Surg Gyn Obst 132:780–782
25. Crile G (1972) Breast Cancer. Am J Surg 124:35–38
26. Crile G, Esselstyn CB, Hermann RE, Hoerr SO (1973) Partial mastectomy for carcinoma of the breast. Surg Gyn Obst 136:929–933
27. Crile G (1975) Multicentric breast cancer. The incidence of new cancers in the homolateral breast after partial mastectomy. Cancer 35:475–477
28. Cutler SJ, Axtell LM, Schottenfeld D, Farrow JH (1970) Clinical assessment of lymph nodes in carcinoma of the breast. Surg Gyn Obst 41–52
29. Dudley H (1981) Radical mastectomy with preservation of the pectoral muscles (Patey) In: Rob & Smith (ed) Atlas of General Surgery, Butterworth, London Boston, pp 130–138
30. Dahl-Iversen E, Tobiassen T (1963) Radical mastectomy with parasternal and supraclavicular dissection for mammary carcinoma.. Ann Surg 157:170–173
31. Dana M, Koskas-Uhry A, Koskas Y (1978) Traitement du cancer du sein. Résultats de l'association télécobalthérapie-chirurgie chez 156 malades. La Nouvelle Presse Médicale 7:4115–4118

32. Dargent M, Mayer M, Hallonet Ph (1972) Nos tendances thérapeutiques pour les formes opérables du cancer du sein. Ann Chir 26:275–295
33. McDivitt RW, Stewart FW, Berg JW (1968) Tumors of the breast. Atlas of tumor pathology second servies, fascile 2. Armed Forces Institute of Pathology. Bethesda, MD
34. Eddy DM (1980) Letter to the editor. JNCI 64:1277
35. Eggert A, Kirschner H, Schröder HJ, Wittmann DH (1977) Das lymphostatische Ödem des Armes nach der Brustkrebsbehandlung. Med Klin 72:2106–2113
36. Esselstyn CB (1975) A technique for partial mastectomy. Surg Clin North Am 53:1065–1071
37. Fisher B, Slack NH (1970) Number of lymph nodes examined and the prognosis of breast carcinoma. Surg Gyn Obst 79–88
38. Fisher B, Montague E, Redmond C, Barton B, Borland D, Fisher ER, Deutsch M, Schwarz G, Margolese R, Donegan W, Volk H, Konvolinka C, Gardner B, Cohn I, Lesnick G, Cruz AB, Lawrence W, Nealon T, Butcher H, Lawton R (1977) Comparison of radical mastectomy with alternative treatments for primary breast cancer. Cancer 39:2827–2839
39. Fisher B, Glass A, Redmond C, Fisher ER, Barton B, Such E, Carbone P, Economou S, Foster R, Frelick R, Lerner H, Levitt M, Margolese R, MacFarlane J, Plotkin D, Shibata H, Volk H (1977) L-Phenylalanine mustard (L-PAM) in the management of primary breast cancer. Cancer 39:2883–2903
40. Fisher B (1977) United States Trials of Adjuvant Therapy. World J Surg 1:331–335
41. Fisher B (1977) United States trials of conservative surgery. World J Surg 327–330
42. Fisher B, Redmond C, Fisher ER (1980) The contribution of recent NSABP clinical trials of primary breast cancer therapy to an understanding of tumor biology – An overview of findings. Cancer 46:1009–1025
43. Fisher ER, Taylor M (1973) Changing pattern of some pathologic parameters of mammary carcinoma. Cancer 32:1380–1384
44. Fisher ER, Gregorio RM, Fisher B (1975) The pathology of invasive breast cancer. Cancer 36:1–85
45. Fisher ER, Redmond C, Fisher B (1980) Pathologic findings from the National Surgical Adjuvant Breast Project (protocol no 4) VI. Discriminants for five-year treatment failure. Cancer 46:908–918
46. Fletcher GH, Montague E, Nelson AJ (1976) Combination of conservative surgery and irradiation for cancer of the breast. Cancer 126:216–222
47. Forrest APM (1977) Conservative local treatment of breast cancer. Cancer 39:2813–2821
48. Forrest APM, Roberts MM, Cant ECM, Henk MB, Hykes LE, Eng CS, Hulbert M, Dudley HA, Champell H (1977) Simple mastectomy and pectoral node biopsy. The Cardiff-St.Mary's Trial. World J Surg 1:320–323
49. Forrest APM (1980) Conservative management of breast cancer: A review of British controlled trials. Ann R Coll Surg Engl 62 (1):41–43
50. Forrest APM (1981) Total mastectomy and pectoral node biopsy. In: Rob & Smith (eds) Atlas of general surgery, Butterworth, London Boston, pp 123–129
51. Gallager HSt, Leis HP (1978) The breast. The Mosby, Saint Louis
52. Haagensen CD (1971) Diseases of the breast. 2nd Edition – Revised Reprint, Saunders
53. Haagensen CD (1974) Behandlung des operablen Mammakarzinoms. Gyn Rdsch 14:41–79
54. Halsted WS (1895) The results of operations for the cure of cancer of the breast performed at the Johns Hopkins Hospital from June 1889 to January 1894. Johns Hopkins Hospital Reports IV:297–350
55. Handley RS, Thackray AC (1963) Conservative radical mastectomy (Patey's Operation). Ann Surg 157:162–164
56. Harder F, Hünig R (1983) Brusterhaltende therapeutische Maßnahmen beim operablen Mammacarcinom. Chirurg 54:255–259
57. Hayward JC, Eng FR CS (1977) The Guy's trial of treatment of "early" breast cancer. World J Surg 1:314–316
58. Hayward JC (1981) The surgeon's role in primary breast cancer. Breast Cancer Research and Treatment 1:27–32
59. Hellmann S, Harris JR, Levene MB (1980) Radiation therapy of early carcinoma of the breast without mastectomy. Cancer 46:988–994
60. Henderson IC, Canellos GP (1980) Cancer of the breast. The past decade. N Engl J Med 302:17–30
61. Henderson IC, Canellos GP (1980) Cancer of the breast. The past decade. N Engl J Med 302:78–90
62. Herfarth Ch (1979) Ziele der operativen Therapie. MMW 121:1438–1441
63. Herfarth Ch (1982) Die Bedeutung der Radikalität für die operative Therapie des Mammakarzinoms. In: Frischbier H-J (ed) Die Erkrankungen der weiblichen Brustdrüse. Thieme, Stuttgart New York
64. Hermann RE, Steiger E (1978) Modified radical mastectomy. Surg Clin N Am 58:743–754
65. Hermann RE, Esselstyn CB, Crile G (1978) Conservative surgical treatment of potentially curable breast cancer. In: Gallager A, St. Leis HP (eds) The breast, Mosby, St. Louis, Chapt 17:219–231
66. Høst H (1979) The role of postoperative radiotherapy in breast cancer. Second Breast Cancer Working Conference EORTC, May 31–June 2 1979 Copenhagen
67. Hughes LE (1981) Operations for benign breast disease. In: Rob & Smith (ed) Atlas of General Surgery, pp 108–122
68. Hutter RVP (1980) The influence of pathologic factors on breast cancer management. Cancer 46:961–976
69. Feiereis, Grewe HE, Johannigmann J, Kaiser P, Schmid MA, Siebert W (1983) Brustkrebs der Frau. Marseille Verlag, München
70. Johansen H (1982) Die einfache Mastektomie mit Nachbestrahlung gegenüber der erweiterten radikalen Mastektomie bei der Nachbehandlung des Mammakarzinoms. In: Frischbier H-J (ed) Die Erkrankungen der weiblichen Brustdrüse. Thieme, Stuttgart New York
71. Johnstone FRC (1972) Results of treatment of carcinoma of the breast based on pathologic staging. Surg Gyn Obst 134:211–217
72. Lacour J, Bucalossi P, Cacers E, Jacobelli G, Kosza-

rowski T, Le M, Rumeau-Rouquette C, Veronesi U (1976) Radical mastectomy versus radical mastectomy plus internal mammary dissection. Cancer 37:206–214
73. Lacour J, Le M, Caceres E, Koszarowski T, Veronesi U, Hill C (1983) Radical mastectomy versus radical mastectomy plus internal mammary dissection. Cancer 51:1941–1943
74. Langlands AE, Pocock ST, Kerr GR, Gore SHM (1979) Long-term survival of patients with breast cancer: a study of the curability of the disease. Br med J 2:1247–1251
75. Langlands AO, Prescott RJ, Hamilton T (1980) A clinical trial in the management of operable cancer of the breast. Br J Surg 67:170–174
76. Lattes R (1980) Lobular neoplasia (lobular carcinoma in situ) of the breast – A histological entity of controversial clinical significance. Path Res Pract 166:415–429
77. McLaughlin CW, Coe JD, Adwers JR (1978) A thirty year study of breast cancer in a consecutive series of private patients. Is axillary nodal study a valuable index in prognosis? Am J Surg 136:250–253
78. Letton AH, Mason EM (1980) The treatment of nonpalpable carcinoma of the breast. Cancer 46:980–982
79. Lewison EF (1980) Changing conceps in breast cancer. Cancer 46:859–864
80. Madden JL, Kandalaft S, Bourque R-A (1971) Modified radical mastectomy. Southern Surgical Association Meeting Virginia:624–634
81. Malt RA (1980) Surgical techniques illustrated, vol 4/1. Little Brown & Company Boston Massachusetts
82. Nemoto T, Vana J, Bedwani RN, Baker HW, McGregor FH, Murphy GP (1980) Management and survival of female breast cancer. Cancer 45:2917–2924
83. Nissen-Meyer R, Kjellgren, Manson B (1982) Adjuvant chemotherapy in breast cancer. In: Mathé G, Bonadonna G, Salmon S (eds) Recent results in cancer research. Springer, Berlin Heidelberg New York
84. Nixel E (1980) Mammographiebefunde bei voroperierten Brüsten. Röntgenblätter 33:632–637
85. Peltokallio P, Kalima T, Frilander M (1969) Results of breast cancer treatment. Acta Chir Scand 135:585–590
86. Peters TG, Donegan WL, Burg EA (1977) Minimal breast cancer: A clinical appraisal. Ann Surg 186:704–710
86a. Radovan Ch (1982) Breast reconstruktion after mastectomy using the temporary expander. Plast Reconst Surg 69:195–206
86b. Rader D, Lemperk G (1984) Der muskulokutane Rectuslappen für Strahlenulcera der Brustwand und der Leiste. In: Lemperle G, Koslowski L (Hrsg) Chirurgie der Strahlenfolgen. Urban u. Schwarzenberg, München Wien Baltimore S 124–130
87. Pichlmayr R (1966) Das Mammakarzinom – Diagnose, Prognose, Therapie. Bruns Beitr klin Chir 213:40–76
88. Priestman T, Baum M, Jones V, Forbes J (1978) Treatment and survival in advanced breast cancer. Brit Med J 2:1673–1674
89. Robinson R, Montague ED (1982) Treatment results in males with breast cancer. Cancer 49:403–406
90. Rosen PP (1980) Axillary lymph node metastases in patients with occult noninvasive breast carcinoma. Cancer 46:1298–1306
91. Shah JP, Rosen PP, Robbins GF (1973) Pitfalls of local excision in the treatment of carcinoma of the breast. Surg Gyn Obst 136:721–725
92. Shingleton WW, Shingleton AB (1980) Ethical considerations in the treatment of breast cancer. Cancer 46:1031–1034
93. Simon S, Dancot H, Feremans W (1970) Le traitement du cancer du sein au stade I par radiothérapie exclusive précedée de tumorectomie simple. Etude de l'évolution des méthodes et de leurs résultats. Acta Chir Belg 5:348–364
94. Southwick HW, Slaughter DP, Humphrey LJ (1973) Chirurgie der weiblichen Brust. Schattauer, Stuttgart New York
95. Spiessl B, Scheibe O, Wagner G (1982) TNM Atlas. UJCC. Springer, Berlin Heidelberg New York
96. Schrudde J (1980) Eine Methode zur Verbesserung des Lymphabflusses. Zschr Plast Chir 4:133–141
97. Schwartz F, Patchesfsky AS, Feig StA, Shaber GS, Schwartz AB (1980) Multicentricity of non-palpable breast cancer. Cancer 45:2913–2916
98. Stewart HJ (1977) Controlled trials in the treatment of "early" breast cancer: A review of published results. World J Surg 1:309–313
99. Taylor H, Baker R, Afortt RW, Hermon-Taylor J (1971) Sector mastectomy in selected cases of breast cancer. Brit J Surg 58:161–163
100. Thomsen K, Stegner H-E, Frischbier H-J (1980) Grundlagen und Grenzen der brusterhaltenden Therapie kleiner Mammakarzinome. Gynäkologe 13:56–66
101. Turnbull AR, Chant ADB, Buchanan RB, Turner DTL, Shepherd JM, Fraser JD (1978) Treatment of early breast cancer. The Lancet 1:7–9
102. Ungeheuer E, Lüders K (1978) Chirurgische Behandlung des Mammakarzinoms. Dt Ärzteblatt 4:161–168
103. Urban JA (1980) Surgical management of palpable breast cancer. Cancer 46:983–987
104. Valagussa P, Bonadonna G, Veronesi U (1978) Patterns of relapse and survival following radical mastectomy. Cancer 41:1170–1178
105. Veronesi U, Banti A, Saccozzi R, Salvadori B, Zucali R, Uslenghi C, Greco M, Luini A, Rilke F, Galtan L (1977) Conservative treatment of breast cancer. Cancer 39:2822–2826
106. Veronesi U, Saccozzi R, Del Vecchio M, Banfi A, Clemente C, De Lena M, Gallus G, Greco M, Luini A, Marubini E, Muscolino G, Rilke F, Salvadori B, Zecchini A, Zucali R (1981) Comparing radical mastectomy with quadrantectomy, axillary dissection, and radiotherapy in patients with small cancers of the breast. N Engl J Med 305:6–11
107. Vorherr H (1980) Breast cancer. Urban & Schwarzenberg, Baltimore Munich
108. Witte ChL (1981) Limited role of mastectomy in treatment of primary carcinoma of the breast. Surg Gyn Obst 152:75–76

F. Operations on the Lung and Tracheobronchial System

Th. Junginger

CONTENTS

1 General Part

1.1 Surgical Aspects of Pulmonary Anatomy

The lung is divided anatomically into lobes and segments. The three lobes of the right lung and two lobes of the left lung are separated by fissures of variable prominence. Each lung presents an oblique fissure which passes through the costal, diaphragmatic, and mediastinal surfaces as far as the hilar structures. The oblique fissure of the right lung runs parallel to the sixth rib and at the level of the midaxillary line crosses the transverse fissure separating the middle and upper lobes. In the left lung the oblique fissure begins at the level of the third thoracic vertebra and terminates anteriorly at the costochondral junction of the sixth rib.

The lobes of the lung are invested by visceral pleura, which lines the interlobar fissures and also envelops the structures that enter or emerge at the hilum. The downward prolongation of the pleural duplicature extending to the diaphragm is called the pulmonary ligament. It unites the lower pulmonary lobes and pericardium and contains lymph nodes, blood vessels (usually of small caliber), and rarely an anomalous branch of the abdominal aorta feeding a pulmonary sequestration (see p. 185).

The right lung is divided into ten bronchopulmonary segments and the left lung into nine, each of which generally has its own segmental bronchus and artery and constitutes a functional and morphologic unit. While the arteries and bronchi course in close proximity to each other, there are intra- as well as intersegmental veins which drain the parenchyma across intersegmental planes. These veins should be preserved in segmentectomies, since their loss may lead to infarction in the adjacent segment.

1.1.1 Bronchial System

The bronchial system begins at the larynx with the trachea, which divides distally at the carina into the right and left main bronchi (see also p.175). The *right* main bronchus passes obliquely downward and gives rise to its first division, the right upper lobe bronchus, which trifurcates into apical, posterior, and anterior segments (S1 to S3). From the continuation of the bronchus, termed intermediate bronchus, the middle lobe bronchus arises anteriorly and divides into a pair of segmental bronchi (S4 and S5) entering the middle lobe. Another segmental bronchus (S6) arises posteriorly, opposite S4 and S5, and distributes to the superior segment of the lower lobe. The remainder of the bronchus divides into the four basal segments of the lower lobe (S7 to S10).

The *left* main bronchus is longer and narrower than the right and arises from the trachea at a more acute angle. The upper lobe bronchus divides into a superior branch with three segmental bronchi for the apical, posterior, and anterior segments (S1 to S3) and an inferior branch for the lingula, which ramifies further into two segmental bronchi (S4 and S5). A true intermediate bronchus is absent, for the superior segmental bronchus to the lower lobe (S6) emerges directly below the upper lobe bronchus. The seventh of these lower lobe segments (S7 to S10) may be absent or may exist only as a subsegment.

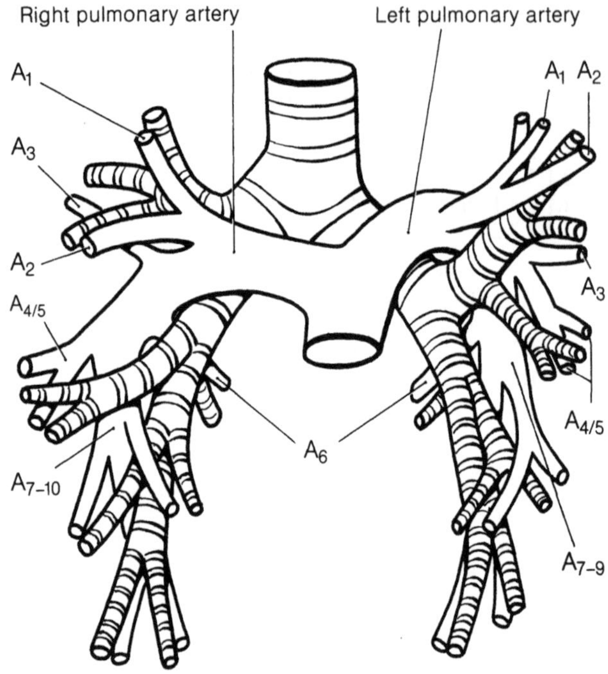

Fig. 1. Arterial supply of the lung

1.1.2 Pulmonary Arteries

The pulmonary trunk arises from the base of the right ventricle, coursing within the pericardium on the left side of the aorta, and divides into right and left pulmonary arteries (Fig. 1). The *right* pulmonary artery extends to the root of the right lung, passing behind the aorta and vena cava and in front of the right main bronchus. It splits into superior and inferior divisions, the former supplying the upper lobe and the latter arching downward and backward between the upper and middle lobe bronchi, distributing branches to the middle and lower lobes. The intrapericardial segment of the *left* pulmonary artery is longer than the right. After leaving the pericardium below the aorta, the vessel arches over the left main bronchus and descends behind it. In the upper lobar region the artery runs lateral to the bronchus; in operations on the laterally recumbent patient, it is the first structure to be encountered in the oblique fissure. The further distribution of the pulmonary arteries is described in connection with lobectomies and segmentectomies (q.v.).

1.1.3 Pulmonary Veins

Venous blood is carried to the hilum by deep intra- and intersegmental vessels lying in the parenchyma and also by superficial veins that run beneath the pleura. Whereas the arteries display an axial arrangement within segments and are closely related to the bronchi, the peripheral veins occupy the pulmonary septa, where they collect blood draining from adjacent lobules. As a rule, two venous trunks enter the left atrium on each side, the veins from the upper lobe and lingula or from the middle lobe forming the superior pulmonary vein, and the veins from the lower lobe forming the inferior vessel (Fig. 2). In rare cases only one venous trunk may be present on each side.

1.1.4 Bronchial Vessels

The bronchial walls, vessels, lymph nodes, and pleura are supplied by the systemic circulation through vessels which usually originate from the aortic arch or intercostal arteries, and rarely from an esophageal artery, the internal thoracic artery, or from the subclavian [35]. Sometimes there is only one artery which splits into two branches shortly after its origin, but usually two to four arteries can be found. The branches run past the esophagus to the bifurcation, where anastomoses are established between the right and left sides. From the bifurcation, the bronchial arteries can be traced as far as the bronchioles. Venous drain-

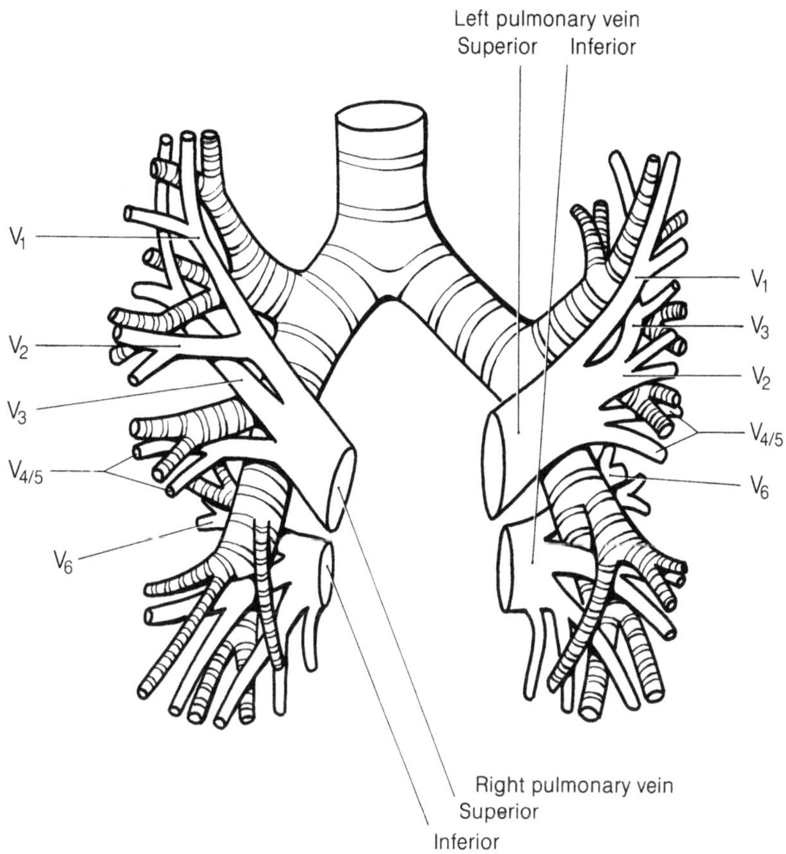

Fig. 2. Venous supply of the lung. (After Kubik [50])

age is by the pulmonary veins and the azygos or hemiazygos system. With absence or hypoplasia of the pulmonary arteries, the bronchial arteries may be hypertrophic.

1.1.5 Lymphatic System

The lung possesses a dense network of lymph capillaries and vessels that occur ubiquitously in the connective tissue: subpleural (identified by their anthracotic pigmentation), interlobular, intersegmental, perivascular, peribronchial, and below the mucosa in the bronchial wall. The subpleural vessels communicate with a deep network which accompanies the bronchi, arteries, and veins and is distributed to the regional lymph nodes. Valves in the lymph vessels direct the flow of lymph toward the hilum. If an obstruction exists in the hilar region, the lymph will drain beneath the pleura or through the pulmonary ligament into the mediastinum [20]. The regional lymph nodes of the lung are divided into two groups: intrapulmonary and extrapulmonary (mediastinal) [30]. The nomenclature is not standardized. Table 1 compares the nomenclatures applied by the TNM system, by Japanese and American authors, and in the Nomina Anatomica.

1.1.5.1 Intrapulmonary Lymph Nodes

The *intrapulmonary lymph nodes* are located beneath the pleura in the angles between the segmental bronchi and arteries (lobular nodes), in the interlobar fissures (interlobar nodes), and among the hilar structures (hilar nodes). The hilar nodes form the connection between the intra- and extrapulmonary nodes. The lymph nodes of the interlobar fissures constitute a "lymphatic sump" [8, 71] that receives afferents from all the pulmonary lobes of that side (Fig. 3 a,b). The *right intrapulmonary lymphatic sump* consists of lymph nodes surrounding the intermediate bronchus. Interlobar nodes that are distal to the origin of the middle lobe bronchi and the superior segment of the lower lobe are rarely involved by carcinoma of the upper lobe.

Table 1. The lymph nodes of the lung. Comparison of the nomenclatures of the TNM system, the National Cancer Center Hospital of Tokyo (Naruke et al. [65]), and the Nomina Anatomica 1975

TNM	Code no. [65]	Designation, location	Nomina Anatomica
		Intrapulmonary lymph nodes	
N1	14	Subsegmental lymph nodes	Pulmonary lymph nodes
	13	Segmental lymph nodes	
	12	Lobar lymph nodes	
	11	Interlobar lymph nodes	
		Hilar lymph nodes	
	10	Hilar lymph nodes	Broncho pulmonary (hilar) lymph nodes
		Mediastinal lymph nodes	
N2	1	Superior mediastinal lymph nodes (para-pretracheal)	Paratracheal lymph nodes
	3	Pretracheal lymph nodes (middle and lower third)	
	2	Superior paratracheal lymph nodes	
	4	Inferior paratracheal lymph nodes (superior tracheobronchial lymph nodes)	Superior tracheo-bronchial lymph nodes
	7	Subcarinal lymph nodes (inferior tracheobronchial lymph nodes)	Inferior tracheo-bronchial lymph nodes
	3a	Anterior mediastinal lymph nodes	Anterior mediastinal lymph nodes
	5	Subaortic lymph nodes	
	6	Paraaortic lymph nodes	
	8	Paraesophageal lymph nodes	Posterior mediastinal lymph nodes
	9	Lymph nodes in the pulmonary ligament	
	3b	Retrotracheal lymph nodes	

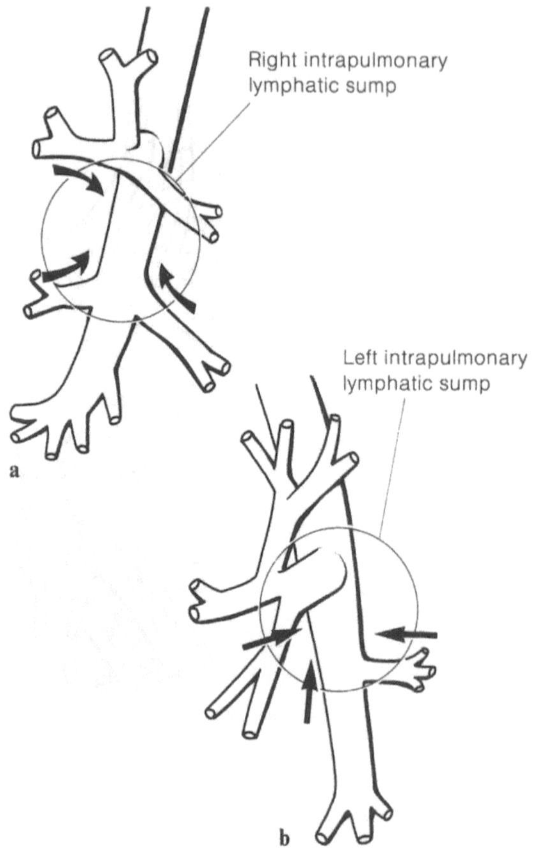

Fig. 3a, b. Intrapulmonary lymphatic sump of the right (**a**) and left (**b**) lung. (Modified from Nohl-Oser et al. [70, 71])

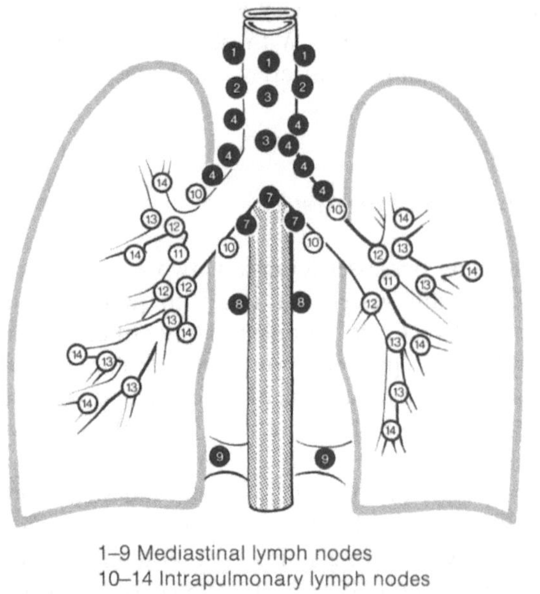

Fig. 4. Major groups of lymph nodes about the trachea and lungs [66]. *Light:* Intrapulmonary and hilar lymph nodes; *dark:* mediastinal lymph nodes

On the *left* side the lymphatic sump is placed in the interlobar fissure and consists of lymph nodes located at the interface of the upper and lower lobes and on the pulmonary artery and its branches. Removal of these nodes is of major importance in carcinoma resections, because 55% (left) and 70% (right) of nodal metastases occur in those areas [37].

1.1.5.2 Extrapulmonary Lymph Nodes

The *extrapulmonary lymph nodes* consist of:
a) the anterior mediastinal lymph nodes
b) the tracheobronchial and pretracheal lymph nodes, and
c) the posterior mediastinal lymph nodes (Fig. 4).

In diseases of the lung, the hilar nodes tend to become involved before the mediastinal nodes. There is no "representative" lymph node that could provide an indication for lymphadenectomy on the basis of intraoperative frozen section, although there have been reports of false-negative frozen section results [11, 61].

1.1.5.2.1 Anterior Mediastinal Lymph Nodes. The *anterior mediastinal lymph nodes* are arranged in a superior and inferior group. The *inferior group* is located at the sternocostal angle and in the area of insertion of the phrenic nerve. It receives afferents from the diaphragm, pleura, and upper abdominal viscera. The *superior group* is located in the upper half of the thorax. On the right side the nodes are arranged medial and parallel to the phrenic nerve and accompanying vessels on the superior vena cava and innominate vein, and on the left side they are placed on the aortic arch. The highest nodes of this group are close to the origin of the recurrent nerve from the vagus nerve on the right side, and level with the origin of the carotid artery on the left side. The lowest node of the left chain is anterior to the ligamentum arteriosum (Botallo's node). Connecting channels exist between the groups. Afferents are derived from the pericardium, trachea, and from the apical portions of the upper lobes, especially the left upper lobe, through lymph nodes around the azygos vein or Botallo's node. Tumors of the left upper lobe can metastasize to these lymph nodes without involving the tracheobronchial nodes [9, 71, 72]. The efferents of the anterior mediastinal nodes mostly join with the right lymphatic duct and thoracic duct.

1.1.5.2.2 Tracheobronchial Lymph Nodes. These lymph nodes are of special importance due to their frequent involvement by bronchogenic carcinoma. The superior group (*paratracheal lymph nodes*) lie on the upper half of the trachea on the right side and in the groove between the esophagus and trachea on the left side. They unite with the cervical lymph nodes. The inferior *tracheobronchial lymph nodes* are arranged in three groups around the tracheal bifurcation: the inferior paratracheal, the superior tracheobronchial, and the inferior tracheobronchial (subcarinal) lymph nodes. The *inferior paratracheal* nodes are continuous with the *superior tracheobronchial group* (lateral tracheobronchial nodes). This largest group is bounded on the *right* side by the azygos vein from above, medially by the aorta, posteromedially by the trachea, anterolaterally by the superior vena cava, and inferiorly by the pulmonary artery and right main bronchus. The group can be reached from below the azygos vein by incising the pleura along the course of the vena cava and retracting the vena cava to the left. On the *left* side these lymph nodes lie in the "aortic window," which is bounded by the aortic arch and left pulmonary artery and is divided into halves by the ligamentum arteriosum. This band to the pulmonary artery may be transected, and pericardial extensions removed, to aid surgical access. The *inferior tracheobronchial* (subcarinal) lymph nodes are placed in the angle between the two main bronchi and form an important connection between the lymphatic systems of both lungs.

The tracheobronchial lymph nodes drain through the paratracheal nodes and separate lymphatic trunks (bronchomediastinal trunks) to the junction of the subclavian and internal jugular veins or through the anterior mediastinal lymph nodes and the nodes around the innominate vein on the right side (innominate route) and through the nodes in front of the aortic arch on the left side (aortic route).

1.1.5.2.3 Posterior Mediastinal Lymph Nodes. This group consists of periesophageal and periaortic lymph nodes as well as nodes in the pulmonary ligament that receive afferents from the basal segments of the lower pulmonary lobes. The posterior mediastinal nodes have connections with the paraesophageal and paratracheal nodes and drain into the cisterna chyli. The numbering system for the lymph node groups customarily used in the Japanese and American literature is shown in Fig. 4.

1.1.5.3 Lymphatic Drainage of the Pulmonary Lobes

Generally the lymphatic drainage of the lungs proceeds from the intrapulmonary nodes to the hilar nodes and then to the extrapulmonary nodes. The drainage route may skip individual groups. Close connections exist among the different nodal groups. On the right side, efferents from the upper lobe pass to the right superior and inferior [29] tracheobronchial nodes. The middle lobe is drained by the superior and inferior tracheobronchial nodes, whose efferents pass to the right paratracheal nodes [71, 72, 74]. The right lower lobe is drained by the inferior tracheobronchial nodes and by the posterior, paraesophageal mediastinal nodes in the pulmonary ligament.

On the left side, efferents from the upper lobe are distributed to the anterior mediastinal group and to the superior and inferior tracheobronchial nodes [71, 72, 74], which also receive afferents from the lingula. The left lower lobe drains first to the inferior tracheobronchial and posterior nodes in the pulmonary ligament.

Mediastinoscopy has contributed much to our understanding of the mediastinal spread of bronchogenic tumors (Fig. 5 a–e). At one time it was thought that the basal segments of the left lower lobe led exclusively to contralateral lymphogenous spread, while the upper lobe segments led exclusively to ipsilateral spread, and both routes were possible in the intermediate region [47, 86]. However, more recent studies [29, 71, 72] utilizing mediastinoscopy indicate that tumors anywhere in the lung can metastasize ipsilaterally as well as contralaterally, with right-sided tumors producing contralateral metastases less frequently than left-sided disease. It appears that right-sided tumors with mediastinal lymph node involvement will produce contralateral metastases in 5%–9% of cases, although the results of Greschuchna and Maassen [29] suggest that basal tumors of the lower lobe segments are capable of ipsilateral metastasis only. In left-sided neoplasms with positive lymph nodes, the incidence of contralateral spread varies between 28% (upper lobe segments 1 to 3), 25% (lingula), 33% (basal lower lobe segments), and 42% (superior lower lobe segment). Tumors of the right upper lobe seed to the subcarinal nodes frequently (20%) according to Greschuchna and Maassen [29] and rarely (1%) according to Nohl-Oser [71]. These figures should be considered approximations only and will vary in individual cases according to the size, location, and histology of the neoplasm.

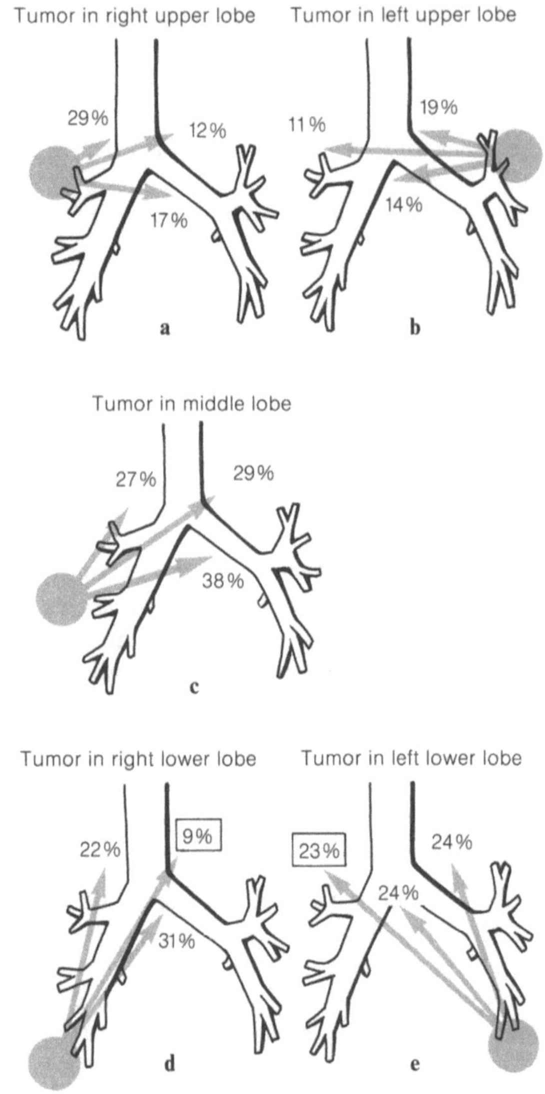

Fig. 5a–e. Ipsi- and contralateral lymph node involvement as a function of tumor location (percentage of tumor-positive excisions relative to total number of specimens taken, after Greschuchna and Maassen [29])

1.2 Introductory Remarks on Operative Technique

Regardless of the indication for pulmonary resection, the initial step after opening the chest is to check the pathology and define the extent of the resection. Before describing the various types of resective procedures, we shall first review some technical aspects relating to exploration of the chest cavity, management of the pulmonary vessels and bronchi, and drainage of the chest.

1.2.1 Exploration of the Chest Cavity

1.2.1.1 Mobilization of the Lung

It is not uncommon to find pleural adhesions when the chest is entered, regardless of the underlying disease. Inflammatory processes generally incite stronger tissue reactions than tumors, which in turn may have infiltrated the chest wall. These tumor extensions should not be divided, but removed en bloc with the rest of the specimen, assuming that an indication exists for resective surgery. In most cases adhesions are less pronounced in the mediastinal and hilar regions than over the rest of the pulmonary surface, especially in the region of the thoracic apex and diaphragm. Adhesions may be separated on the intrapleural or extrapleural plane. Fine adhesive strands may be sharply divided with scissors followed by the coagulation of any present vessels. Blunt dissection with the finger or flat hand is dangerous, as it may traumatize the parenchyma. Heavier adhesions are progressively divided under vision with the scissors while applying counterpressure to the lung with the hand or lung retractor. Bleeding points are controlled with the electrocautery, and diffuse bleeding by temporary compression with warm surgical sponges and the application of fibrin glue. The surgeon must work carefully to avoid provoking heavy bleeding in the hilar region. If adhesions are such that the correct plane of dissection cannot be developed between the pleural layers, as evidenced by the presence of multiple parenchymal fistulas, extrapleural mobilization of the lung is usually a simpler and less traumatizing option. For this the pleura is incised with the scissors and mobilized at the edge of the thoracotomy along with the endothoracic fascia, using first sharp dissection and then blunt dissection with the flat hand. With this technique there is a risk of separation on the wrong plane, with associated heavy bleeding, and of injury to extrapulmonary structures such as the mammary artery, the aortic arch and its branches, the esophagus, and the thoracic duct; hence separation of the pleura in these areas must be done with extreme care. The lung should be mobilized sufficiently to permit the insertion of a self-retaining intercostal retractor.

For pneumonectomies and upper lobectomies, it is necessary to free the entire pulmonary surface. For a lower lobectomy, it is not essential that the upper lobe be mobilized.

1.2.1.1.1 Upper Lobes. The upper lobes of the lungs are frequently adherent to the apex and posterior chest wall. If the pleural space is completely obliterated, the heart is used as a landmark, and the lung is separated from the pericardium below the azygos vein on the right side and below the aortic arch on the left side, where adhesions are usually less dense. Then the pleura is incised above the azygos vein on the right side and above the aorta on the left and bluntly dissected from the vessels until a tunnel is formed that extends to the posterior limit of the thoracotomy. From this channel, the lung is freed from the thoracic apex on the extrapleural plane, proceeding gradually upward from below. An indwelling gastric tube aids orientation and helps to avoid esophageal injury.

1.2.1.1.2 Lower Lobes. Before removal of the lower lobes, it may be necessary to separate paravertebral adhesions with the parietal pleura, adhesions with the diaphragm and costophrenic sinus, or with the pericardium. Anterior adhesions between middle lobe or lingula and pericardium usually are relatively easy to separate, making it possible to mobilize the lung downward along the pericardium until the diaphragm is reached. While the lung is retracted upward and posteriorly, the rest of the upper surface of the diaphragm is cleared by blunt or sharp dissection. Posterior adhesions of the lower lobe may have to be cleared extrapleurally in some instances. Mobilization of the lung initially requires division of the pulmonary ligament, which is located below the inferior pulmonary vein and anterior to the esophagus. The latter is identified from the indwelling gastric tube, and the pulmonary ligament is divided in stepwise fashion from the anterior or posterior side. As exposure of the inferior lung surface proceeds, the remaining connections with the costophrenic sinus can be divided.

1.2.1.2 Assessment of Disease and Resectability

Preoperative diagnostic studies can tell us much about the nature and extent of the underlying disease and the probable extent of the resection. However, the surgeon should carefully confirm these points before dividing a major vessel or bronchus so that he can avoid intraoperative corrections and minimize the operative risk by following a standardized procedure. Resection is always preceded by careful inspection of the pleura, the lung parenchyma, and the hilar and mediastinal structures. The *pleura* is explored for tumor infiltration or metastasis, and the extent of pleural tumors is ascertained, using frozen section confirmation as required. Evaluation of the *lung parenchyma* centers on the extent and localization of the primary disease and its relation to the lobes. The lung should be deflated at this stage and examined bimanually. If a morphologic diagnosis cannot be made, an intraoperative frozen section study is advised and is a necessary preliminary to pneumonectomy. Finally the surgeon assesses the involvement of the *hilar structures and adjacent organs* including the lymph nodes, esophagus, and liver (by transdiaphragmatic palpation). Often an exploratory dissection of the vessels, bronchi, and neighboring organs will have to be performed before operability can be assessed and the type of resection determined.

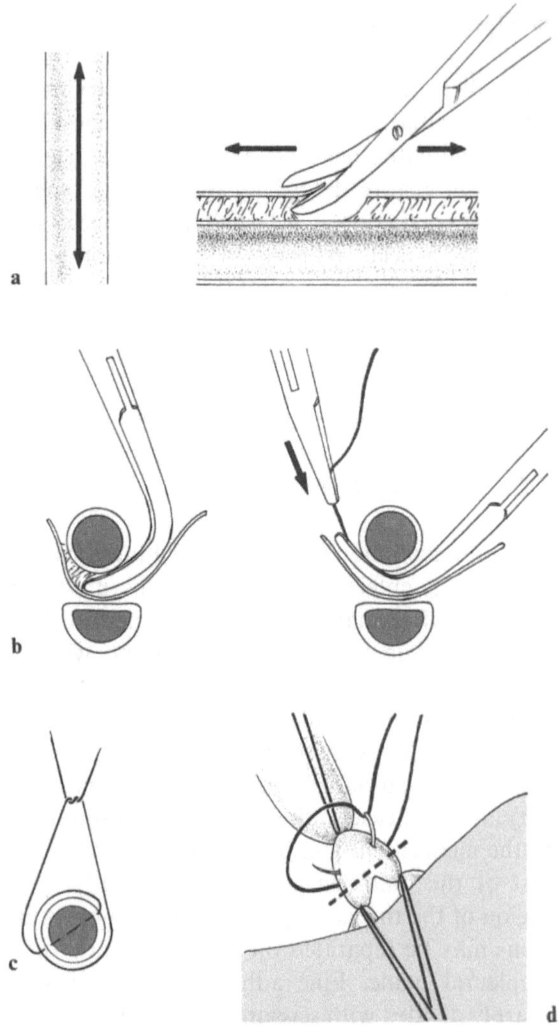

Fig. 6a–d. Technique for dissection, ligation, and division of blood vessels. **a** Incision of the vascular sheath. **b** Encircling the vessel and passing the ligature. **c, d** Placement of transfixion ligature proximal to line of transection

1.2.2 Management of the Pulmonary Vessels

1.2.2.1 Exposure of the Vessels

The arteries of the lung, unlike those of the systemic circulation, are muscular vessels that are easily injured. This fact must be considered during dissection and ligation of the vessels, especially when dense adhesions are present. The pulmonary vascular anatomy is such that the vessels may be exposed at the hilum, in the interlobar fissure, or at their entry into the lung tissue. Often the vessels are surrounded by enlarged lymph nodes, which provide useful landmarks but can also cause bleeding when they are dissected off the vessels. To expose the vessel wall, and in preparation for encircling it, the perivascular tissue is incised along the course of the vessel, and the anterior circumference is exposed using a combination of patty dissection and sharp dissection with a scissors. The pulmonary vessels are relatively short, and usually they have to be exposed to their lobar divisions for confident identification and ligation. Next we pass increasing sizes of blunt, angled dissecting forceps beneath the vessel (Rumel A to D) and carefully open the jaws in preparation for encircling the vessel with a ligature (Fig. 6 a–d).

1.2.2.2 *Division of the Vessels*

After the vessel has been circumferentially cleared, the ligatures are passed around the vessel with the aid of the dissecting forceps and are tied. Initially the ends of the ligature are left long, as traction on the threads can be helpful in dissecting any vascular branches that require separate ligation. The ligatures on these branches are also left long. Slippage of the proximal circular ligature can be prevented by placing a transfixion ligature through the vessel wall. To reduce hemorrhage, this stitch is not placed until the proximal and distal ligatures have been tied. The end of the transfixion ligature is passed around the vascular trunk and through the vessel wall on an atraumatic needle and tied. Care is taken at this stage to avoid unnecessary pressure or tension on the threads that could disrupt the fragile, muscular vessel wall. The transfixion ligature having been tied, the vessel is divided, and the ends of the threads are clipped. We have found that bleeding from major vessels after lung resections is rare when this type of transfixion ligature is employed (Fig. 6).

We prefer an absorbable suture material with a polyglycolic acid base for closure of the pulmonary vessels. Heavier sutures are less apt to cut through the vessel wall, so we close the hilar vessels with a No. 0 ligature and the peripheral vessels with a 2-0 ligature. Alternatively, closure of the pulmonary veins may be accomplished with the stapling instrument (TA 30 V, 2.5 mm). This is an especially good technique when the vascular trunks are short.

If the segment available for ligation is too short because of adhesions or tumor infiltration, space can be gained by dividing the vessel between vascular clamps. The proximal stump is closed with a double row of continuous 5-0 monofilament sutures, and the distal stump, which is to be discarded, is simply ligated (Fig. 7 a–d). With the hilar vessels, additional space can be gained by dissection within the pericardium (see pp. 134).

If tumor extends to a vessel that is to be preserved, the vessel should be isolated above and below the area of tumor involvement before it is cleared. This may be done by applying vascular clamps at two levels and placing a tourniquet round the trunk of the pulmonary artery before proceeding to dissect the tumor off the vessel. The latter step may require sacrificing a portion of the vessel wall. Occasionally it is possible simply to clamp off the vessel with a curved vascular clamp

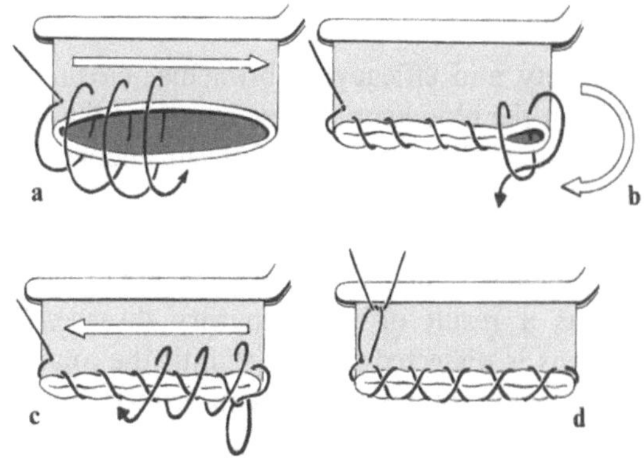

Fig. 7 a–d. Vascular closure with a double row of over-and-over continuous sutures

(Satinsky) before clearing it of tumor. Any defect in the vessel wall is repaired by continuous suture (5-0 atraumatic monofilament). If it was necessary to resect a segment of the pulmonary artery, continuity can generally be restored by an end-to-end anastomosis (see p. 174).

1.2.2.3 *Intraoperative Bleeding*

One cannot always avoid intraoperative bleeding associated with dissection of the vessels or traction on the lung. To control arterial bleeding during lobectomies or segmentectomies, we recommend snaring the pulmonary trunk on the affected side with a tourniquet at the start of the operation. Once the operation is underway, the tourniquet may be tightened as needed to give rapid control of intraoperative hemorrhage.

Temporary manual compression is preferable to blind clamping or ligation for the control of intraoperative bleeding. While the compression is applied and the field is cleared of blood, an attempt is made to isolate the vessel and clamp it proximal and distal to the bleeding site. This exposure may require opening the pericardium, or in rare cases it may necessitate extension of the thoracotomy. After the vessel has been clamped off, the defect is oversewn in a deliberate and unhurried fashion with an atraumatic, absorbable monofilament suture material. In the very rare cases where this is not successful, it will be necessary to extend the procedure to a pneumonectomy.

1.2.3 Closure of the Bronchus

The safety and efficacy of bronchial closure depends on the blood supply, the length of the bronchial stump, the condition of the bronchial wall, and the tension of the closure.

The bronchus is exposed by freeing it from the peribronchial tissue, which may be greatly thickened as a result of inflammatory disease. The bronchus is dissected free only until the anatomy of the region of interest is appreciated and the proposed level of transection is reached. Dissection beyond that point can deprive the bronchial wall of much of its blood supply. If possible, the bronchial arteries are ligated at the level of the bronchial transection. It is conceivable that the bronchial clamps used in various methods of bronchial closure (Klinkenbergh) may compromise the blood supply, but this has not been proved. Long bronchial stumps predispose to infection and suture leak, so the bronchus should be divided as close to its origin as possible. The risk of stump leak is also increased by tumor infiltration. Anderson states that the bronchus should be transected 1.5 cm proximal to visible or palpable tumor, but we have found cancer tissue in peribronchial tissue located 2 cm from the gross tumor margin. Severe inflammatory change associated with, say, tuberculosis or bronchiectasis likewise predisposes to stump leak and underscores the importance of resecting healthy margins or preceding the resection by appropriate therapy. A perfect suture technique is of fundamental importance for bronchial healing. The particular technique that is used is less critical than a tension-free approximation of the cut edges. Numerous methods have been described (Craford, Sturzenegger, Klinkenbergh, Rienhoff, Overholt, Zenker, etc.), and no single method has shown definite superiority. Two methods will be described here: staple closure and closure with simple interrupted sutures.

1.2.3.1 Staple Closure (Fig. 8)

The advantages of staple closure are the good tissue compatibility of the staples, the uniformity and aerostasis of the staple line, the rapidity of the closure (requiring only a short interruption of asepsis, eliminating the danger of aspiration, and causing no interference with ventilation), the relative ease of use in areas poorly accessible to manual suturing, and sparing of the tissue between the

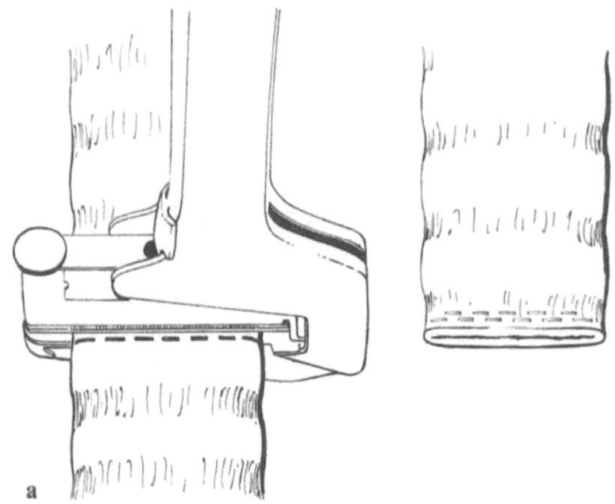

a b

Fig. 8a, b. Staple closure of a bronchus

double row of staggered staples. On the negative side, it is possible for the instrument to crush the bronchial tissue, especially if it is applied incorrectly. Forrester-Wood [24] found in two consecutive series that the incidence of bronchopleural fistula after pneumonectomy declined from 11.1% with manual sutures to 2.6% with stapling. Either the TA 30 instrument (producing staple rows 30 mm long) or the TA 55 (producing 55-mm staple rows) may be used. The cartridges are color-coded to indicate staple size, with 4.8-mm staples (green cartridge) used for the main bronchus and 3.5-mm staples (blue cartridge) for the lobar bronchi. The instruments are applied close to the origin of the bronchus, parallel to the cartilage rings and perpendicular to the bronchial axis, in such a way that the membranous and cartilaginous portions of the wall will be apposed (Fig. 8). If space is limited, a dissecting forceps can be used to direct the instrument to the proper site. After the staples have been inserted and a clamp has been applied distally, the bronchus is transected by cutting along the edge of the instrument with a scalpel, and antiseptic solution is applied to the stump. At that point the stapler is opened and removed (Fig. 8). Sutures do not need to be placed distal to the staple line. Before closing, the stump is checked for air leak by immersing the staple line in irrigating fluid (Ringer's solution warmed to body temperature) and inflating the lung. Technical errors in the use of stapling instruments most commonly result from failure to approximate the membranous and cartilaginous portions of the bronchial wall, leading to undesired tension and crushing of tissues. This usually makes it necessary to repeat the bronchial closure or reinforce it with interrupted sutures. If the integrity of the closure is questionable, it is safer to increase the extent of the resection.

1.2.3.2 Bronchial Suture

When sutures are used for closure, the edges of the bronchus are cut in a fish-mouth fashion, leaving a somewhat longer lip of membranous tissue. The stump is then closed with interrupted sutures placed external to the mucosa and perpendicular to the cut edges. The sutures are placed at the corners first, then at the center, and finally at other sites around the circumference. The sutures are passed around the cartilaginous ring (Fig. 9 a–c). When suturing in a deep field, it is helpful first to immobilize the bronchial wall with a pair of stay sutures. The sutures should be spaced 3 mm apart and also 3 mm from the cut edge of the bronchus. The needle is inserted into the mucosa from the outside, brought out through the cut edge, than passed through the opposite wall in a reverse fashion. This produces an airtight inversion and approximation of the mucosal surfaces, avoids intraluminal threads, and thus prevents the formation of suture granulomas with consequent stenosis, which develops in 7%–17% of cases when the suture is inside the lumen [19]. With the suture passed around the cartilage in this way, the cartilaginous ring forms a bolster that keeps the suture from cutting the tissue. After all sutures have been placed, they are individually tied and clipped.

For ten years we have used absorbable suture material (polyglycolic acid) exclusively for bronchial closures. The recently developed absorbable monofilament sutures (PDS) are also acceptable. It is our experience and that of other authors [91] that the use of absorbable material has significantly lowered the incidence of suture fistulas. The suture technique described above is derived from the technique for bronchial anastomosis.

1.2.3.3 Coverage of the Bronchial Stump

Covering the sutured or stapled bronchial stump with a tissue flap has been widely recommended, especially in resections for inflammatory disease. Although this practice has become less frequent, it continues to be justified in some cases, especially when there is evidence of stump leak. We do not

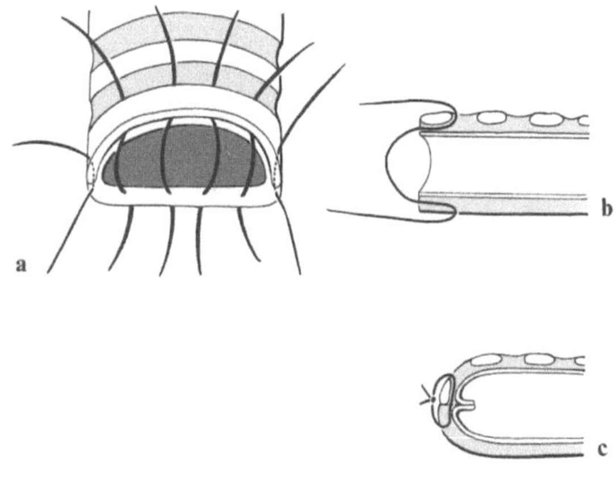

Fig. 9 a–c. Bronchial closure with extramucous sutures

cover the bronchial stump following lobectomy for carcinoma, but we do feel that coverage of the bronchus may have value after pneumonectomy in cases where an extensive lymph node dissection has been performed. There is still diversity of opinion on this issue [30].

The bronchial stump may be covered with a flap from the pleura or pericardium, mediastinal organs, or intercostal muscle. The azygos vein and surrounding pleura may be utilized after a right pneumonectomy, while a pericardial flap is recommended after a left pneumonectomy. A vascularized strip of intercostal muscle has been advocated for difficult cases [71]. This flap is created after the chest is entered by dividing the periosteum and adjacent intercostal muscle, prior to insertion of the rib spreader. The flap is based posteriorly to preserve its blood supply. After the lung resection is completed, the flap is tacked over the bronchial stump with sutures (Fig. 10).

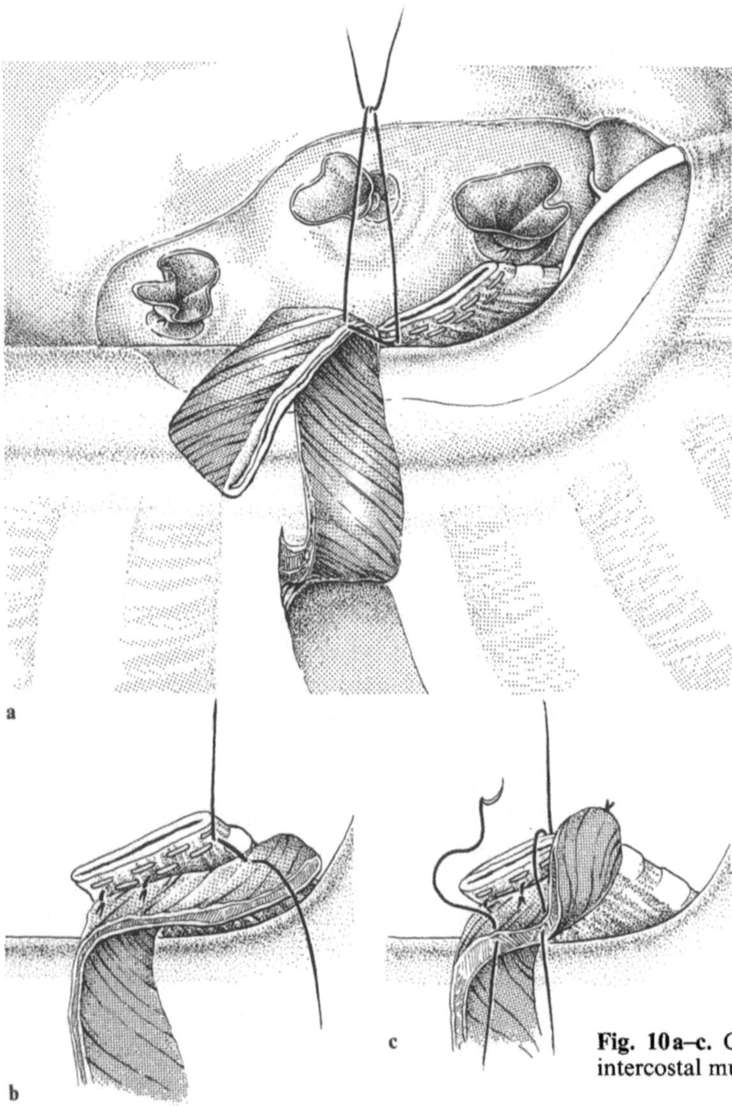

a

b

c

Fig. 10a–c. Coverage of the bronchial stump with an intercostal muscle flap. (After Nohl-Oser et al. [71])

1.2.4 Sequence of Management of the Hilar Structures

In all lung resections the bronchi, arteries, and veins must be dealt with separately. The sequence depends on the individual preference of the surgeon. Clamping of the bronchus may be advised as a primary measure in the presence of heavy secretion or traumatic hemorrhage that cannot be managed preoperatively with a catheter or endotracheal tube. The advantage of performing the arterial ligation first is that it interrupts the blood supply to the lung, whereas primary venous ligation might cause engorgement of the lung, although there is no direct experimental evidence of this [62]. On the other hand, primary ligation of the veins is reasonable from an oncologic standpoint, as it minimizes the dissemination of tumor cells. That is why we generally begin all our resections for bronchogenic cancer with the pulmonary vein before turning to the pulmonary artery and lastly to the bronchus, although this sequence is subject to modification depending on circumstances.

1.2.5 Drainage of the Chest Cavity

In all operations where the pleural space is entered, drainage is necessary for removing accumulations of air, fluid, and blood and monitoring their extent. Besides catheters for air drainage, large-gauge tubes with multiple side openings are best for providing complete drainage of fluid material and preventing clot formation in the tube.

Generally two tubes are inserted: an anterior tube to drain air from the apex of the chest, and a posterior tube to drain fluid from the most dependent point of the costophrenic sinus. The tubes are brought out through separate skin incisions before the thoracotomy is closed. With one hand placed against the inner surface of the chest wall for guidance, a skin incision is made over the intended site with the other hand, the opening is enlarged with a scissors, and a dressing forceps is introduced bluntly through the interspace below the thoracotomy to grasp the end of the tube and deliver it through the incision (Fig. 11). It is best to tunnel obliquely through the tissue layers, as this will allow the layers to close and create an effective seal when the tube is withdrawn.

The posterior drain site is in the midaxillary line so that it will not cause discomfort in the supine patient. Tube kinking and erosive lesions in the chest can be avoided by fixing the end of the tube to the inside of the chest wall with surgical gut. The tubes are also sutured to the skin externally. A horizontal mattress suture is placed about the incision and is used for wound closure at the time of tube removal.

The tubes are connected separately to a waterseal apparatus to promote air and fluid drainage and prevent reflux. Because the negative pressure dwindles as the collecting vessel fills, the vessels should be changed regularly and the tubes evacuated. Suction is necessary only in the presence of unexpanded residual lung and, when used, should always be applied to both tubes equally. The apical tube is usually removed after 24 h following expansion of the remaining lung and the exclusion of pulmonary fistulae. The posterior drain may be removed when the volume of secretions falls below 200 ml in a 24-h period.

1.2.5.1 Drainage after Pneumonectomy

A single chest tube is placed after pneumonectomy for the purpose of monitoring postoperative blood loss and providing a relief valve for the drainage of fluids that collect too rapidly. It is essential to avoid mediastinal shift. This is best accomplished by allowing pressures to equalize spontaneously through the tube, which is connected to a waterseal, for a maximum of one hour after the patient is extubated while close clinical observation is maintained. Then the chest tube is clamped and removed within the next 12 h. The normal position of the mediastinum should be watched very carefully in the initial period after pneumonectomy. With rapid collection of serum or blood, it may be necessary to drain some of the fluid through the tube or remove fluid by needle aspiration. Intrathoracic hemorrhage after an extensive pleural resection constitutes a grave situation in which early reintervention is necessary. Active suctioning through the tube is contraindicated after pneumonectomy. Monitoring of the mediastinal position after pneumonectomy requires experience and is a major factor in the success of the operation.

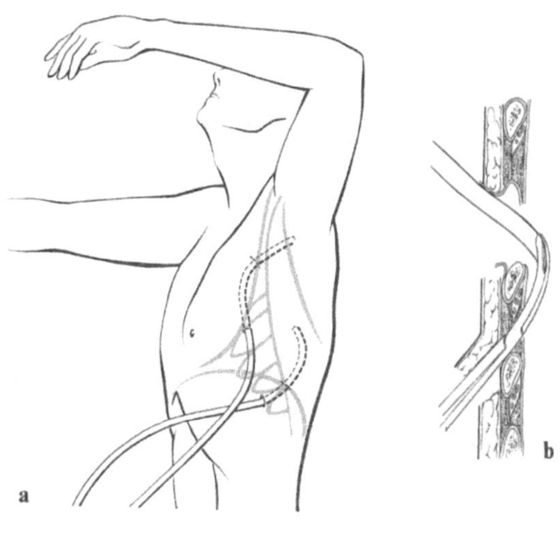

Fig. 11 a, b. Drainage of the chest cavity

1.3 **Pneumonectomy** [28, 70, 85]

1.3.1 Indications

Pneumonectomy carries a higher operative risk than lobectomy and causes a greater limitation of pulmonary function. It is indicated for tumors that cannot be removed by lobectomy, lobectomy with sleeve resection, or wedge resection, i.e., tumors that involve the mainstem bronchus or multiple lobes, tumors with extensive mediastinal lymph node involvement (necessitating an extensive lymph node dissection), and pleural tumors that are resectable by pleuropneumonectomy. Pneumonectomy is contraindicated if it appears that a resection will become necessary on the contralateral side with progression of the disease.

Pneumonectomy is justified in certain benign conditions, such as chronic obstructive lung disease resulting in widespread destruction or suppuration of the lung parenchyma, long-standing inflammatory diseases of the pleura with irreversible shrinkage of the lung, and bronchopulmonary malformations.

1.3.2 Right Pneumonectomy

1.3.2.1 Intubation

The patient is intubated with a spiral endotracheal tube. Selective intubation for one-lung anesthesia may be indicated in special cases.

1.3.2.2 Position and Approach

Left lateral decubitus, anterolateral thoracotomy in the bed of the fifth rib.

1.3.2.3 Instruments

Basic set II, extra thoracic set.

1.3.2.4 Anatomy of the Right Hilum

The right pulmonary hilum is bounded anteriorly by the right atrium and vena cava and by the phrenic nerve with its accompanying vessels; it relates posteriorly to the azygos vein, esophagus, and vagus nerve. Superiorly it is bounded by the arch of the azygos vein and the tracheobronchial lymph nodes. The most anterior of the hilar structures is the superior pulmonary vein, which is adjoined posteriorly by the pulmonary artery and then the right main bronchus. In the craniocaudal direction, the structure just below the arch of the azygos vein is the right main bronchus, followed by the pulmonary artery and finally the superior pulmonary vein. The inferior pulmonary vein is situated below and posterior to the superior pulmonary vein, at the upper end of the pulmonary ligament and cranial to one or more lymph nodes. Fibers from the pericardium radiate anteriorly and posteriorly into the wall of the vein, separated from the vessel by connective tissue. These fibrous extensions must be incised close to the pericardium before the vessels can be exposed.

Variations in the number of pulmonary veins are more common on the left side than on the right [40]. There may be only one pulmonary vein on each side, or there may be more than two, in which case the middle lobe vein empties directly into the left atrium.

1.3.2.5 Technique

Steps in procedure:

(1) Dissection of the lung
(2) Incision of the pleura over the hilum from the inferior hilar border anteriorly to the center of the hilum posteriorly
(3) Exposure, ligation and division of the superior pulmonary vein
(4) Division of the pulmonary ligament and completion of the pleural incisions
(5) Exposure, ligation and division of the inferior pulmonary vein from the posterior side
(6) Exposure, ligation and division of the pulmonary artery from the anterosuperior side after division of pericardial extensions
(7) Exposure, ligation and division of the right main bronchus from the posterior side
(8) Lymph node dissection (encompassing superior and inferior tracheobronchial, paratracheal, anterior and posterior mediastinal nodes)

After the chest cavity has been entered and explored (see p. 115), the pleura over the hilum is divided in circumferential, stepwise fashion prior to the vascular and bronchial dissections. The key landmarks posteriorly are the esophagus, which can be identified by an indwelling tube in the presence of dense adhesions, and the azygos vein, whose site of entry into the superior vena cava marks the superior border of the right main bronchus. While the lung is retracted downward and posteriorly, the pleura over the hilum is divided in curved fashion with a scissors below the azygos vein, starting anteriorly at the inferior border of the hilum and sparing the phrenic nerve. The incision is carried posteriorly to about the center of the hilum. In the absence of lymph node metastases, it is unnecessary to sever the azygos vein.

The loose connective tissue below the pleura can be reflected off the hilar structures by patty dissection. It may be necessary to free individual lymph nodes and divide the pericardial extensions parallel to the pleural incision before the pulmonary vessels can be visualized. The pericardial

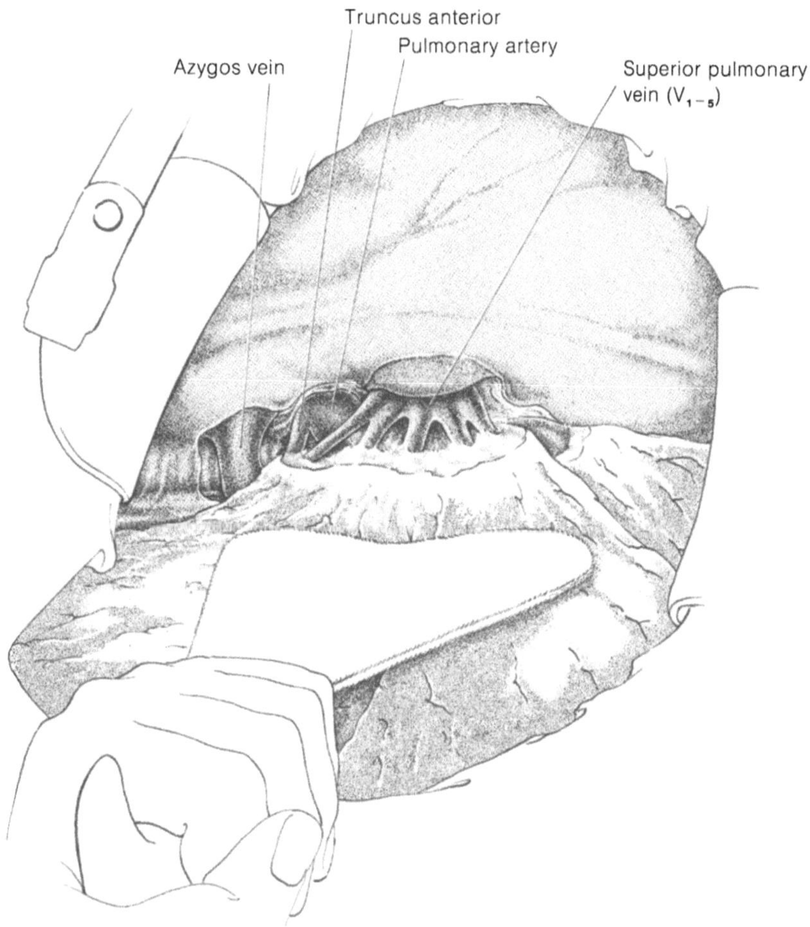

Fig. 12. Exposure of the right superior pulmonary vein

fibers extend from the lateral border of the superior vena cava to the anterior surfaces of the pulmonary artery and superior pulmonary vein and may pass deeply between the individual branches. These fibers are divided to expose the superior pulmonary vein with its segmental divisions V1 through V3. Behind this broadest and most anterior of the pulmonary vessels lies the pulmonary artery, which pulsates synchronously with the right ventricle (Fig. 12). Generally these vessels are ligated and divided outside the pericardium; intrapericardial dissection may be necessary with tumor infiltration of the vessels or in cases of intraoperative bleeding (see p. 134).

1.3.2.5.1 Venous Dissection. First the anterior wall of the superior pulmonary vein is exposed over its entire width, then a Rumel or Overholt forceps is passed around the vessel, proceeding in small steps and avoiding injury to the pulmonary artery (Fig. 13). Adhesions may be present and usually are most dense posteriorly. We use small dissecting patties and incremental sizes of blunt dissecting forceps (Rumel A–D) to isolate the vein; finger dissection is also acceptable. The cleared vein is ligated by encircling it with a No. 0 absorbable suture, which is tied as proximally as possible. With traction on the ligature, the vein is dissected farther into the parenchyma and, depending on the length of the venous trunk, the distal ligature is placed central to or beyond the origins of the segmental veins. The proximal and distal ligatures should be spaced at least 5–8 mm apart to prevent slippage. The proximal ligature is secured with a transfixion ligature (0 absorbable monofilament on an atraumatic needle) before the vessel is divided and the ends of the ligatures are clipped. With a short venous trunk, the vessel may be divided between clamps and the proximal stump

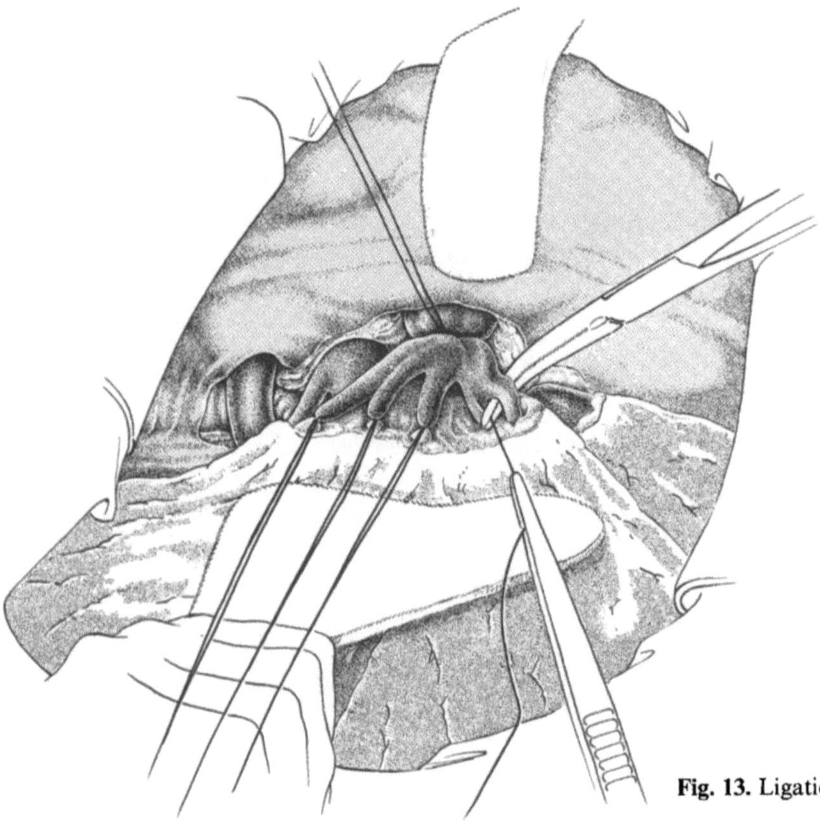

Fig. 13. Ligation of the right superior pulmonary vein

closed with a double row of continuous sutures (4-0 or 5-0 monofilament). Attention is now turned to the inferior pulmonary vein (Fig. 14). It is found at the upper border of the pulmonary ligament, which additionally contains important lymph nodes of the lower lobe that must be removed in carcinoma resections. The lung is pulled upward and forward to make the pulmonary ligament tense, and, starting at the diaphragm, the ligament is dissected from the posterior aspect and divided. Smaller blood vessels are coagulated, and larger vessels are divided between clamps. In rare cases an anomalous branch may be found passing from the abdominal aorta to a "sequestered" segment of lung (see p. 185). Following division of the pulmonary ligament, the pleura is incised upward on the posterior and anterior sides of the hilum (if this has not already been done), and the inferior pulmonary vein is cleared and divided between ligatures using the technique described for the superior pulmonary vein. As an alternative to ligatures, the pulmonary veins may be occluded with a double row of staples (TA 30 V, white cartridge, 2.5 mm).

1.3.2.5.2 Arterial Dissection. Exposure of the right pulmonary artery is facilitated by the prior ligation of the pulmonary veins. The lung is retracted inferiorly and posteriorly. If the pericardial extensions have not been divided, usually only the truncus anterior will be visible from the front. With the vena cava retracted medially, the pericardial extensions are divided until the adventitia of the pulmonary artery is widely exposed. The vessel is dissected free from the connective tissue using blunt forceps and very small sponge sticks. The proximal ligature is applied (0 or 1 absorbable suture), whereupon the artery is dissected farther distally and ligated on the trunk or, preferably, beyond its initial point of division (truncus anterior and interlobar artery). The proximal circular ligature is secured with a transfixion ligature (0 atraumatic absorbable monofilament) before the vessel is transected and the threads are clipped. When space is limited, the vessel may be divided between clamps (Fig. 15) or intrapericardially (see p.134).

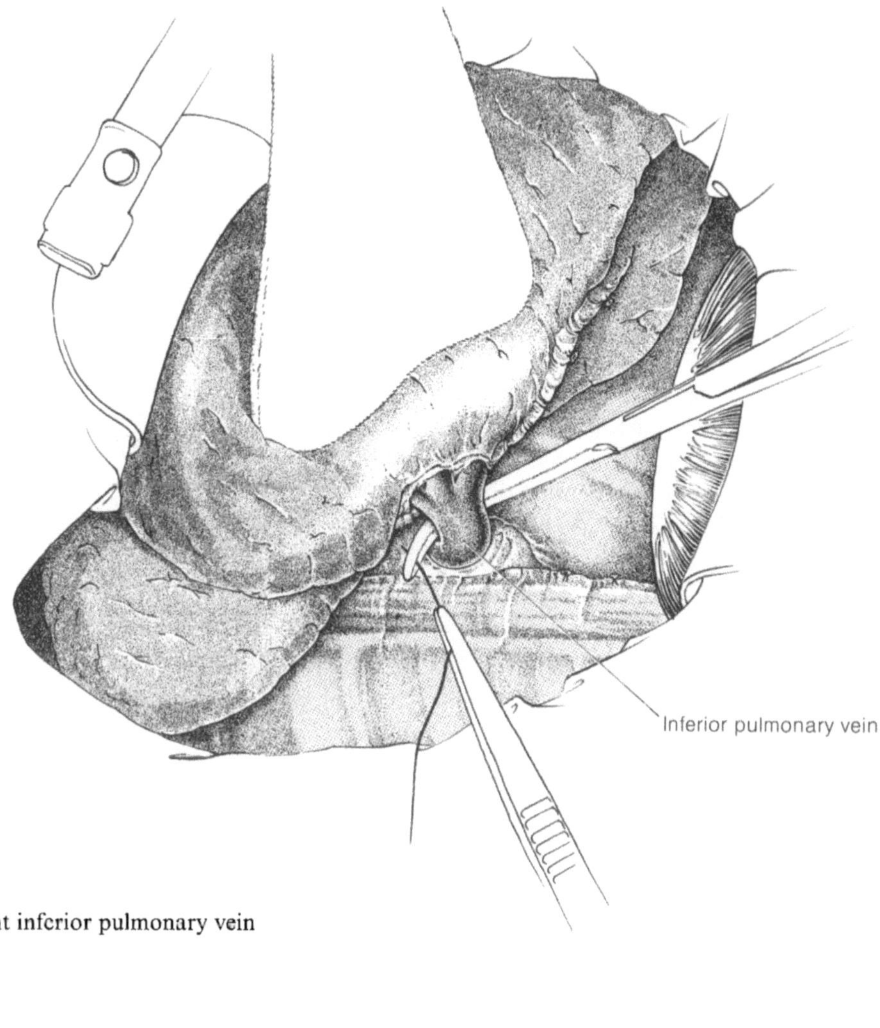

Fig. 14. Ligation of the right inferior pulmonary vein

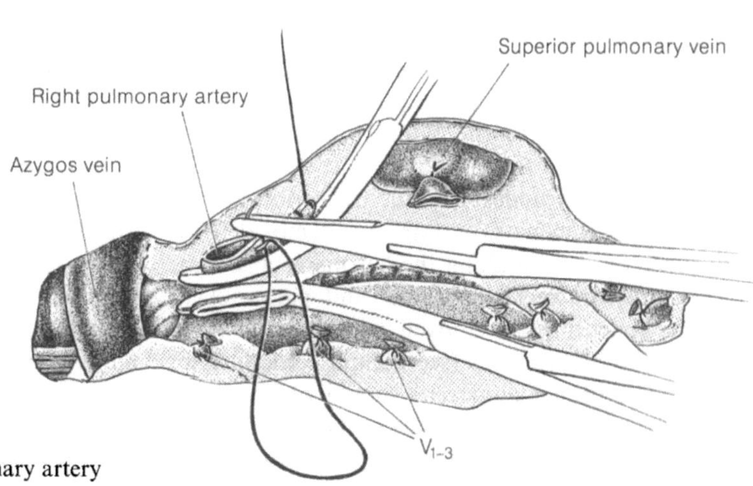

Fig. 15. Suture closure of the right pulmonary artery

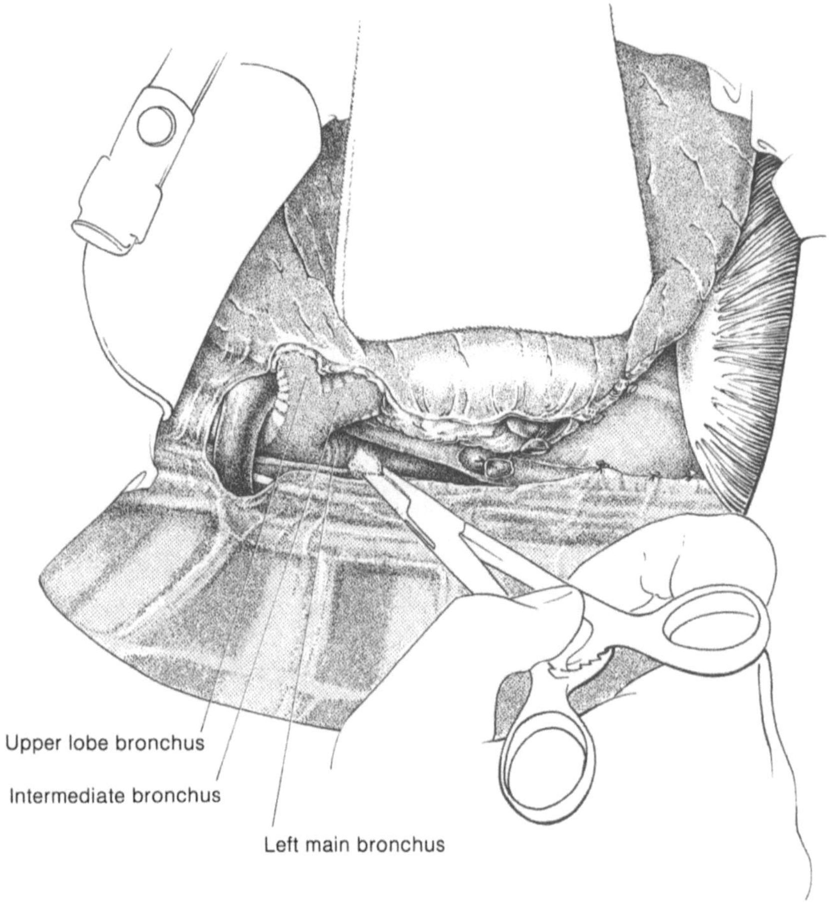

Fig. 16. Exposure of the right main bronchus and bifurcation

1.3.2.5.3 Bronchial Dissection. After the vessels have been secured, the lung can be retracted forward to give good posterior exposure of the mainstem bronchus. The peribronchial connective tissue may be thickened, especially in inflammatory diseases, and this tissue is incised below the azygos/vena cava junction at the superior border of the bronchus until reaching the cartilaginous portion of the bronchial wall, which is further exposed by progressive blunt dissection (Fig. 16). To avoid creating a blind pouch, the bronchus should be severed as close to the bifurcation as possible. With alternating traction applied to the lung, the regional lymph nodes (inferior tracheobronchial) are removed en bloc, carrying the removal for a distance of 3–5 cm along the left main bronchus. The superior tracheobronchial and paratracheal lymph nodes may be removed before or after transection of the bronchus (see Lymph Node Dissection). The bronchial arteries should be ligated at the level of the proposed transection.

Access to the bifurcation can be facilitated and vision improved by dividing the right main bronchus close to the origin of the upper lobe bronchus between two clamps and removing the lung. After further proximal dissection has been carried out, the resection of the bronchus is completed and the stump closed in standard fashion.

Stapling provides a simple and effective means of closing the bronchus (TA 30 instrument, 4.8 mm, green cartridge). To avoid creating a blind pouch, the instrument is applied across the origin of the main bronchus from the trachea, at right angles to the long axis of the bronchus, such that the membranous portion of the bronchial wall is apposed to the cartilaginous portion. The bronchus is clamped distally, transected with a scalpel along the edge of the stapler, and the stump is treated with antiseptic solution (Fig. 17). If a stapling instrument is not available, the bronchus may be closed over a clamp, or an open suturing technique may be used (see p. 118). In the open

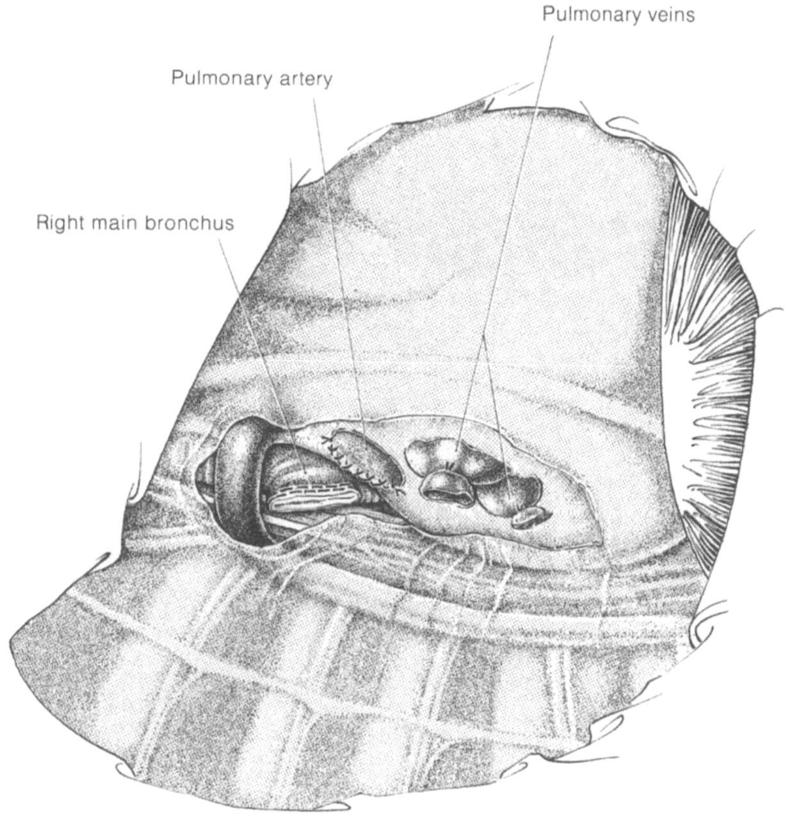

Fig. 17. Status following division of the hilar structures

technique the bronchus is transected, and the indwelling endotracheal tube is advanced under digital guidance into the left main bronchus to isolate the bronchial system. After the stump has been sutured, the tube is withdrawn into the trachea, and the integrity of the suture line is tested by saline immersion. The specimen is examined to determine the distance of the tumor from the cut edge and assess the need for additional resection.

1.3.2.5.4 Lymph Node Dissection. In accordance with the regional lymphatic drainage of the lung (see above), the lymph node dissection in pneumonectomy encompasses the superior tracheobronchial and paratracheal lymph nodes, the inferior tracheobronchial (subcarinal) nodes, the posterior mediastinal nodes in the pulmonary ligament and around the esophagus, and the anterior mediastinal nodes. The subcarinal nodes are accessible when traction is applied to the lung during the bronchial dissection and can be removed at that time; the posterior mediastinal nodes are similarly accessible during division of the pulmonary ligament and inferior pulmonary vein. After the pneumonectomy has been completed, it remains to dissect the superior tracheobronchial, paratracheal, and anterior mediastinal nodes (Fig. 18). This requires extending the incision in the parietal pleura up to the highest point of the thoracic apex at the level of the subclavian vein. Division of the azygos vein is acceptable where lymph node involvement is extensive, but otherwise an attempt may be made to isolate and preserve the vessel. The phrenic nerve also may be divided in the thoracic apex and removed with a 1- to 2-cm-wide strip of pleura as far as the hilum. This gives access for removing the lymph nodes on the vena cava and brachial vessels and clearing the paratracheal and superior tracheobronchial nodes between the vena cava and trachea while sparing the vagus nerve. Anterior retraction of the vena cava is necessary for this maneuver. The paratracheal dissec-

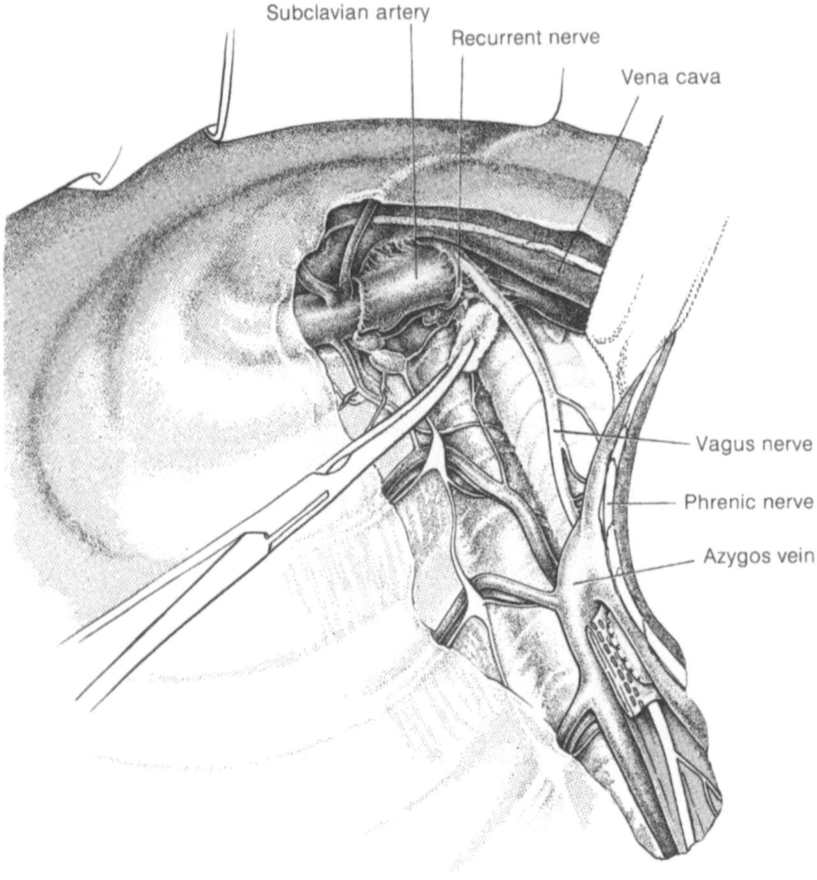

Fig. 18. Removal of the paratracheal and superior tracheobronchial lymph nodes

tion is carried toward the opposite side until the loop of recurrent nerve about the aortic arch is visualized. The dissection is carried inferiorly as far as the diaphragm. Finally the paraesophageal region and hilar vessels are inspected for remaining lymph nodes.

Drainage and closure of the chest are described on p. 121.

1.3.2.6 Right Pneumonectomy with en bloc Removal of the Lymph Nodes

As an alternative to the standard procedure of dividing the pulmonary veins first, it is possible to perform an en bloc excision of the right lung in continuity with the mediastinal lymph nodes. This procedure, described by Brock and Whytehead [10], is appropriate in cases of extensive lymph node involvement by central neoplasms. First the apical parietal pleura is incised over the subclavian vein and innominate vein. After division of the phrenic nerve and its accompanying vessels, a strip of pleura 1–2 cm wide is resected on both sides of the nerve as far as the hilum, and the azygos vein is divided between ligatures. This gives access to the lymph nodes distal to the origin of the recurrent laryngeal nerve on the great vessels as well as the paratracheal nodes between the superior vena cava and trachea. Both pleural cavities are closely adjacent in this area, so care must be taken not to enter the left pleural space. The next step is dissection of the superior tracheobronchial lymph nodes in the angle between the trachea and the upper border of the right main bronchus. With anterior traction on the vena cava, this dissection is carried medially to the aortic arch, stopping short of the loop of the recurrent nerve. Next the pulmonary artery is transected, and the hilar nodes are removed. The phrenic nerve is divided at the diaphragm with the surrounding connective tissue, and a strip of pleura 1–2 cm wide is dissected toward the hilum from the pericardium to the existing pleural incision. This is followed by division of the pulmonary ligament and removal of the lymph nodes around the inferior pulmonary vein, the remaining hilar nodes, and the paraesophageal depots. After both pulmonary veins have been ligated and divided as close to the pericardium as possible, the main bronchus and the subcarinal nodes are the only remaining hilar structures to be dealt with. Removal of the subcarinal nodes is aided by alternating traction on the lung, extending the dissection as far along the left main bronchus as possible. The presence of ramifying bronchial arteries in that area requires a meticulous dissection employing hemostats and ligatures. Finally the right main bronchus is amputated at its origin and closed, and the specimen is removed.

1.3.3 Left Pneumonectomy

1.3.3.1 Intubation

The patient is intubated with a spiral endotracheal tube. Selective intubation for one-lung anesthesia may be indicated in special cases.

1.3.3.2 Position and Approach

Right lateral decubitus, anterolateral thoracotomy in the bed of the fifth rib.

1.3.3.3 Instruments

Basic set II, extra thoracic set.

1.3.3.4 Anatomy of the Left Hilum

The left hilum is bounded anteriorly by the left phrenic nerve, which courses more anteriorly than on the right, posteriorly by the aorta, esophagus, and left vagus nerve, superiorly by the aortic arch, and inferiorly by the pericardium. The left vagus nerve runs closer to the lung than its right-sided counterpart. It crosses the aortic arch, runs backward over the pulmonary artery, and passes to the esophagus over the posterior surface of the left main bronchus. The recurrent laryngeal nerve arises from the vagus nerve at the level of the aortic arch, winds around that vessel distal to the ligamentum arteriosum, and ascends between the esophagus and trachea.

As on the right, the most anterior structure of the left hilum is the superior pulmonary vein, adjoined posteriorly by the pulmonary artery and bronchus. After crossing the left main bronchus, the pulmonary artery forms the most superior of the hilar structures and is adjoined inferiorly by the left main bronchus and pulmonary vein. The inferior pulmonary vein is located below and posterior to the superior pulmonary vein in the region of the pulmonary ligament. Fibrous bands project from the pericardium to the superior pulmonary vein, to the pulmonary artery, and pass in front of the ligamentum arteriosum to the aorta.

Variations in vascular anatomy are less common on the left side than on the right. Supernumerary pulmonary veins from the lingula have been described as well as a single venous trunk.

1.3.3.5 Operative Technique

The chest cavity having been explored (see p. 115), the hilum is identified, and the lung is retracted inferiorly to expose the aortic arch and the vagus nerve crossing it. Below the origin of the recurrent nerve, the pleura is opened anteriorly to posteriorly with a curved incision, sparing the phrenic nerve. The vagus nerve provides a useful landmark in the presence of dense adhesions or tumor infiltration. Dissecting downward or upward along the course of the nerve will lead to the major hilar structures (Fig. 19).

1.3.3.5.1 Venous Dissection. After incision of the pleura, the lung is retracted posteriorly and the pericardial extensions are divided to expose the most anterior of the hilar structures, the superior pulmonary vein. Once the vessel wall has been identified, it is cleared circumferentially by forceps or finger dissection. Proximal to the site of entry of the lingular vein, a circular ligature (0 absorbable) is passed around the common venous trunk with the aid of a dissecting forceps and tied. If the lingular vein enters the trunk too far proximally, it will require a separate ligature. Because of the shortness of the proximal vein, it is usually necessary to ligate the tributary veins separately; these are freed from connective tissue and lung parenchyma by patty dissection. Generally a trans-

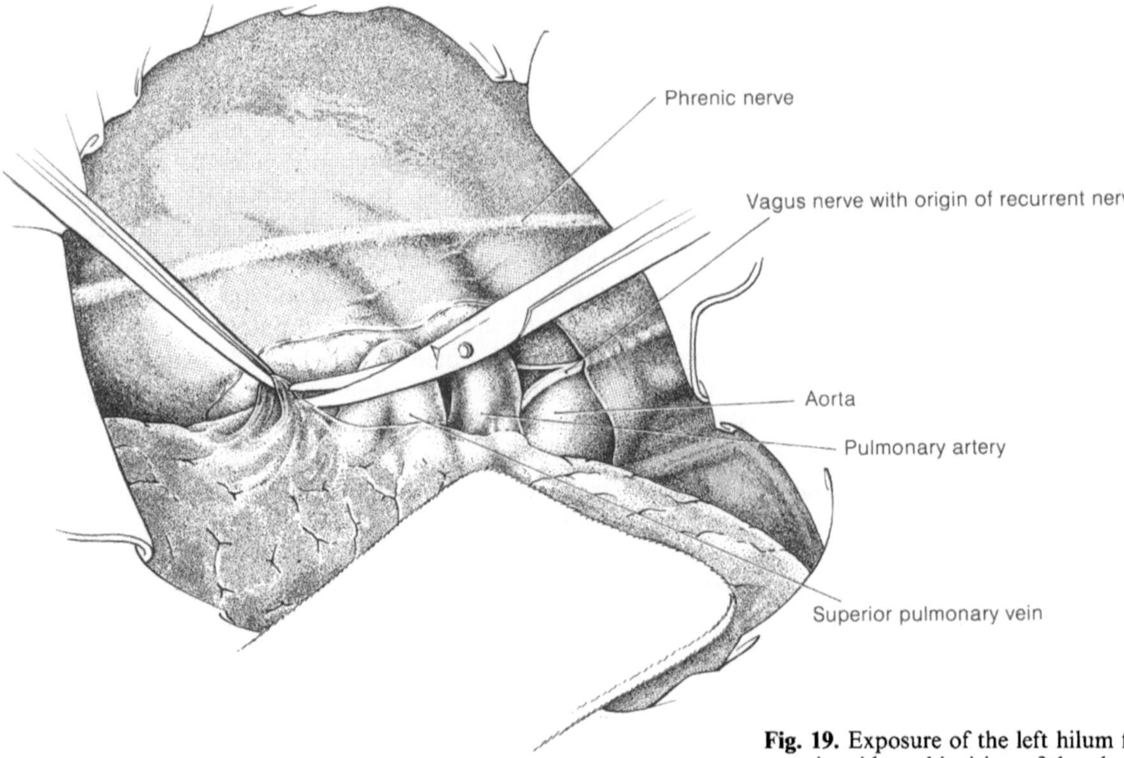

Fig. 19. Exposure of the left hilum from the anterior side and incision of the pleura

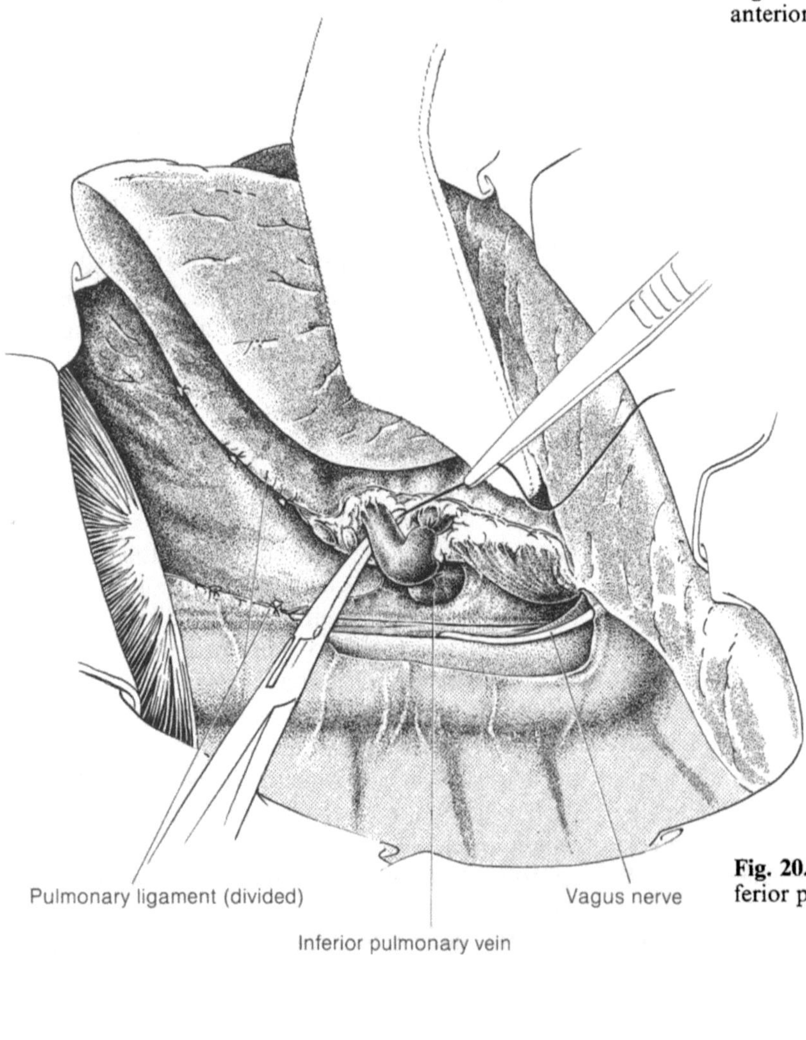

Fig. 20. Exposure and ligation of the left inferior pulmonary vein

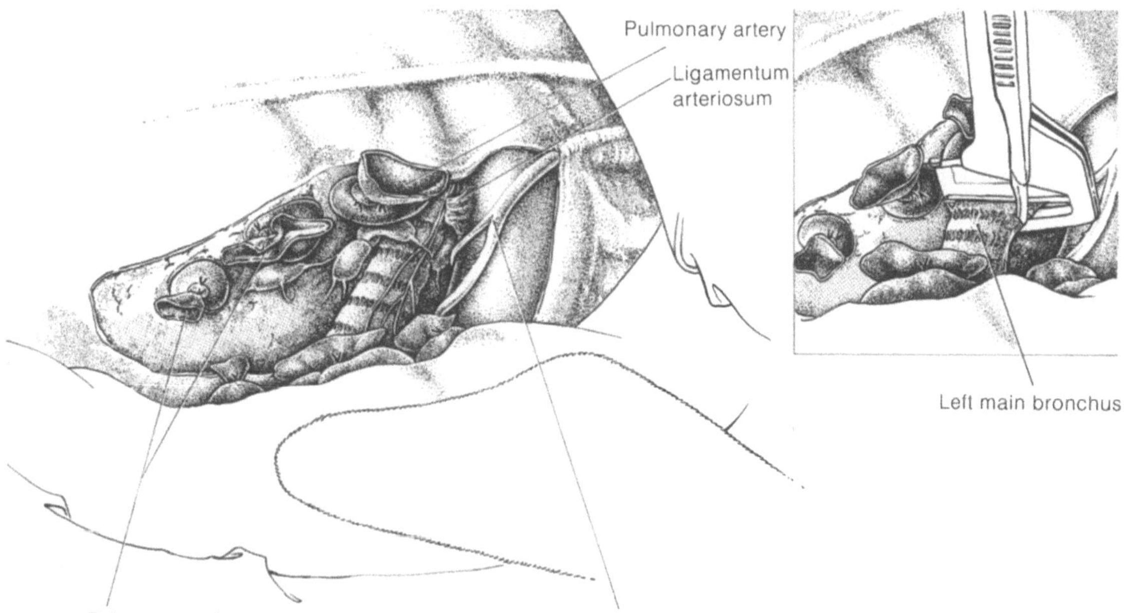

Fig. 21. a Status following division of the left pulmonary artery and left pulmonary veins. **b** Staple closure of the left main bronchus

fixion ligature (0 atraumatic absorbable suture) is placed adjacent to the proximal circular ligature before the vessel and the ligatures are cut. If only a short vascular trunk is available, it is divided between a proximal vascular clamp and distal Overholt clamp, whereupon the proximal stump is closed with continuous sutures and the distal stump with a suture ligature. When space is limited, it may be necessary to employ an intrapericardial ligature (see p. 134). The inferior pulmonary vein (Fig. 20) is exposed by retracting the lung upward and anteriorly to place tension on the pulmonary ligament, followed by division of the ligament proceeding from the diaphragm; the small vessels in the ligament are coagulated or ligated. In operations for carcinoma, it is necessary to take the lymph nodes below the vein as well as the paraesophageal nodes. Next the pleura anterior and posterior to the hilum is incised upward to the existing incision, and the inferior pulmonary vein is ligated and divided after severing any pericardial extensions, as described for the superior pulmonary vein. Alternatively, the vein may be divided between staple rows (TA 30 V 2.5 mm, white cartridge).

1.3.3.5.2 Arterial Dissection. The left pulmonary artery is longer than the right and therefore is somewhat easier to dissect. With the upper lobe retracted inferiorly, the vessel (which pulsates synchronously with the heart) can be palpated below the aortic arch. All projections of pericardium on the surface of pulmonary artery must be divided before the vessel wall can be seen, and it may also be necessary to remove lymph nodes below the aortic arch. Special attention is given to branches of the bronchial arteries in this region. The recurrent nerve may be obscured by dense adhesions or enlarged lymph nodes but can be identified by tracking the vagus nerve from both directions. The recurrent nerve should be resected only if infiltrated by tumor. After its wall has been exposed, the vessel is cleared by forceps dissection on the perivascular plane and is separated from the anterior surface of the left main bronchus. This should present no difficulties when the dissection is performed gently and on the correct plane. Alternatively, the artery may be cleared from above with the index finger, using the bronchial wall posteriorly as a guide. When the posterior wall has been cleared, a forceps is placed against the tip of the finger and is passed around the artery as the finger is withdrawn. This forceps is used to encircle the vessel with a ligature, which is tied proximally as close to the ligamentum arteriosum as possible. Usually the distal ligature can also be placed on the trunk; otherwise the first division is ligated first, followed by the rest of the vessel. The proximal ligature is always secured with a transfixion ligature (0 atraumatic absorbable suture) before cutting the vessel and the threads. Often it is safer to grasp the proximal part of the artery with a curved vascular clamp and close the stump with a double row of continuous sutures (000 atraumatic monofilament). With extensive tumor infiltration, it is best to divide the ligamentum arteriosum and ligate the left pulmonary artery close to its origin, taking care to preserve patency of the right vessel (Fig. 21).

1.3.3.5.3 Bronchial Dissection. In pneumonectomy for carcinoma, the lymphatic drainage areas below the aortic arch (in the aortic window) are removed as far as the trachea and right main bronchus at the time the left main bronchus is divided. This should include removal of the lymph nodes on the aorta (superior anterior mediastinal nodes) and the tracheobronchial nodes. While the former usually are easily accessible between the ligamentum arteriosum and vagus nerve, the deeper areas are more difficult to reach than on the right side. Division of the ligamentum arteriosum facilitates access. During removal of the lymph nodes, the feeding arteries should be carefully ligated to avoid postoperative bleeding.

While the lung is retracted anteriorly, the bronchus is dissected free from the posterior side. Often the peribronchial tissue is thickened, especially in the presence of inflammatory disease, and it must be divided down to the cartilaginous bronchial wall before the bronchus can be cleared first in its cartilaginous portion and then in its membranous portion. Access to the bifurcation can be aided if necessary by dividing the main bronchus between clamps above the origin of the upper lobe and removing the lung. With traction on the proximal clamp, the bronchus can be dissected toward the trachea, resected proximally, and closed. Special attention is given to arterial vessels arising from the aortic arch, which are ligated as required. Vagus nerve branches that pass forward to the hilum may be divided. The bronchus should be sectioned as close to the trachea as possible to avoid the formation of a blind pouch. The stapling instrument (TA 30, 4.5 mm, green cartridge) provides a simpler and more effective closure in this

Fig. 22a–c. Left supraaortic pneumonectomy

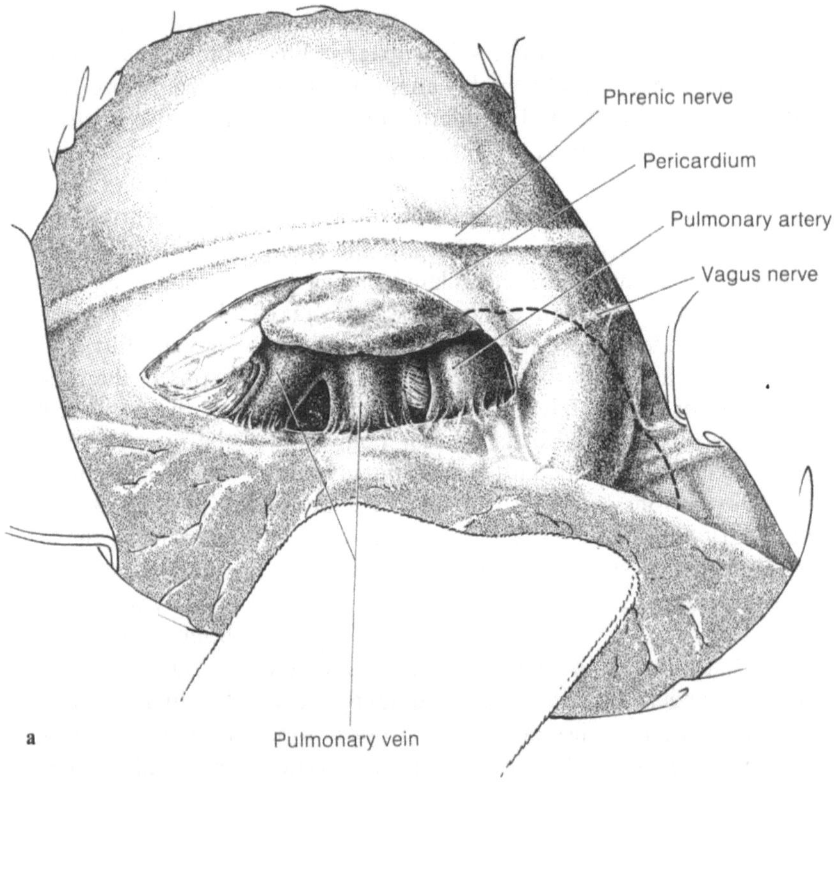

a

region, which can be difficult to suture manually. With brief retraction of the aorta and esophagus, the stapler is passed to the trachea with a vein hook and applied across the bronchus such that the membranous and cartilaginous portions of the wall are coapted. After the stapler has been fired, the bronchus is transected along the edge of the instrument with a scalpel, and the specimen is removed. If this technique is not available, the bronchus may be divided in stepwise fashion and simultaneously closed with simple interrupted sutures after first advancing the endotracheal tube into the right main bronchus for temporary occlusion of the bronchial system. Stepwise division and suturing of the bronchus facilitates placement of the sutures inasmuch as traction can be applied to the specimen as the closure is carried out.

1.3.3.5.4 Supraaortic Pneumonectomy [94]. Generally it is possible to occlude the left main bronchus with the stapling instrument below the aorta. But if this cannot be done because of the proximity of the tumor to the bifurcation, the supraaortic approach proposed by Smith and Nigam in 1979 may be used. In this approach the arch of the aorta is mobilized and retracted inferiorly (Fig. 22 a–c), and the hilar vessels are ligated intrapericardially. The mediastinal pleura is incised over the course of the aorta to expose the aorta and subclavian artery, and the vagus nerve with the origin of the recurrent nerve is isolated. The ligamentum arteriosum, the vagus nerve segment distal to the origin of the recurrent nerve, and the first three aortic branches distal to the origin of the subclavian artery are divided between ligatures. Next the aorta is dissected free on all sides and encircled from the posterior side, central to the tumor, until the bifurcation can be seen. Then the tumor is dissected from the aortic wall and esophagus, and the origin of the main bronchus is exposed. After advancing the endotracheal tube into the right main bronchus and with temporary traction on the aorta, subclavian artery, and esophagus, the left main bronchus is divided from above close to its origin, and the specimen is removed below the aortic arch. Negative margins are confirmed by frozen section, and the bronchus is closed with manual sutures. A potential exists for spinal cord ischemia due to division of the aortic branches, but the authors of the technique did not observe this complication.

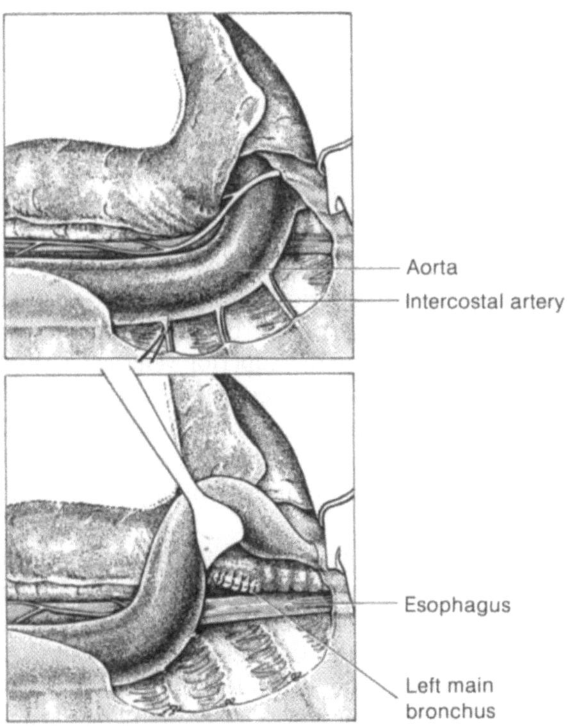

b
c

1.3.3.5.5 Lymph Node Dissection. The lymph node dissection encompasses the anterior and posterior mediastinal nodes, the superior and inferior tracheobronchial nodes, and any paratracheal nodes that were not removed during the bronchial dissection (Fig. 23).

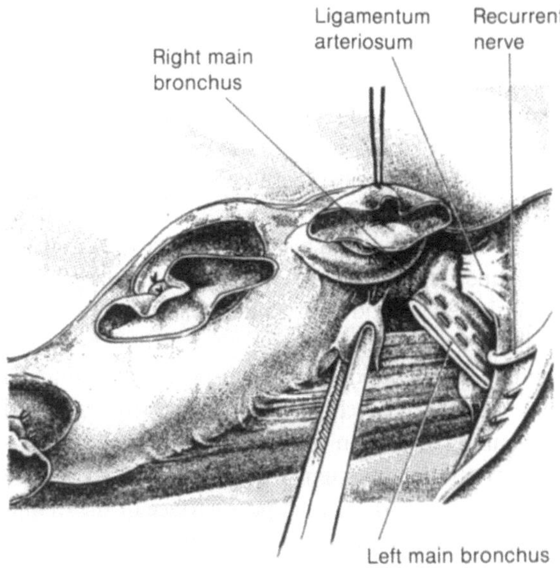

Fig. 23. Dissection of the subcarinal lymph nodes after left pneumonectomy

After incision of the pleura from the apex of the chest to the hilum, the anterior mediastinal nodes are freed from the region of the left carotid artery, left subclavian artery, innominate vein, and aortic arch. Meticulous control of all arterial and venous bleeding is necessary to avoid postoperative complications. With extensive lymph node involvement, the phrenic nerve should be resected with a strip of pleura 1–2 cm wide. The superior paratracheal nodes situated deeply between the left carotid artery and trachea are also taken while sparing the portion of the recurrent nerve ascending in that region. The superior tracheobronchial nodes are placed deeply in the "aortic window," and meticulous dissection in this area may require division of the ligamentum arteriosum. The dissection is carried inferiorly to the upper surface of the diaphragm, and extensive tumor involvement may necessitate a second division of the phrenic nerve at that level.

1.3.3.6 Left Pneumonectomy with en bloc Removal of the Lymph Nodes

On the left side the aortic arch poses an obstacle to en bloc removal of the mediastinal nodes. The lymph node dissection begins at the thoracic apex, where the phrenic nerve is identified with its accompanying vessel and divided between ligatures. A strip of pleura 1–2 cm wide over the nerve is incised as far as the hilum, and the underlying tissue on the carotid artery, subclavian artery, innominate vein, and anterior side of the aortic arch is removed. The dissection is carried above the aortic arch as far as the trachea and encompasses the "aortic window" inferiorly, which is accessible after division of the ligamentum arteriosum between clamps. The vagus nerve and recurrent laryngeal nerve are identified and preserved unless involved by tumor. The pulmonary artery and superior pulmonary vein are exposed and dealt with as previously described. Further dissection proceeds from the diaphragm to the hilum. First the phrenic nerve is divided at the diaphragm with its accompanying vessels, and it is resected with the surrounding tissue all the way to the hilum. This is followed by stepwise division of the pulmonary ligament, removal of the posterior mediastinal lymph nodes around the inferior pulmonary vein and esophagus, and ligation and division of the vessels. At that point the hilum is free except for the bronchus. As alternating traction is applied and the subcarinal nodes are dissected free, an attempt is made to expose as much of the right main bronchus as possible so that the lymph nodes in that region can be adequately cleared. The left bronchus is amputated close to its origin, and the specimen is removed.

1.3.4 Pneumonectomy with Intrapericardial Dissection of the Pulmonary Vessels

Intrapericardial dissection of the great pulmonary vessels is indicated when the extrapericardial vascular segments are involved by tumor or for the control of acute hemorrhage following injury to these vessels.

1.3.4.1 Intrapericardial Anatomy of the Great Vessels

The outer fibrous pericardium is continuous with the adventitia of the great vessels as they emerge from the pericardial sac. The inner serous pericardium is reflected onto the vessel walls and invests them to their site of origin from the heart. Both pericardial layers are separated by connective tissue at the sites of emergence of the vessels (Fig. 24). The aorta and the pulmonary trunk possess a common serosal coat, as do the pulmonary veins and atria. The resulting connections between the vessels must be divided before a particular vessel can be cleared and ligated intrapericardially. The aorta and pulmonary trunk leave the pericardium together in their common serosal sheath, their adjacent surfaces bound together by connective tissue. The *right pulmonary artery* runs transversely and emerges from the pericardium at the level of the right lateral border of the vena cava, passing between the serous and fibrous layers. Thus the vessel is covered anteriorly by a serosal coat that is crossed and interrupted by the perpendicular serosal reflection of the superior vena cava (Fig. 24). This serosa-covered segment of the right pulmonary artery forms the roof and posterior wall of the transverse sinus, a slitlike space behind the aorta and pulmonary artery within the pericardium.

The course of the *left pulmonary artery* within the pericardium is somewhat more prolonged. The anterior surface of the vessel is covered by serosa, which extends to the ligamentum arteriosum. A crescent-shaped fold of endocardium (the rudiment of a left superior vena cava) passes from

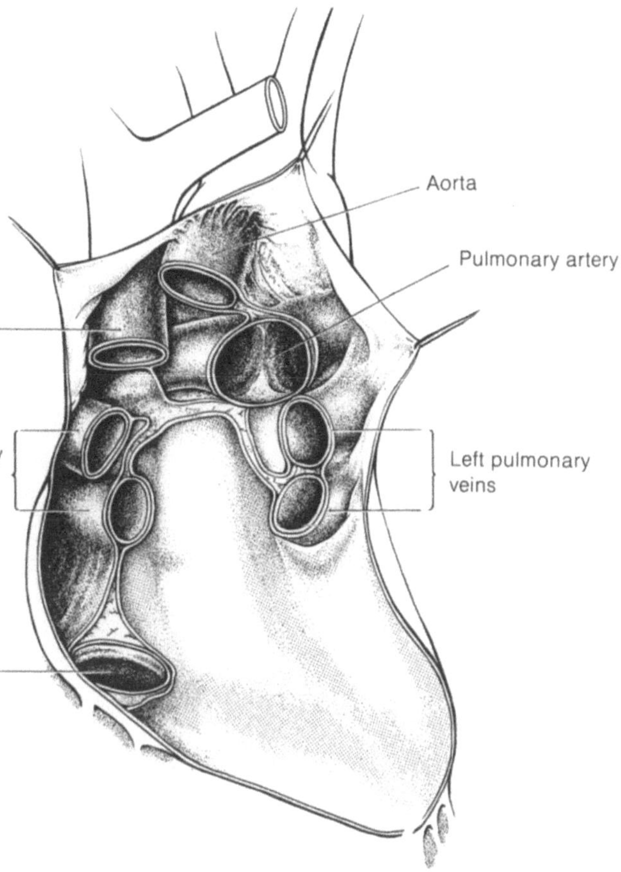

Fig. 24. Intrapericardial anatomy of the great vessels after removal of the heart

the anterior surface of the left pulmonary artery to the left atrium. The pulmonary veins and venae cavae are partially covered by serosa and are interconnected by corresponding folds. The vessels are separated from one another by small recesses. Because of the shorter intrapericardial course of the vessels on the right side, there is usually room for only one proximal ligature, requiring that the distal ligature be placed extrapericardially.

1.3.4.2 Intrapericardial Dissection of the Right Pulmonary Vessels

Steps in procedure:

(1) Pericardotomy, incision of the serosa over the pulmonary artery at the lateral border of the superior vena cava or between the aorta and superior vena cava; artery is cleared and ligated
(2) Incision of the serosal connections between the pulmonary veins parallel to course of the vessels
(3) Encircling of the superior pulmonary vein after division of the posterior serosal connections
(4) Encircling of the inferior pulmonary vein after incision of the serosal folds to the inferior vena cava and superior pulmonary vein

The pericardium behind the phrenic nerve is picked up on a needle in a needle holder, incised longitudinally with a knife or scissors, and opened superiorly and inferiorly to expose the right atrium and intrapericardial segment of the vena cava (Fig. 25). The serosa-covered pulmonary veins present behind the vena cava, and the pulmonary artery above it.

The *pulmonary veins* pass separately, or rarely as a single trunk, to the left atrium. Their dissection begins by dividing the serosal connections in the recesses between the adjacent vessels, keeping the incisions parallel to the vascular long axis. The serosa is reflected onto the superior pulmonary vein from its posterior side. As the vessel is cleared with the fingertip or dissecting forceps, this serosa must be incised before a ligature can be applied. The inferior pulmonary vein is connected to the superior pulmonary vein and to the inferior vena cava by serosal folds, both of which must be di-

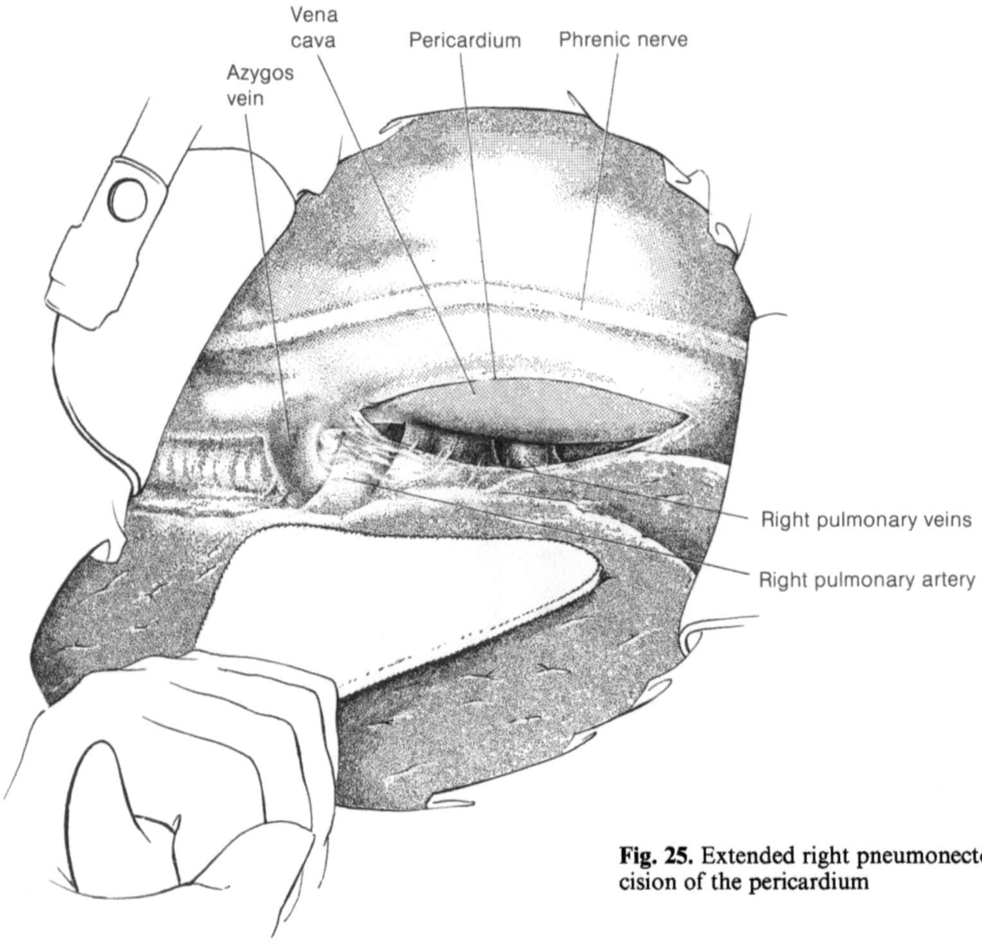

Fig. 25. Extended right pneumonectomy, status after incision of the pericardium

vided to avoid injury to the left atrium. After the vessel has been encircled, it is ligated and divided as in a standard pneumonectomy.

The *right pulmonary artery* is exposed by retracting the vena cava medially, a maneuver which unfolds the retrocaval recess over the artery. The vessel is identified by its pulsations and by the bulge of the serosa. The latter is incised along the upper and lower border of the vessel, the arterial wall is dissected free, and the artery is cleared with the forefinger or dissecting forceps. Alternatively, the pulmonary artery may be approached between the aorta and the superior vena cava. With opposite traction applied to both vessels, the serosa over the pulmonary artery is incised, and the vessel is exposed. A proximal circular ligature is applied and secured with a transfixion ligature, the distal ligature is applied (usually extrapericardially), and the artery is transected.

The pericardial incision is left open. Larger defects should be partially closed with interrupted sutures or patched with a strip of dura.

1.3.4.3 Intrapericardial Dissection of the Left Pulmonary Vessels

Steps in procedure:

(1) Exposure of the pulmonary artery after division of the ligamentum arteriosum (sparing the recurrent nerve) and the connective tissue fibers extending to the left atrium
(2) Ligation and division of the artery
(3) Incision of the serosal connections between the pulmonary veins; veins are cleared, ligated, and divided

The pericardium is picked up in front of the lung and behind the phrenic nerve and incised longitudinally with a knife or scissors. Using digital guidance, the incision is extended superiorly to the level of the aortic arch and downward to the level of the inferior pulmonary vein (Fig. 26)

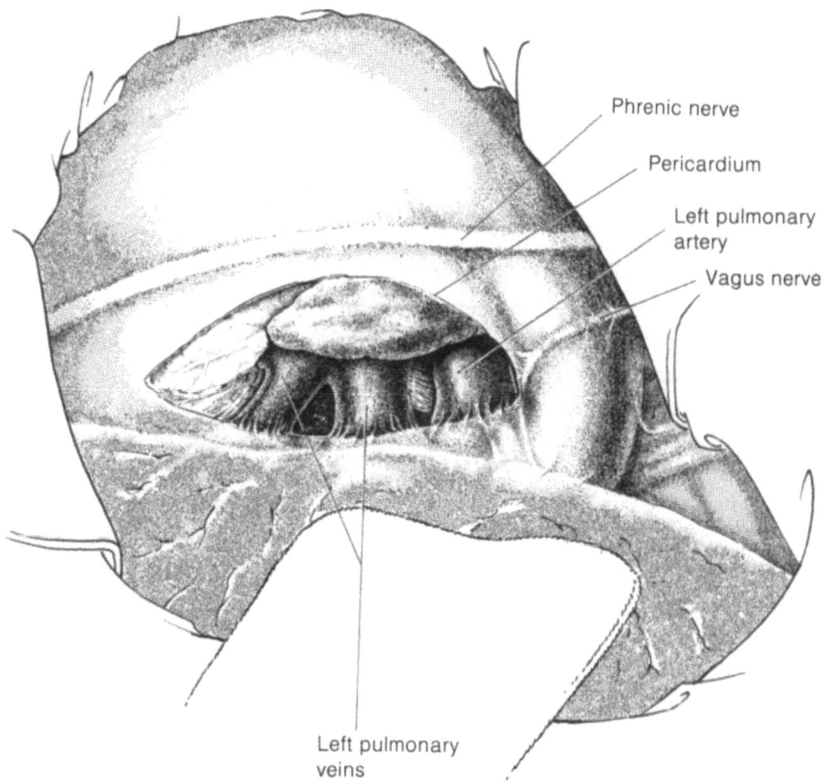

Fig. 27. Extended left pneumonectomy, status after incision of the pericardium

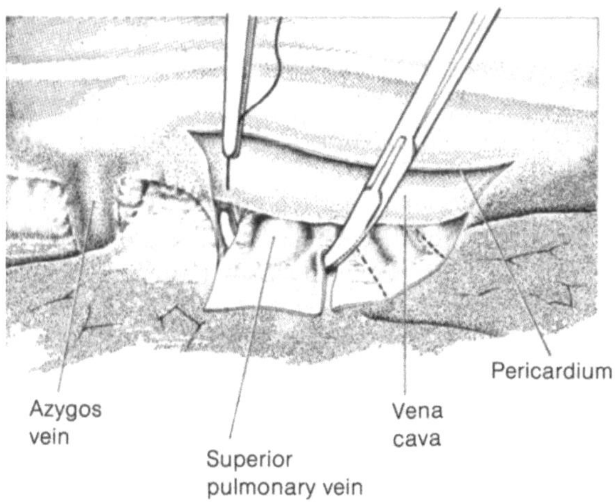

Fig. 26. Extended right pneumonectomy. Technique for encircling the superior pulmonary vein

As on the right side, the *left pulmonary veins* are interconnected by serosa, although no connection exists on the left between the inferior pulmonary vein and inferior vena cava. The serosal folds become tense when the vein is encircled and can be divided on the fingertip or open forceps. Ligation and division of the vessels is performed in standard fashion. Instead of dealing with both veins separately, their site of entry into the left atrium may be divided between clamps (Satinski) and thc proximal stump closed with a double row of continuous sutures (3-0 atraumatic monofilament).

Exposure of the *pulmonary artery* is aided by dividing the ligamentum arteriosum (sparing the recurrent nerve) so that the pericardial cavity is opened from above. The pericardial fibers at the upper margin of the vessel and the connective tissue fibers extending from the lower margin to the left atrium are also incised to a point where the vessel can be bluntly cleared with a finger or forceps and snared with a suture. Division of the ligamentum arteriosum also helps to avoid kinking and potential thrombosis of the right pulmonary artery. Owing to the long vascular trunk of the pulmonary artery, it is usually possible to place both arterial ligatures intrapericardially on the left side.

The pericardium is left open. Larger incisions are closed or partially closed with interrupted sutures or a dural graft (Fig. 27).

1.3.4.4 Pneumonectomy with Intrapericardial Dissection of the Pulmonary Vessels and en bloc Resection of the Lymph Nodes

Brock and Whytehead [10], Cahan et al. [11], and others routinely dissect the pulmonary vessels intrapericardially in pneumonectomies on the strength of observations that central carcinomas frequently spread along the adventitia of the great vessels to the pericardial reflection. Factors that do not favor routine intrapericardial dissection are the higher complication rates and the current lack of proof that it benefits the prognosis. The procedure combines the en bloc resection with intrapericardial dissection of the great pulmonary vessels (see above).

1.4 Lobectomy

1.4.1 Indications

Lobectomy has gained wide acceptance on the grounds that, by preserving healthy lung parenchyma, the risks and late sequelae of pulmonary resection are diminished. Lobectomy is appropriate for malignant tumors that are confined to one lobe of the lung. While pneumonectomy offers no advantages over lobectomy in terms of removal of the *intrapulmonary* lymph nodes, the potential for eradicating the *extrapulmonary* nodes is judged to be different in lobectomy and pneumonectomy, especially with regard to the subcarinal group. However, these nodes, too, are accessible in lobectomy, so there should be no basic objection to this operation even when the mediastinal lymph nodes are found to be involved by metastasis.

The indication for lobectomy can be extended to proximal, bilateral upper lobe tumors and left upper lobe tumors by including a bronchial sleeve resection and removing a segment of the pulmonary artery (see pp. 170ff.).

1.4.2 Right Upper Lobectomy

1.4.2.1 Intubation

Spiral endotracheal tube. The tube should be long enough to be advanced into the left main bronchus if necessary.

1.4.2.2 Position and Approach

Left lateral decubitus, anterolateral thoracotomy in the bed of the 4th–5th rib.

1.4.2.3 Instruments

Basic set II, extra thoracic set.

1.4.2.4 Basic Surgical Anatomy

The *pulmonary artery* typically sends a large anterior branch, the truncus anterior, to the right upper lobe. It divides into a superior branch for the apical segment (A1) and an interior branch for the anterior segment (A3). Farther distally, in the interlobar region, one or two smaller branches are distributed to the posterior segment (A2). Often this segment is additionally supplied by vessels that cross the oblique fissure from the superior segment of the lower lobe (A6). In rare cases a common trunk will exist for all three segments (Fig. 28).

The *veins of the right upper lobe* (Fig. 2) unite to form three collecting vessels: the apical vein (V1), the anterior vein (V3) coursing between the middle and upper lobes, and the posterior vein (V2) coursing in the interlobar fissure between the posterior segment and lower lobe. The veins from the upper lobe unite with the middle lobe veins to form the superior pulmonary vein. The apical vein and anterior vein often are the first structures encountered during dissection from the mediastinum. The posterior vein arises more deeply and runs anterior to the interlobar portion of the pulmonary artery and posterior to the anterior segmental bronchus. Generally the three veins form an obvious trifurcation; they may unite close to the junction of the middle lobe veins. In 15%–20% of cases [40] the anterior vein drains into a middle lobe vein, or a middle lobe vein drains into an upper lobe vein. Rarely, the superior and inferior pulmonary veins merge outside the pericardium to form a common trunk.

The short trunk of the right *upper lobe bronchus* generally trifurcates into three segmental divisions. In anomalous cases the upper lobe bronchus may arise directly from the trachea or bifurcation, the middle lobe bronchus may originate from the upper lobe bronchus, or the upper lobe bronchus may show only two divisions, with a third segmental division arising from the trachea or middle lobe bronchus.

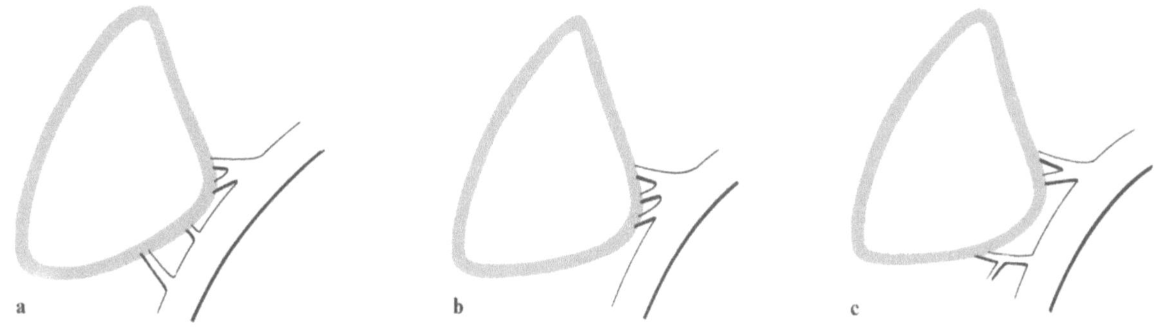

Fig. 28 a–c. Variations of arterial supply to the right upper lobe

1.4.2.5 Operative Technique

Steps in procedure:

(1) Separation of adhesions
(2) Incision of the pleura anteriorly below the arch of the azygos vein to the lower margin of the superior pulmonary vein
(3) Snaring of right pulmonary artery (tourniquet)
(4) Exposure, ligation and division of the superior (three) branches of the pulmonary vein from the anterior side, sparing the tributaries from the middle lobe
(5) Exposure, ligation and division of the upper lobe arteries from the anterior side (truncus anterior) and interlobar aspect (A2), sparing the superior segmental branch to the lower lobe (A6)
(6) Exposure and transection of the upper lobe bronchus from the posterior side; division of additional vessels to the upper lobe
(7) Division of parenchymal connections with the middle lobe and the superior segment of the lower lobe
(8) Removal of lymph nodes (intrapulmonary sump, mediastinal nodes)

The first step is to free the lobe from the apex of the chest in stepwise fashion, taking care to preserve the superior vena cava and azygos vein, especially when extensive adhesions are present (see p.115). The pleura is opened with a curvilinear incision over the hilum starting anteriorly at about the lower border of the superior pulmonary vein and extending posteriorly to a point below the arch of the azygos vein. If bleeding is anticipated during further dissection, it is wise to encircle the pulmonary artery with a tourniquet so that bleeding can be controlled promptly. The artery is found at the upper pole of the hilum by identifying the pulsating truncus anterior below the azygos vein and following it centrally. Pericardial extensions may have to be divided before the vessel can be dissected free.

1.4.2.5.1 Venous Dissection. For the anterior phase of the dissection, the lung is retracted posteriorly so that the superior pulmonary vein can be

Fig. 29. a Exposure of the superior pulmonary vein. **b** Ligation and division of the right upper lobe veins and truncus anterior

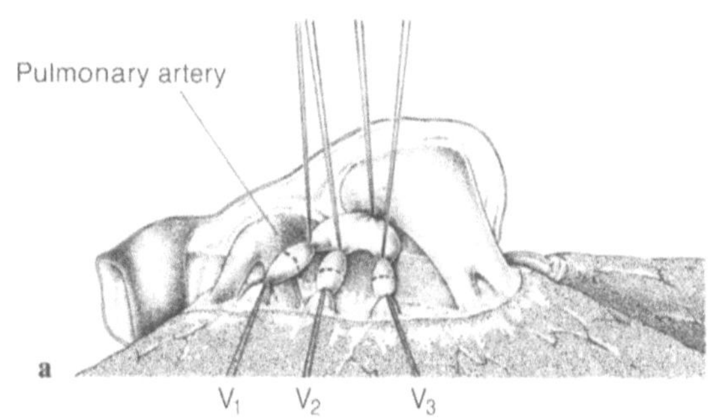

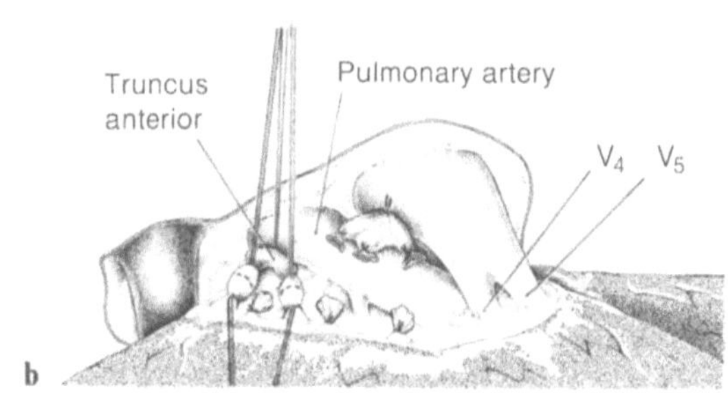

seen. After the connective tissue over the vessel has been incised and any intervening lymph nodes have been freed, the vein is traced distally to its tributaries (Fig. 29 a). Special attention is given to the course of the posterior vein (V2). It passes forward over the interlobar segment of the pulmonary artery, which may be injured if the dissection is carried too deeply. At the same time, it is necessary to preserve the venous drainage of the middle lobe, which should present no difficulties if the transverse fissure is well developed and the venous branches can be dissected. If the middle lobe cannot be positively identified, the inferior branches of the pulmonary vein are not ligated until the end of the operation, by which time the upper lobe will be clearly defined. After the vein has been cleared, the common venous trunk is ligated close to the pericardium (0 absorbable suture), and distal ligatures are placed on the individual branches. Before the vessel is transected, a proximal transfixion ligature (0 absorbable thread) is applied to prevent slippage of the proximal ligature (Fig. 29 b,c).

1.4.2.5.2 Arterial Dissection. Generally the arterial branches to the right upper lobe are dissected from both the anterior aspect (truncus anterior) and the interlobar aspect (branches to the posterior segment, A2). The lung is retracted inferiorly for ligation of the truncus anterior. This vessel is the first pulsating structure to be encountered below the azygos vein. It is directly anterior to the upper lobe bronchus and may be covered by the apical vein (V1), which is divided in the initial step. Pericardial fibers usually project onto the truncus anterior and have to be divided. The truncus anterior and its two branches to the anterior (A3) and apical (A1) segments are ligated, and the vessel is transected.

The remaining arterial branches are most easily approached through the interlobar fissure (Fig. 30). If the pulmonary fissures are well developed, the pulmonary artery will be found at about the point of convergence of the transverse and oblique fissures and can be palpated in that area. The middle lobe is retracted anteriorly and the lower lobe posteriorly. The connective tissue at the base of the fissure can then be incised longitudinally in small steps. Lymph nodes signify proximity of the vessel and usually have to be freed before the artery, recognized by its pulsations and the pale color of its wall, can be visualized. The perivascular sheath is incised over the course of the vessel, and

Fig. 30. Interlobar exposure of the right pulmonary artery

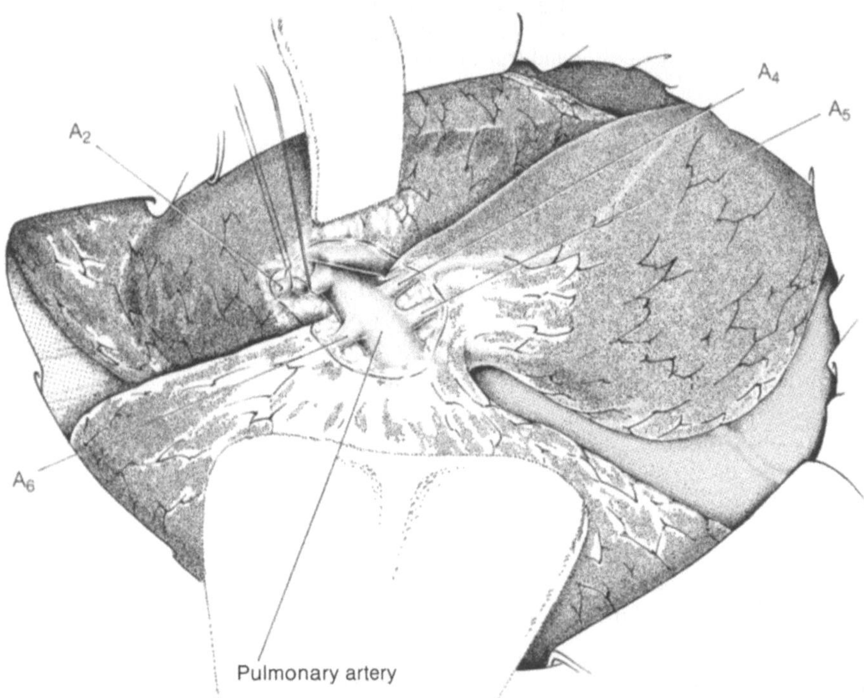

the arterial branches are exposed: One or two branches pass anteriorly to the middle lobe (A 4,5), and one branch at the same or lower level (or occasionally at a higher level!) passes posteriorly to the superior segment of the lower lobe (A6). The posterior segmental branch to the upper lobe (A2) arises at once from the main trunk and runs posteriorly; it is divided between ligatures after the other branches have been identified. In some cases the arteries to the posterior upper lobe segment or accessory branches (25%) are not seen until dissection of the main bronchus and are dealt with at that time.

The interlobar artery can be difficult to identify if the fissures are not well developed. If the boundary between the upper and lower lobes is obscure, the subpleural anterior branch to the lower lobe segments can be identified in the fissure between the middle and lower lobes and traced toward the hilum until the pulmonary artery and its branches are visualized. Alternatively, the posterior segmental artery may be approached from the posterior aspect [72] after exposure of the bronchus (see below).

1.4.2.5.3 Bronchial Dissection. The upper lobe bronchus is exposed from the posterior side. The lung is reflected anteriorly, and the pleura is incised posterior to the hilum. The upper margin of the right main bronchus is palpable posteriorly, below the azygos vein. The bronchus travels a short distance before giving rise to the upper lobe bronchus, whose superior border is usually well defined. Generally there is a lymph node in the peribronchial tissue at the inferior border of the upper lobe bronchus which marks the origin of the intermediate bronchus and the upper end of the oblique fissure [40, 72]. After incision of the peribronchial tissue, the upper lobe bronchus is cleared circumferentially by blunt dissection with the finger or forceps, staying on the bronchial wall to avoid injuring the pulmonary artery, which is directly anterior to the bronchus. Large bronchial arteries are occasionally found in close proximity to the bronchus, especially in inflammatory lung diseases, and these need to be ligated before the bronchus is severed. After the bronchus has been cleared on all sides, it is occluded with the TA 30 stapling instrument (3.5 mm, blue cartridge) (Fig. 31 a). Finally the bronchus is clamped distally and transected along the edge of the stapling instrument with a scalpel (Fig. 31 b,c). The bronchus also may be divided between clamps or in open fashion, in which case the endotracheal tube is temporarily advanced into the left main bronchus, or the divided bronchus is directly occluded through the operative field (Fig. 32 a,b). After the bronchus has been divided, the pulmonary artery can be seen in its interlobar course, and the posterior segmental artery and any accessory branches to the upper lobe may be ligated, if this has not already been done.

If the fissures are incomplete, the residual lung can be inflated slightly to define the boundaries of the atelectatic upper lobe. Parenchymal connections usually exist with the middle lobe and the superior segment of the lower lobe; these are most easily divided by stapling with the TA 30 instrument, preserving essential vessels (Fig. 33). Dissection along the interlobar venous branches is a more tedious process that often results in parenchymal fistulas. At the end of the operation the bronchus and parenchyma are immersed in saline to exclude air leak. Larger pulmonary fistulas are oversewn (2-0 or 3-0 atraumatic absorbable monofilament), and smaller fistulas are sealed with fibrin glue. The margins of the specimen are examined to assess the need for additional resection.

1.4.2.5.4 Lymph Node Dissection. The major areas of concern in the lymph node dissection are the "intrapulmonary sump" around the right intermediate bronchus and the extrapulmonary nodes (superior mediastinal, paratracheal, and superior and inferior tracheobronchial nodes). The posterior mediastinal nodes generally are not involved by upper lobe tumors. Following the lobectomy, all the lymph nodes surrounding the intermediate bronchus and pulmonary artery are removed, if possible carrying the dissection distally to the origin of the middle lobe bronchus. As described for right pneumonectomy, the extrapulmonary lymph node groups are exposed by incising the pleura from the thoracic apex to the hilum and are cleared as far as the right tracheobronchial angle and the left main bronchus below the bifurcation. Postoperative bleeding from these areas is not uncommon, so very careful attention is given to hemostasis. We do not recommend dividing the pulmonary ligament to aid expansion of the residual lung, as this may lead to kinking of vessels in the remaining lobes.

Chest tube insertion is described on p. 120.

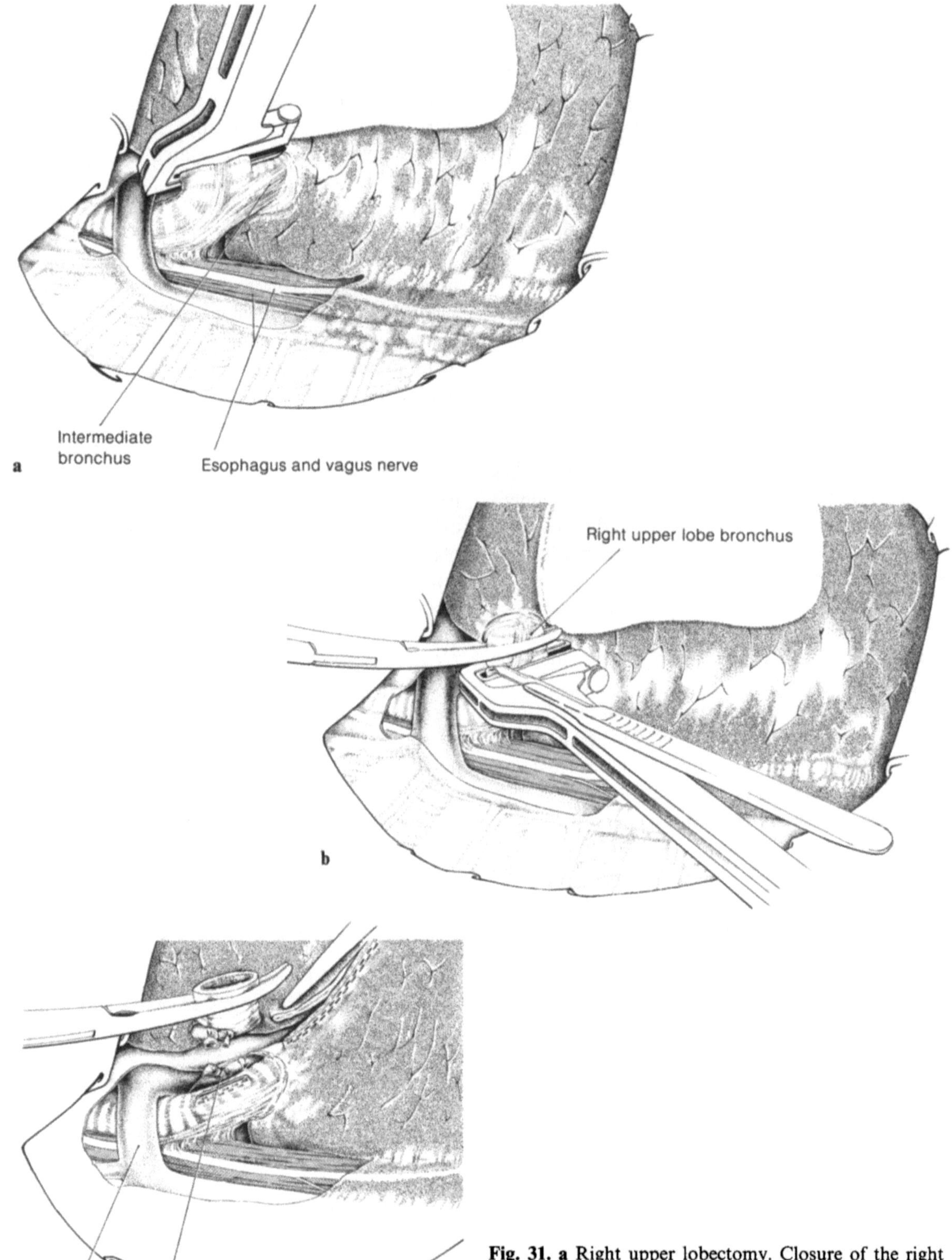

Fig. 31. a Right upper lobectomy. Closure of the right upper lobe bronchus with the TA stapling instrument. **b** Right upper lobectomy. Division of the bronchus after insertion of the staples. **c** Right upper lobectomy. Status following transection of the bronchus

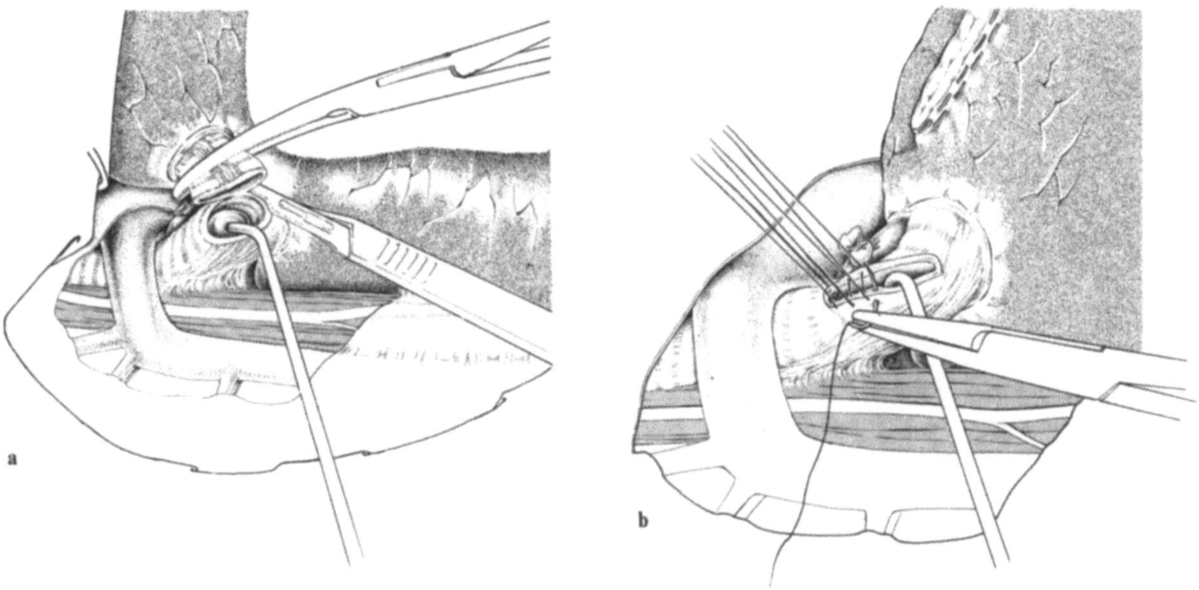

Fig. 32. a Right upper lobectomy. Occlusion of the bronchus through the operative field. **b** Right upper lobectomy. Open transection of the bronchus and closure with manual sutures

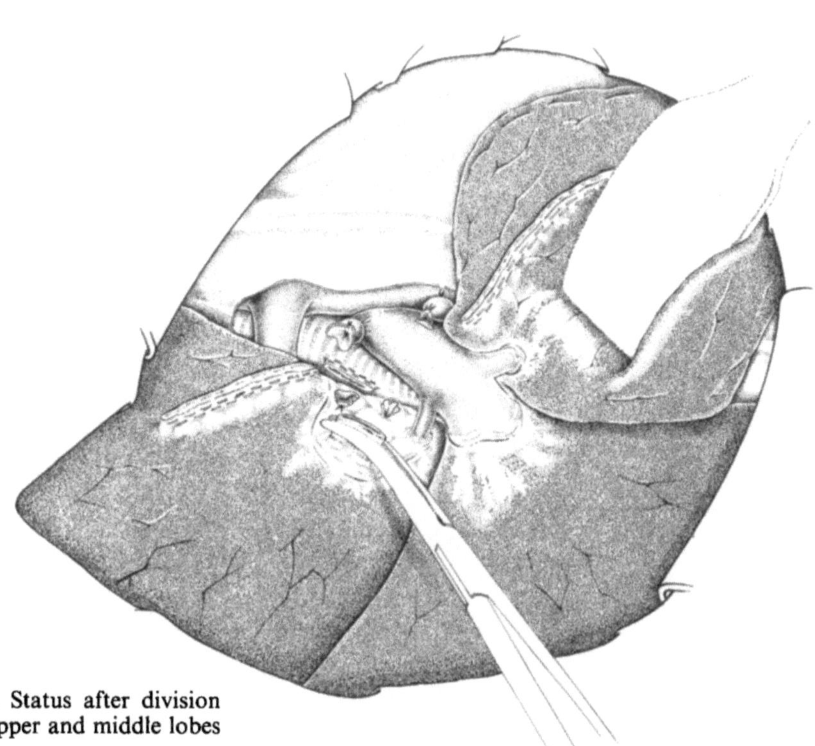

Fig. 33. Right upper lobectomy. Status after division of the parenchyma between the upper and middle lobes with the stapling instrument

1.4.3 Middle Lobectomy

1.4.3.1 Indications

Lobectomy is not considered an adequate operation for carcinoma of the middle lobe because 1) centrally located tumors frequently involve the bronchial divisions of the lower lobe and 2) the lymph node dissection would pose a significant risk of vascular injury if only the middle lobe were removed. Elimination of the lymphatic sump is accomplished more simply and effectively by combining middle lobectomy with removal of the upper or lower lobe.

Removal of the middle lobe alone is acceptable for benign tumors and inflammatory diseases that cannot be managed by a wedge resection. Dissection is often made difficult in these cases by the presence of dense adhesions and enlarged lymph nodes. The lobe may be best approached anteriorly or through the interlobar fissure, depending on circumstances. Especially when dense adhesions are present, it is a good precaution to encircle the pulmonary trunk with a tourniquet before beginning the dissection.

1.4.3.2 Intubation

Spiral endotracheal tube.

1.4.3.3 Position and Approach

Left semilateral position, anterolateral thoracotomy in the bed of the fifth rib.

1.4.3.4 Instruments

Basic set II, extra thoracic set.

Steps in procedure:

(1) Exposure of the arteries and bronchus through the interlobar fissure
(2) Occlusion and division of the arteries and bronchus, sparing A6 and the lower lobe bronchus
(3) Exposure, ligation and division of middle lobe veins in the depths of the interlobar fissure
(4) Division of parenchymal connections with the upper and lower lobes
(5) With dense interlobar adhesions: dissection of the veins, bronchus, and artery from the anterior side

1.4.3.5 Basic Surgical Anatomy

The middle lobe consists of a lateral (S4) and a medial segment (S5), which usually are supplied by two equal-size branches of the middle lobe bronchus. The segments are not delimited by septa, which can make isolated removal difficult unless a stapling device is used. The middle lobe is supplied with equal frequency by one or two arterial branches arising from the interlobar portion of the pulmonary artery. One branch arises opposite the origin of the superior segmental artery of the lower lobe (A6), and the second branch, if present, arises at a more proximal level, covered by the parenchyma of the upper lobe. In rare cases an atypical branch arises from the middle lobe arteries and passes to the upper lobe; it should be preserved. In half the population the superior pulmonary vein receives one tributary vessel from the middle lobe. In the remaining half there are two or more branches, which may drain into a segmental vein of the upper lobe (14%), into the inferior pulmonary vein (8%), or in rare cases may communicate directly with the left atrium [40].

1.4.3.6 Interlobar Approach

In this approach the arterial and bronchial dissections are carried out via the interlobar fissure. The vein also may be exposed through this approach or from the anterior side. As in the upper lobectomy, the pulmonary artery is exposed in the interlobar space at the level of the transverse fissure, its sheath is incised, and the vessel is followed into the upper lobe (Fig. 34 a). If dense adhesions are present, it may be easiest to locate the anterior branch of the basilar artery (A8) and follow it toward the hilum. The superior segmental artery (A6) is seen running posteriorly from the parent vessel. Opposite and anteriorly are one or two arterial branches to the middle lobe, and at a more proximal level the posterior segmental artery may be seen coursing upward and backward to the upper lobe. It is common for scarred lymph nodes to hamper the dissection. If the anatomic relations are absolutely clear, the surgeon may proceed with ligation of the middle lobe arteries; otherwise he should change to the anterior approach (see below). Division of the arterial vessels between ligatures gives access to the underlying middle lobe bronchus, which presents deep in the interlobar fissure. The bronchus may be temporarily clamped

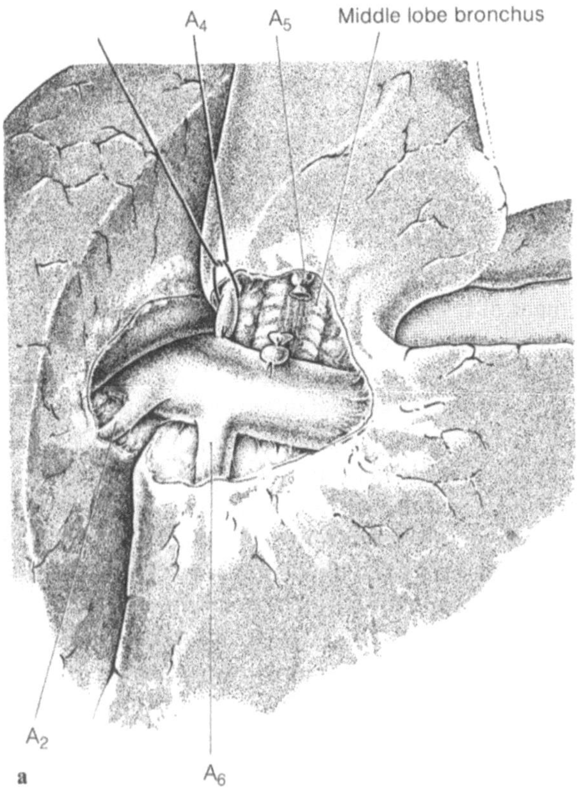

a

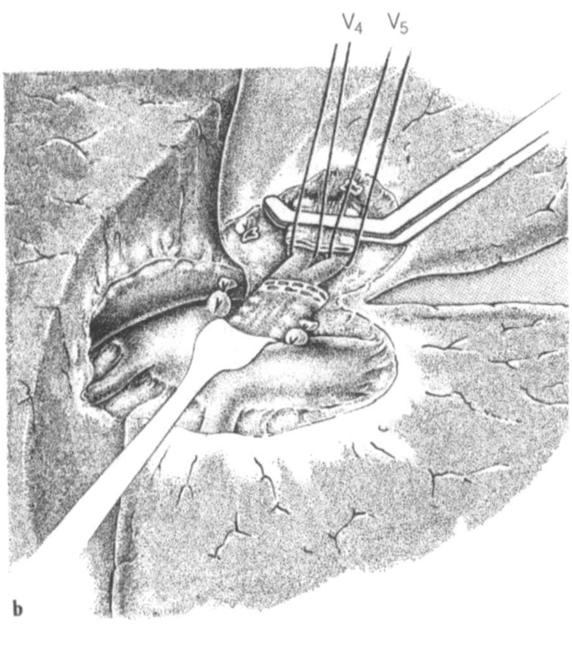

b

Fig. 34. a Middle lobectomy. Interlobar exposure of the arteries. **b** Middle lobectomy. With the bronchus divided, the veins of the middle lobe bronchus are snared

to determine whether it is in fact the lobar bronchus or merely a segmental bronchus. The lower lobe bronchus also should be clearly identified at this time. The middle lobe bronchus is clamped distally, transected close to its origin, and closed with an interrupted suture line (2-0 absorbable); usually there is not enough room for stapling. Next the middle lobe vein is identified farther anteriorly (Fig. 34 b). It is divided between ligatures at this time, assuming this was not done initially from the anterior side.

Because the transverse fissure is rarely complete, it is usually necessary to inflate the residual lung slightly before the middle lobe can be distinguished from the rest of the lung, especially from the upper lobe. Division of the incomplete fissure with thc TA stapling instrument is recommended. By contrast, the middle lobe generally has only minimal connections with the lower lobe, and these may be divided between clamps or rows of staples. After removal of the specimen, the bronchial stump and parenchyma are checked for air leak, and fibrin glue is applied as necessary to secure aerostasis.

1.4.3.7 Anterior Approach

An anterior hilar exposure (Fig. 35 a,b) can be employed for all dissections when adhesions preclude the interlobar approach. The pleura anterior to the hilum is incised, the upper lobe vein is identified, and thc vcsscls draining the middle lobe are divided between ligatures. The branches of the superior pulmonary vein must be clearly exposed at this stage so that anomalies and atypical connections with the veins of the upper and lower lobe can be recognized. The middle lobe bronchus or its segmental divisions are identified posterior to the middle lobe vein. The bronchus is temporarily clamped to verify that the superior segmental bronchus and lower lobe bronchus are not constricted. Then the bronchus is transected close to its origin and closed with simple interrupted sutures. The distal stump is retracted to give access to the more deeply situated pulmonary artery and its branches to the middle lobe. The pulmonary artery is easiest to identify when the middle lobe is well defined and the vessels entering the parenchyma can be visualized. The remaining steps in the procedure are like those in the interlobar dissection.

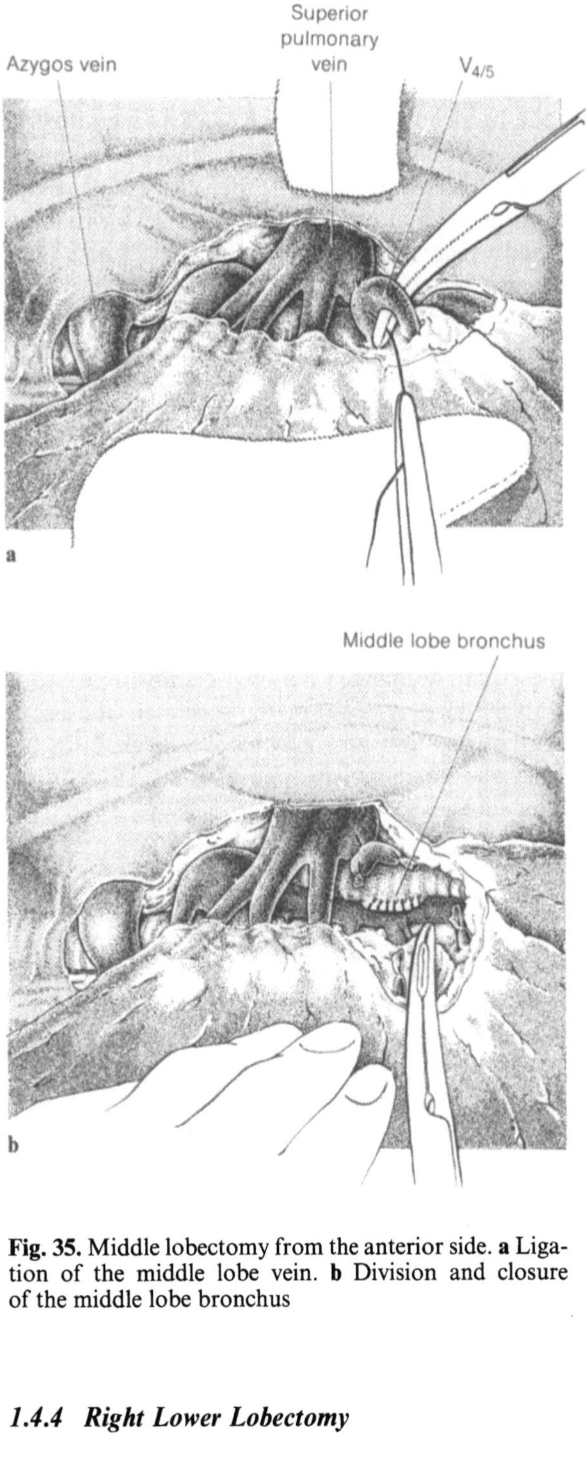

Fig. 35. Middle lobectomy from the anterior side. **a** Ligation of the middle lobe vein. **b** Division and closure of the middle lobe bronchus

1.4.4 Right Lower Lobectomy

1.4.4.1 Intubation

Spiral endotracheal tube.

1.4.4.2 Position and Approach

Left lateral decubitus, posterolateral or anterolateral thoracotomy in the bed of the fifth rib.

1.4.4.3 Instruments

Basic set II, extra thoracic set.

1.4.4.4 Basic Surgical Anatomy

The right *lower lobe bronchus* splits into five segmental bronchi. The bronchus to the superior segment of the lower lobe (S6) arises posteriorly from the intermediate bronchus, opposite the middle lobe bronchus or at a slightly lower level. Occasionally an accessory fissure is present which separates the superior segment of the lower lobe from the basal segments. The absence of this fissure implies an absence of interlobar septa [35], so that resection of this segment must be performed through lung parenchyma. In rare cases (5%–6% [40]) the superior segment is supplied by two segmental bronchi.

As the lower lobe bronchus continues distally, it gives origin to the medial basal bronchus (No. 7) and the anterior basal bronchus (No. 8) before bifurcating into the terminal branches for the laterobasal (S9) and posterobasal (S10) segments.

The *pulmonary artery* descends lateral to the main bronchus and is the first structure to be encountered in the interlobar fissure. The segmental arteries usually arise superior to the corresponding bronchi. The superior segment of the lower lobe is supplied by one arterial branch in 80% of cases and by two or more branches in 20% [40]. A common artery may supply the posterior segment of the upper lobe (10% [40]), in which case it is necessary to preserve that branch when ligating the arteries of the superior lower lobe segment. Often this anomaly is not appreciated until the lymph nodes in the interlobar fissure have been freed, and it must be excluded before vascular ligatures are applied. Artery A7 is the first branch given off by the basilar artery after it enters the lower lobe; it may possess a common trunk with A8. Finally the artery divides into branches A9 and A10, which, because of their relations, are commonly regarded as a unit [106].

The *inferior pulmonary vein* generally receives three major tributaries from the right lower lobe. The apical vein enters from above; its horizontal branch runs between segment S6 and the basal segments and receives blood from both sides. The basal vein passes between segments S7/8 and S9/10 to the hilum, and the paramediastinal vein is between segments S7 and S10.

1.4.4.5 Operative Technique

Steps in procedure:

(1) Separation of adhesions
(2) Placement of tourniquet around the pulmonary artery
(3) Division of pulmonary ligament from the posterior side, incision of the pleura posteriorly over the lower hilum as far as the upper lobe bronchus and anteriorly to the superior pulmonary vein
(4) Exposure, ligation and division of the inferior pulmonary vein from the posterior side
(5) Interlobar exposure of the arteries; separate ligation and division of A6 and the basilar artery, protecting A4 and A5
(6) Exposure and division of the bronchus in the interlobar fissure, sparing the middle lobe bronchus
(7) Division of parenchymal attachments with the posterior upper lobe segment and middle lobe
(8) Lymph node dissection (subcarinal, posterior, mediastinal)

It is occasionally necessary, after opening the chest, to separate adhesions between the lower lobe and the parietal pleura posteriorly, in the costophrenic angle, and toward the pericardium (see p. 115). If the anatomy is obscure, especially in the interlobar fissure, the pulmonary trunk should be encircled with a tourniquet before further dissection is carried out to provide immediate control of any bleeding that may occur.

1.4.4.5.1 Venous Dissection. The veins of the right lower lobe are exposed by retracting the lung anteriorly and superiorly and dividing the pulmonary ligament between clamps or after vascular cautery, beginning at the diaphragm. All lymph nodes that are encountered, including the paraesophageal nodes, are removed. The pleura is then incised over the posterior hilum to the level of the upper lobe bronchus and anteriorly to the superior pulmonary vein, so that the wall of the inferior pulmonary vein can be dissected free and the tributaries from the superior and basal segments can be identified (see Fig. 14). The main trunk is cleared circumferentially with incremental sizes of dissecting forceps. Before ligatures are applied, it is necessary to exclude anomalous drainage of the middle lobe vein into the lower lobe vein or the presence of only one pulmonary vein. The proximal ligature is placed as close to the pericardium as possible, and distally the individual branches are isolated and ligated, leaving a sufficiently long vascular stump. The proximal ligature is secured with a transfixion ligature (2-0 absorable atraumatic suture), and the vein is divided.

1.4.4.5.2 Arterial Dissection. The arteries of the right lower lobe are approached through the interlobar fissure (Fig. 36). The key landmark in this region is the juncture of the oblique and transverse fissures, where the pulmonary artery is palpable, and perivascular nodes indicate the course of the vessel. The lymph nodes are dissected free, and the perivascular sheath is incised. If the anatomy is obscured by adhesions, the surgeon may dissect centrally along the anterior branch (A8) of the basilar artery, or he may enter the oblique fissure from the posterosuperior aspect: The lymph node at the inferior margin of the upper lobe bronchus marks the upper end of the oblique fissure. Immediately below that is the superior segmental artery of the lower lobe (A6). It leads to the interlobar portion of the pulmonary artery, which may be followed toward the hilum and also peripherally until the typical branching pattern is recognized. Directly opposite A6 one or two arteries arise to supply the middle lobe (A4 and A5). At a more cranial level the segmental artery A2 passes posteriorly to the upper lobe, while distally, below the origin of A6, the arterial trunk splits into three or four basilar divisions. The importance of preserving atypical branches from A6 to the upper lobe was previously noted (Fig. 28). Given the pattern of branching of the lower lobe arteries, it generally is not possible to interrupt the arterial supply to the lower lobe with a single ligature. To preserve the blood supply to the middle lobe, the segmental artery A6 must be divided separately between ligatures. If the vessel gives off an upper lobar branch (which is often covered by lymph nodes), the ligature is placed distal to the origin of the atypical branch. The basilar trunk of the pulmonary artery is cleared and ligated in the perivascular plane, while two to four separate ligatures are placed farther distally, regardless of the branching pattern. A proximal transfixion ligature is applied, the vessel is transected, and the ends of the ligatures are cut (Fig. 36).

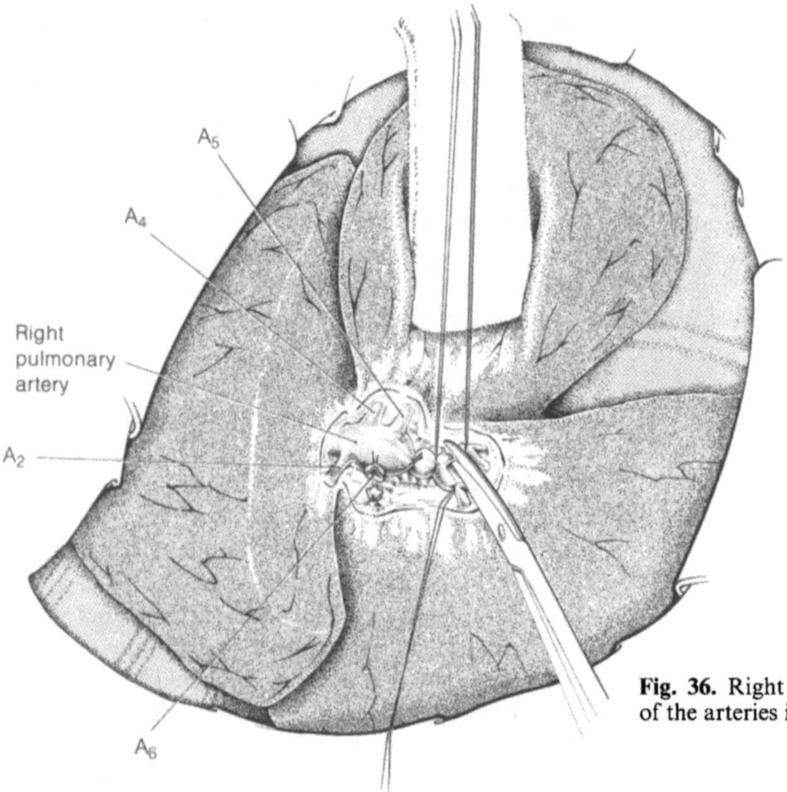

Fig. 36. Right lower lobectomy. Ligation and division of the arteries in the interlobar fissure

1.4.4.5.3 Bronchial Dissection. The right lower lobe bronchus presents in the interlobar fissure below and medial to the divided pulmonary artery. It is freed from surrounding connective tissue from the interlobar and posterior sides, simultaneously removing all accessible lymph nodes. Bronchial arteries in proximity to the bronchus are ligated at the level of the proposed point of transection. Analogous to the ligation of the lower lobe arteries, it is usually necessary to handle the superior segmental bronchus and the basilar bronchus separately in order to preserve ventilation of the middle lobe. The superior segmental bronchus is transected about 3 mm distal to its origin and closed with simple interrupted sutures (2-0 or 3-0 absorbable atraumatic), and the rest of the bronchus is occluded with the TA 30 stapler (3.5 mm, blue cartridge). If the superior segmental bronchus originates below the level of the middle lobe bronchus, the stapler can be applied obliquely above its origin, and the entire lower lobe bronchus can be occluded with one staple line (Fig. 37 a,b). Before the staples are inserted, it is recommended that the patency of the middle lobe bronchus be confirmed by observing its ventilation (Fig. 38).

After the vessels and bronchus have been divided, it remains to separate the superior segment of the lower lobe from the posterior segment of the upper lobe. This is done by means of traction on the hilar structures and blunt dissection. After careful inflation of the residual lung, the lobar boundaries are identified, and the pleura is incised. Thick parenchymal connections are most easily divided with the TA 90 stapler (4.8 mm, green cartridge), dividing the tissue on the lower lobe side with the scalpel. Finally the operative site is immersed in saline to check for air leaks, which are repaired as necessary with fibrin glue.

1.4.4.5.4 Lymph Node Dissection. Dissection of the regional lymph nodes following the lobectomy includes the nodes of the intrapulmonary lymphatic sump around the right intermediate bronchus. The structures to the middle lobe are preserved, even though this makes for a less radical excision. The dissection is carried to the bifurcation, taking the subcarinal nodes; the posterior mediastinal nodes in the pulmonary ligament and the paraesophageal nodes are additionally removed. Careful consideration should be given to a lower lobectomy when the superior tracheobronchial and paratracheal nodes are found to be involved by tumor. In these cases it is appropriate to weigh the risks of pneumonectomy, which provides clearance of

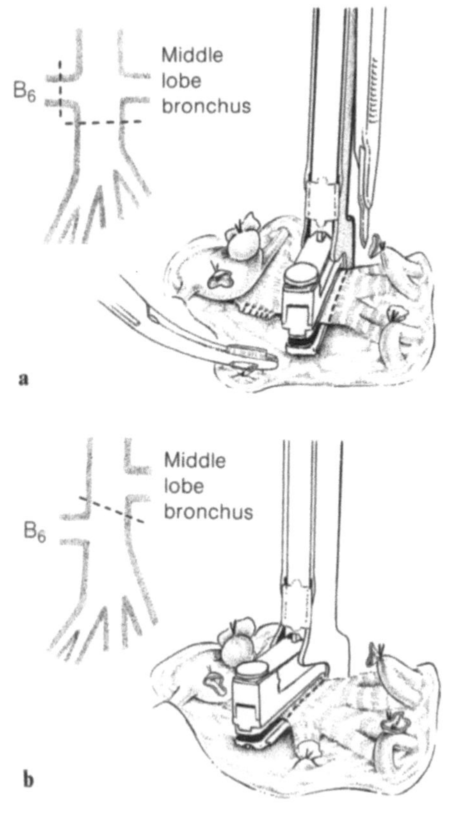

Fig. 37 a, b. Right lower lobectomy. Separate (**a**) and common (**b**) occlusion of the segmental bronchus B6 and the basal segmental bronchi

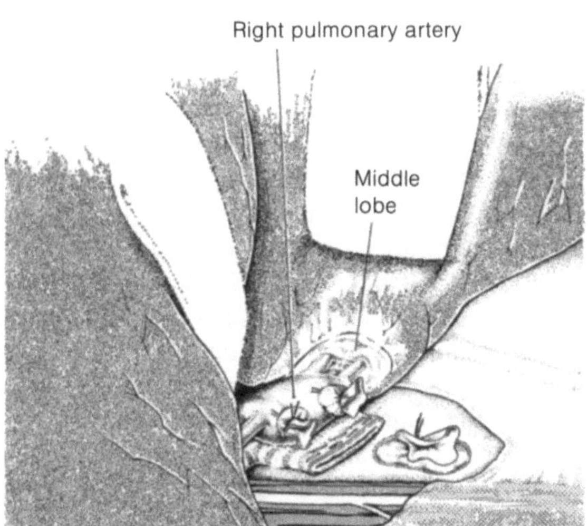

Fig. 38. Right lower lobectomy. Status after removal of the right lower lobe

all accessible nodes, against the functional advantages of lobectomy.

Drainage and closure of the chest are described on p. 120.

1.4.5 Upper Bilobectomy

1.4.5.1 Indications

Upper bilobectomy is appropriate for tumors or inflammatory diseases involving the upper and middle lobes or the intermediate bronchus in cases where pneumonectomy is not acceptable.

1.4.5.2 Operative Technique

The extent of disease is established by venous dissection from the anterior side, arterial dissection in the interlobar fissure, and bronchial dissection from the posterior side. This is especially important in cases where extension to a right pneumonectomy is not an acceptable option. The possibility of extending the procedure to a sleeve resection, with or without segmental resection of the pulmonary artery, is also assessed (see p. 174).

The technique of operation corresponds to that described for the resection of individual lobes. Ligation of the inferior pulmonary vein is sufficient, barring anomalies, to occlude the venous drainage of the upper and middle lobes. The interlobar dissection reveals the typical branching pattern of the pulmonary artery, and ligatures are placed in a way that preserves the blood supply to the lower lobe, especially to its superior segment. The middle lobe bronchus is generally handled through the interlobar fissure, while the upper lobe bronchus is transected from the posterior side.

1.4.5.3 Lymph Node Dissection

As in upper lobectomy, the lymph node dissection includes the paratracheal, superior and inferior tracheobronchial, and anterior mediastinal nodes. All accessible nodes about the intermediate bronchus and pulmonary artery are additionally removed to eradicate most of the intrapulmonary lymphatic sump.

Chest tube insertion is described on p. 120

1.4.6 Lower Bilobectomy

1.4.6.1 Indications

Removal of the middle and lower lobes is indicated for tumors or inflammatory diseases that involve both lobes. It is appropriate for lower lobe tumors with extensive metastasis about the intermediate bronchus to ensure removal of the intrapulmonary lymphatic sump.

1.4.6.2 Approach

Anterolateral thoracotomy in the bed of the fifth or sixth rib or posterolateral thoracotomy in the bed of the sixth rib.

1.4.6.3 Operative Technique

The advantage of lower bilobectomy over lower lobectomy is that it ensures concomitant removal of the right intermediate bronchus, thus eliminating the intrapulmonary lymphatic sump. The posterior approach to the bronchus is more favorable than dissecting from the interlobar or anterior aspect. Even in resections for benign disease, preliminary ligation and division of the veins and arteries facilitates the dissection of the intermediate bronchus.

As in the technique for individual lobectomy, the middle lobe tributary to the superior *pulmonary vein* is exposed and ligated from the anterior side, while the inferior pulmonary vein is exposed and ligated posteriorly after division of the pulmonary ligament.

The *pulmonary artery* is exposed in the interlobar fissure, and its typical branches to the three pulmonary lobes are identified. If there is a sufficiently long trunk between the posterior segmental artery (A2) and the arteries passing anteriorly to the middle lobe, the proximal ligature is placed at that site, and the common vessel for the middle and lower lobes is transected after distal ligation of the individual branches (Fig. 39 a). Otherwise the middle lobe arteries, the superior segmental artery, and the trunk of the basilar artery will have to be ligated and divided separately (Fig. 39 b). In all cases atypical branches to the upper lobe arising from A6 or a middle lobe artery should be identified and preserved.

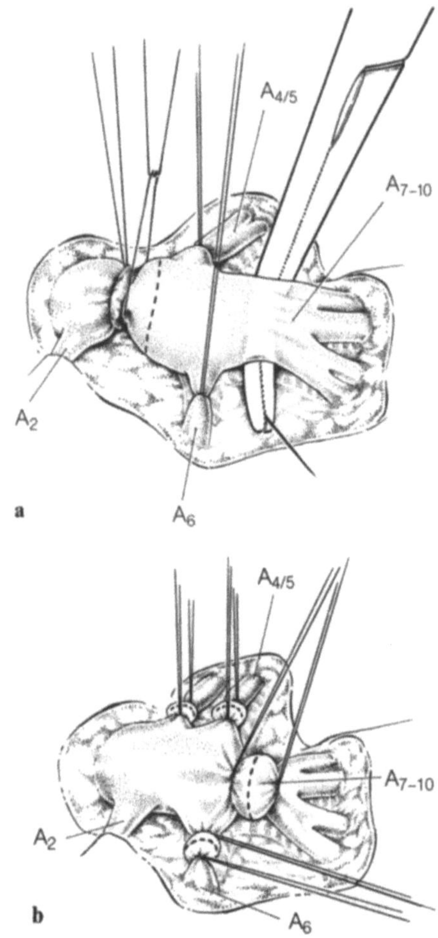

Fig. 39 a, b. Right lower bilobectomy. Options for vascular ligation. **a** Common ligation of the segmental arteries. **b** Separate ligation of the segmental arteries

The *intermediate bronchus* is generally exposed through the interlobar fissure, or it may be approached from the posterior aspect of the hilum (Fig. 16). The start of the intermediate bronchus distal to the origin of the upper lobe bronchus is marked with reasonable consistency by a lymph node at the bifurcation; this node is in close proximity to a bronchial artery. The peribronchial tissue is incised, and the bronchus is carefully cleared circumferentially with dissecting forceps. The pulmonary artery is in direct contact with the bronchus, so the plane of the dissection must be kept on the bronchial wall to avoid trauma to that vessel. Previous isolation of the artery through the interlobar field is also helpful in this regard.

Dissection of the bronchial wall is carried inferiorly until the stapling instrument can be applied just below the origin of the upper lobe bronchus.

The instrument is fired, and the bronchus is transected at that level (Fig. 40). The distal portion is occluded with a clamp. If the fissures are incomplete, the residual lung is carefully inflated to define their boundaries, and parenchymal connections are divided with the TA stapler.

Chest tube insertion is described on p. 120.

1.4.7 Left Upper Lobectomy

1.4.7.1 Intubation

Spiral endotracheal tube. The tube should be long enough to be advanced into the right main bronchus if necessary.

1.4.7.2 Position and Approach

Lateral position, anterolateral thoracotomy in the bed of the fourth rib or (rarely) posterolateral thoracotomy in the bed of the fifth rib.

1.4.7.3 Instruments

Basic set II, extra thoracic set.

Steps in procedure:

(1) Separation of adhesions
(2) Curved incision of the pleura over the hilum below the aortic arch, sparing the phrenic nerve
(3) Snaring of the pulmonary artery (tourniquet)
(4) Exposure, ligation and division of the superior pulmonary vein from the anterior side
(5) Arterial dissection from the superior and interlobar aspect, preserving the superior segmental artery
(6) Bronchial dissection from the interlobar aspect; with a short trunk, separate division of the branches to the upper lobe and lingula
(7) Division of the parenchymal connections with the lower lobe
(8) Lymph node dissection (intrapulmonary lymphatic sump, superior and inferior tracheobronchial nodes, paratracheal nodes, anterior mediastinal nodes)

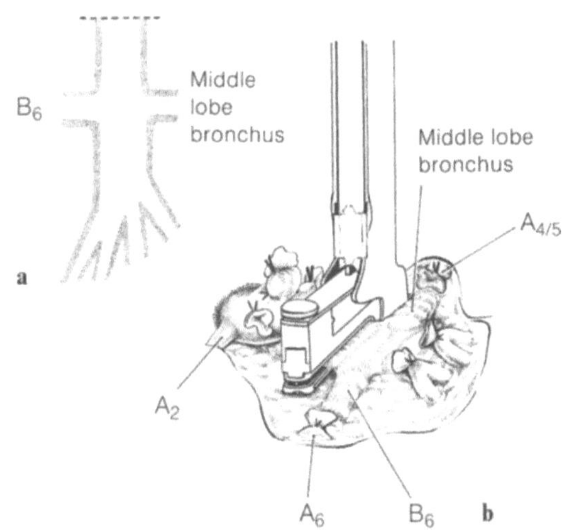

Fig. 40a, b. Right lower bilobectomy. Staple closure of the intermediate bronchus

1.4.7.4 Basic Surgical Anatomy

The left *upper lobe bronchus* arises from the anterolateral surface of the left main bronchus and divides into a superior and inferior branch. The superior branch sends a twig to the anterior segment of the upper lobe (S3) and a common twig to the apical (S1) and posterior segments (S2). The inferior branch is the lingular bronchus, which itself divides into superior and inferior divisions (S4 and S5). The bifurcational pattern predominates; trifurcation of the left main bronchus or upper lobe bronchus is seen rarely.

The left *pulmonary artery* crosses the left main bronchus and passes behind the upper lobe bronchus to the posterior surface of the lower lobe. Between four and eight segmental arteries (usually five or six) arise from the arch of the pulmonary artery and are distributed to the individual segments of the upper lobe, entering them from the anterior or posterior side (Fig. 41 a). There is no exact counterpart of the truncus anterior on the left side, although the first branch of the pulmonary artery is larger than on the right, and it supplies the anterior segment (A3) and usually a neighboring segment as well. The lingular segmental arteries frequently arise from a common trunk that originates opposite or distal to the superior segmental artery of the lower lobe. In 20%–30% of the population the lingular branches arise directly from the arch of the pulmonary artery, and in 8% the lingula is supplied entirely by one ascending branch [40]. Atypical arteries may traverse

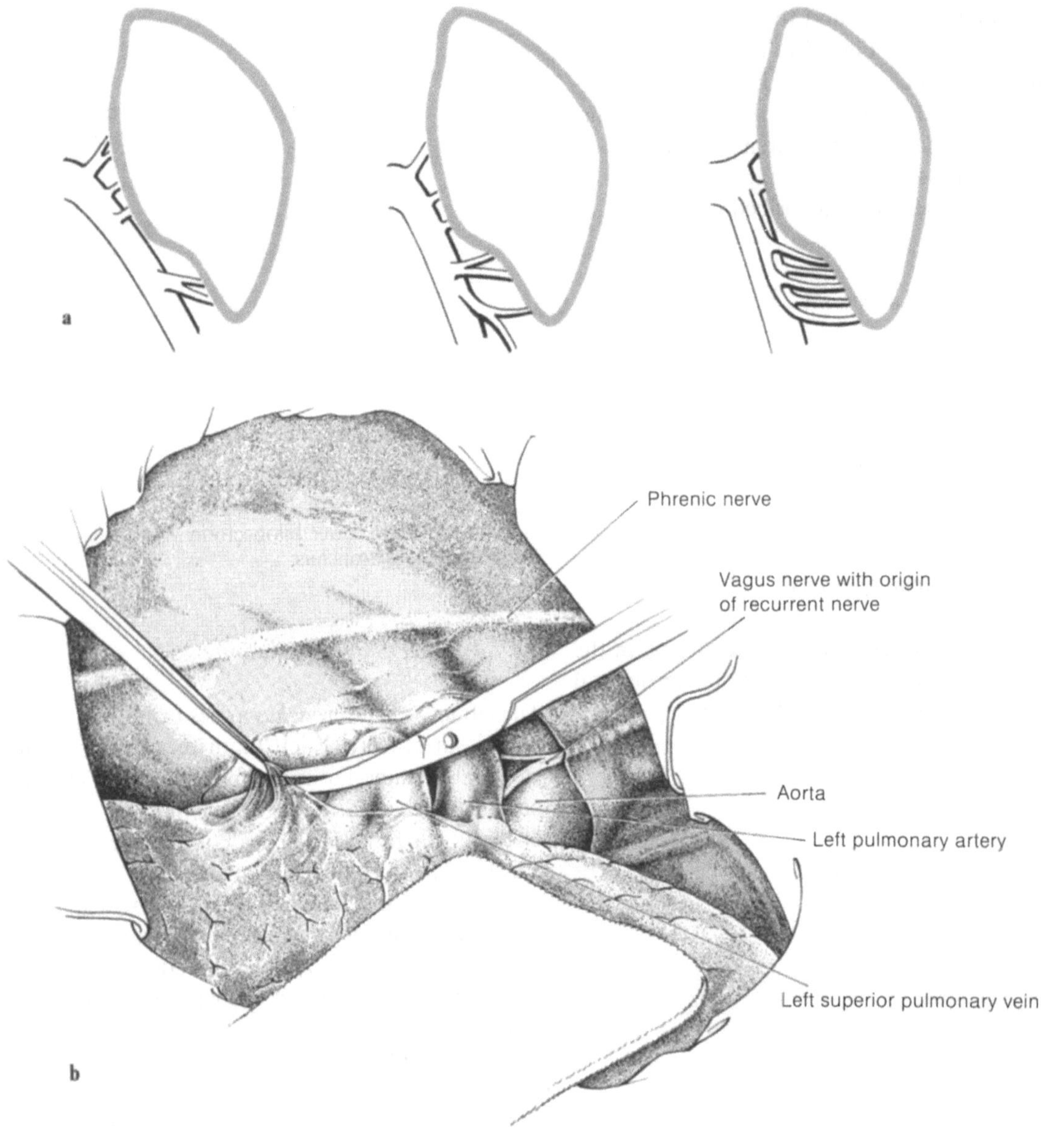

Fig. 41 a, b. Left upper lobectomy. **a** Variations of arterial supply. **b** Incision of the pleura over the hilum from the anterior side

the parenchymal tissue between the apex of the lower lobe and the posterior upper lobe (see Fig. 41 a).

The *four veins* of the left upper lobe (apical posterior veins V1 and V2, anterior vein V3, lingular veins V4 and V5) merge to form the superior pulmonary vein. These are accompanied in one-third of cases by a superior hilar vein that courses on the pulmonary artery and must be divided before the artery can be dissected free. The lingular veins may also drain into the inferior pulmonary vein, and the superior and inferior pulmonary veins may form a common extrapericardial trunk.

1.4.7.5 Operative Technique

Steps in procedure:

(1) Separation of adhesions
(2) Placement of tourniquet around the pulmonary artery
(3) Division of the pulmonary ligament from the posterior side, incision of the pleura from the front of the hilum posteriorly to the center of the hilum
(4) Exposure, ligation and division of the inferior pulmonary vein from the posterior side
(5) Exposure, ligation and division of the arteries through the interlobar fissure, sparing the branches to the lingula
(6) Exposure of the bronchus from the posterior or interlobar aspect, transection below the origin of the upper lobe bronchus
(7) Division of parenchyma between the upper lobe and lingula
(8) Lymph node dissection (intrapulmonary sump, subcarinal nodes, posterior mediastinal nodes)

Following thoracotomy, separation of adhesions (see p. 115, and assessment of local disease, the hilum is exposed, and the vagus nerve is identified on the aortic arch along with the loop of recurrent nerve arising from the vagus. The pleura is opened with a curved incision that starts on the anterior side of the hilum (sparing the phrenic nerve) and extends posteriorly between the lung and vagus nerve, below the aortic arch.

1.4.7.5.1 Venous Dissection. Primary ligation and division of the pulmonary vein facilitates subsequent exposure of the arterial vessels. The pulmonary vein, which may be covered by lymph nodes, is the most anterior hilar structure and lies within connective tissue that is reflected off the vessel wall by patty dissection. After incision of the vascular sheath, the vein is carefully encircled with incremental sizes of dissecting forceps and then ligated close to the pericardium (No. 0 absorbable suture). The vessel may have dense posterior connections with the bronchus, so the dissection in that area must be done with extreme care. With traction placed on the ligature to make the vein tense, the tributary vessels are dissected free. The second ligature may be placed proximal to the tributaries, or the latter may be ligated separately, depending on the length of the trunk. A transfixion ligature is carefully placed to secure the proximal tie, and the vessel is divided. Alternatively, the vein may be divided between two rows of staples applied with the TA 30 instrument (2.5 mm, white cartridge).

1.4.7.5.2 Arterial Dissection. Before the individual arterial branches of the left upper lobe are exposed, the pulmonary trunk should be encircled with a tourniquet to allow for immediate control of hemorrhage (Fig. 42). For this purpose the apex of the lung is retracted inferiorly. The pulmonary artery is palpable following reflection of the connective tissue. Any pericardial extensions are divided with a scissors, and the vascular sheath is entered. Dissecting forceps are used to further isolate the vessel and separate it from the underlying bronchus until it can be encircled with a tourniquet. This maneuver also may be done with the index finger, which then serves as a guide for passing a dissecting forceps around the vessel and introducing the tourniquet, which is placed distal to the recurrent nerve and proximal to the origin of the first branch of the pulmonary artery.

The interlobar fissure is entered from above by incising the pleura over the artery, and the plane between the lobes is progressively developed by scissors dissection until the arterial branches are

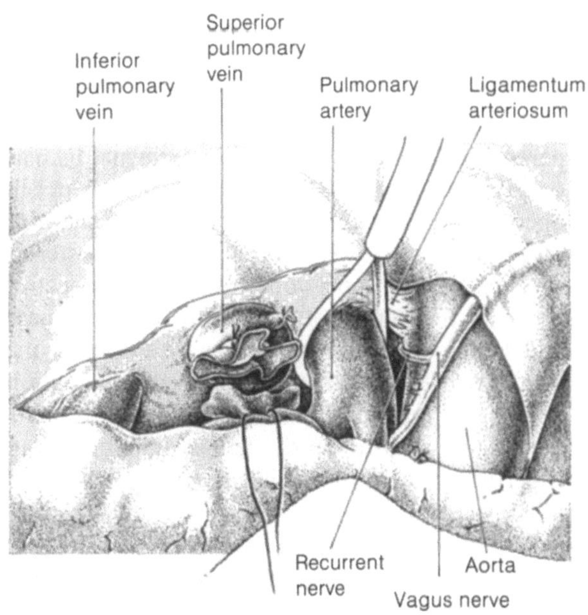

Fig. 42. Left upper lobectomy. A tourniquet has been placed around the left pulmonary artery

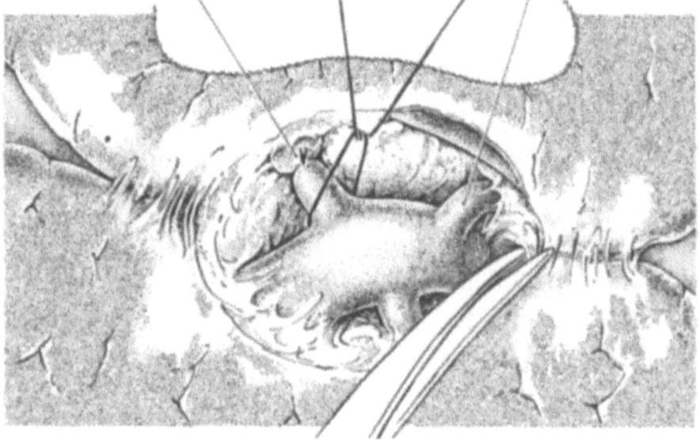

Fig. 43. Left upper lobectomy. Interlobar exposure of the segmental arteries

visualized. The first segmental branch to the upper lobe is large. It may bifurcate immediately after its origin and is closely related to the apical branch of the superior pulmonary vein. This vessel is easily injured because of its position in the arch of the pulmonary artery. It must be freed from the connective tissue and carefully encircled on the perivascular plane with dissecting forceps, which may be guided by the index finger introduced from above. If the vessel is short, it may be easier to divide it between clamps and oversew the proximal stump than divide the vessel between ligatures. If further arterial branches to the upper lobe are accessible in this region, they are divided between ligatures, watching for any atypical branches passing to the lingula (Fig. 43).

Separation of the interlobar fissure is difficult in the presence of extensive inflammation or fused parenchyma and will result in parenchymal fistulas or hemorrhage if the correct plane is not developed. By applying opposite traction to the superior segment of the lower lobe and to the posterior segment of the upper lobe, the loose connective tissue in the depths of the fissure is made tense and can be divided in small steps with the scissors. The presence of the artery is disclosed by palpation and by the presence of perivascular nodes. Usually the fissure is more clearly defined inferiorly than superiorly, so the artery is easier to palpate and identify in that area.

When dense adhesions are present, it is helpful first to undertunnel the fused parenchyma on the pulmonary artery from above and from below. For this purpose the vascular sheath is opened at the superior margin of the fissure and below the fused parenchyma. The dissection then proceeds from both sides along the upper surface of the vessel until a tunnel has been formed over the artery. The parenchymal connections over the interlobar fissure are then divided between clamps or staple rows without injuring the artery. At this point the pulmonary artery is exposed from its trunk to the superior segmental artery (A6).

In the inferior portion of the interlobar fissure, the anterior basilar segmental arteries (A7, A8) that enter the side of the lower lobe facing the lingula can serve as guides for locating the interlobar segment of the pulmonary artery. As traction is placed on the lingula and the adhesions passing to the lower lobe are divided, the fissure is opened from below, and the artery can be identified and traced hilarward.

When the fissure is completely obliterated, Nohl-Oser [70] suggest the anterior approach as an alternative: After upward retraction of the lung, the pulmonary ligament is divided, and the anterior wall of the inferior pulmonary vein is dissected free. The lower lobe bronchus is palpable above the vein. The dissection is carried superiorly to the origin of the upper lobe bronchus. Often a lymph node is found at that site and must be removed; a bronchial artery also may be encountered. Lateral to the division of the bronchus is the trunk of the pulmonary artery and also the inferior point of the fissure, from which access can be gained to the remainder of the interlobar fissure.

The interlobar branches to the lingula are identified opposite the superior segmental artery of the lower lobe; they may arise at the same level as the superior segmental artery or more distally. All the more proximal, anterior upper lobe arteries are divided between ligatures; it is unnecessary to establish the exact segmental distribution of the vessels. Finally the lingular arteries are ligated and divided.

1.4.7.5.3 Bronchial Dissection. When the pulmonary artery has been dissected free as far as its basilar divisions, the interlobar exposure can additionally be used for dissection of the bronchus, which is in close proximity to the artery.

The origin of the upper lobe bronchus can be visualized by applying alternate posterior and medial traction to the vessel. All accessible peribronchial and periarterial lymph nodes in the interlobar fissure are taken as in a radical operation. Generally the TA 30 stapling instrument (3.5 mm, blue

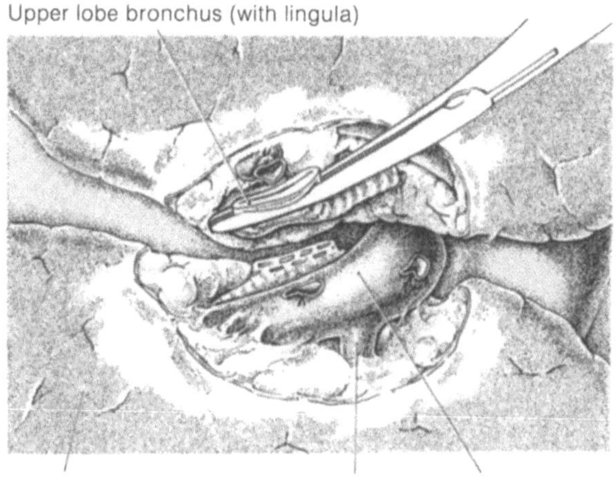

Fig. 44. Left upper lobectomy. Division of the bronchus

cartridge) can be applied across the origin of the upper lobe bronchus, close to the mainstem bronchus, whereupon the staples are driven in and the bronchus sectioned with a scalpal following distal application of a clamp (Fig. 44). Care is taken that the anterior and posterior walls are accurately apposed, and that the carina is not caught in the staple line. With a very short trunk, it will be necessary to deal with the lingular and upper lobe branches separately.

If an open transection is preferred, the endotracheal tube can be advanced into the right main bronchus until the balloon occludes the bifurcation, or a small-gauge Fogarty catheter can be inserted proximally through the bronchial opening to isolate the site of the transection from the respiratory circuit while the stump is being closed (Fig. 32 a).

After closure of the bronchus, remaining parenchymal connections with the lower lobe are divided with the TA instrument. Finally the bronchus and parenchyma are immersed to confirm aerostasis, and any leaks are sealed with fibrin glue. Although division of the pulmonary ligament has been advocated to aid expansion of the residual lung, we do not consider this advisable, as unrestrained upward movement of the lower lobe can cause kinking of the vessels.

1.4.7.5.4 Lymph Node Dissection. The lymph node dissection in left upper lobectomy includes removal of the intrapulmonary nodes about the main bronchus and the origin of the left upper lobe and around the interlobar portion of the pulmonary artery. It also encompasses the anterior superior mediastinal nodes and the superior and inferior tracheobronchial and paratracheal nodes. These groups are removed following incision of the pleura from the thoracic apex to the hilum. Dissection in the aortic window and below the main bronchus is done with particular care, avoiding injury to the recurrent nerve. The dissection should be carried as far as possible along the contralateral mainstem bronchus (Fig. 23).

Drainage and closure of the chest are described on p. 120

1.4.7.6 Preservation of the Lingula

Preservation of the lingula is possible only if its parenchyma is not involved by disease, and the lingular segmental bronchus has a well-defined, proximal origin from the upper lobar bronchus. If doubt exists, only the venous tributaries from the upper three segments are ligated initially, and the lingular arteries are left intact until the bronchus has been dissected and the potential for sparing the lingula can be assessed.

The origin of the upper lobe bronchus is exposed in the interlobar fissure (see above). The bronchus is temporarily clamped in atelectasis and the remaining segments reinflated to assess the distribution of ventilation and confirm that the proposed line of transection is correct. Then the superior division of the upper lobe bronchus is resected with or without use of the stapling instrument, depending on its length. The boundary beween the lingula and the remaining upper lobe segments can be identified on the pulmonary surface by careful inflation of the lung. The pleura over that site is incised superficially in small steps. With traction on the distal bronchus and vessels, the upper lobe segments are pulled away from the lingula, preserving the intersegmental veins. Tense venous branches to the upper lobe are divided between clamps, and any parenchymal fistulas are sealed with fibrin glue. Division of the parenchyma is easier when the stapling device is used (TA 90, 4.8 mm, green cartridge).

1.4.8 Left Lower Lobectomy

1.4.8.1 Intubation

Spiral endotracheal tube.

1.4.8.2 Position and Approach

Anterolateral thoracotomy in the bed of the fifth rib or, more rarely, posterolateral thoracotomy in the bed of the sixth rib [72].

1.4.8.3 Instruments

Basic set II, extra thoracic set.

1.4.8.4 Basic Surgical Anatomy

The portion of the left lower lobe bronchus between the origins of the upper lobe bronchus and superior segmental bronchus is usually longer than on the right side, so it is not necessary to transect the superior segmental bronchus (B6) separately. Beyond the origin of the superior segment, the basilar bronchus usually splits into two segmental branches of equal size: an anterior branch to the anterior basal segment (S8) and a posterior branch to segments S9 and S10 (lateral basal segmental bronchus and posterior basal segmental bronchus). Bronchus B7 is a side branch of the anterior basal segmental bronchus (B8) and, in contrast to the right side, does not ventilate a separate segment.

The superior segment of the lower lobe (S6) is supplied in 60% of cases by a single artery that originates slightly above the origin of the lower lingular artery (A5) (Fig. 45 a–d). In the remaining cases two or more arteries are present [30], the inferior vessel arising at the level of the lingular artery and the superior vessel arising close to or conjointly with the branch to the posterior segment of the upper lobe. The rest of the pulmonary artery continues on as the basal artery, which generally divides first into two branches and then into four, which are highly variable in their course.

Venous drainage is accomplished by two tributaries to the left inferior pulmonary vein. The superior tributary receives blood from the superior segment of the lower lobe, while the inferior tributary drains the remaining segments. A horizontal branch of the superior segmental vein runs be-

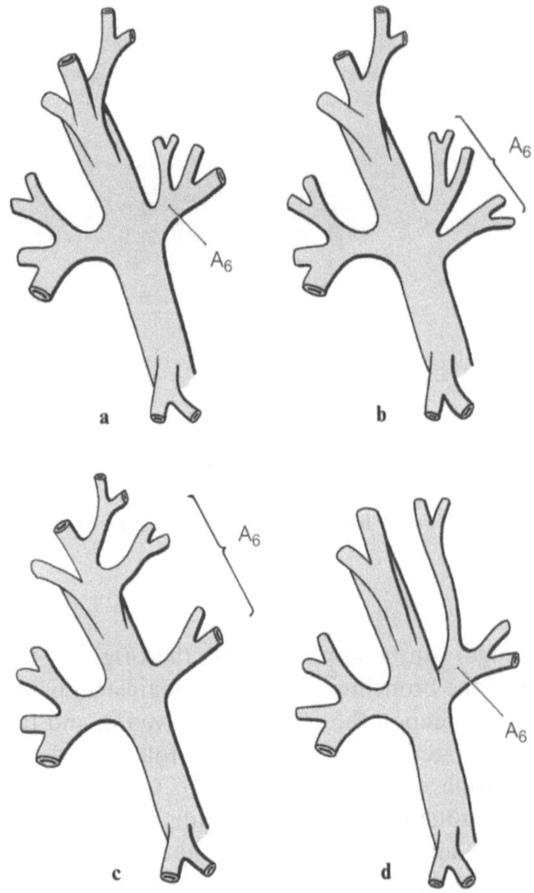

Fig. 45a–d. Left lower lobectomy. Variations of arterial supply. **a** Normal arterial supply. **b** Two arteries supply the superior segment of the lower lobe (30%). **c** An accessory branch A2 supplies the superior segment of the lower lobe (40%). **d** An accessory branch from the superior segment of the lower lobe supplies the upper lobe (S2) (rare)

tween the superior and basal segments of the lower lobe. In rare cases vessels from the lingula or a retrohilar vein from the pulmonary apex empty into the left inferior pulmonary vein. The superior and inferior pulmonary veins form an extrapericardial trunk in 8%–25% of the population [40], and this must be excluded before ligation of the vein is undertaken.

1.4.8.5 Operative Technique

After thoracotomy, adhesions between the left lower lobe and pleura are freed in stepwise fashion, avoiding injury to the esophagus and to the phrenic nerve coursing on the pericardium. As a precaution, we recommend encircling the pulmonary artery with a tourniquet after incising the pleura below the arch of the aorta (Fig. 42).

1.4.8.5.1 Venous Dissection. The inferior pulmonary vein is found at the upper end of the pulmonary ligament, which is divided from below upward between clamps while the lung is retracted superiorly. Occasionally a pulmonary sequestration is present on the left side, supplied by vessels in the pulmonary ligament; dividing these vessels without ligation can cause massive intraabdominal bleeding (see p. 185). Next, with the lung retracted anteriorly, the pleura is incised anteriorly and posteriorly to about the center of the hilum, and the inferior pulmonary vein with its two major branches is dissected free, isolated, and divided between ligatures in standard fashion (No. 0 absorbable sutures), preserving any atypical tributary vessels from the upper lobe. In resections for carcinoma, all lymph nodes in this region and about the esophagus are removed.

1.4.8.5.2 Arterial Dissection. The arterial branches are exposed in the interlobar fissure between the upper lobe, which is retracted anteriorly and superiorly, and the lower lobe, which is retracted posteriorly. The pleura in the fissure is incised in small steps until the artery is visualized; this may require the freeing of several lymph nodes. Identification of the artery is aided by palpation, and if necessary by exposing the subpleural anterior segmental artery of the lower lobe and dissecting it proximally to the interlobar artery (see p. 153). The vessel is exposed until its typical branching pattern is appreciated. One or two branches pass anteriorly to the lingula (A4, A5), and superior or inferior to that point a branch arises posteriorly to the superior segment of the lower lobe (superior segmental artery, A6). Farther up the vessel, segmental branches are distributed to the upper lobe, while distally a basilar trunk of variable length ramifies into the basal segmental arteries. Atypical branches from the superior segmental artery to the upper lobe (Fig. 45) can be recognized after the interlobar fissure has been completely dissected free. As a rule, separate ligation of the superior segmental artery and of the basilar vessels is necessary to occlude the arterial supply to the lower lobe while preserving the total blood supply to the lingula (Fig. 46). Usually the basilar artery is ligated proximally while the basilar segmental branches are ligated individually.

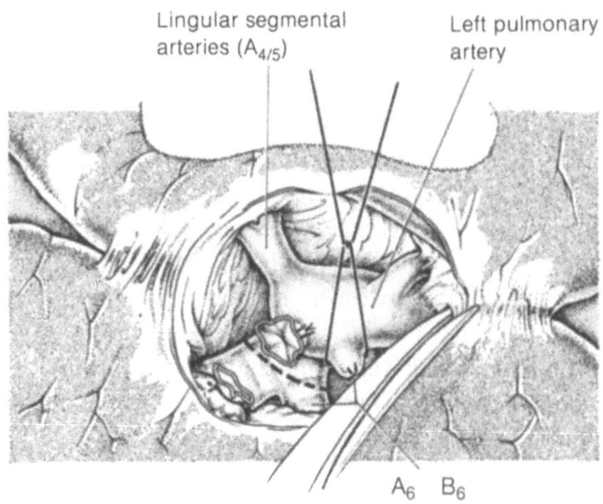

Fig. 46. Left lower lobectomy. Exposure, ligation, and division of the arteries. The line of bronchial transection is shown

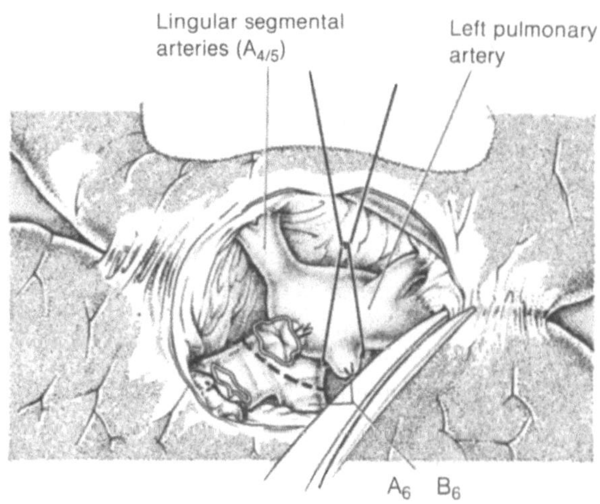

Fig. 47. Left lower lobectomy. Exposure of the arteries and transection of the lower lobe bronchus through the interlobar fissure

1.4.8.5.3 Bronchial Dissection. After the appropriate arterial branches have been secured, the upper lobe bronchus is exposed in the interlobar field, and the origin of the upper lobe bronchus is identified (Fig. 47). The bronchial dissection also may be performed from the posterior aspect. On the left side more often than on the right, it is possible to occlude the common trunk of the lower lobe bronchus with one staple line placed obliquely below the origin of the upper lobe bronchus and above the origin of the superior segmental bronchus. If the trunk is so short that a single staple line might compromise the upper lobar orifice, the superior segmental bronchus is closed separately with simple interrupted sutures (2-0 absorbable). The lower lobe bronchus may be occluded with the TA 30 stapling instrument (3.5 mm, blue cartridge) or by traditional technique. The boundaries of the lower lobe can be defined at this stage by careful inflation of the residual lung. Usually there is considerable parenchyma between the lower lobe and the lingula, and these connections may contain atypical veins that must be separately ligated before the fissure is divided with the TA instrument.

1.4.8.5.4 Lymph Node Dissection. The extent of the lymph node dissection in a lower lobectomy is necessarily more limited than in an upper lobectomy. The dissection encompasses the intrapulmonary nodes in the interlobar fissure and the extrapulmonary posterior mediastinal nodes in the pulmonary ligament, around the inferior pulmonary vein, and around the esophagus. The subcarinal nodes can be located and removed by following the left main bronchus to the bifurcation. The trunk of the pulmonary artery prevents a more extensive dissection. Exposure of the paratracheal and superior tracheobronchial nodes is described in the section on Left Pneumonectomy (p. 133).

Chest tube insertion is described on p. 120.

1.4.8.6 Resection of the Lower Lobe and Lingula

In this operation the decision whether to resect the lingula concurrently with the lower lobe or as a separate procedure will depend on pathoanatomic circumstances and on the course of the operation.

In a combined lower lobectomy and lingulectomy, it is unnecessary to separate the lower lobe from the lingula. The arterial dissection is performed through the interlobar fissure. The lingular tributary to the superior pulmonary vein is ligated from the anterior side, while the inferior pulmonary vein is ligated from the posterior side after severing the pulmonary ligament. Both the lingular bronchus and the lower lobe bronchus are accessible through the interlobar field (see p. 153); they are divided below the arterial stumps after temporarily clamping the bronchi to confirm that the remaining segmental bronchi are not compromised. The divided bronchi are closed with staples or interrupted sutures (Fig. 48). When dense adhesions are present, the lingular bronchus can be isolated and divided from the anterior side after severing the veins, and the lower lobe bronchus can be divided from the posterior side (Fig. 49).

Chest tube insertion and closure of the chest are described on p. 120.

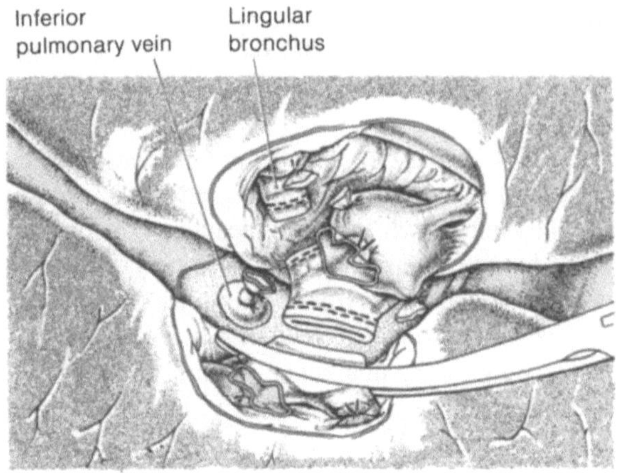

Fig. 48. Lower lobectomy with lingulectomy. Division of the arteries and bronchi

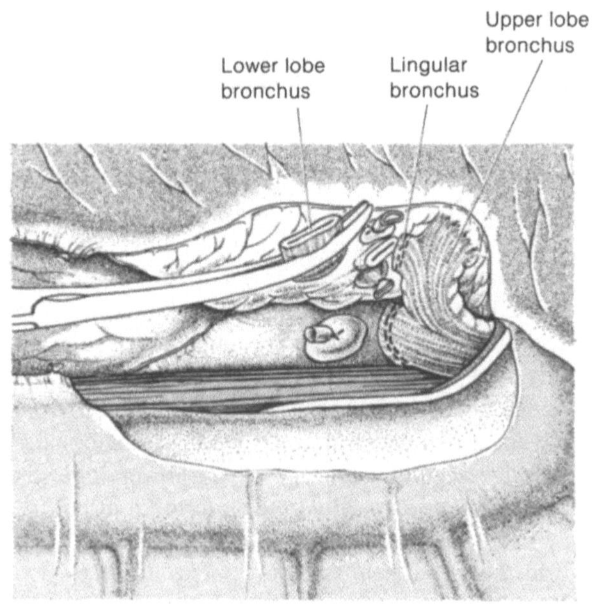

Fig. 49. Lower lobectomy with lingulectomy. Division of the bronchi from the posterior side

1.5 Segmentectomy

The anatomic subdivision of the lung into bronchoarterial units has led to operative procedures whose goal is the isolated removal of pulmonary segments [15, 75]. However, anatomic studies and clinical experience have shown that not every segment can be removed without compromising the residual lung because of intimate connections with the adjacent parenchyma. The importance of segmentectomy has been further diminished by the practice of wedge resections, which depend less on anatomic boundaries than on pathologic findings, and which have become simpler and safer in recent years owing to the use of stapling devices. Nevertheless, a detailed knowledge of the segmental anatomy of the lung is essential even in wedge resections to avoid vascular or bronchial damage in the residual lung.

1.5.1 Indications

Segmentectomy is appropriate for bronchiectasis, which affects mainly the basal segments of the lower lobe and lingula (or middle lobe), and for tuberculomas, which are most common in the apical and posterior segments of the upper lobe and in the superior segment of the lower lobe. However, segmentectomy in these cases has been performed less frequently in recent years owing to the availability of drug therapies. Other potential indications for segmentectomy are pulmonary abscess, arteriovenous aneurysms, benign neoplasms, cysts, bronchial adenomas, intrapulmonary foreign bodies, and unidentified coin lesions of the lung. Segmentectomy has proven less favorable than lobectomy for many cases of stage I bronchogenic carcinoma [5, 61], suggesting that segmentectomy may be justified as a palliative measure in rare instances where lobectomy is contraindicated on functional grounds.

Whenever a segmentectomy is proposed, the appropriateness of a wedge resection, which leads to fewer postoperative complications, should be considered. The more peripheral the lesion, the greater the preference for this type of resection.

1.5.2 Introductory Remarks on Operative Technique

Segmentectomy is facilitated by intubating the patient with a double-lumen endotracheal tube (e.g., a Robert Shaw tube). This makes it possible to define the segmental boundaries by clamping the segmental bronchus in atelectasis and then reinflating the lung. The artery, vein, bronchus, and visceral pleura are dealt with separately in segmental resections. The sequence of the dissections may vary, and primary dissection of the bronchus [52, 69], artery [17], or vein [106] has been advocated by various authors. Differentiation of the *segmental vein* from the veins coursing between the segments cannot always be accomplished at the hilum. It may be best, therefore, to deal with the artery and bronchus first and defer ligation of the vein until its identify can be established with greater certainty.

The *segmental bronchus* is generally identified by following the lobar bronchus peripherally in the deflated lung. A clamp is applied, and the residual lung is carefully inflated so that the occluded, nonaerated segment can be idenfitied. Air may drift from adjacent segments into the occluded segment through Cohn's pores, but this process is delayed and can even aid identification of the occluded segment. Another means of identifying the segment to be resected is to inflate the lung and watch for the delay in the deflation of the clamped segment.

Overholt et al. [74] recommend that transection of the segmental bronchus be deferred until just before the segment is removed so that the anatomic relationships can be more clearly appreciated.

The *arteries* are exposed through the interlobar fissure, except for the apical posterior segmental artery of the left upper lobe (A1, A2) and the apical and anterior segmental arteries of the right upper lobe (A1, A3). Given their close proximity to the bronchi, the vessels also can be found close to the retracted distal bronchial stump following identification and division of the segmental bronchus.

After the artery and bronchus have been divided, the segment is removed by blunt dissection while traction is applied to the distal bronchial stump. The residual lung is carefully inflated to define the intersegmental boundary. On the surface of the lung, the pleura at the segmental interface is divided with scissors in small steps, and the intersegmental plane is developed further by finger dissection while traction is applied to the bronchus. The dissection is continued until the entire segment is clear. The correct plane is signified by a lack of resistance and also by the presence of intersegmental veins, which should be left intact on the adjacent parenchyma. Branches draining the segment to be resected are divided between small clamps (Fig. 50).

Bleeding after removal of the segment comes mostly from smaller veins and is controlled by compression and cautery. Parenchymal fistulas may be oversewn, although most can be adequately sealed with fibrin glue. We do not recommend approximating the edges of the remaining lobe over the raw surface, as this can lead to the formation of parenchymal leaks and cavities that are prone to infection.

1.5.3 Resection of the Apical Posterior Segment of the Right Upper Lobe (S1, S2)

The approach, position, instrumentation, and surgical anatomy are the same as described for right upper lobectomy (see p. 138).

The apical segment of the right upper lobe is supplied by the superior division of the truncus anterior. In more than half of cases the trunk also sends a branch to the posterior segment, which usually (80%, [40]) receives additional vessels from the interlobar fissure or from the superior segment of the lower lobe. The common vascular supply of the two segments (S1, S2) underlies the recommendation that they be removed together, although separate resection is also possible.

The upper lobe is dissected free, the pathology is checked, and the pleura is incised below the arch of the azygos vein from the front of the hilum posteriorly to about the center of the hilum.

1.5.3.1 Bronchial Dissection

The upper lobe is retracted anteriorly and inferiorly to expose the posterior aspect of the right main bronchus below the azygos vein. The right main bronchus is followed to the upper lobe bronchus, whose branches are dissected free from the lung parenchyma. Usually an adjacent bronchial artery must be ligated at this time, and a lymph node in the angle between the upper lobe bronchus and intermediate bronchus must be removed. This lymph node marks the superior end of the oblique fissure, which is entered for dissection of the pulmonary artery. Deep to the angle between the upper lobe bronchus and intermediate bronchus is the superior segmental artery of the lower lobe (A6), and above the angle are the bronchial divisions to the posterior segment of the upper lobe (S2). Only the apical segmental bronchus (B1), which runs superiorly, and the posterior segmental bronchus (B2) arising at right angles to it are visi-

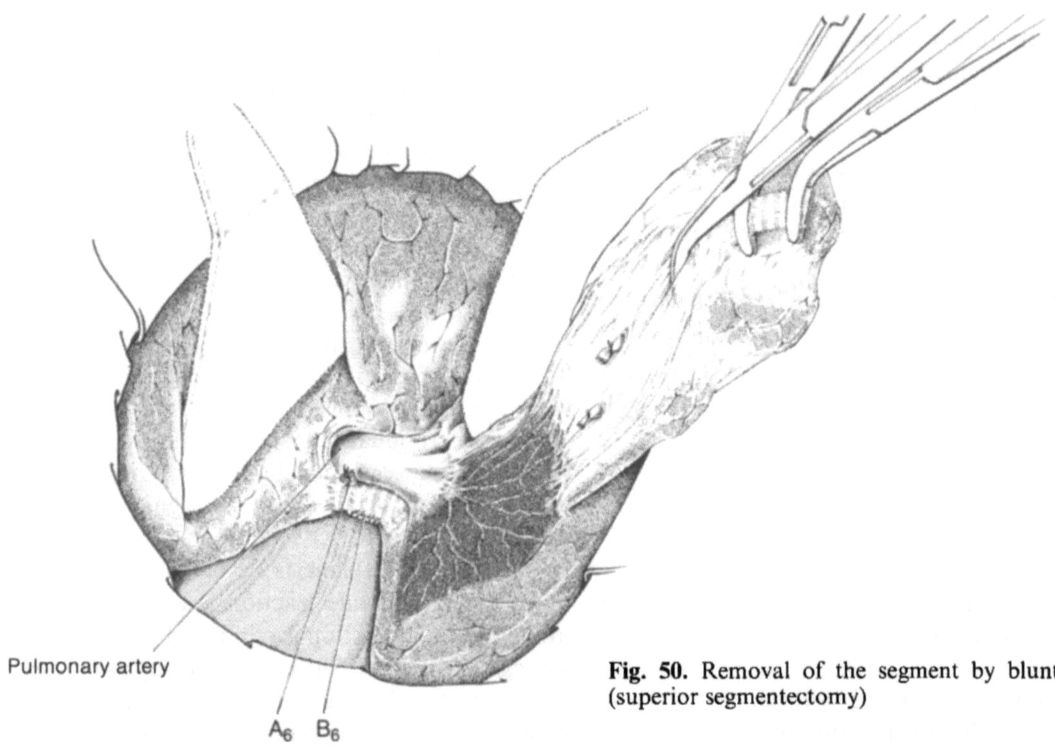

Fig. 50. Removal of the segment by blunt dissection (superior segmentectomy)

ble from the posterior side. The anterior segmental bronchus (B3) arises anteriorly at the same level (Fig. 51). Care is taken not to restrict the lumen of B3 during division of the apical and posterior segmental bronchi, and this should be checked beforehand by temporarily clamping the bronchi before they are severed. The proximal bronchial stumps are closed with interrupted sutures (2-0 or 3-0 absorbable atraumatic monofilament).

1.5.3.2 Arterial Dissection

The segmental arteries become tense when traction is placed on the distal segmental bronchi, and they can be divided between ligatures at that time. Usually it is easier to expose the apical segmental artery anteriorly at its origin from the truncus anterior. Resection of the posterior segment facilitates orientation and vascular ligation if first the superior portion of the oblique fissure is opened to expose the posterior segmental artery, which is divided after first identifying the adjacent vessels, most notably the superior segmental artery to the lower lobe. During proximal dissection of the interlobar artery, the first structure encountered in the parenchyma is the posterior division of the upper lobe vein, which overlies the pulmonary artery.

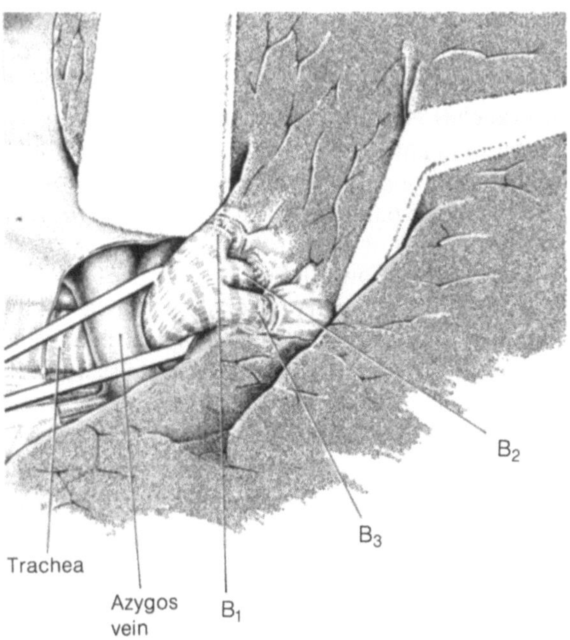

Fig. 51. Segmentectomy of the right lower lobe. Exposure of the divisions of the upper lobe bronchus from the posterior side

1.5.3.3 Venous Dissection

Only veins that obviously drain the segments to be removed, i.e. the apical and posterior segmental veins, are divided. The intersegmental branches of both these veins should be left on the raw surface of the anterior pulmonary segment.

For removal of the segment, the upper lobe is retracted inferiorly. The lobe is inflated, and the boundary between the aerated and nonaerated segments is observed. Traction is applied to the bronchus and artery, and the segments are separated while following the intersegmental veins and ligating the intrasegmental vessels. If the course of the intersegmental veins can be seen, the residual lung tissue can be divided with the TA stapler. This instrument is especially useful for dividing connections with the superior segment of the lower lobe.

1.5.4 Resection of the Anterior Segment of the Right Upper Lobe (S3)

The approach, position, instrumentation, and surgical anatomy are the same as described for right upper lobectomy (see p. 138).

Resection of the anterior segment (S3) is technically more difficult than removal of the apical or posterior segment due to the relatively poor accessibility of the anterior segment and the many vascular anomalies that can occur there. In most cases it is simpler to perform a wedge resection using a stapling instrument, so this segmentectomy is rarely indicated.

1.5.4.1 Arterial Dissection

The anterior segment of the right upper lobe usually receives its arterial supply from the inferior division of the truncus anterior. This may be supplemented by branches ascending from the interlobar fissure or rarely from the middle lobe artery. The first step in ligating the feeding arteries is to dissect the truncus anterior free anteriorly and from above. The most cranial branch of the superior pulmonary vein (the apical segmental vein, V1) is mobilized until the major divisions of the truncus anterior are visualized. The superior division to the apical and posterior segments is left alone; the inferior division to the anterior segment is divided between ligatures. Additional feeding vessels are located by entering the upper third of the interlobar fissure and exposing the arterial branches to the middle lobe, to the superior segment of the lower lobe, and possibly to the anterior segment. The latter also are divided after they have been positively identified.

1.5.4.2 Venous Dissection

The anterior vein (V3) is usually the largest vein draining the upper lobe and can be recognized by its intersegmental branch, which runs horizontally between the upper and middle lobes. The intersegmental branch of the apical vein (V1) is on the interface between the anterior and apical segments and drains blood from both segments. The anterior vein is dissected from the anterior side, and its intersegmental branch is followed into the parenchyma, thus marking the boundary of the middle lobe. As the anterior vein receives blood exlusively from the anterior segment, it may be divided between ligatures. Next the intersegmental branch of the apical vein is dissected free, and its branches to the anterior segment are ligated.

1.5.4.3 Bronchial Dissection

The anterior segmental bronchus (B3) can be dissected free from the posterior aspect between the apical and posterior segments (see p. 160). After the upper lobe bronchus has been dissected free, it is encircled with the index finger and thumb, which can then feel anteriorly for the palpable anterior segmental bronchus. The bronchus is exposed by incision of the overlying lung parenchyma. It is occluded distally with a small clamp, transected, and closed proximally with an interrupted suture line.

A more favorable technique is to expose the bronchus in the interlobar fissure. The pulmonary artery is dissected free at the juncture of the oblique and transverse fissures and is followed toward the hilum. The segmental bronchus (B3) is identified above the posterior upper lobe vein, which crosses the pulmonary artery. The close proximity of the bronchus to the vein requires very careful dissection in this area. The bronchus is temporarily clamped to confirm its identification, divided, and closed with interrupted sutures. Finally the anterior segment is dissected free as previously described, preserving the intersegmental branch of the apical vein.

1.5.5 Resection of the Apical Posterior Segment of the Left Upper Lobe (S1, S2)

The approach, position, instrumentation, and surgical anatomy are the same as described for left upper lobectomy (see p. 151).

The individual segments of the left upper lobe can be removed separately. However, the common bronchial trunk of the apical posterior segments provides a rationale for the combined removal of these areas. As in the procedure for upper lobectomy, the pleura is opened with a curved incision over the pulmonary artery on the anterior and posterior sides of the hilum extending to the level of the lingula or the apex of the lower lobe; care is taken to spare the vagus and phrenic nerves. As a precaution, the pulmonary artery is snared with a tourniquet before further dissections are carried out (see Fig. 42).

1.5.5.1 Arterial Dissection

The apical posterior segment of the left upper lobe is supplied by at least two separate vessels that originate from the arch and interlobar portion of the pulmonary artery. Given the variability of the arterial supply, the individual branches should be dissected well into the parenchyma to avoid confusion. The first branch of the pulmonary artery is usually distributed to the anterior segment (S3). This vessel may be quite large and may give off branches to neighboring segments. The next arterial branches generally are distributed to the apical posterior segment. The upper lobe segments may receive additional branches from the interlobar portion of the pulmonary artery–possibly from the lingular vessels or even from the superior segmental artery of the lower lobe.

First the pulmonary artery is exposed at the hilum, if necessary dividing the apical hilar vein, and is followed into the interlobar fissure. The fissure is next opened distally to expose the whole arterial arch as far as the origin of the superior segmental artery (A6). After the individual vessels have been identified, the branches to the apical posterior segment are divided between ligatures.

1.5.5.2 Bronchial Dissection

The common apical posterior bronchus is accessible after division of the arteries (Fig. 52). Primary

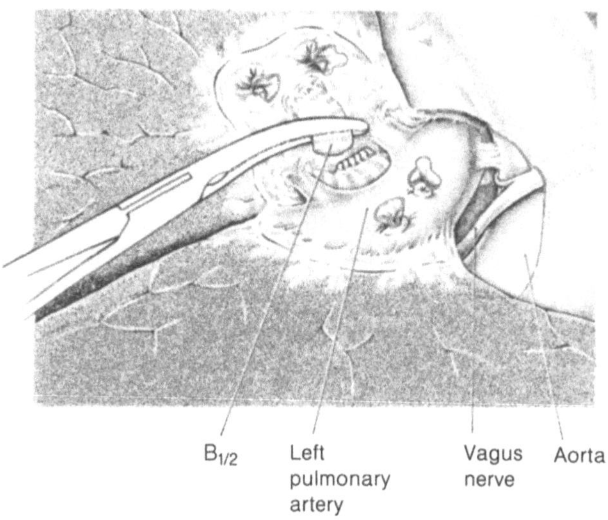

Fig. 52. Segmentectomy of the left upper lobe. Transection of the apical posterior segmental bronchus (S1, S2) through the interlobar field

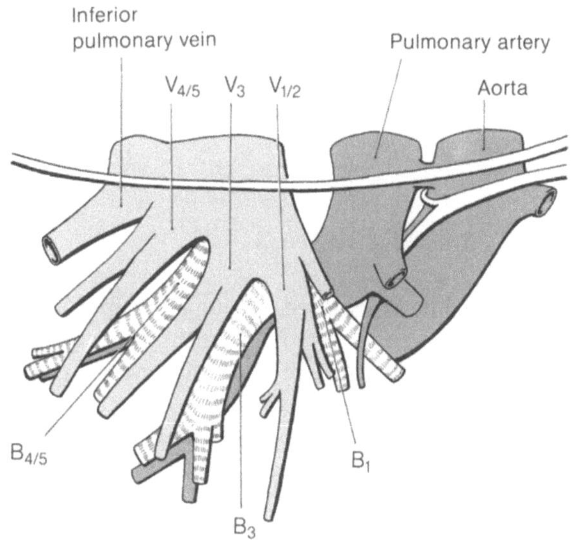

Fig. 53. Divisions of the left superior pulmonary vein, anterior view

exposure and division of the bronchus from the posterior aspect, as may be done on the right side, is not advised on the left side due to the overlying pulmonary artery. The left upper lobe bronchus is palpable deep to the divided arteries in the interlobar field. Its branches are exposed by retracting the pulmonary artery, freeing any intervening lymph nodes, and incising the peribronchial tissue. The short trunk of the upper lobe bronchus divides into the lingular bronchus and also into a superior branch that ventilates the first three segments. The trunk for the apical posterior segment is continuous with the superior border of the upper lobe bronchus. The anterior segmental bronchus (S3) can be seen coursing anteriorly. When the apical posterior bronchus is clamped to delineate the atelectatic segment, the clamp must not restrict the lumen of S3. After this has been confirmed, the bronchus is transected and the proximal stump closed with simple interrupted sutures (2-0 or 3-0 absorbable material).

1.5.5.3 Venous Dissection

The upper lobe vein is dissected free from the anterior side. Its most superior division is the apical posterior vein (V1/2), adjoined inferiorly by the anterior vein (V3) and then by the lingular vein group (V4/5) (Fig. 53). The intersegmental branch of the apical posterior vein is left intact on the plane of separation from the anterior segment, and only the branches that actually enter the apical posterior segment are divided. The segment is removed by applying traction on the divided bronchus from the interlobar aspect, carrying the dissection along the intersegmental vein to the anterior segment. Once this venous branch has been identified, the remaining parenchyma may be divided, using the TA instrument if desired.

1.5.6 Resection of the Anterior Segment of the Left Upper Lobe (S3)

The approach, position, instrumentation, and surgical anatomy are the same as described previously for left upper lobectomy (see p. 151).

1.5.6.1 Arterial Dissection

The anterior segment of the left upper lobe might be supplied by the first branch of the pulmonary artery, by a separate branch from the interlobar fissure, or by a branch from the lingular arteries. The most common pattern is one branch from the superior portion of the pulmonary artery and one from the interlobar portion. The supply is determined by exposing the pulmonary artery from above and in the oblique fissure as far as the origin of the lingular vessels. The arterial branches are followed into the lung parenchyma to establish their segmental identities. Only then may the vessels to the anterior segment be divided between ligatures.

1.5.6.2 Bronchial Dissection

The bronchus is exposed through the interlobar fissure after ligation of the segmental artery and adequate mobilization of the pulmonary artery. We recommend that a snare be used for this purpose. The upper lobe bronchus is exposed at the base of the interlobar fissure. The lingular bronchus is identified, and the anterior branch of the three higher segmental bronchi is isolated in the anterior bifurcation of the superior pulmonary vein. The bronchus is clamped distally and divided close to its origin, maintaining the patency of the apical posterior segmental bronchus. The stump is closed with simple interrupted sutures.

1.5.6.3 Venous Dissection

The superior pulmonary vein is exposed from the anterior aspect, and its branches (apical posterior, anterior, lingular) are identified. The anterior segmental vein may pass directly to the superior pulmonary vein, or it may open into the apical or lingular veins. The branches draining the parenchyma of the anterior segment are transected; the intersegmental veins on the planes between the anterior segment and the apical and lingular segments are preserved when the anterior segment is removed. With traction on the distal bronchial stump, the atelectatic segment is bluntly separated from the upper lobar parenchyma, starting at the hilum and proceeding toward the periphery. Once the intersegmental veins have been exposed and the plane of the dissection clearly defined, the residual parenchyma may be divided with the TA instrument.

1.5.7 Lingulectomy ([15], see also p. 155)

The approach, position, instrumentation, and surgical anatomy are the same as described for left upper lobectomy (p. 151).

The frequency of involvement of the lingula by bronchiectasis has declined, so surgical resection is infrequently performed. With involvement of the inferior segment (S5), isolated removal is feasible. However, a simpler procedure is wedge resection with the stapling instrument, and we have come to prefer that option in the majority of cases.

When the lingula is removed concurrently with the upper lobe segments or with the lower lobe, the arterial and bronchial dissections are performed via the interlobar fissure. For resection of the lingula alone, or if the fissure is obscured by adhesions, all the structures may be dissected from the anterior side.

1.5.7.1 Venous Dissection

The lingular veins generally drain separately or as a common trunk into the superior pulmonary vein, and less frequently into the inferior pulmonary vein. In exceptional cases a venous branch from the inferior segment may pass to the lower lobe through a fused portion of the interlobar fissure. The superior pulmonary vein and its branches are exposed from the anterior side following incision of the pleura. The most inferior tributaries are from the lingula; these are isolated, identified, and divided between proximal and distal ligatures. The horizontal branch of the anterior vein marks the boundary of the anterior segment of the upper lobe. Removal of the lingula is facilitated by first identifying the course of this vessel.

1.5.7.2 Arterial Dissection

The interlobar fissure is opened to expose the typical branching pattern of the pulmonary artery: one or two vessels pass anteriorly to the lingula opposite or below the origin of the superior segmental artery, and distally is the common trunk that supplies the basilar segments (Fig. 54). In rare cases the lingula is supplied by branches that arise from the arch of the pulmonary artery and descend between the lingular bronchus and the superior pulmonary vein (see p. 153). After the lingular vessels have been divided, the bronchus is palpable in the depths of the field.

1.5.7.3 Bronchial Dissection

The lingular bronchus is sought below the divided artery in the interlobar fissure. Either the trunk of the lingular bronchus or its bifurcation into in-

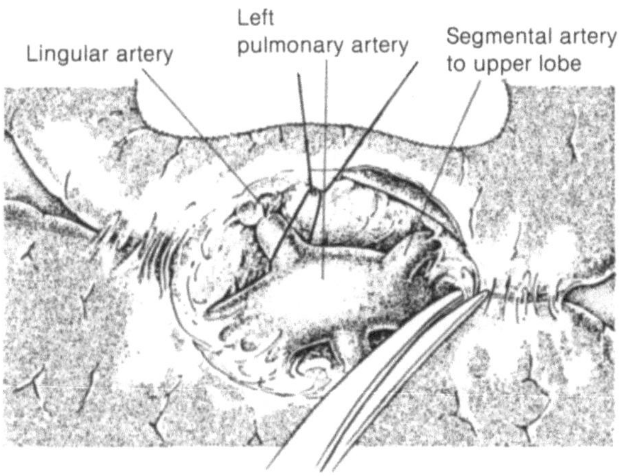

Fig. 54. Lingulectomy. Ligation of the lingular artery

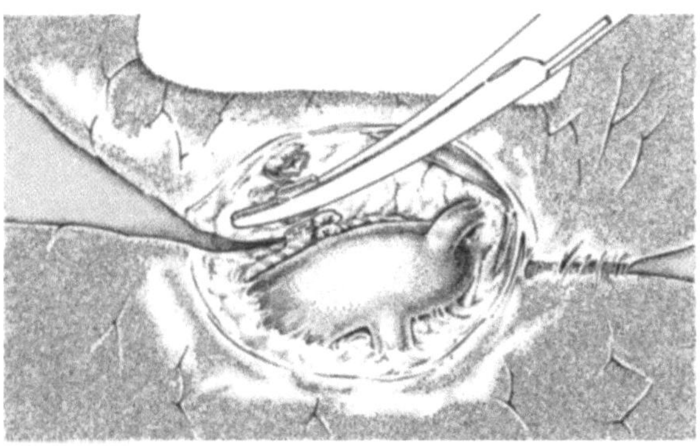

Fig. 55. Lingulectomy. Transection of the bronchus

ferior and superior divisions may be visualized (Fig. 55). Large lymph nodes and thickened bronchial arteries may have to be dissected free or ligated to gain clear exposure, especially in bronchiectasis. The bronchus is transected between clamps at the trunk or in its segmental divisions, depending on the situation. The proximal stump is closed with staples or with simple interrupted sutures (2-0 or 3-0 atraumatic absorbable material). With traction on the distal stump, the lingula, whose boundaries are defined by the area of atelectasis, is separated from the residual upper lobe and also from the lower lobe while preserving the intersegmental vein to the anterior segment of the upper lobe (see above), and the visceral pleura is divided. With a well-defined plane of dissection, the TA instrument may be used to divide the bridging parenchyma. If it is necessary to dissect the lingula from the lower lobe, one should watch for an anomalous division of the anterior basal segmental bronchus passing to the lingula or a tributary vessel passing to the inferior pulmonary vein (see above). These structures generally have a small caliber and are easily ligated.

1.5.7.4 Lingulectomy from the Anterior Side

The anterior approach is prefered for isolated lingulectomy when the interlobar fissure is obscured by dense adhesions. First the lingular branches of the upper lobe vein are divided, and the intersegmental branch of the anterior vein, which marks the transverse fissure, is exposed. The bronchus is dissected free posterior to the lingular vein and divided. As traction is placed on the distal bronchial stump and separation of the lingula is begun, the feeding arteries below the venous branches to the upper lobe are visualized and divided. The lingula is then removed in standard fashion.

1.5.8 Superior Segmentectomy of the Lower Lobe

This procedure begins by dividing the pulmonary ligament and mobilizing the lower lobe. The pleura is incised over the posterior aspect of the hilum (see pp. 146 and 156).

1.5.8.1 Arterial Dissection

The interlobar fissure is opened posteriorly, dividing any connections between the upper and lower lobes, and the superior segmental artery is exposed. In the right lung, a lymph node at the inferior border of the upper lobe bronchus consistently marks the superior end of the fissure; in the left lung, orientation may be gained by following the pulmonary artery from the hilum into the lung parenchyma. If dense adhesions are present, the oblique fissure may be entered inferiorly (see Left Upper Lobectomy and p. 153).

The superior segmental artery (A6) arises posteriorly from the pulmonary artery, roughly opposite the origin of the middle-lobe or lingular arteries. In 20% of cases multiple vessels are present, the most superior of which usually arises close to the branches passing to the upper lobe [25]. Orientation is facilitated by exposing the pulmonary artery proximally to the origin of these vessels and distally to the basilar segmental divisions. Branches from the superior segmental artery to the posterior segment of the upper lobe are identified and left intact (Fig. 56 a).

1.5.8.2 Venous Dissection

The inferior pulmonary vein and its branches are exposed from the posterior aspect after division of the pulmonary ligament. The most superior tributary is from the superior segment (Fig. 57 a,b). It runs posterior to the lower lobe bronchus and inferior to the superior segmental bronchus. The horizontal twig of the superior branch of the inferior pulmonary vein marks the boundary of the basal segments. As it contributes little to the drainage of the basal segments, it may be divided between ligatures along with the superior branch of the inferior pulmonary vein. The horizontal twig is dissected free in the parenchyma to define the segmental boundary.

1.5.8.3 Bronchial Dissection

The bronchus is best approached from the posterior side. It is palpable following division of the segmental veins and arteries. On the right side the superior segmental bronchus arises opposite the middle lobe bronchus, whose patency must not be compromised. This danger does not exist on the left side, because the lingular bronchus originates at a higher level. An alternative approach is through the interlobar fissure, where the bronchus is accessible below and medial to the divided segmental artery (Fig. 58 a,b). After the bronchus has been clamped, the residual lung is inflated slightly to confirm nonaeration of the segment to be removed. The bronchus is isolated for a length of 1–2 cm, transected about 3 mm distal to its origin, and closed with simple interrupted sutures (2-0 or 3-0 atraumatic absorbable material). Traction is applied to the distal bronchial stump, and the segment is separated from the basal segments. The plane of separation corresponds to the horizontal branch of the apical vein, which has previously been dissected free. Since no interlobar septa exist on this plane, separation of the segment opens the parenchyma, and the stapling instrument should be used to produce an airtight closure.

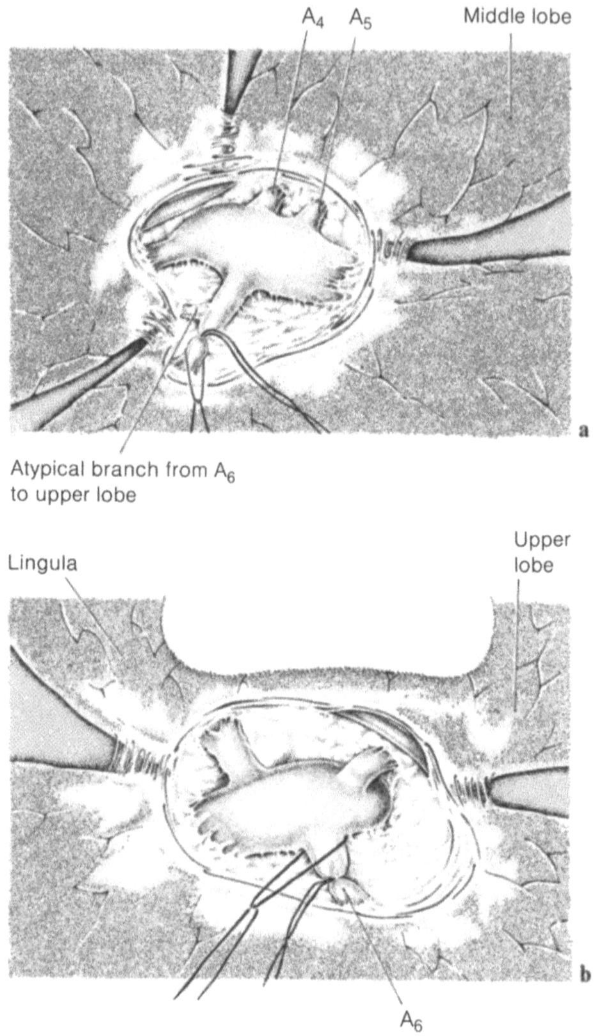

Fig. 56. a Ligation of the superior segmental artery of the right lower lobe, preserving an accessory branch to the upper lobe. **b** Ligation of the superior segmental artery of the left lower lobe

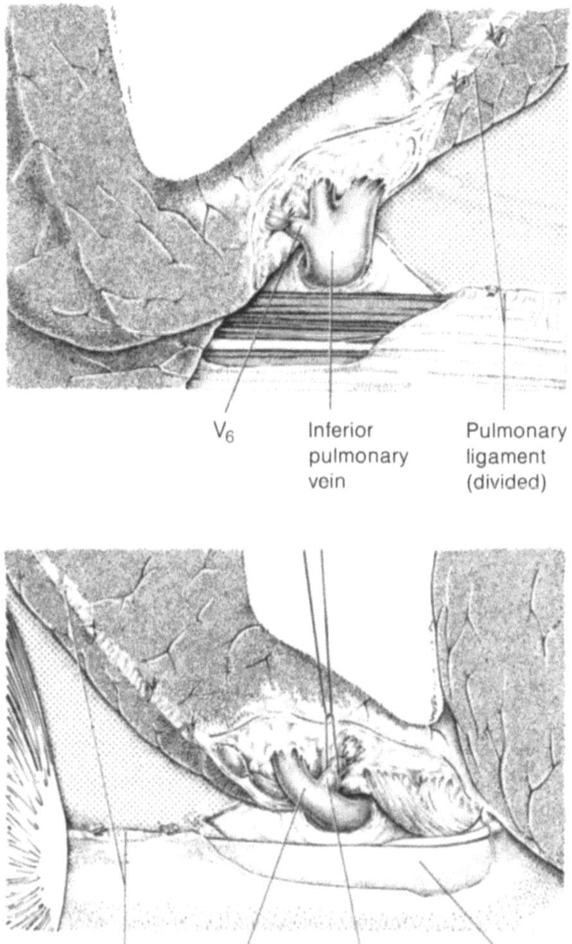

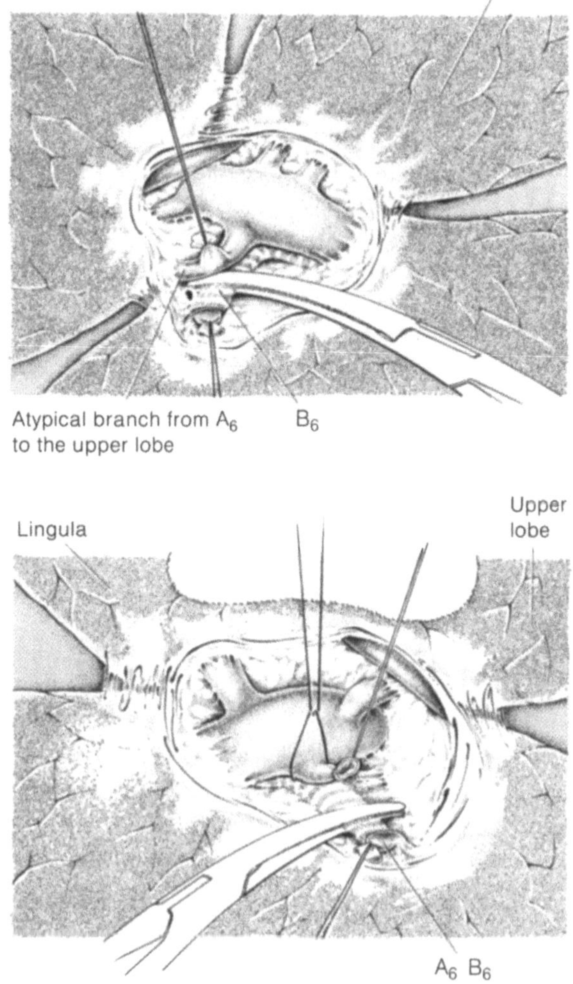

Fig. 57. a Superior segmentectomy of the right lower lobe. Exposure of the vein from the posterior side. **b** Superior segmentectomy of the left lower lobe. Ligation of the vein

Fig. 58. a Superior segmentectomy of the right lower lobe. Occlusion of the segmental bronchus. **b** Superior segmentectomy of the left lower lobe. Occlusion of the segmental bronchus

1.5.9 Basal Segmentectomy of the Lower Lobe

The position, instrumentation, and surgical anatomy are the same as described for lower lobectomy (pp. 146 and 156).

1.5.9.1 Arterial Dissection

As in the procedure for lower lobectomy, the pulmonary artery and its branches are exposed in the interlobar fissure. Key landmarks are the superior segmental artery, which arises posteriorly, and the middle-lobe or lingular arteries that arise anteriorly. Distal to these branches is the basilar artery, which is ligated (Fig. 59 a,b). Generally the segmental divisions of the basilar artery also have to be individually ligated before the vessel is divided after placement of a proximal transfixion ligature.

1.5.9.2 Venous Dissection

The pleura is incised over the hilum, and the inferior pulmonary vein and its branches are exposed by dividing the pulmonary ligament and reflecting the lung anteriorly (Fig. 60 a,b). Generally the vein from the superior segment (apical or superior segmental vein, V6) is definable as a separate branch from the basilar tributaries. This superior branch is relatively constant, whereas the remaining branches of the inferior pulmonary vein are quite variable, especially on the right side. It should be noted that the superior segmental vein crosses the lower lobe bronchus posteriorly, while the basilar veins may run anterior to the bronchus. There may also be tributary veins from the lingula or middle lobe, or from the upper lobe. The superior segmental vein, including its horizontal branch marking the boundary of the basal segments, must be preserved. The basilar veins are divided between ligatures individually or at their trunk.

1.5.9.3 Bronchial Dissection

The basilar bronchus may be approached posteriorly, but usually it is more easily accessible below the divided artery in the interlobar field (Fig. 61 a,b). In inflammatory diseases the bronchial arteries may be greatly enlarged and must be divided between clamps. Before the bronchus is sectioned,

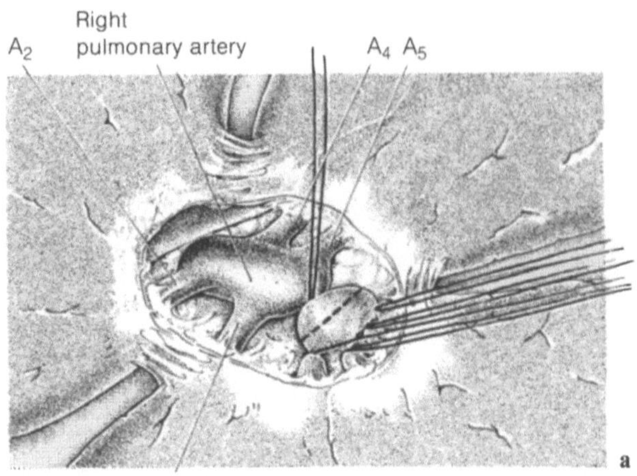

a

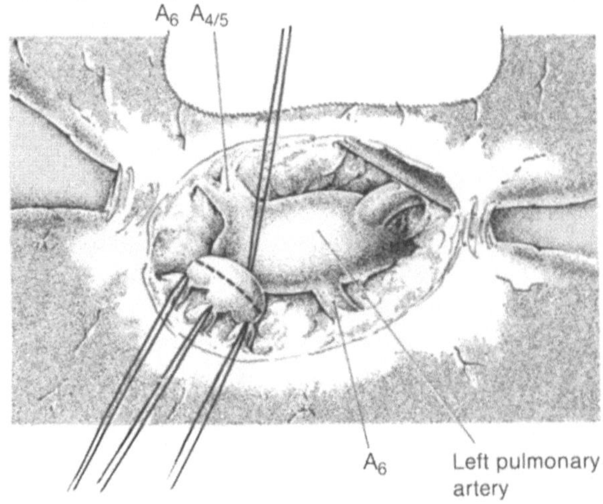

b

Fig. 59 a, b. Basal segmentectomy of the right (top) and left lower lobe. Ligation of the arteries

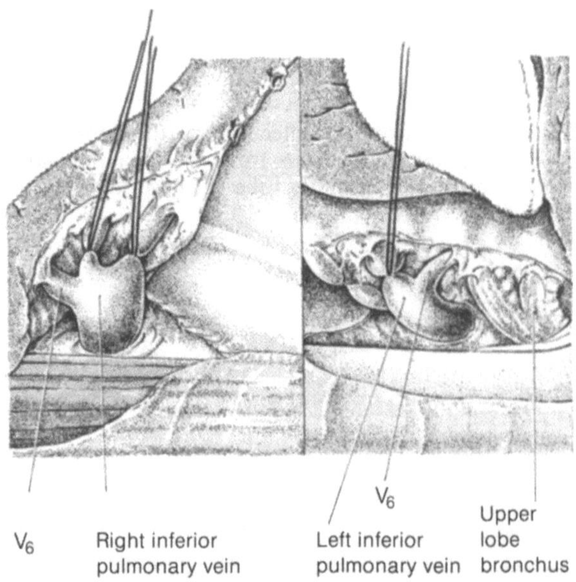

Fig. 60. Basal segmentectomy of the right and left lower lobe. Ligation of the veins, sparing the superior segmental vein of the lower lobe

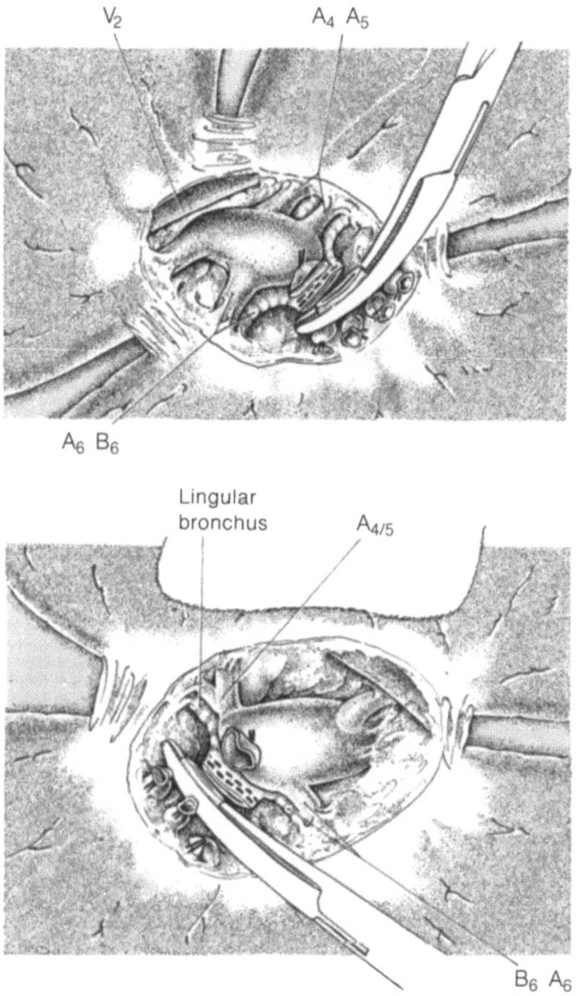

a
b

Fig. 61a, b. Basal segmentectomy of the lower lobe. Transection of the right (top) and left segmental bronchus

the superior segmental bronchis should be exposed by further arterial dissection so that its patency can be preserved. The basilar bronchus is occluded distal to its origin with the stapling device or by a conventional suture technique.

The basal segments of the lower lobe are removed along the course of the intersegmental branch of the superior segmental vein, which runs transversely posterior in the right lung and obliquely posterior in the left lung. Besides blunt dissection, we recommend use of the stapling instrument for division of the parenchyma once the intersegmental plane has been defined. Any parenchymal leaks are oversewn or sealed with fibrin glue.

1.5.9.4 Resection of Individual Basal Segments of the Lower Lobe

Individual basal segments can be resected from the lower lobe, although the variability of the arterial supply and bronchial arborization and the frequent concomitant involvement of adjacent segments have lessened the importance of these procedures in favor of wedge resections using a stapling instrument. The procedure follows the general guidelines for segmentectomies (see p. 159). The segmental arteries are exposed through the interlobar fissure. Their division gives access to the segmental bronchus. The veins are not ligated until the segment is freed so that intersegmental tributaries can be preserved.

1.6 Wedge (Local) Resection

1.6.1 Indications

A local pulmonary resection is appropriate for peripherally located inflammatory diseases, benign tumors, metastases, for the biopsy or frozen-section examination of peripheral round lesions, and for biopsy in chronic diffuse lung disease (sarcoidosis, pneumoconiosis, interstitial pneumonia). The value of wedge resection for peripheral carcinoma remains controversial. The low surgical risk, as well as reports of survival rates comparable to those achieved with lobectomy [39], support use of the procedure in suitable cases–especially in patients who have severe pulmonary dysfunction.

The line of resection is chosen in accordance with pathologic findings and local anatomy, while avoiding the division of major bronchi or blood vessels. The lobe containing the lesion is delivered into the thoracotomy incision, and the lesion may be resected between clamps or stapled off (see below).

For open lung biopsy, we prefer for cosmetic reasons to make a small (5–8 cm) left anterior inframammary incision in the fourth interspace for access to the lingula. Gaensler and Carrington [26] recommend a thoracotomy in the second interspace, 2 cm lateral to the sternal margin, using the inferior border of the anterior segment of the upper lobe as the biopsy site. This approach gives a better view of the mediastinum; also, it is claimed that tissue from the lingula or middle lobe often is not representative of disease processes in the remainder of the lungs [40]. Following palpation of the lung tissue, a sufficiently large piece of lung (3 × 4 cm) is excised, or several specimens may be taken from multiple sites for various diagnostic studies (light and electron microscopy, immunohistology, bacteriologic and virologic studies, testing for fungal disease). The resection of inflated lung tissue will enable a better pathohistologic evaluation of the specimen.

1.6.2 Resection between Clamps

Two clamps with Glover jaws (or one curved clamp) are applied to outline the wedge of lung to be excised, leaving about a 2-cm margin of normal tissue around the lesion. The specimen is removed peripheral to the clamps with a scalpal (Fig. 62). A basting stitch (2-0 atraumatic absorbable monofilament) is placed behind the clamps, the clamps are removed, and the cut edge is oversewn with a simple over-and-over suture. The needle holes are sealed with fibrin glue.

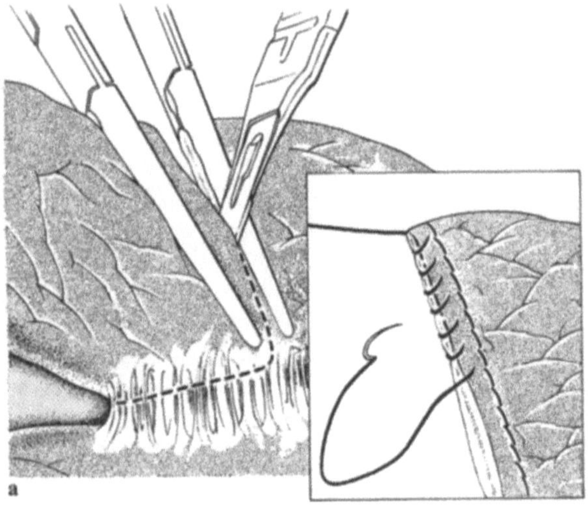

a b

Fig. 62 a, b. Pulmonary wedge resection between clamps

1.6.3 Resection with the Stapling Instrument

A simpler technique of pulmonary wedge resection involves the use of a stapling instrument (TA 30 to 90, 3.5 mm to 4.8 mm). The affected area is wedged out with two rows of staples applied in a V-shaped fashion. The unstapled area at the apex of the V is oversewn with interrupted sutures (2-0 or 3-0 atraumatic absorbable monofilament) (Fig. 63).

After the wedge has been excised, any bleeding points or parenchymal fistulas are secured with ligating sutures, or fibrin glue may be applied to the cut surface. If frozen section confirms adequate margins, the closure is checked for air leak by saline immersion, a drain is inserted, and the chest is closed in layers.

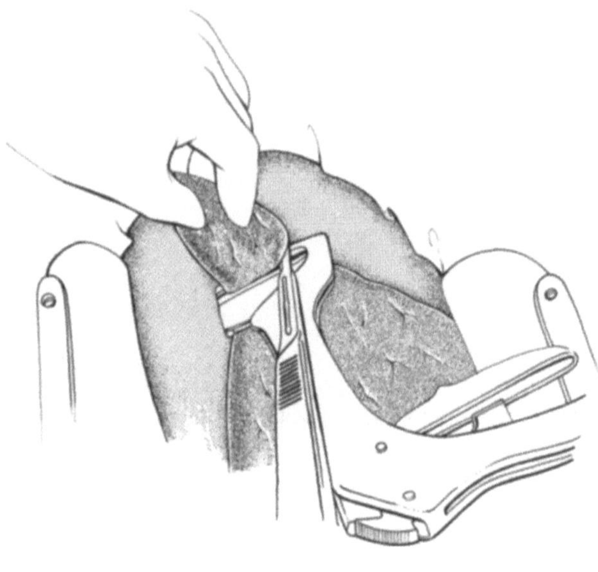

Fig. 63. Pulmonary wedge resection with the stapling instrument

1.7 Extensions of Pulmonary Resection

1.7.1 Resection of the Bronchi [77, 82]

1.7.1.1 Indications

Bronchial sleeve resection is mainly indicated for malignant tumors at the origin of the right upper lobe bronchus, for pneumonectomy in these cases is associated with a relatively high mortality and morbidity. Sleeve resections are also used for tumors at the origin of the left upper lobe, and rarely for tumors of the left lower lobe that have spread to the mainstem bronchus, in which case the upper lobe is anastomosed to the trachea or left main bronchus. There is diversity of opinion concerning the operative risk of sleeve resection (1.8%–19%, [80, 92, 102, 103]), but in patients with comparable prognoses, the more conservative sleeve resection results in a substantially smaller loss of pulmonary function than pneumonectomy.

Sleeve resection for carcinoma is appropriate only if the tumor is confined to one lobe and can be excised with a rim of healthy tissue. Incomplete tumor resections are associated with a high incidence of local recurrence and a correspondingly poor prognosis, so in doubtful cases the adequacy of the excision should be confirmed by frozen section. The value of sleeve resection in patients with mediastinal lymph node metastases is controversial. While Weisel [102] claims that peribronchial and tracheobronchial lymph node metastases do not contraindicate sleeve resection since the nodes can be removed as in a pneumonectomy, Maasen [53] categorically rejects sleeve resection in the presence of mediastinal involvement. Involvement of the pulmonary artery is not a strict contraindication to sleeve resection, for a segment of this vessel can be resected in suitable cases and continuity restored by reanastomosis (see p. 174). On the other hand, infiltration of the veins of the adjacent lobes generally is regarded as a contraindication for the procedure. There is also disagreement as to the value of preoperative irradiation in reducing tumor size and eliminating nodal metastases [91, 103].

Other, more frequent indications for sleeve resections are benign tumors close to the mainstem bronchus and inflammatory stenosis of a main bronchus leading to constriction of the lobar bronchus with loss of function of the pulmonary lobe. The partial resection of a bronchus without concurrent lobectomy may be appropriate for posttraumatic or tuberculous stenosis.

The type of procedure selected will depend on preoperative endoscopic findings, which the surgeon should personally check if possible, and on intraoperative findings. The definitive procedure is not decided upon until the chest has been entered, keeping in mind that an uncomplicated pneumonectomy can pose less danger to the patient than a lesser resection with a prolonged, complicated postoperative course.

1.7.1.2 Intubation

All resective procedures on the bronchi require temporary ventilation through the opposite lung. This is most easily accomplished by having the anesthetist advance the endotracheal tube temporarily into the contralateral main bronchus under the visual and digital guidance of the operator. After the anastomosis has been completed, the tube is withdrawn, and the integrity of the suture line is checked. It is further recommended that the pulmonary artery be clamped while the lung is isolated to prevent the admixture of unoxygenated blood. An alternative, available at some centers, is high-frequency jet ventilation, which provides adequate oxygentation even with an open airway system.

1.7.1.3 Wedge Resection of the Main Bronchus

Especially with benign tumors at the origin of the right or left upper lobe bronchus that show minimal involvement of the lumen, a wedge resection of the main bronchus combined with upper lobectomy can ensure a complete removal. The procedure is used less frequently for malignancies. Removing the tumor with adequate margins would create a relatively large defect whose direct closure might lead to kinking of the main bronchus with a restriction of ventilation. A sleeve resection is usually more appropriate in these cases.

The initial steps in the procedure correspond to those for a right or left upper lobectomy (see pp. 146 or 151). The veins and arteries should be divided first to facilitate subsequent handling of the bronchus, which is exposed from the posterior side. Adequate space can be gained by mobilizing the pulmonary artery, snaring it with a tape, and retracting it anteriorly to expose the origin of the lobar bronchus. The resection should be made as close as possible to the origin of the bronchus to minimize the size of the defect and should not exceed half the circumference of the main bronchus (Fig. 64). Also, care should be taken to resect equal portions from the anterior and posterior walls of the bronchus to enable a smooth, symmetrical closure without excessive angulation.

The wedge resection is closed from the angles toward the center with simple interrupted sutures (2-0 atraumatic absorbable monofilament) placed around the cartilage, preferably outside the mucosa, and perpendicular to the anastomotic line. After all the sutures have been placed, they are tied, proceeding from the ends of the anastomosis toward its center.

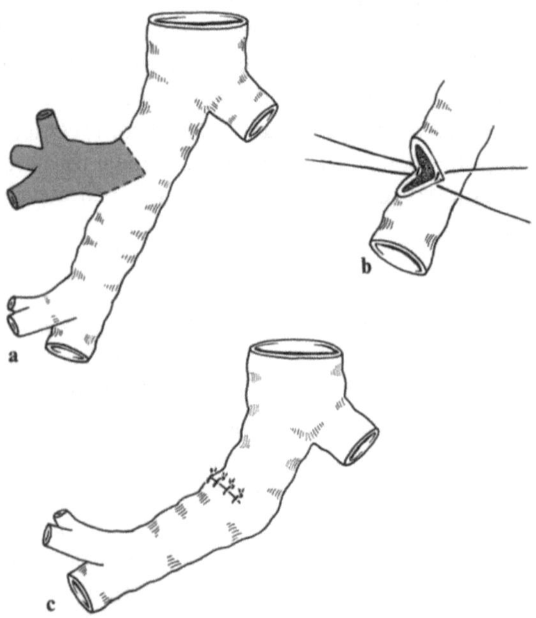

Fig. 64a–c. Wedge resection of the right main bronchus

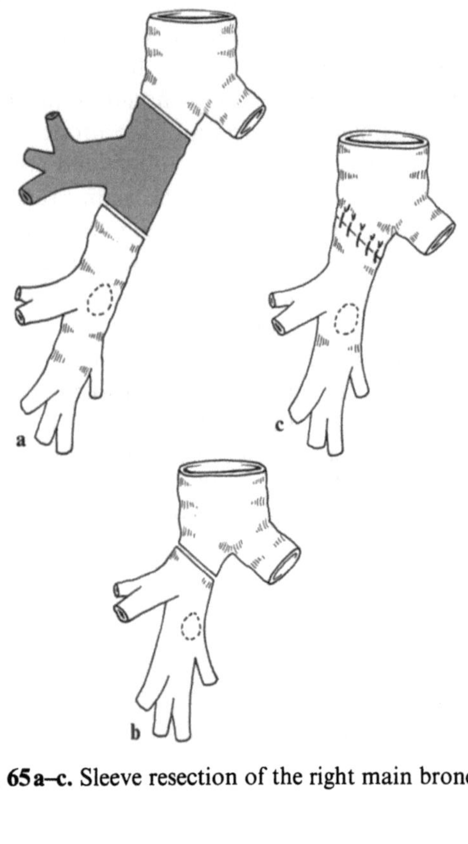

Fig. 65a–c. Sleeve resection of the right main bronchus

1.7.1.4 Sleeve Resection of the Right Main Bronchus

This procedure encompasses a right upper lobectomy, sleeve resection of the right main bronchus, and end-to-end anastomosis of the intermediate bronchus to the stump of the main bronchus or trachea (Fig. 65). The procedure is like that described for lobectomy up until division of the bronchus (see p. 138). It is easier to perform on the right side than on the left because of better access and the availability of the intermediate bronchus for anastomosis. After incision of the pleura as far as the azygos vein and isolation of that vein (which may have to be divided), the right main bronchus is exposed to the bifurcation and mobilized until the pulmonary artery can be snared and completely separated from the main bronchus. Partial resection of the pulmonary artery may be indicated if the vessel is involved by tumor (see p. 174). The bronchus is dissected free distally to the origins of the middle lobe bronchus and superior segmental bronchus. If findings warrant a sleeve resection after the bronchus has been dissected free, the endotracheal tube is advanced into the left main bronchus by the anesthetist. If this cannot be done, the resection may be performed by an open technique and the tube placed under direct vision after the segment has been excised. This maneuver is unnecessary when jet ventilation is employed.

The proximal bronchotomy is performed close to the trachea with a scalpel (Fig. 66). If the tumor has spread to the trachea but does not involve the left main bronchus or carina, a portion of the tracheal wall may additionally be removed. The distal division is made a sufficient distance from the origins of the middle-lobe and superior segmental bronchi to avoid stenosing the orifices of those segments. In rare cases where tumor has spread to the middle lobe, the latter may be removed concurrently with the upper lobe, followed by anastomosis of the lower lobe bronchus to the mainstem bronchus.

The anastomosis must make allowance for the different sizes of the lumina. The fit can be optimized by beveling or incising the distal bronchus to expand its lumen or by reducing the proximal lumen before the anastomosis is performed. The opening in the trachea or main bronchus can be made smaller by longitudinal suturing or by making a small wedge excision and closing it transversely. Usually the luminal discrepancy is minor

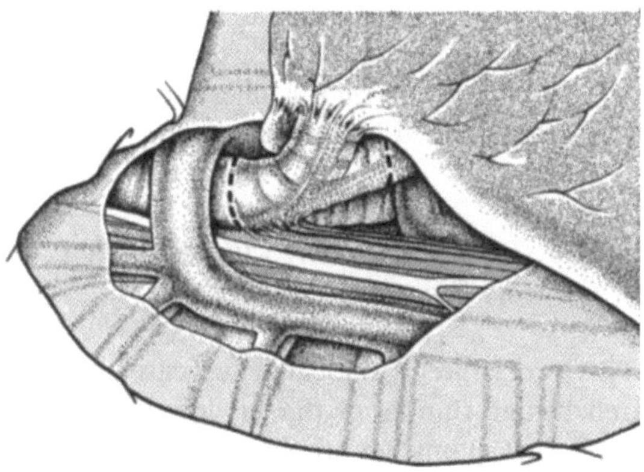

Fig. 66. Upper lobectomy with sleeve resection of the right main bronchus. The lines of resection are shown

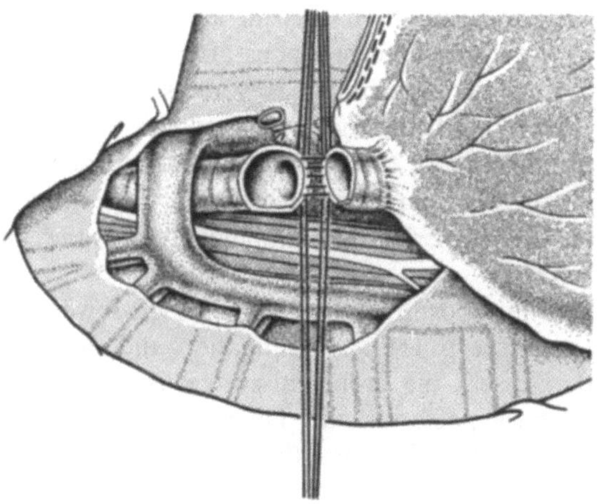

Fig. 67. Upper lobectomy with sleeve resection of the right main bronchus. Anastomosis of the bronchial stumps

and can be corrected by appropriate spacing of the sutures (Fig. 67). We perform the anastomosis with 2-0 atraumatic absorbable monofilament sutures, which are placed extramucosally with the knots outside the lumen. At least a portion of the adjacent cartilage rings are included in the suture line. The sutures on the side away from the surgeon (pars cartilaginea) are placed first and are tied after the stumps have been apposed. Then the rest of the circumference is closed, the ventilating tube is withdrawn into the trachea, and the integrity of the anastomosis is tested by immersion. Marked respiratory movements of the residual lung, especially on expiration, confirm adequate ventilation. Division of the pulmonary ligament is recommended to assist expansion of the residual lung. We do not cover the suture line with a flap of pleura or other tissue.

Keszler [45] described a rare procedure in patients with right lower lobe tumors and impaired pulmonary function, in which the lower lobe bronchus and intermediate bronchus are resected and the middle lobe is preserved by anastomosing the middle lobe bronchus to the proximal stump of the intermediate bronchus.

Lymph node dissection, drainage and closure of the chest are described on p. 148.

1.7.1.5 Sleeve Resection of the Left Main Bronchus

A spiral endotracheal tube is used that can be advanced temporarily into the right main bronchus. Given the shortness of the right main bronchus, we recommend using a double-lumen tube (e.g., Robert Shaw) to avoid occlusion of the right upper lobe bronchus.

Sleeve resection for tumors of the left upper lobe that involve the mainstem bronchus is more difficult than on the right side due to the constraints imposed by the aortic arch, the absence of an intermediate bronchus, and the proximity of the pulmonary artery. Björk [6] suggested mobilizing the aortic arch by dividing the superior four pairs of intercostal arteries and the ligamentum arteriosum and retracting the aorta far enough anteriorly that the left lower lobe can be sutured to the tracheal bifurcation. However, with careful technique it should be possible to perform the anastomosis without this extensive mobilization of the aorta, which carries a risk of spinal cord ischemia.

Because of its close relation to the upper lobe bronchus, the pulmonary artery may be infiltrated by tumor and require partial resection (see p. 174). After division of the veins and arteries of the upper lobe, the bronchus is mobilized from the posterior side while the snared pulmonary artery is pulled anteriorly. Division of the ligamentum arteriosum facilitates the central approach. Before the sleeve resection is performed, the endotracheal tube is advanced into the right main bronchus, at which time the left pulmonary artery may be occluded with a tourniquet. The extent of the sleeve resection is defined, the resection is performed with a scalpel or scissors, and the upper lobe is removed (Fig. 68). The origin of the superior segmental bronchus (B6) is left intact. Finally the lower lobe

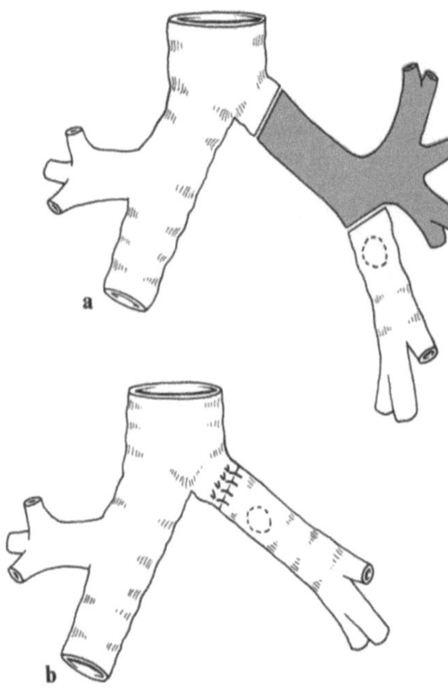

Fig. 68 a, b. Sleeve resection of the left main bronchus

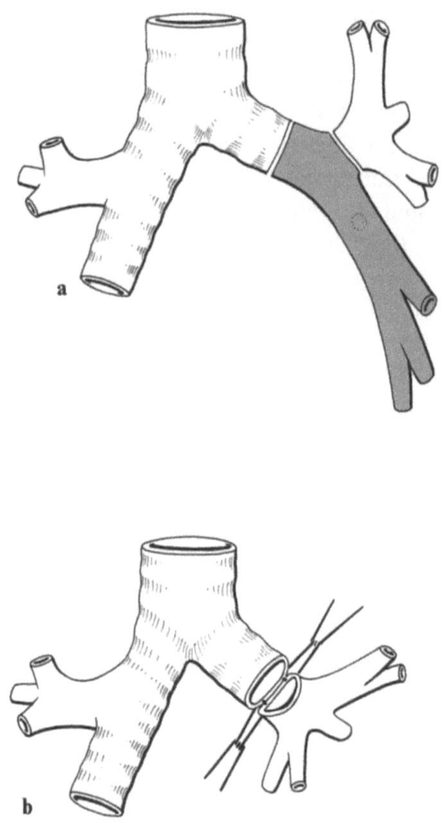

Fig. 69 a, b. Lower lobectomy with sleeve resection of the left main bronchus ("reverse" sleeve resection)

bronchus is reanastomosed to the proximal stump of the main bronchus.

Lymph node dissection, chest drainage and closure are described on p. 155.

1.7.1.6 Lower Lobectomy with Sleeve Resection of the Main Bronchus

This procedure is indicated for carcinoid lesions and benign tumors of the left lower lobe that involve that mainstem bronchus. Carcinomas of the left lower lobe that have spread to the main bronchus require pneumonectomy to eradicate the lymphatic drainage area.

The procedure is used mainly on the left side because of the greater length of the mainstem bronchus, which enables the stump to be sutured to the upper lobe bronchus after resection of the tumor-bearing segment (reverse sleeve resection) (Fig. 69). On the right side it would be necessary to anastomose the upper lobe to the trachea following the mainstem resection, which would require intrapericardial mobilization of the great vessels.

The exposure is like that for a left lower lobectomy (see p. 156). After ligation and division of the vessels, the bronchial system is dissected free from the posterior side. The pathology is checked, and in suitable cases the ventilator tube is advanced into the right main bronchus to immobilize the left lung. The upper lobe bronchus is divided close to its origin, preserving its vascular supply. The tumor-bearing lower lobe is removed with a segment of the left main bronchus, placing the line of resection so that a sufficient stump of main bronchus is left, yet adequate margins are obtained. The upper lobe bronchus is anastomosed to the mainstem stump with simple interrupted sutures (2-0 atraumatic absorbable monofilament), beginning on the cartilaginous portion of the bronchial wall on the side away from the operator (see p. 172 for suture technique).

1.7.2 Partial Resection of the Pulmonary Artery

If an upper lobe carcinoma situated close to the mainstem bronchus involves a segment of the pulmonary artery, that segment can be excised as part of the bronchial sleeve resection, and pneumonectomy can be avoided. Because of its anatomic relations, the left pulmonary artery is involved more frequently by upper lobe tumors than is the right artery (Fig. 70). The need for a pulmonary artery resection is assessed intraoperatively after the bronchial system and pulmonary artery have been dissected free. The pulmonary trunk should be encircled with a tourniquet before the dissection is begun.

The extent of the pulmonary artery resection (tangential or circumferential resection) is dependent on pathologic findings. If tumor infiltration precludes the ligation of segmental arteries, their site of origin on the parent vessel can be excised between vascular clamps or with a Satinsky clamp and the vessel closed transversely or longitudinally with interrupted sutures (5-0 atraumatic nonabsorbable monofilament), using a patch graft as required. If the whole circumference of the pulmonary artery is involved by tumor, the involved segment is occluded proximally with the tourniquet and distally with a vascular clamp after other dissections have been completed. The tumor-bearing segment of the pulmonary artery is then excised at the time of the bronchial sleeve resection. On completion of the bronchial anastomosis, the vascular stumps are approximated with a double row of continuous atraumatic sutures (6-0 atraumatic nonabsorbable monofilament). Care is taken during suturing not to exert undue tension on the delicate, muscular vessel wall.

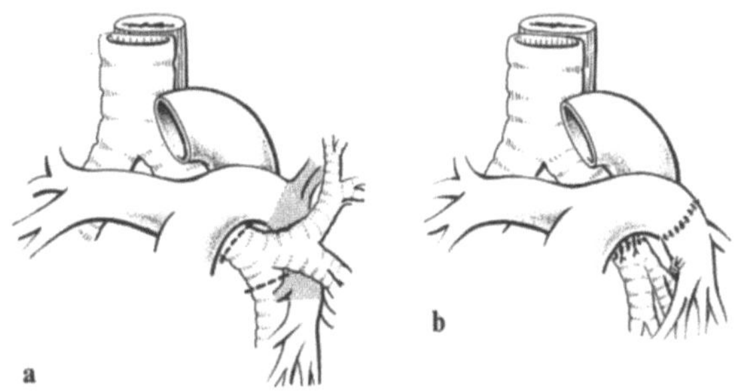

Fig. 70 a, b. Extended pulmonary resection. Partial resection of the left pulmonary artery and sleeve resection of the bronchus

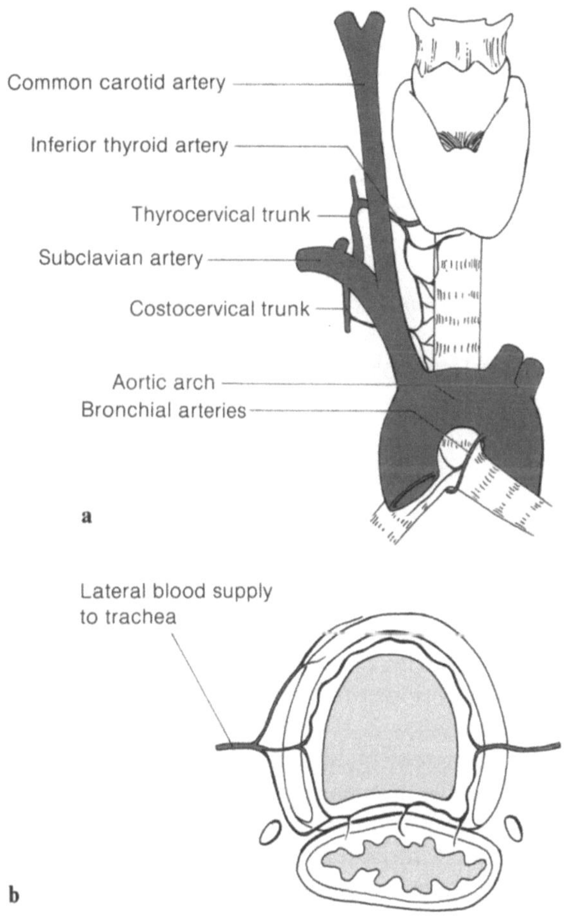

Fig. 71 a, b. Arterial supply to the trachea

1.7.3 Resection of the Distal Trachea and Carina

Steps in procedure:

(1) Accurate preoperative localization of the disease and determination of its extent
(2) Sparing mobilization to preserve the blood supply to the remaining trachea
(3) Anastomosis of healthy wall with absorbable suture material

1.7.3.1 Basic Surgical Anatomy

The trachea in adults measures about 12 cm (10–13 cm) from the inferior border of the cricoid cartilage to the carina, of which about 5 cm is cervical and 7 cm intrathoracic. The trachea contains between 17 and 22 [40, 72] cartilaginous rings, or about 2 per cm of its length.

The cervical part of the trachea is supplied by branches of the inferior thyroid artery, and the thoracic part by tracheoesophageal vessels from the subclavian artery, internal mammary artery, and the superior intercostal arteries. The bifurcation is supplied by bronchial arteries originating from the aorta (Fig. 71). The vessels interanastomose on both sides of the traches, which they enter laterally. It is best, therefore, to mobilize the trachea from its anterior and posterior sides, which are relatively avascular.

1.7.3.2 Mobilization

Depending on the patient's age, up to 3 cm of the trachea can be removed, and approximation effected, without the need for extensive mobilization. Where a greater length of trachea must be resected, the mobilization of adjacent structures is required. For resections of the distal trachea, additional length can be gained by dissecting out the hilum and dividing the pulmonary ligament, by intrapericardial mobilization of the pulmonary vessels, and even by transecting the left main bronchus, which is fixed below the aortic arch, and implanting it in the intermediate bronchus, although this compounds the operative risk.

1.7.3.3 Instruments

Basic set II, endobronchial tubes and extension.

1.7.3.4 Indications

Because the right main bronchus is shorter than the left, the bifurcation is more commonly involved by right-sided tumors than left-sided tumors. The high postoperative mortality following tracheal resections has been reduced somewhat by improved perioperative management, although it still approaches 22%–30% in large series [101]. It can be extremely difficult to preserve the blood supply to the bronchial system when mobilizing the trachea, which is why open surgery in carcinoma patients should always be weighed against other treatment options (irradiation, endoscopic tumor removal). Resection of the distal trachea and carina is indicated for tumors (benign tumors or slow-growing malignancies) that have spread from the mainstem bronchi and also for recurrent tumors of the bronchial stump that are not associated with extensive mediastinal or hematogenous spread. Even when the tumor has spread to the trachea, it may not be necessary to resect the entire bifurcation, and so the type of anastomosis required will depend on the individual case.

1.7.3.5 Wedge Resection of the Trachea and Carina

In rare cases a carcinoma of the right upper lobe may spread along the upper border of the right main bronchus to involve the distal trachea while sparing the bifurcation. These cases can be managed by a pneumonectomy with partial resection of the trachea, and the defect repaired by using the uninvolved medial portion of the main bronchus as a flap [44, 95] (Fig. 72). A portion of the upper lobe bronchus can be used for a similar purpose after excision of the carina [44, 96]. Pneumonectomy can be avoided in some cases by anastomosing the intermediate bronchus to the tracheal lumen, which is appropriately reduced to accommodate the smaller bronchial orifice (Fig. 73 a,b). The transplantation of a bronchial flap has been successful in isolated cases [55].

1.7.3.6 Right Sleeve Pneumonectomy with Removal of the Bifurcation

When the bifurcation is removed as part of a right pneumonectomy, the patient must be ventilated across the operative field until the tracheobronchial anastomosis is completed. Before the resection is performed, appropriate airway tubes and a sterile ventilator connector are prepared and are available on the field. The trachea and the tumor-bearing right main bronchus are dissected free, and two traction sutures are placed through the tracheal wall above the proposed line of resection. Similar sutures are placed in the left main bronchus distal to the line of resection. After adequate oxygenation has been established, the trachea is divided transversely in its distal third about 1 cm above the lesion, and the left main bronchus is obliquely divided close to its origin so that the bifurcation can be removed along with the tumor-bearing right lung.

The patient is now ventilated through a tube inserted directly into the left main bronchus. Before the bifurcation is reconstructed, it is wise to obtain frozen-section confirmation of the margins to avoid a palliative resection. The luminal disparity between the trachea and left main bronchus can generally be corrected by beveling the end of the bronchus and by spacing the sutures differently in the tracheal and bronchial stumps. The anastomosis is performed with simple interrupted sutures (2-0 or 3-0 absorbable monofilament) placed exter-

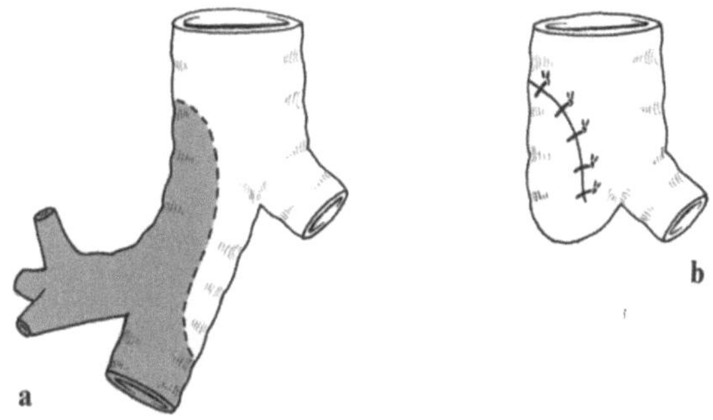

Fig. 72a, b. Right pneumonectomy with partial resection of the trachea, closed with a medial flap of bronchus

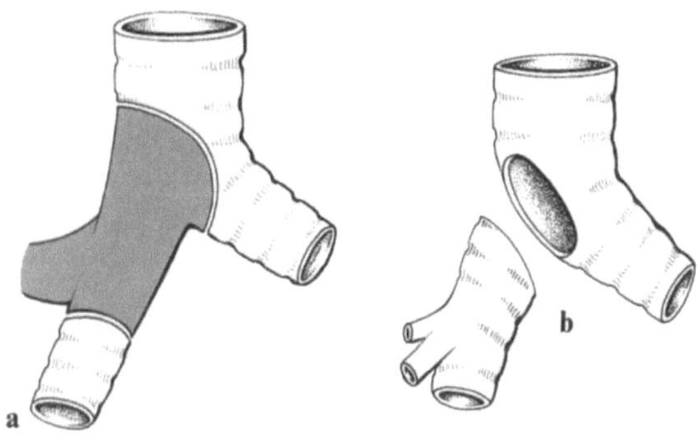

Fig. 73a, b. Right upper lobectomy with partial resection of the trachea and implantation of the right intermediate bronchus

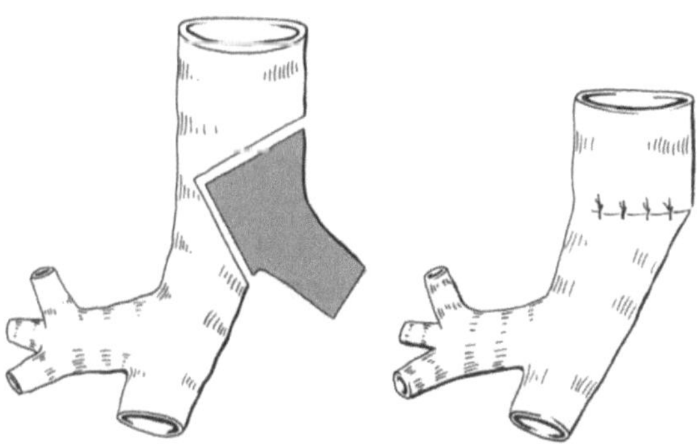

Fig. 74a. Left pneumonectomy with wedge resection of the trachea

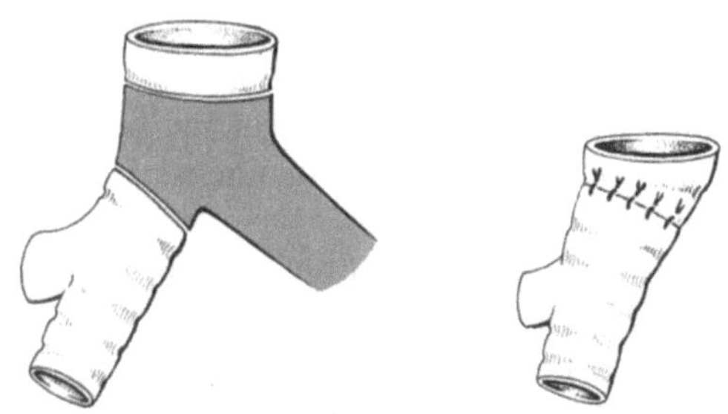

Fig. 74b. Left pneumonectomy with resection of the bifurcation

nal to the mucosa and around the cartilage, starting on the side of the trachea away from the operator. The central suture is placed first, and additional threads are placed outward from it and tied. The traction sutures are used to maintain approximation of the bronchus and trachea. When half the anastomosis has been completed, the traction sutures are removed, and the anastomosis is manipulated by the two corner threads. The distal ventilating tube may be removed, and the endobronchial tube may be advanced into position until all the anastomotic sutures have been placed and tied. The tube is then withdrawn into the trachea and the integrity of the suture line assessed. The procedure is completed in the fashion of a standard pneumonectomy. The patient should be extubated as soon after surgery as possible. If ventilatory support is required, the tube should be positioned above the anastomosis to avoid pressure injury. Tracheotomy should be avoided.

1.7.3.7 Left Sleeve Pneumonectomy with Removal of the Bifurcation

Dissection of the bifurcation is more difficult through a left-sided approach than a right-sided approach due to the presence of the aortic arch. Left-sided, centrally located bronchogenic carcinomas that extend to the bifurcation tend to infiltrate adjacent structures and the aorta, so resection of the bifurcation is rarely appropriate. With less invasive tumors, the bifurcation and distal trachea are accessible after pneumonectomy even with a left-sided approach (Fig. 74 a,b). Björk's technique of aortic mobilization [6] was mentioned previously (see p. 133), but we consider it to be unnecessary in most cases.

Formerly a two-stage, bilateral procedure was recommended for the removal of left-sided pulmonary tumors involving the bifurcation, but this has become obsolete owing to positive experience with a single-stage operation [89]. Some authors have also recommended a transsternal approach.

The dissection, resection, and anastomosis are the same as described for right-sided neoplasms (see p. 176).

1.7.3.8 Resection of the Bifurcation

1.7.3.8.1 Intubation. The patient is intubated with a spiral endotracheal tube long enough to be advanced into the left main bronchus. A sterile airway tube and extra ventilator are required for temporary ventilation of the left lung through the operative field.

1.7.3.8.2 Position and Approach. Lateral decubitus, posterolateral thoracotomy in the bed of the fourth rib on the right side. The carina also may be resected from a left-sided approach in diseases that necessitate a left pneumonectomy (see above).

1.7.3.8.3 Instruments. Basic set II.

1.7.3.8.4 Operative Technique. The carina is dissected free on all sides, preserving the blood supply to the healthy trachea. The extent of the resection will depend on the extent of disease, but every effort should be made to preserve uninvolved portions of the tracheal or bronchial walls (Fig. 75).

Next traction sutures are placed proximally in the trachea and distally in both main bronchi. After the left bronchus has been opened distal to the lesion, an airway tube is introduced for temporary ventilation of the left lung. The right lung is not ventilated while the anastomosis is performed. Clamping of the right pulmonary artery is also recommended. Additional ventilation of the right lung through the operative field may be necessary in patients with significant preexisting pulmonary dysfunction. After resecting the carina, we first suture the adjacent portions of the bronchial walls together. We then suture the posterior wall of the trachea to the posterior walls of both main bronchi. At that point the distal tube may be removed, and the endobronchial tube may be passed into the left main bronchus while the anterior part of the anastomosis is completed. After all sutures have been placed and tied, the tube is withdrawn into the trachea, and both lungs are inflated. Coverage of the anastomosis with a pedicled pleural flap has been recommended [72].

When extensive resection of the left main bronchus is necessary, the stump cannot be anastomosed to the trachea because of its fixation below the aortic arch. One solution in these cases is to anastomose the right main bronchus to the trachea, whose lumen is appropriately reduced, and then bring the left main bronchus across the mediastinum for anastomosis to the intermediate bronchus [2]. As the latter sutures are placed, the bronchial system is sealed off digitally or with sponges to secure ventilation.

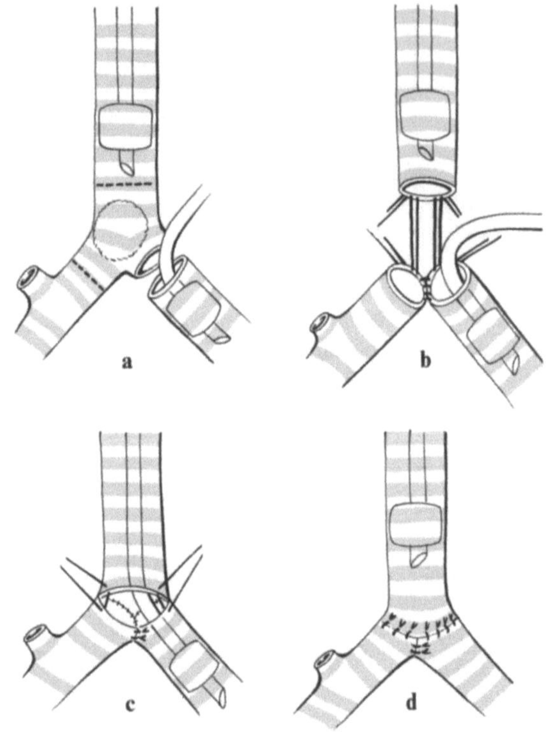

Fig. 75a–d. Resection of the bifurcation (see text)

1.7.3.9 Resection of the Distal Trachea

1.7.3.9.1 Indications. Stenosis of the distal trachea secondary to intubation or neoplastic disease.

1.7.3.9.2 Intubation. Spiral endotracheal tube. Sterile tube for temporarily ventilation through the operative field.

Mobilization of the Trachea

- Without mobilization: up to 3 cm can be resected and the ends approximated.
- Extrapericardial mobilization of the hilum and division of the pulmonary ligament: 3 cm gain in length
- Intrapericardial mobilization of the hilum: 1 cm gain in length
- Division of the left main bronchus and implantation of stump into intermediate bronchus: 2.5 cm gain in length

1.7.3.9.3 Instruments. Basic set II.

1.7.3.9.4 Position and Approach. Posterolateral thoracotomy in the bed of the fourth rib on the right side. Lateral decubitus position with the head free to move so that length can be gained by cervical flexion.

1.7.3.9.5 Operative Technique. Since it it not always possible to push an endotracheal tube past the site of the stenosis, the patient should be fully prepped for surgery at the time anesthesia is induced, as it may be necessary to expose the trachea and carina quickly, open the stenosis distally, and ventilate the patient through a tube passed distally into the right main bronchus. If the patient's ventilatory status permits, the resection should be delayed until the trachea and adjacent mainstem bronchi can be dissected free and mobilized, and the reconstructive technique is determined.

The thoracotomy incision is made, and the pleura is incised between the trachea and esophagus from the superior border of the hilum to the innominate vein. The azygos vein is divided between ligatures. The anterior and posterior surfaces of the trachea are adequately dissected from the vena cava and esophagus. If the extent of the resection requires it, the pleura is incised over the hilum, the pulmonary ligament is severed, and the main bronchi are exposed as far as the pulmonary artery on the right side and 2–3 cm below the aortic arch on the left side. Additional length can be gained by incising the pericardium and circumferentially dissecting the hilar vessels.

Before the trachea is divided, traction sutures are placed above and below the lesion, and a suitable airway tube and connecting equipment are made available. The trachea is now divided below the site of the stenosis. If the lowermost level of the pathology cannot be established by palpation or from the position of the tube, the trachea is opened close to the principal lesion, and additional tissue is resected as necessary. Care is taken not to remove too much trachea, although the trachea should be divided where the tissue appears normal (Fig. 76). At this point the distal trachea is intubated, and the tube is passed into the left main bronchus and connected to a separate anesthesia machine. Dissection is now carried farther up the trachea, which is transected above the stenosis.

The first suture for reapproximating the trachea is placed in the midline posteriorly. The sutures (2-0 or 3-0 atraumatic absorbable monofilament)

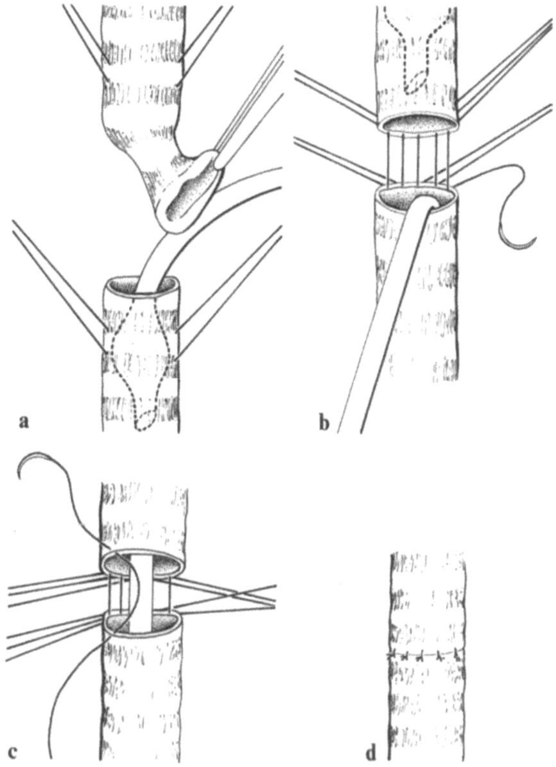

Fig. 76a–d. Resection of tracheal stenosis, reconstruction by end-to-end anastomosis

are placed around the cartilage and external to the mucosa in simple interrupted fashion. Animal studies have shown a correlation in the trachea between anastomotic tension and anastomotic strength, so the declining tensile strength of absorbable sutures has the effect of increasing the strength of the anastomosis [8]. Starting from the center, the remaining sutures for the posterior part of the anastomosis (pars membranacea) are placed and then tied while the cut ends of the trachea are approximated with the traction sutures and the patient's head is flexed forward. When the posterior sutures have been placed, the distal tube is removed, and the endotracheal tube is advanced through the anastomosis. Next the anterior anastomotic sutures are applied. Luminal disparities generally can be corrected by adjusting the suture spacing. After all sutures have been placed and tied, the tube is withdrawn into the upper trachea, the anastomosis is tested for leakage, and the chest is closed over a drainage catheter. The patient should be extubated as soon as possible, and tracheotomy should be avoided due to the risk of infection in the operative area.

1.7.4 Tracheal Reconstruction

Attempts to bridge large defects in the trachea with prosthetic materials are still mostly in the experimental stage. Long-term results with the use of a Marlex patch sutured to the outside of the trachea and covered with a pedicled pericardial flap are not yet available [63]. Neville [67] employed a silicone prosthesis as a substitute for the trachea or bifurcation. The prosthesis is introduced transluminally, and the wall of the trachea or bronchus is tacked to plastic rings on the implant. Results to date are inconclusive, but the procedure may offer an acceptable option in borderline situations (tumor obstruction with impending asphyxiation, lack of therapeutic alternatives) [102].

1.7.4.1 Partial Resection of the Superior Vena Cava

Tumors widely encasing the superior vena cava generally signify inoperability. However, if only a circumscribed area of the vein is infiltrated by tumor or a lymph node metastasis with an otherwise localized and resectable primary tumor, partial resection of the superior vena cava may be indicated.

Due to the risk of cerebral injury, it has been recommended that a temporary bypass be established between the vena cava and right atrium, but we do not believe that this is necessary routinely. In cases with limited tumor growth and involvement of the vena cava, we separate the tumor from the vena cava while temporarily clamping the vessel without opening it. We then dissect more of the vessel wall free and excise portions that show tumor infiltration. Smaller defects are repaired with a venous, xenogenous, or allogenous patch. If a longer segment of vessel is resected, continuity is restored with an allogenous vascular or plastic prosthesis of equal luminal diameter. We recommend establishing an arteriovenous fistula in the arm to increase the flow velocity through the vessel and reduce the danger of thrombosis.

1.7.4.2 Partial Removal of the Left Atrium

Partial removal of the left atrium may be indicated for tumor that has spread along the pulmonary vein to the left atrium, and also for the intrapericardial ligation and division of the pulmonary vein. The procedure corresponds to that described previously for intrapericardial dissection of the pulmonary vessels (see p. 134). The site of entry of both pulmonary veins is clamped off (Satinsky) along with portions of the left atrium, and the clamped area is excised. The defect is closed with a double row of continuous over-and-over sutures (3-0 atraumatic monofilament).

1.7.4.3 Concomitant Removal of Other Organs

The extent of disease may require that the pulmonary resection be combined with removal of other structures such as the chest wall (q.v.) or diaphragm (q.v.). Wide infiltration of the *esophagus* with involvement of the mucosa generally implies that the disease has progressed to an inoperable stage. On the other hand, tumor that has infiltrated the muscular coat of the esophagus locally without invading the mucosa can be removed without opening the lumen. If the extent of disease required that the esophagus be opened at operation, it will be necessary to perform an esophagectomy, occlude the pouch distally, establish a cervical esophagostomy, and construct a feeding gastrostomy. When the patient has recovered from the procedure and there is no evidence of tumor progression, esophageal replacement (colon reconstruction) may be undertaken in a second stage.

1.8 Complications Following Pulmonary Resection

1.8.1 Atelectasis

Atelectasis is avoided by carefully inflating the lung intraoperatively before the chest is closed. Before the patient is extubated, a chest X-ray is taken to assess the status of the contralateral lung and hemithorax, and bronchoscopic suctioning is performed as required. A program of intensive physiotherapy is instituted after surgery and is supported by nasotracheal or bronchoscopic suction. A rare cause of postoperative atelectasis is torsion of a pulmonary lobe, usually the middle lobe or the isolated lingula. This can be prevented by stapling or suturing these segments to the adjacent lung. The torsion of a lobe with hemorrhagic infarction implies disruption of the bronchopulmonary vessels. Blood gas data can be misleading in these cases due to the absence of an intrapulmonary shunt [43]. Pulmonary torsion is manifested clinically by a progressive downhill course with persistent opacity of the twisted lung. Treatment consists in early reoperation and removal of the atelectatic area.

1.8.2 Postoperative Bleeding

Postoperative bleeding from the major hilar vessels is rare following standard resective procedures on the lung. It is more common to encounter bleeding from the pleura after the separation of adhesions, from intercostal vessels, or from bronchial arteries following lymph node dissection. The main factor in the prevention of postoperative hemorrhage, besides meticulous intraoperative hemostasis, is complete expansion of the residual lung. Viereck [100] recommends that this be accomplished by pressure-adapated drainage through a double-catheter system that enables a negative pressure of 6 to 20 cm H_2O to be applied postoperatively, depending on the extent of existing parenchymal fistulas. The indication for reexploration is acute in the face of a massive hemorrhage or a sustained blood loss exceeding 250 ml/h for more than 4 h. Removal of intrathoracic clot is indicated when the clot enlarges to the size of a fist or exceeds more than one-fourth the volume of the hemithorax in the first days after surgery. After 4–6 weeks decortication is recommended, since by that time the organization phase of the clot will be complete [100].

1.8.3 Parenchymal Fistula

A distinction is drawn between postoperative parenchymal fistula and bronchial stump leak. Most parenchymal fistulas can be closed intraoperatively by suture ligation with absorbable monofilament threads or with fibrin glue. High postoperative ventilatory pressures are avoided by extubating the patient as soon after surgery as possible. If air leakage still occurs, an expectant approach may be taken if the fistula is small. The parenchymal openings should close spontaneously with progressive expansion of the residual lung. Occasionally this expansion can be induced by temporarily increasing the suction on the chest tubes (8–12 h, -20 to -40 cm H_2O). If the leak persists beyond the seventh postoperative day, the drainage tube should be partly withdrawn (as its openings permit) while maintaining a moderate suction so that the lung can fuse with the pleura. A refractory fistula is an indication for reoperation.

A mild residual pneumothorax after pulmonary resection generally will become absorbed and requires no special treatment.

1.8.4 Bronchial Stump Leak

Leakage from the bronchial suture or staple line may occur at any time during the initial days or months after a pulmonary resection. It is more common after pneumonectomy than after a lobectomy or segmentectomy. Causes include infection of the suture line, excessive bronchial stump length, excessive dissection of the bronchial wall, and faulty suturing technique. A stump leak can also result from tumor infiltration of the resection line. The condition is manifested clinically by the expectoration of pleural contents and radiographically by an expanding collection of air in the pleural cavity. Diagnosis is confirmed by bronchoscopy.

If continuous air leak from the chest tube is noted in the early postoperative period, an urgent indication exists for reexploration. If a bronchial stump leak develops later in the postoperative course, management depends on the type of primary operation. In the lobectomized patient the incompetent stump is resected, and the freshened stump is resutured and covered with a vascularized flap of intercostal muscle (see p. 119). In the pneumonectomized patient, the primary treatment measure for leakage from a mainstem bronchial stump is drainage of the pleural space and systemic antibiotic therapy. Generally these patients, too, will require reoperation with closure of the bronchus, which may be done transmediastinally in conjunction with an adequate thoracoplasty for treatment of empyema. The technique of bronchial closure will depend on circumstances. If sufficient wall can be mobilized, the stump may be restapled; otherwise simple interrupted sutures are used.

Bronchopleural fistulas following surgery for tuberculosis are particularly serious. Again, primary treatment consists of drainage, although this measure alone usually cannot effect closure of the fistulas. This requires a thoracoplasty, at which time the stump may be covered with a pedicled flap of intercostal or pectoralis muscle.

1.8.5 Esophagopleural Fistula

At one time this rare condition was seen mostly after pneumonectomy for tuberculosis and following the separation of massive adhesions. Its incidence after pneumonectomy for carcinoma is approximately 0.5%, with the majority of cases occurring on the right side [23]. A communication between the esophagus and pleural space can result from intraoperative injury to the esophagus during the removal of mediastinal lymph nodes, a disturbance of the blood supply at the level of the carina, or an infection of the pleural space spreading to the esophagus. Late cases may be caused by recurrent tumor. Treatment depends on the time of occurrence and underlying cause. Measures include antibiotic therapy, parenteral hyperalimentation, drainage of empyema, and definitive closure of the fistula. The sooner the fistula develops after surgery, the more urgent the indication for its closure. This can be done by oversewing the defect, covering the fistula with a pedicled flap of muscle or pleura, or by performing an esophagectomy and reconstructing the esophagus in a second stage. Thoracoplasty may follow if required. In some cases symptoms can be improved by the placement of an endoesophageal tube, especially when the fistula is caused by a tumor.

2 Special Part

2.1 Tumors

2.1.1 Benign Lung Tumors

The goal of surgery is to remove the benign tumor with a margin of healthy tissue. Peripheral lesions are removed by wedge resection, while centrally located tumors are managed by segmentectomy or lobectomy. Subpleural hamartomas can be shelled out. With benign tumors of the bronchial system, bronchoscopic resection is adequate only for the rare lesions that are pedunculated. Operative excision of the tumor-bearing bronchial wall is usually required. The defect may be closed directly if it is small enough, or a bronchoplastic sleeve resection and reanastomosis may be performed. Healthy lung parenchyma should be preserved if at all possible. If it is unclear whether the tumor is benign or malignant, an intraoperative frozen section examination is advised.

2.1.2 Arteriovenous Aneurysms [14]

Arteriovenous aneurysms are rare, usually congenital malformations that may be solitary (1/3) or multiple (2/3). Most are asymptomatic and are detected incidentally on chest X-rays [40]. Before a patient is selected for operation, a pulmonary arteriogram must be obtained to establish the diagnosis and determine the number of malformations that are present.

Surgical treatment is indicated:

(1) in patients who are symptomatic due to a large shunt volume,
(2) when enlargement is noted,
(3) in the presence of multiple lesions to reduce the shunt volume, and
(4) when lesions communicate with the systemic circulation [18].

When changes are diffuse and involve both lungs, surgical treatment is not feasible.

The procedure of choice is a wedge resection, segmental resection, or lobectomy so that parenchyma can be conserved. Embolization may be attempted as an alternative to open surgery [81].

2.1.3 *Malignant Tumors*

2.1.3.1 *Bronchogenic Carcinoma*

2.1.3.1.1 Indications for Surgery. Surgery is the treatment of choice for bronchogenic carcinoma unless contraindications exist. These include:

(1) Distant hematogenous, lymphogenous (contralateral, cervical) or pleural metastases.

Hematogenous spread can be detected preoperatively with a high degree of confidence. For assessing mediastinal lymph node involvement, CT has largely replaced mediastinoscopy among our patients as a routine preoperative study. However, experience to date is not yet adequate to prove inoperability, so suspicion of contralateral lymph node involvement should be checked by mediastinoscopy if the patient appears to be operable on the basis of other findings.
Pleural effusion contraindicates surgery in patients with cytologic proof of malignancy. In the absence of pleural effusion, the indication for surgery depends on other findings.

(2) Small cell anaplastic carcinomas. These tumors generally are managed by a combination of radiotherapy and chemotherapy. Exceptions are peripheral tumors without mediastinal lymph node metastases (T1 N0 M0), for which surgical resection followed by adjuvant chemotherapy is increasingly recommended [38].

(3) Involvement of nonresectable adjacent structures. Wide infiltration of the esophagus, aorta, vena cava, cardiac wall, trachea, and contralateral mainstem bronchus generally contraindicate a local excision. Sites of limited infiltration may be removed, however (see above). Recurrent or phrenic nerve palsy due to tumor infiltration also signifies inoperability. But if the recurrent nerve palsy is due to lymph node enlargement, eradication of the tumor may still be possible in selected cases. If preoperative studies are unable to establish the extent of disease, this should be clarified by exploratory thoracotomy.

(4) Patients at risk. Preexisting cardiopulmonary disease may prohibit resectional surgical. The decision to operate will depend on the results of pulmonary function tests, perfusion scan, tumor staging, and the extent of the proposed resection [48].

2.1.3.1.2 Procedure. Lesions of undetermined histology are removed by wedge resection or less frequently by a segmentectomy or lobectomy and evaluated intraoperatively by frozen section. A histologic diagnosis is required before a pneumonectomy may be undertaken for tumor removal. The procedure of choice for the treatment of bronchogenic carcinoma is lobectomy. Pneumonectomy offers no added benefit in terms of life expectancy for a tumor that is confined to one lobe and surrounded by healthy parenchyma [4, 13, 78] yet is associated with a two-fold higher mortality rate and a greater morbidity than lobectomy. Segmentectomy is considered by some to be an adequate procedure for stage I disease [42], but high rates of local recurrence [5] and unfavorable long-term results [61] do not appear to justify its routine use, especially when one considers the marked decline in the risk of lobectomy. Like wedge resection, the procedure may be appropriate in borderline situations.
Surgical treatment of bronchogenic carcinoma includes eradication of the ipsilateral lymphatic drainage tract [66, 84] both to assess the extent of disease and to improve the prognosis. Although prospective randomized studies on this point are lacking, clinical results even in N2 disease (with mediastinal node involvement) justify an attempt at radical resection, which may be combined with postoperative radiation (49% 3-year survival [58]).

2.1.3.2 *Pancoast Tumor*

Apical lung tumors associated with erosion of the ribs and infiltration of the brachial plexus and stellate ganglion [75] remain localized for some time, are prone to local infiltration, and tend to produce nodal and distant metastases as a late event. The combination of radiotherapy and surgical resection appears to give better results than radiation or surgery alone [59]. The prognosis is most favorable in the absence of lymph node metastasis and distant spread (up to 50% 5-year survival [97]).

Martini et al. [56, 57] recommend a combined modality in which the diagnosis of carcinoma is first established by transthoracic needle biopsy under fluoroscopic control. Then the patient is given external radiation in a dose of 4000 rad administered over a period of 4 weeks. Four weeks following irradiation the extent of the disease is reevaluated. If the tumor is still localized, thoracotomy is performed, and if possible an en bloc excision of all involved tissues, including the chest wall and arm, is carried out. Residual tumor is treated by the implantation of iodine-125 seeds. Masaoka et al. [58] recommend approaching the tumor through an upper sternotomy with an anterolateral thoracotomy in the fourth interspace supplemented by a transverse cervical incision above the clavicle. This is said to provide better exposure than the posterolateral thoracotomy [90].

2.1.3.3 Pulmonary Metastases [19, 98]

2.1.3.3.1 Indications for Surgery. The surgical removal of pulmonary metastases is acceptable only when employed as part of a scientifically founded, combined treatment modality concept.

Several criteria must be met before the resection of pulmonary metastases may be considered:

(1) an eradicated primary tumor with no local recurrence, or complete removal of the primary tumor in a synchronous procedure;
(2) absence of metastases in other organs;
(3) resectability of all pulmonary metastases; and
(4) lack of therapeutic alternatives.

The presence of bilateral or multiple metastases, a short interval between the primary operation and detection of metastases, the spread of metastases to the chest wall or mediastinum, and a short tumor doubling time are poor prognostic signs [65, 83] but do not necessarily contraindicate surgery as long as the other criteria are satisfied. Surgical resection may also be appropriate in borderline cases if it would have a reasonable chance of improving the efficacy of nonsurgical therapies. The decision whether to recommend surgery also depends on the primary tumor and the pattern of metastases. With tumors that tend to seed to multiple organs (e.g., malignant melanoma), surgery is preceded by a more extensive diagnostic workup and is elected less frequently than in patients whose tumors tend to produce isolated pulmonary metastases (e.g., hypernephroma, sarcoma).

2.1.3.3.2 Procedure. The goal of surgery is excision of the metastatic lesions with a margin of healthy tissue. Enucleation is not adequate and predisposes to recurrence. Most pulmonary metastases are peripheral and subpleural, and a wedge resection with a stapling instrument may be acceptable for these lesions. Centrally located tumors will require a lobectomy or segmentectomy. Pneumonectomy is very rarely justified. Before the resection is begun, the hilar and mediastinal lymph nodes should be evaluated (e.g., by frozen section), and the entire lung should be carefully palpated in both the inflated and deflated condition. Ramming [82] stresses the importance of marking all metastases at the start of the operation to avoid later confusion with atelectatic areas or sites of intrapulmonary hemorrhage.

Generally it is recommended that bilateral metastases be resected in one sitting through a median sternotomy [60]. Metastases in the left lower lobe are not easily accessible by this route and are managed more effectively by a single-stage [65] or two-stage bilateral thoracotomy, beginning on the less involved side so that the indication for resection on the contralateral side can be more accurately assessed.

2.2 Cystic Lung Diseases (Table 2)

Cystic diseases of the lung encompass a variety of conditions for which a uniform nomenclature does not exist. A cyst in the true sense is a pathologic cavity lined by epithelium. This must be distinguished from the emphysematous bulla, which is covered by visceral pleura and lacks an epithelial lining, and from the pseudocyst (pneumatocele), which can develop in the wake of a necrotizing pneumonitis. Depending on their etiology and relation to the bronchial system, the cysts may be air- or water-filled, may remain stationary or increase in size, or may be asymptomatic or incite complications (compression of the surrounding parenchyma, hemorrhage, infection, rupture). It is important surgically to distinguish congenital and acquired cystic diseases in infants and newborns from cystic lesions that develop in later life [95].

Table 2. Morphologic classification of congenital cystic malformations of the lung. (After Spencer [94])

I.	Congenital cysts a) Central type b) Peripheral type
II.	Cystic malformation in pulmonary sequestration
III.	Adenomatoid cystic malformation
IV.	Cystic lymphangiectasis
V.	Enterogenic cysts

2.2.1 Congenital Malformations

2.2.1.1 Lobar Emphysema [67]

Lobar emphysema is characterized by massive overdistention of a lobe of the lung, usually the left upper lobe. In newborns it produces a mediastinal shift and atelectasis of the residual lung, leading to acute respiratory distress. Coexistence with cardiac anomalies is not uncommon. The treatment of choice is immediate lobectomy.

2.2.1.2 Pulmonary Cysts

Pulmonary cysts may be single or multiple and may or may not communicate with the bronchial system (Fig. 77 a–d). The indication for surgery is undisputed when symptoms and complications exist. Even in asymptomatic cases, the danger of later complications and the relatively low operative risk justify surgical treatment, whose goal is the complete removal of the cystic wall. Larger cysts can occasionally be shelled out or, if pedunculated, surgically ablated. Lobectomy is usually required because of changes in the surrounding lung parenchyma or the presence of additional cysts. Partial excision or reefing of the cyst wall invites recurrence, especially if adhesions develop with the chest wall.

2.2.1.3 Cystic Adenomatoid Malformation [12]

Cystic adenomatoid malformation is a rare condition based on an anomaly of pulmonary development and generally affecting one lobe, which contains numerous air- or water-filled cysts or solid areas. Indications for surgery in infants are progressive respiratory distress due to distention of the affected lobe, and compression of the residual lung; older patients may require surgery due to recurring infections. Treatment consists of removal of the diseased lobe [32].

2.2.1.4 Bronchogenic Cysts

Bronchogenic cysts most commonly occur in the mediastinum between the esophagus and trachea. They can produce bronchial stenosis in children, and in adults they can enlarge and give the impression of a mediastinal tumor. Generally the cysts can be removed by enucleation [32].

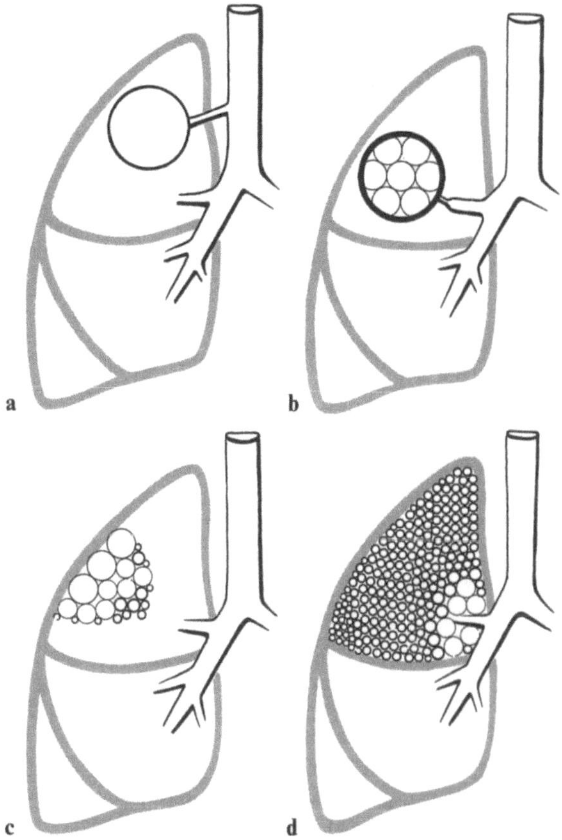

Fig. 77. a Monolocular bronchogenic cyst with bronchial communication. **b** Multilocular bronchial cyst with bronchial communication. **c** Congenital cystic disease, localized form. **d** Congenital cystic disease, diffuse form. (Modified from Doerr and Seifert [20])

2.2.1.5 Pulmonary Sequestration

Pulmonary sequestration is the term applied to a nonfunctioning area of lung tissue showing cystic degeneration and deriving its blood supply from the systemic circulation. In the more common intralobar form, the sequestered tissue is situated within the normal lung parenchyma; the extralobar form has its own pleural covering and is separate from the normal lung (Fig. 78 a,b). Both forms are more common on the left side than on the right, and most occur in the lower lobe or posterior mediastinum. Between 80% and 90% of pulmonary sequestra derive their blood supply from branches of the thoracic aorta, and the rest from infradiaphragmatic vessels that can cause massive intraabdominal hemorrhage if inadvertently severed without prior ligation. Venous

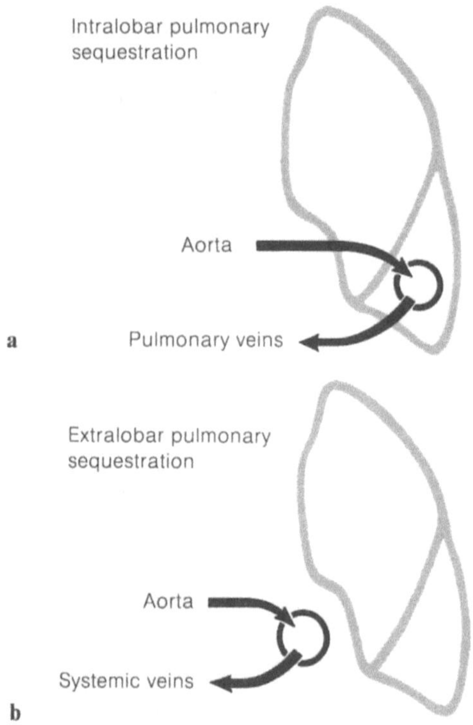

Fig. 78a, b. Intra- and extralobar pulmonary sequestration. (Modified from Doerr and Seifert [20])

drainage is into the azygos or hemiazygos vein in the intralobar form and into the inferior pulmonary vein in the extralobar form. Intralobar sequestra frequently communicate with the bronchial system; extralobar sequestra rarely do [40, 46].

Surgical treatment is indicated in symptomatic cases (recurring infections, left-to-left shunt) or if neoplasia is suspected. The treatment for extralobar sequestration is excision, while the intralobar form is usually managed by lobectomy. An essential part of surgery is ligation and division of the anomalous vessels [32].

2.2.2 Acquired Cystic Malformations

2.2.2.1 Bullous Emphysema

Emphysematous bullae usually develop in the setting of chronic bronchitis and, unlike pulmonary cysts, are not lined by epithelium. The roof of the bulla is formed by visceral pleura and the base by lung parenchyma. The bullae may remain clinically silent, or they may incite local complications and, by enlarging, cause deterioration of respiratory function due to compression of lung tissue or mediastinal organs.

2.2.2.1.1 Indications for Surgery. Surgery is indicated when complications arise (bleeding, pneumothorax, infection) or when there is increasing compression of the surrounding lung tissue, a situation marked clinically by progressive respiratory failure and radiographically by a bulla occupying more than one-third of the chest cavity, and by a marked lateral disparity on perfusion scans. Surgery is not appropriate in cases of severe recurring bronchitis or for cysts occurring in association with a progressive lung disease (alpha$_1$-antitrypsin deficiency, vanishing lung). The indication for surgery in asymptomatic patients is controversial, with views ranging from categorical rejection of surgery to recommendations for early removal to avoid complications [49].

2.2.2.1.2 Procedure. The goal of surgery is removal of the bulla while sparing as much functioning lung tissue as possible. Pedunculated bullae can be ligated and ablated. Wide-based lesions are incised at their junction with the lung parenchyma, and the cut surface is oversewn with continuous sutures (4-0 absorbable monofilament). The pleural margins are approximated to produce a reefing effect and control air leak. Deep suturing should be avoided due to the risk of injury to the delicate parenchyma. Bullae also may be stapled off and excised. A wedge resection may even be considered for smaller, peripheral cysts. Lobectomy is not advised, as it sacrifices too much functioning lung. Intracavitary transthoracic drainage of emphysematous bullae has been employed in severely dyspneic patients but has not gained wide acceptance [49].

2.2.2.2 Echinoccosis (Hydatid Disease)

Hydatid cysts consist of the actual parasite–a fluid-filled "endocyst" containing brood capsules and scoleces–and an external capsule of compressed, fibrous lung tissue (pericyst). Pulmonary hydatid cysts tend to grow rapidly and may rupture into the bronchial system or pleural cavity, resulting in tension pneumothorax, pleural empyema, or anaphylactic shock. Surgical removal is advised even in asymptomatic cases to avoid complications. The rupture of a cyst can produce a life-threatening situation that requires immediate intervention.

2.2.2.2.1 Surgical Treatment. Uncomplicated cysts can generally be removed by enucleation [3]. In rare cases where complications exist or lung tissue has been destroyed, a segmental resection or lobectomy may be required. In all cases the surgeon should avoid opening the cyst to prevent intrapleural dissemination and anaphylactic shock. The prophylactic administration of cortisone is recommended prior to dissection of the cyst. After thoracotomy, pleural adhesions are separated, and the pleural cavity is packed off with towels soaked in 10% saline. The tissue overlying the cyst is incised until the endocyst is visualized. At that point the incision is extended, the lung is inflated, and the cyst is delivered into a waiting spoon or basin [3]. The projecting edges of the pericyst are resected down to normal lung and oversewn with a continuous suture line. Bleeding points in the bed of the cyst and bronchial openings are secured with suture ligatures. We feel it is unnecessary to remove the pericyst completely or to suture the cyst bed from the inside, starting at the deepest point of the cavity.

2.3 Inflammatory Lung Diseases

2.3.1 Lung Abscess

Lung abscess is a localized area of suppuration with associated tissue destruction caused by aerobic or anaerobic organisms. Etiologic distinctions are drawn between abscess resulting from the aspiration of septic debris, usually during unconsciousness; postpneumonic abscess; and abscess secondary to the bacterial colonization of existing pulmonary lesions (carcinoma, cysts, tuberculous cavities, infarct, septic emboli) or the spread of a subphrenic abscess [1].

Treatment includes several weeks of selective antibiotic therapy and drainage of the abscess through the bronchial system, which is usually accomplished by physiotherapeutic measures, by bronchoscopy [41], and sometimes by means of a coronary angiography catheter introduced transbronchially [16]. A bronchoscopic examination is also indicated to exclude bronchogenic carcinoma or a foreign body. Transthoracic abscess drainage [69] is important only as an emergency measure in patients who are very ill or have a very large abscess that is displacing the mediastinum (see below).

2.3.1.1 Surgical Resection

Resection is indicated in about 10%–30% of patients [22, 104] who have chronic abscess cavities. Factors warranting open surgery are persistence of the cavity after four to six weeks of conservative therapy, the demonstration of fungal infection, massive hemoptysis, bronchopleural fistula, the presence of a foreign body, suspicion of tumor, or septic abscess formation in other organs. At the start of the operation the infected bronchial tract should be occluded with a Carlens tube or balloon catheter. During removal of the abscess, care is to avoid disseminating septic material and to avoid injury to healthy tissue with consequent parenchymal fistulas that could prevent expansion of the remaining lung tissue. The bronchus should be closed in an area where the tissue is normal. Lobectomy is the procedure of choice for abscesses close to the hilum [22], and wedge resection for peripheral abscesses.

2.3.1.2 Transthoracic Drainage

Transthoracic drainage [64] may be performed safely when the pleural layers over the abscess are fused. Otherwise there is a danger of pleural empyema.

The abscess is localized by radiologic means, and the skin over the designated drainage site is incised under general anesthesia. About a 3-cm segment of overlying rib is resected subperiosteally, and the intercostal vessels are ligated [51]. After confirmatory aspiration, the abscess cavity is opened and aspirated to obtain material for bacteriologic and histologic examination. Then a suction drain is inserted whose end should project freely into the abscess cavity to avoid vascular erosion. The incision is closed over the drainage tube, through which continuous suction (-10 cm H_2O) is applied. The tube is removed at the earliest opportunity after evacuation of the abscess [51].

2.3.1.3 Amebiasis of the Lung

Amebiasis of the lung almost invariably results from the transdiaphragmatic erosion of an hepatic abscess into the right pleura, lung, or pericardium. Transabdominal drainage of the hepatic abscess and chemotherapy are first-line measures and usually provide resolution of pulmonary changes, especially bronchobiliary fistula [100].

2.3.2 Bronchiectasis

Bronchiectasis has become rare owing to the early initiation of effective antibiotic treatment for bronchopulmonary infections. It may develop in the setting of systemic diseases (e.g., mucoviscidosis) or may be secondary to a local intra- or extrabronchial obstruction (foreign body, enlarged lymph nodes). The disease most commonly affects the basal segments of the lower lobe, the lingula, and the middle lobe [27].

2.3.2.1 Indications for Surgery

Surgery is indicated following a trial of medical therapy if significant symptoms persist (especially recurring bouts of pneumonia) or if complications arise such as abscess formation or massive bleeding. Surgery will be of no benefit if the scope of the involvement is extensive (more than two lobes) or minimal (less than one segment), although the disease should be limited enough to be resectable. Surgery is in appropriate in the presence of systemic disease due to the potential for bronchiectasis to develop in the remainder of the lung. Surgery must be preceded by an accurate diagnostic evaluation that includes bronchoscopy, bronchography of all lobes, pulmonary function studies, as well as careful physiotherapeutic preparation.

2.3.2.2 Procedure

Surgery should not be undertaken in the acute inflammatory stage, and a two-stage approach is advised when the disease is bilateral. A meticulous operating technique is essential for an uncomplicated postoperative course. All involved segments must be removed in order to alleviate complaints and avoid the high risk of reoperation. The procedure of choice may be lobectomy, segmentectomy, wedge resection (with a stapling device), or a combination of these techniques, depending on the extent of disease. Healthy segments should not be injured, as parenchymal fistulae will hinder expansion of the residual lung.

2.3.3 Pulmonary Tuberculosis

The development of new chemotherapeutic agents has reduced the need for surgical procedures (2%–15%) [53, 105] and has also made them more successful. Collapse therapy for pulmonary tuberculosis (pneumothorax, extrapleural pneumolysis, collapse thoracoplasty) has become obsolete.

2.3.3.1 Indications for Surgery

Surgical treatment is indicated after an unsuccessful trial of medical therapy (drug resistance, atypical mycobacteria), in patients with a destroyed lobe or lung, and when significant complications exist [105]. The specific indications for resection are [53]:

(1) life-threatening hemoptysis,
(2) tuberculomas larger than 2–3 cm,
(3) destroyed lobe or lung,
(4) bronchial stenosis refractory to endoscopic treatment,
(5) persistent cavitary disease.

The decision to operate will also depend on other organic manifestations of tuberculosis, coexisting diseases, and the patient's age and social situation. With disseminated or extrathoracic tuberculosis, preference will be given to medical rather than surgical treatment.

2.3.3.2 Preoperative Preparation

In the absence of massive, life-threatening hemoptysis, surgery must be preceded by several weeks of treatment. Immediately before surgery it is recommended that a new drug be added to the chemotherapeutic agents already in use to prevent intraoperative bacteremia and local contamination [36]. Preoperative preparations include breathing exercises, pulmonary function studies, and a perfusion scan. Patients with bronchiectasis should undergo bronchography and bronchoscopy to exclude bronchial tuberculosis, bronchial stenosis, and malignant disease. General preperations also include the correction of nutrutional deficits.

2.3.3.3 Operative Technique

With some experience, a double-lumen endotracheal tube can be placed in a way to keep pus and blood from entering the healthy bronchial system during intraoperative manipulations. If the placement proves difficult, the diseased bronchial system can be occluded preoperatively with a balloon catheter introduced bronchoscopically.

The thoracotomy must be large enough to give sufficient exposure and access in the presence of dense adhesions. When adhesions are extensive, it may be less traumatizing to free the lung extrapleurally than to attempt an intrathoracic exposure that could cause significant bleeding and parenchymal injury. Lymphadenopathy can make exposure of the blood vessels far more difficult than in resections for carcinoma. When a lobectomy is proposed, the trunk of the pulmonary artery should be snared with a tourniquet if possible before further dissections are performed. It may be necessary in some cases to ligate and divide the vessels peripheral to the hilum at the segmental level, leaving the central lymph nodes alone [36]. When dissecting and dividing the bronchi, it is essential to preserve their blood supply, avoid creating a blind pouch, and obtain a secure closure to forestall later complications such as bronchopleural fistula. Closure with the stapling device is particularly recommended [36, 105].

Perifocal reactions, especially around areas of bronchial stenosis, can produce a mass effect about the hilum which makes it difficult to clear individual structures without opening them. The bronchus may be thin and cordlike. The extent of wall changes can be determined by making a diagnostic bronchotomy proximally and then distally, and by making an additional incision farther out if wall changes are discovered. If excision of the scar tissue is not possible, pneumonectomy may be considered as an alternative to a reconstructive procedure.

Of the resectional procedures, segmentectomy is associated with a relatively high rate of postoperative complications [34]. The preferred procedure is a lobectomy or possibly the wedge resection of stapled-off lung. Both procedures may be necessary due to the frequency of translobar extension. Complete expansion of the residual lung is essential for an uncomplicated recovery. Except in lower lobectomies, this will require wide mobilization of the residual lung, meticulous hemostasis, and closure of all larger parenchymal fistulas. When loss of parenchyma is extensive, a partial thoracoplasty with preservation of the first rib may be performed at the end of the resective procedure or 3–6 weeks thereafter [36].

2.3.3.4 Hemoptysis

With improvements in antituberculous therapy, there has been a decline in the frequency of hemoptysis severe enough to warrant surgery. Even so, immediate surgical treatment remains the only effective option for massive bleeding and is the only means to avoid severe complications due to aspiration. Preoperative localization of the bleeding site is essential. The finding of a typical cavity on roentgenograms is suggestive. A more accurate localizing procedure is bronchoscopy, which should precede operation if bleeding is not too severe. Besides localizing the bleeding site, the flexible bronchoscope can be used to introduce a ventilating tube into the healthy lung. This is often simpler and faster than the attempt to place a double-lumen tube. If hemoptysis is mild and the source of the bleeding remains unclear, the patient may be sedated and managed expectantly while serial roentgenograms are obtained at frequent intervals (1–4 h). Since erosion of the bronchial arteries is causative in most cases, the first step at operation should be to divide and occlude the appropriate lobar or mainstem bronchus prior to ligation of the pulmonary vessels.

2.3.4 Fungal Infections of the Lung

Fungal diseases are an infrequent indication for thoracic surgery. But given the rising incidence of these infections, at least in the United States [33], it is appropriate to consider the major types of infection and the role of surgery in their management.

2.3.4.1 Histoplasmosis

Chronic histoplasmosis affects emphysema patients preferentially. The infection causes a caseating necrosis of the lung and regional lymph nodes with subsequent calcification. Thick-walled cavities may develop in the lung parenchyma and are a frequent source of hemorrhage. Adenopathic changes lead to bronchial stenosis and may penetrate the bronchial wall, causing hemorrhage.

Surgical treatment is indicated for:

(1) persistence of thick-walled cavities after several trials of medical therapy, if the patient's pulmonary function is such that he can tolerate an operation;
(2) establishing the nature of a solitary round lesion in the lung;
(3) hemoptysis from cavities or secondary to bronchial erosion of the lymph nodes;
(4) bronchial stenosis due to extrabronchial lymph node enlargement, with recurring infections of the atelectatic lung tissue.

Findings may warrant a lobectomy or a wedge resection, possibly combined with a sleeve resection of the bronchus. Intracapsular removal of the necrotic lymph node tissue also has been described [40]. The mediastinal manifestations of histoplasmosis (fibrosing mediastinitis, constrictive pericarditis) are discussed in the next chapter.

2.3.4.2 Coccidioidomycosis

Coccidioidomycosis is a rare disease that is most prevalent in South America and the southwestern part of the United States. Surgery may be indicated for diagnostic reasons (solitary round lesion [88]) and for persistent cavitary disease posing a risk of pyopneumothorax, hemoptysis, or secondary infection.

The type of surgical procedure depends on the pathology. Cavities are excised with a margin of surrounding tissue. Lobectomy is not performed routinely, since lesser resections are associated with low rates of recurrence and complications, provided the lesion is not opened [88]. Perioperative treatment with amphotericin B has been found to lower the risk of dissemination and postoperative complications, at least in immune-compromised patients.

2.3.4.3 Cryptococcosis

Infection with *Cryptococcus neoformans* causes pneumonia in rare cases and may progress to a generalized (e.g., meningeal) form in patients with an impaired immune response. Roentgenograms usually show a solitary, rounded density in the lower lobe and occasionally a cavity with calcifications. The diagnosis is established by the resection of a solitary round lesion of the lung. Special stains and cultures are needed to identify the infecting organisms. In positive cases treatment with amphotericin B and 5-fluorocytosine is indicated to prevent meningeal cryptococcosis, which develops in up to 10% of surgically treated patients [33]. This therapy may be omitted only if a small, calcified, inactive focus has been removed intact from healthy parenchyma. The drug treatment is especially indicated for debilitated patients, patients with diabetes mellitus, and patients receiving high doses of cortisone or immunosuppressive drugs.

2.3.4.4 Aspergillosis

Only the intracavitary form of aspergillosis, with saprophytic infestation of preexisting pulmonary cavities or cysts, is of surgical interest. The resulting aspergilloma (fungus ball) is a rounded, necrotic mass of hyphae, fibrin, and inflammatory cells lying freely in the cavity. More than half of these patients will develop hemoptysis [21].

As systemic medical treatment is ineffective, resection is indicated in symptomatic patients. In most cases the patient's general condition and cardiopulmonary status are seriously compromised as a result of the underlying pulmonary disease. Surgery should be performed under amphotericin protection, and the lesion should be removed by a lobectomy or wedge resection to conserve healthy lung tissue. In patients who are poor candidates for operation, the instillation of amphotericin via a percutaneous or transbronchial catheter may be tried [21], although it is unclear whether and for how long such treatment may be successful.

References

1. Alexander JC, Wolfe WG (1980) Lung abscess and emphyema of the thorax. Surg Clin North Am 60:835
2. Barclay RS, Mc Swan N, Welsh TM (1957) Tracheal reconstruction without the use of grafts. Thorax 12:177
3. Barrett NR (1949) Removal of simple univesicular pulmonary hydatid cyst. Lancet 2:234
4. Beattie EJ (1957) The surgical treatment of lung tumors: Pneumonectomy or lobectomy. Surg 42:1124
5. Bennett WF, Smith RA (1979) Segmental resection for bronchogenic carcinoma: A surgical alternative for the compromised patient. Ann Thorac Surg 27:169
6. Björk VO (1955) Left-sided bronchotracheal anastomosis. J Thorac Surg 30:493
7. Blum U, Schröder D, Ungeheuer E (1981) Zystische Mißbildungen der Lunge. Fortschr Med 99:521
8. Borrie J (1952) Primary carcinoma of the bronchus; prognosis following surgical resection. Ann Coll Surg Engl 10:165
9. Bowen TE, Zajtchuk R, Green DC, Brott WH (1978) Value of anterior mediastinotomy in bronchogenic carcinoma of the left upper lobe. J Thorac Cardiovasc Surg 76:269
10. Brock R., Whytehead LL (1955) Radical pneumonectomy for bronchial carcinoma. Br J Surg 43:8
11. Cahan WG, Watson WL, Pool IL (1951) Radical pneumonectomy. J Thorac Surg 22:449
12. Chin KY, Tang MY (1949) Congenital adenomatoid malformation of one lobe of a lung with general anasarca. Arch Pathol 48:221
13. Churchill ED, Belsey R (1939) Segmental pneumonectomy in bronchiectasis. Ann Surg 109:481
14. Churton J (1978) Multiple aneurysm of pulmonary artery. Brit Med J 1:1223
15. Churchill ED, Sweet RH, Soutter L, Scannell JG (1950) The surgical management of carcinoma of the lung: A study of the cases treated at the Massachusetts General Hospital from 1930 to 1950. J Thorac Surg 20:349
16. Connors JP, Roper CL, Ferguson TB (1975) Transbronchial catheterisation of pulmonary abscesses. Ann Thorac Surg 19:254
17. Derra E, Franke H, Rink H (1951) Technik und Anwendung der segmentalen Resektion bei Lungentuberkulose. Zentralbl Chir 76:1155
18. Dines DE, Arms RA, Bernatz PE, Gomes MR (1974) Pulmonary arteriovenous fistulas. Mayo Clin Proc 49:460
19. Divis G (1927) Ein Beitrag zur operativen Behandlung der Lungengeschwülste. Acta Chir Scand 62:329
20. Doerr W, Seifert G (Hrsg.) (1983) Spezielle pathologische Anatomie, Bd. XVI: Pathologie der Lungen I/II. Springer, Heidelberg New York Tokyo
21. Eastridge CE, Young JM, Cole F, Gowley R, Pate JW (1972) Pulmonary aspergillosis. Ann Thorac Surg 13:397
22. Estera AS, Platt MR, Mills LJ, Shaw RR (1980) Primary lung abscess. J Thorac Cardiovasc Surg 79:275
23. Evans JP (1972) Postpneumonectomy oesophageal fistula. Thorax 27:674
24. Forrester-Wood CP (1980) Bronchopleural fistula following pneumonectomy for carcinoma of the bronchus. J Thorac Cardiovasc Surg 80:406
25. Franke H, Irmer W (1958) Die Technik der Lungenresektionen. In: Derra E (Hrsg) Handbuch der Thoraxchirurgie 3. Band, Spezieller Teil II. Springer, Berlin Göttingen Heidelberg
26. Gaensler EA, Carrington CB (1980) Open Biopsy for chronic diffuse infiltrative lung disease: Clinical, roentgenographic and physiological correlations in 502 patients. Ann Thorac Surg 30:411
27. George STA, Leonardi HK, Overholt RH (1979) Bilateral pulmonary resection for bronchiectasis: a 40-year experience. Ann Thorac Surg 28:48
28. Graham EA, Singer JI (1933) Successful removal of an entire lung for carcinoma of the bronchus. J Am Med Assoc 101:1371
29. Greschuchna D, Maaßen W (1973) Die lymphogenen Absiedlungen des Bronchialkarzinoms. Thieme, Stuttgart
30. Haagensen CD, Feind CR, Herter FP, Stanetz ChA, Weinberg IA (1972) The lymphatics in cancer. Saunders, Philadelphia London Toronto, 231 f.
31. Halkier (1978) Surgical improvement of respiratory insufficiency. Scand J Thorac Cardiovasc Surg 12:75
32. Haller JA et al. (1979) Surgical Management of lung bud anomalies: Lobar emphysema, bronchogenic cyst, cystic adenomatoid malformation, and interlobar pulmonary sequestration. Ann Thorac Surg 28:33
33. Hammon JW, Prager RL (1980) Surgical Management of fungal diseases of the chest. Surg Clin North America 60:897
34. Hankins JR, Miller JE, Attar S et al. (1978) Bronchopleural fistula. J Thorac Cardiovasc Surg 76:755
35. Hayek OH (1958) In: Derra E (Hrsg) Handbuch der Thoraxchirurgie, Bd I, Allgemeiner Teil. Springer, Berlin Göttingen Heidelberg
36. Harrison LH (1980) Current aspects of the surgical management of tuberculosis. Surg Clin North Am 60:883
37. Hermanek P, Gall FP (1979) Lungentumoren. Kompendium der klinischen Tumorpathologie, Bd. II. Witzstrock, Baden-Baden Köln New York
38. Higgins GA jr, Shields ThW (1979) Experience of the veterans administration surgical adjuvant group. In: Muggia FW, Rosenzweig M (eds) Lung cancer. Progress in therapeutic research. Raven Press, New York
39. Hoffmann TH, Randsdell HT (1980) Comparison of lobectomy and wedge resection for carcinoma of the lung. J Thorac Cardiovasc Surg 79:211
40. Humphrey EW, Mc Keown DL (1982) Manual of pulmonary surgery. Springer, New York, Heidelberg Berlin
41. Jackson CL, Judd AR (1940) The role of bronchoscopy in the treatment of pulmonary abscess. J Thorac Surg 10:179
42. Jensik RJ, Faber LP, Kittle CF (1979) Segmental resection for bronchogenic carcinoma. Ann Thorac Surg 28:475
43. Kelly MV, Kyger RE, Miller WC (1977) Postoperative lobar torsion and gangrene. Thorax 32:501

44. Kergin FG (1952) Carcinoma of the trachea. J Thorac Surg 26:164
45. Keszler P (1980) Zur Bronchusplastik bei Bronchialkarzinom. Zentralblatt Chir 105:242
46. Kahlil KD, Kilmann JW (1975) Pulmonary sequestration. J Thorac Cardiovasc Surg 70:928
47. Klingenberg I (1964) Histopathologic findings in the prescalene tissue from 1000 post mortem cases. Acta Chir Scand 127:57
48. Konietzko N, Ferlinz R, Lodenkemper R, Magnussen H, Schlimmer P, Toomet H, Wichert PV (1983) Empfehlungen zur präoperativen Lungenfunktionsdiagnostik. Praxis Klin Pneumol 37:1199
49. Krummhaar D, Ramme U, Holtz U (1980) Cysten und Bronchiektasien der Lunge. Chirurg 51:566
50. Kubik St (1969) Klinische Anatomie. Ein Farbphoto-Atlas der Topographie. Thorax. 2. Aufl. Thieme, Stuttgart
51. Lawrence GH, Rubin SL (1978) Management of giant lung abscess. Am J Surg 136:134
52. Lezius A (1953) Die Lungenresektionen. Thieme, Stuttgart
53. Maassen W (1980) Pleuro-pulmonary tuberculosis – Current status of surgical therapy. Thorac Cardiovasc Surg 28:225
54. Maassen W (1981) Commentary. Thorac Cardiovasc Surg 29:45
55. Mac Hale SJ (1974) Techniques in the surgery of the major bronchi. In: Smith RE, Williams WG (eds) Surgery of the lung. Butterworths, London
56. Martini N, Beattie EJ (1980) Current views in primary pulmonary cancer. Int Adv Surg Oncol 3:275
57. Martini N, Flehinger BJ (1980) Prospective study of 445 lung carcinomas with mediastinal lymph node metastases. J Thorac Cardiovasc Surg 80:390
58. Masaoka A, Ho Y, Yasumitsu T (1979) Anterior approach for tumor of the superior sulcus. J Thorac Cardiovasc Surg 78:413
59. Meng RL, Jensik RJ, Kittle CF. Faber LP (1980) Median sternotomy for synchronous bilateral pulmonary operations. J Thorac Cardiovasc Surg 80:1
60. Mc Cormack PM (1980) Primary lung carcinoma (Disc). NY State J Med 80:612
61. Miller EG, Aberg THJ, Gerbode F (1968) Effect of pulmonary vein ligation on pulmonary artery flow in dogs. J Thorac Cardiovasc Surg 55:668
62. Moghissi K (1975) Tracheal reconstruction with a prosthesis of Marlex mesh and pericardium. J Thorac Cardiovasc Surg 69:499
63. Monaldi V (1956) Endocavitary aspiration in treatment of lung abscess. Diseases of the Chest 29:193
64. Morrow CE, Vassilopoulos PP, Grage TB (1980) Surgical resection for metastatic neoplasms of the lung. Cancer 45:2981
65. Naruke T, Snemasu K, Ishihawa S (1978) Lymph node mapping and curability at various levels of metastases in resected lung cancer. J Thorac Cardiovasc Surg 76:832
66. Nelson RL (1933) Congenital cystic diseases of the lung. J Pediatr 1:233
67. Neville WE, Bolanowski PJP, Soltanzadek H (1976) Prosthetic reconstruction of the trachea and carina. J Thorac Cardiovasc Surg 72:525
68. Nissen R (1931) Exstirpation eines ganzen Lungenflügels. Zentralblatt Chir 58:3003
69. Nissen R (1949) Die Technik der Lungenexstirpation. Chirurg 20:577
70. Nohl-Oser HCh (1972) An investigation of the anatomy of the lymphatic drainage of the lungs. Ann R Coll Surg Engl 51:157
71. Nohl-Oser HCh, Nissen R, Schreiber HW (1981) Surgery of the lung. Thieme, Stuttgart
72. Nomina anatomica (1975) 4. Aufl. Tokyo
73. Okada Y, Ito M, Nagaishi Ch (1979) Anatomical study of the pulmonary lymphatics. Lymphology 12:118
74. Overholt RH, Woods FM, Betts RH (1948) An improved method of the resection of pulmonary segments. J Thorac Surg 17:464
75. Pancoast HK (1932) Superior pulmonary sulcus tumor. J A M A 99:1391
76. Paulson DL, Shaw RR (1955) Bronchial anastomosis and bronchoplastic procedures in the interest of preservation of the lung tissue. J Thorac Cardiovasc Surg 29:238
77. Paulson DL (1957) Survival rates following resection for bronchogenic carcinoma. Ann Surg 146:997
78. Perianayagam WJ, Freitas E, Sharma SS, Mulalidharan S, Jairaj PS, John S (1979) Pulmonary hydatic cyst: a 25-year experience. Aust N Z J Surg 49:450
79. Pichlmaier H, Spelsberg F (1971) Organerhaltende Operation des Bronchuskarzinoms. Langenbecks Arch Chir 328:221
80. Porstmann W (1977) Therapeutic embolisation of arteriovenous pulmonary fistulas by catheter technique. In: Eklöf O (ed) Current concepts of pediatric radiology. Springer, Berlin Heidelberg New York
81. Price-Thoams C (1956) Conservative resection of the bronchial tree. J R Coll Surg Edinb 1:169
82. Ramming KP (1980) Surgery for pulmonary metastases. Surg Clin North Am 60:815
83. Ramsey HE, Caham WG, Beattie EJ, Humphrey C (1969) The importance of radical lobectomy in lung cancer. J Thorac Cardiovasc Surg 58:225
84. Rienhoff WF (1933) Pneumonectomy – A preliminary report of the operative technique in two successful cases. Bull Johns Hopkins Hosp 53:390
85. Rouviere H (1932) Anatomie des Lymphatiques de l'homme. Masson, Paris
86. Ruttunen APM, Sikkenk PJH (1982) Stapling devices in pulmonary surgery. Nether J Surg 34:211
87. Salomon NW, Osborne R, Copeland JG (1980) Surgical manifestations and results of treatment of pulmonary coccidioidomycosis. Ann Thorac Surg 30:433
88. Schildberg FW, Valesky A, Nissen R (1982) Anatomische und funktionelle Grundlagen für die Wahl von Nahtmitteln und Nahttechniken in der Lungen- und Trachealchirurgie, In: Thiede A, Hammelmann H (Hrsg) Moderne Nahtmaterialien und Nahttechniken in der Chirurgie. Springer, Berlin Heidelberg New York
89. Sethi GK, Takaro T (1978) Esophagopleural fistula following pulmonary resection. Ann Thorac Surg 25:74
90. Shaw KM, Luke DA (1979) Lobectomy with sleeve resection of the bronchus for malignant disease of the lung and the influence of the suture material used for the bronchial repair. Thorac Cardiovasc Surg 27:325

91. Shaw RR, Paulsen DL, Kee JL (1961) Treatment of the superior sulcus tumor followed by resection Ann Surg 154:29
92. Shields TW (1972) General thoracic surgery. Lea and Febiger, Philadelphia
93. Smith RA, Nigam BK (1979) Resection of proximal left main bronchus carcinoma. Thorax 34:616
94. Spencer H (1977) Pathology of the lung, vol I. Pergamon Press, Oxford New York Paris Frankfurt p 71
95. Spoto G, Rossi NP, Allsbrook WL (1977) Tracheobronchial plasma cell granulome. J Thorac Cardiovasc Surg 73:804
96. Stanfort W (1980) Influence of staging in superior sulcus (Pancoast) tumors of the lung. Ann Thorac Surg 29:406
97. Stocker JT, Madewell JE, Drake RM (1977) Congenital cystic adenomatoid malformatial of the lung – Classification and morphologic spectrum. Hum Pathol 8:155
98. Torek F (1930) Removal of metastatic carcinoma of the lung and mediastinum. Suggestions to the technic. Arch Surg 21:1416
99. Verghese M, Eggleston FC, Handa AK (1979) Management of thoracic amebiasis. J Thorac Cardiovasc Surg 78:757
100. Viereck H-J (1980) Reinterventionen in der Pleura- und Lungenchirurgie. Chirurg 51:85
101. Vogt-Moykopf I, Pierro G, Pertzborn W (1984) Grenzen der Belastbarkeit in der allgemeinen Thoraxchirurgie. Langenbecks Arch Chir 364:181
102. Weisel RD (1979) Sleeve lobectomy for carcinoma of the lung. J Thorac Cardiovasc Surg 78:839
103. Windheim K von, Piendl I (1980) Lungenabszeß. Chirurg 51:562
104. Wolfarth W (1980) Der heutige Stand der chirurgischen Behandlung der Lungentuberkulose. Chirurg 51:549
105. Wurnig P (1967) Technische Vorteile bei der Hauptbronchusresektion rechts und links. Thoraxchirurgie Vask Chir 15:16
106. Zenker R, Heberer G, Löhr HH (1954) Die Lungenresektionen. Springer, Berlin Göttingen Heidelberg

G. Procedures on the Mediastinum

H. HAMELMANN and M. THERMANN

CONTENTS

A number of surgical approaches to the anterior mediastinum have been devised (Fig. 1). The partial or full median sternotomy (a) gives access to the entire anterior mediastinum (see Sect. 4 and 5). The anterior parasternal thoracotomy (b) usually requires the division of one or more costal cartilages. It is especially recommended for the biopsy of laterally situated lesions and can be extended to an anterolateral thoracotomy as required. The cervical or collar mediastinotomy (c) is the standard incision for mediastinoscopy and for entering the anterior mediastinum by blunt dissection (see Sect. 2 and 3).

1 Diagnostic Procedures

1.1 Fine Needle Aspiration

Indication: Cytologic evaluation of mediastinal tumors not of arterial origin.

Preoperative preparation: Patient is fasted and sedated. The aspiration is performed under fluoroscopic or CT guidance.

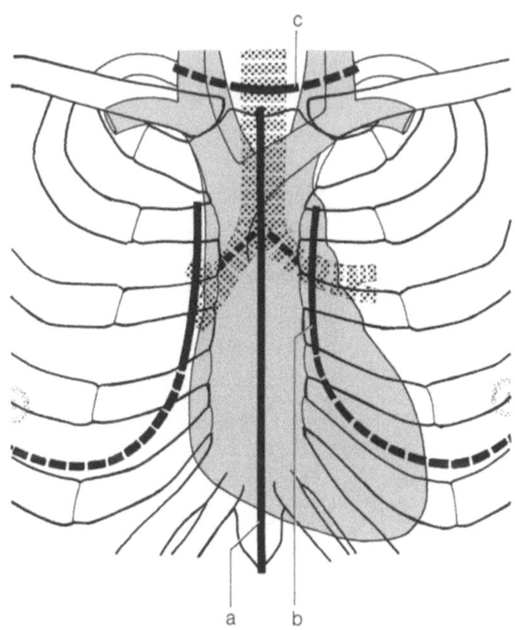

Fig. 1. Surgical approaches to the mediastinum. *a* Median sternotomy (partial or full); *b* anterior parasternal mediastinotomy; *c* collar mediastinotomy

Instruments: Instruments for local anesthesia, stylet, thin aspirating needle, 10-ml syringe; a special syringe holder is helpful.

Position: Usually supine.

Procedure: The lesion is localized by X-ray or CT, the skin is infiltrated with 1%–2% procaine solution without epinephrine, and a stab incision is made in the skin. A needle of suitable length is inserted into the lesion, and the needle tip is moved in and out several times while the plunger is raised. The aspirated material is expelled onto a slide, and a smear is prepared and fixed with an alcohol or spray fixative.

Complications: Vascular injury or pneumothorax. Postoperative radiographs are indicated right away if a complication is suspected; otherwise they may be deferred for up to 2 h after the procedure.

1.2 Obtaining Biopsy Material

Indications: Lesions of the anterior or superior mediastinum.

1.2.1 Mediastinoscopy

This procedure, introduced by Carlens in 1956, enables inspection, palpation, and tissue sampling in the pre- and paratracheal region, the tracheobronchial angles, and the subcarinal area. The procedure may be extended beyond these limits–below the xiphoid process, for example–although the indication for this is controversial.

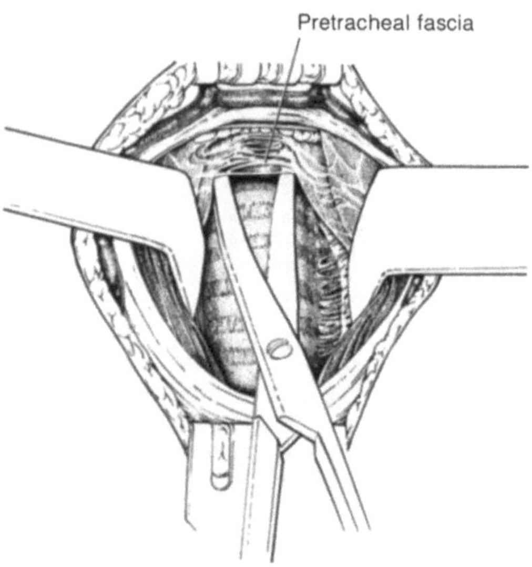

a

Fig. 2. a, b Technique of mediastinoscopy. **a** The anterior tracheal wall is exposed, and the pretracheal fascia is incised. **b** Position of the mediastinoscope after insertion into the mediastinum. **c** Relation of the mediastinoscope to surrounding structures (here the scope is trained on the subcarinal nodes)

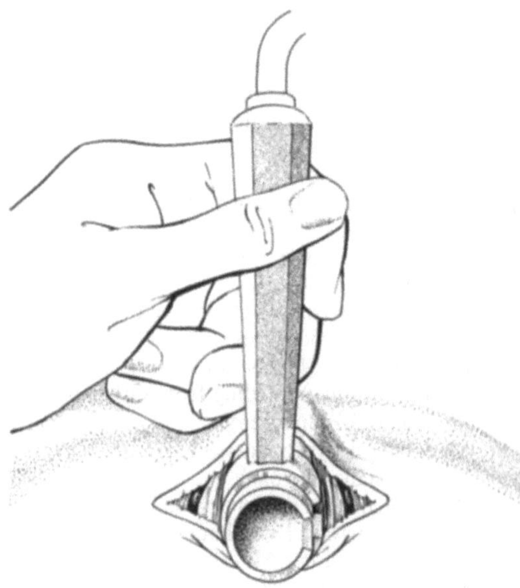

b

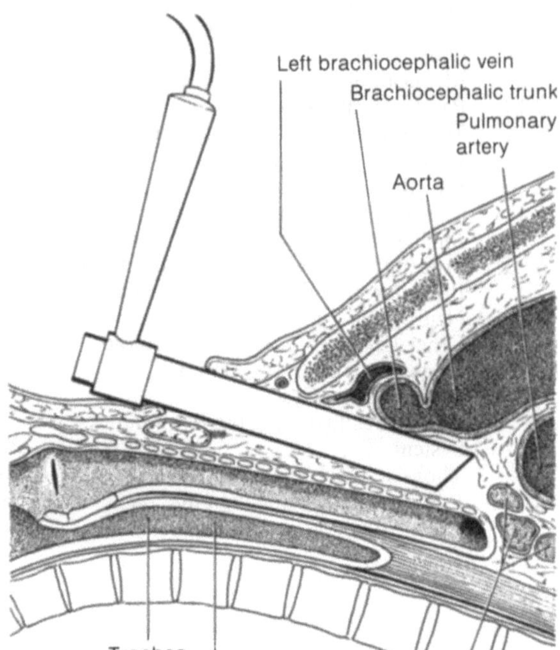

c

Preoperative preparation: Empty stomach, endotracheal anesthesia.

Instruments: Small basic set, mediastinoscopes of varying lengths, metal suction catheters, long biopsy forceps, long sponge sticks. Power source for electrocoagulation.

Position: Supine with the head well extended and a sand bag below the upper thoracic spine.

Approach: Transverse incision in the suprasternal fossa (see Fig. 1).

Steps in procedure:

(1) Transverse incision in the suprasternal fossa
(2) Vertical incision of the strap muscles
(3) Transverse incision of the pretracheal fascia
(4) Exposure of the anterior tracheal wall
(5) Digital exploration of the mediastinum anterior and lateral to the trachea
(6) Insertion of the mediastinoscope
(7) Needle aspiration or biopsy of the tumor or lymph nodes

The skin is incised transversely in the suprasternal fossa, and the subcutaneous tissue and platysma are divided. The strap muscles are separated in the midline by a vertical incision and are retracted laterally with Langenbeck retractors. Usually this can be done without ligating the vena thyreoidea ima, which runs longitudinally. The thyroid gland is retracted superiorly. The lateral walls of the trachea are exposed on both sides with a scissors, and exposure is maintained with Langenbeck retractors. The pretracheal fascia is incised transversely (Fig. 2a), whereupon the finger is passed downward along the anterior wall of the trachea to dissect the pre- and paratracheal space and enlarge it as much as possible. The finger should remain in contact with the anterior tracheal wall as the dissection progresses. The brachiocephalic trunk is palpable anteriorly, and the aortic arch is palpable anterolaterally on the left side. After the dissected space has been palpated and evaluated, the finger is withdrawn, the tissue in front of the trachea is elevated anteriorly with a Langenbeck retractor, and the short mediastinoscope is introduced (Fig. 2 b,c). The instrument should be held against the tracheal anterior wall as it is advanced so that it will not stray from the intended plane. Further blunt dissection of the pre- and paratracheal areas is performed with the suction catheter. If the intent is to explore the mediastinal lymph nodes for the staging of bronchogenic carcinoma, the bronchopericardial membrane should be bluntly divided to give access to the subcarinal nodes, and the dissection extended laterally to the origin of the right upper lobe and to the left pulmonary artery (Fig. 3 a,b). The pulmonary artery should be visualized below the subcarinal nodes.

In older patients the lymph nodes can usually be recognized by their anthracotic discoloration.

Fig. 3a, b. Topography of the anterior mediastinum. **a** Superior view; **b** anterior view

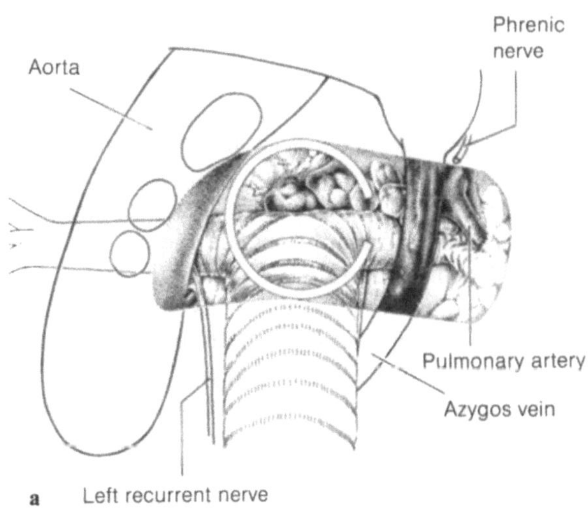

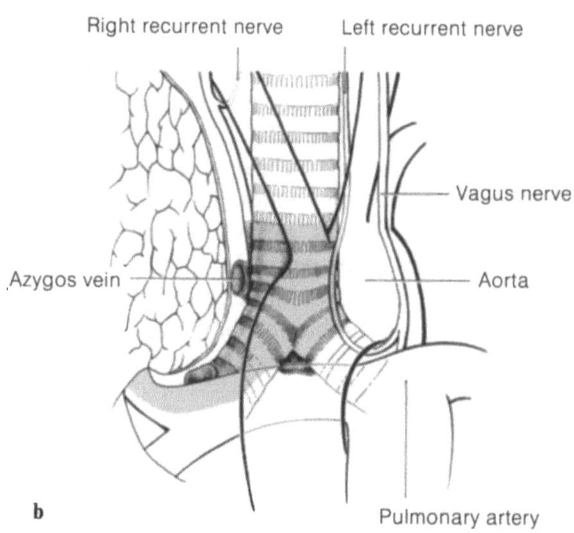

They must be adequately dissected free and cleared on all sides if possible with the suction catheter. If mediastinoscopy is being performed for sarcoidosis, the lymph nodes can be cleared and removed with relative ease. A biopsy is performed only if the tissue has been positively identified as a lymph node or tumor. It can be especially difficult to distinguish a vein from a lymph node in the right tracheobronchial angle (azygos vein, see Fig. 3). If doubt exists, biopsy should be preceded by trial aspiration with a thin needle. This is also recommended for masses not clearly distinguishable from the aortic arch by palpation. Postbiopsy bleeding from smaller vessels (especially lymph node vessels) can be controlled by electrocautery with the isolated tip of the metal suction catheter. Most bleeding points can be controlled by local compression with a sponge stick, which may be soaked in epinephrine solution.

The mediastinoscopic examination should always commence with the short instrument. The long instrument is necessary only for visualizing the tracheobronchial area or the bifurcation.

If complete hemostasis cannot be achieved, the placement of a Redon suction drain is advised.

The wound is closed in layers, using a longitudinal suture line to reapproximate the muscles. An intracutaneous skin suture is preferred.

In the presence of inflow stasis, mediastinoscopy can be performed without troublesome venous bleeding by ligating the dilated subcutaneous veins. Venous distention is usually not encountered in the mediastinum itself.

In the pretherapeutic staging of bronchogenic or esophageal carcinoma, the question of metastasis to the mediastinal lymph nodes is a basic prognostic concern (N2, N3). In contrast to cases where mediastinoscopy is used solely for the biopsy of unidentified lesions (e.g., in sarcoidosis), adequate carcinoma staging requires that the procedure be extended to include the inspection and biopsy of all paratracheal, pretracheal, tracheobronchial, and subcarinal lymph nodes that are accessible through the instrument. Because the nature of tumor spread (intra- or perinodal growth) can also be an important factor in selecting patients for operation, it is desirable to obtain a wide biopsy that includes removal of the lymph node capsule or excision of the entire node.

1.2.1.1 Complications

Recurrent nerve palsy is most likely to occur on the left side as a sequel to lymph node exploration in the paratracheal area or left tracheobronchial angle. Even relatively simple manipulations in these areas or traction on the lymph nodes can cause recurrent nerve injury leading to transient vocal cord paralysis (Fig. 3 b). This complication is most common during mediastinoscopy for staging, where it occurs in up to 1.4% of cases. The patient should be informed of this prior to operation. (See [2, 4].)

The most dangerous complication of mediastinoscopy is *hemorrhage* which may involve systemic arteries (due to tumor infiltration of the arterial vascular system or perforation of an aortic aneurysm). Hemorrhage from a pulmonary artery has been observed following the erroneous biopsy of that structure. Laceration of the azygos vein can also occur (see above). Torn lymph node vessels are the most frequent source of hemorrhage.

Rare complications include *injuries* of the esophagus or cardiac wall by the erroneous biopsy of those structures, and pneumothorax caused by perforation of the parietal pleura or by the biopsy of emphysematous bullae.

Mediastinitis can develop as a result of iatrogenic infection, the opening of infected lymph nodes, or esophageal perforation.

Hemiparesis due to compression of the brachiocephalic trunk has been described in isolated cases.

1.2.1.2 Management of Intraoperative Complications

Massive bleeding from major arterial vessels is an indication for emergency sternotomy with compression of the bleeding site and repair of the vascular lesion. It is common for these hemorrhages to terminate fatally. With hemorrhage from a pulmonary artery or vein, compression of the bleeding site by tamponade (for eight days) usually is sufficient to secure hemostasis. Otherwise the bleeding site must be exposed through a right lateral thoracotomy and definitively closed.

Entry into the pleural cavity in the absence of a lung defect can usually be managed by closing the mediastinoscopy wound after first reinflating the lung. If parenchymal injury exists, a chest tube should be placed. When an esophageal perforation is recognized during the operation, the cervical incision is extended, and the perforation is oversewn. A drain is inserted, and parenteral nutrition is maintained for five to six days. Mediastinitis is managed by opening and draining the mediastinum and administering antibiotics.

1.2.2 Anterior Mediastinotomy

Indication: Paramediastinal lesions of the anterior and superior mediastinum that are inaccessible to mediastinoscopy.

Preoperative preparation: Empty stomach, endotracheal anesthesia.

Instruments: Basic set, small self-retaining sternal retractor, mediastinoscope or thoracoscope as required.

Position: Supine.

Approach: Curved parasternal incision (see Fig. 1)

Steps in procedure:

(1) Vertical parasternal incision
(2) Parasternal resection of the second or third costal cartilage
(3) Ligation and division of the internal mammary artery and vein
(4) If necessary, insertion of a mediastinoscope or thoracoscope
(5) Biopsy or extirpation of the lesion

Following incision of the skin and subcutaneous tissue, the pectoralis muscle is divided across its fibers with an incision 3–4 cm long, and about 3 cm of the 2nd or 3rd costal cartilage is resected (Fig. 4 a,b). The internal mammary artery and vein are divided between ligatures. If the lesion to be biopsied is not directly under the chest wall, a mediastinoscope or thoracoscope should be introduced through the space created by blunt reflection of the parietal pleura or by pleurotomy. If it appears that a more extensive operation is needed, the incision may be extended to an anterolateral thoracotomy (Fig. 1).

Complications: Bleeding from the internal thoracic artery or vein, phrenic nerve palsy, left recurrent nerve injury by dissection about the aortic arch, pneumothorax.

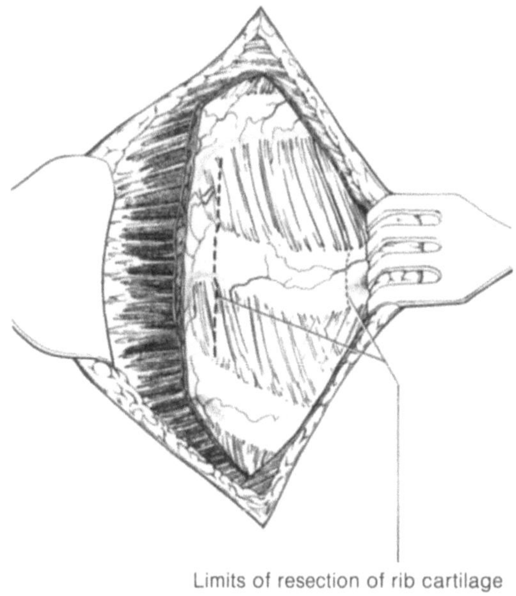

a

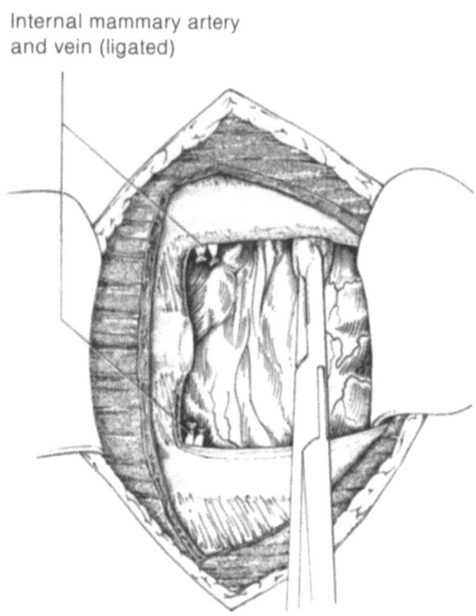

b

Fig. 4. a Division of the pectoralis muscle in preparation for anterior mediastinoscopy. **b** Exposure of the anterior mediastinum after resection of a costal cartilage and ligation of the internal mammary artery and vein

2 Inflammatory Diseases

The mediastinum encompasses several organ systems that can serve as starting points for suppurative or cellulitic processes. Once established, these processes can spread freely in the mediastinal compartment and invade adjacent body cavities. The problem of treatment is compounded by the relative difficulty of surgical access.

2.1 Infections Caused by Operative or Endoscopic Procedures

(1) Infections can result from primarily sterile procedures such as mediastinoscopy, cardiac operations, and the excision of mediastinal tumors. An especially dreaded complication is the infected sternotomy wound, which may progress to osteomyelitis. Drainage with continuous irrigation is recommended in these cases in addition to specific antibiotic therapy. Mechanical stabilization of the sternotomy wound with cerclage wire or metal sutures is of major importance. The use of polymer or felt threads can prolong and compound the problems resulting from the infection.

(2) Results of surgical procedures on the esophagus (anastomotic leak, incompetent esophagotomy, mediastinoscopy with biopsy of the esophageal wall) and instrumental perforations (e.g., with tumors) are a frequent cause of mediastinal abscess (see Chap. I for treatment). Palliative procedures on the trachea, such as the laser coagulation of an obstructing neoplasm, can precipitate a mediastinitis that generally will terminate fatally because of the advanced underlying disease.

2.2 Posttraumatic Mediastinitis

Stab or gunshot wounds can lead to mediastinal infection even when a hollow organ has not been perforated by the injury. Clinical manifestations include fever, inflow stasis, and widening of the mediastinum on X-rays. The detection of air in the mediastinum signifies perforation of the trachea, bronchus, or esophagus. Any posttraumatic mediastinitis requires an endoscopic and radiologic evaluation of the esophageal and bronchial system. Irritative effusion of the pleural cavity and perforation of the parietal pleura are not uncommon. Mediastinitis is treated by eradicating the focus of infection and instituting drainage through a cervical mediastinostomy. The anterior mediastinum is opened in the same way as for mediastinoscopy, and the trachea and paraesophageal tissue are cleared as widely as possible on both sides. Soft drainage tubes are recommended (Penrose, Easy Flow). Mediastinitis secondary to injury of the trachea, bronchial system, or esophagus is discussed in Chapters F and I.

2.3 Inflammations Spreading from Other Sites

Infections of the oropharynx or neck can spread into the loose connective tissue of the mediastinum. The clinical presentation is that of a septic state accompanied by cervical swelling, venous engorgement, dysphagia, and respiratory difficulties. X-rays show widening of the mediastinum. Besides treating the primary focus, it is necessary to perform a wide transverse cervical mediastinotomy (see Mediastinoscopy for technique) and institute drainage with a silicone or Penrose drain. Antibiotic treatment is imperative. If a definite primary focus cannot be found in the oropharynx, the mediastinitis is probably secondary to an esophageal perforation, and this should be confirmed by appropriate X-ray and endoscopic studies.

3 Mediastinal Emphysema

Air or gas can enter the mediastinum from the respiratory or alimentary tract. Mediastinal emphysema can lead to subcutaneous emphysema, and rarely the air may enter the peritoneal cavity, leading to the detection of free air within the abdomen.

Small amounts of air in the mediastinum usually originate from the intestinal tract, whereas large air volumes with pronounced intraabdominal and subcutaneous emphysema result from injury to the trachea or major bronchi. Endoscopy or radiography of the tracheobronchial system or esophagus is necessary to establish the site of the leak.

Mediastinal emphysema in itself is rarely of clinical significance. If it leads to extensive subcutaneous emphysema, a cervical mediastinotomy (q.v.) may be performed with wide dissection of the pre- and paratracheal areas. Usually this is unnecessary, however, and in most cases the air will reabsorb quickly due to spontaneous closure of the leak once positive-pressure ventilation has been discontinued.

A mild degree of mediastinal emphysema may be noted on X-rays following esophageal injury and retroperitoneal rupture of the duodenum.

4 Mediastinal Lymphadenectomy

Lymphadenectomy is performed as part of the staging and possibly the curative resection of bronchogenic and esophageal carcinoma, in which case the lymphatic drainage tracts of the lung or esophagus must be removed.

4.1 Transsternal Approach

Indication: Thyroid carcinoma, bronchogenic carcinoma.

Preoperative preparation: Assessment of vocal cord function and diaphragm motility; general endotracheal anesthesia.

Instruments: Thoracic set, sternal saw, vascular clamps.

Position: Supine.

Approach: Median sternotomy.

Steps in procedure:

(1) The sternum is incised longitudinally from the jugulum to the epigastrium
(2) The sternum is divided with a saw or osteotome
(3) The thymus is pushed aside, and the anterior pericardium is opened, carrying the incision past the aortic arch
(4) The aortic arch, brachiocephalic trunk, and brachiocephalic vein are dissected free
(5) The posterior leaf of the pericardium is opened, and the trachea and bifurcation are exposed
(6) Systematic lymphadenectomy is carried out with division of the left pulmonary artery, left pulmonary veins, and bronchus
(7) The bronchus is closed with staples or sutures
(8) The wound is closed in layers.

Procedure: An incision is made over the sternal midline, and the sternum is splint longitudinally with the sternal saw. Exposure is maintained with a self-retaining retractor. In a lymphadenectomy for thyroid carcinoma, the thymic tissue is excised, and the lymph nodes are removed as far as the pericardium. The great veins are skeletonized (see 5.2 for details). The sternum is reapproximated with wire sutures.

The technique of mediastinal lymphadenectomy with left upper lobectomy or left pneumonectomy (Hata's operation) is described below:

Following median sternotomy, the thymus is dissected free toward the left side without entering the right pleural space. The left pleural space is opened widely so that local operability can be assessed. Next the pericardium is incised vertically upward from the cardiac center, and a lateral extension is made at right angles toward the left side. The aortic arch is snared and dissected free; this step is facilitated by identifying the left recurrent nerve. Lengthy portions of the brachiocephalic trunk and left innominate vein are also cleared and mobilized. The superior vena cava, pulmonary trunk, and left pulmonary artery are visualized. Using padded retractors, the aortic arch is retracted to the left, the brachiocephalic trunk and left innominate vein superiorly, the superior vena cava to the right, and the pulmonary trunk inferiorly, whereupon the posterior layer of the pericardium is incised to expose the tracheobronchial angle and distal trachea. All fat and lymph nodes are progressively dissected free from above downward, aided by exposure of the left recurrent nerve. As the dissection is carried out, care is taken not to enter the right pleural space. Since excessive traction on the aorta can provoke arrhythmias or even cardiac arrest, the heart rate should be closely monitored. After removal of all the lymph nodes in the pre- and paratracheal areas and about the bifurcation, including the subcarinal nodes, the left pulmonary artery is cleared, ligated, and divided, placing an extra suture proximally to secure the stump. Next the pulmonary veins are identified and secured by intra- or extrapericardial ligation and division, depending on local findings. The lung is isolated from the mediastinum, the left main bronchus is dissected free, and it is divided close to its origin using the stapling device or an open technique with suture closure. After division of the ligamentum arteriosum, the left main bronchus is pulled through below the aortic arch, taking the lymph nodes in that area (Botallo's nodes), and the left lung is completely mobilized and removed. A chest tube and mediastinal drain are inserted, and the sternum is closed.

Complications: Entry into the right pleural space. Left recurrent nerve palsy. Arrhythmias or cardiac arrest from aortic displacement.

4.2 Right Mediastinal Lymphadenectomy

Indication: Right-sided bronchogenic carcinoma.

Preoperative preparation: Same as for pulmonary resection.

Instruments: Thoracic set.

Position: Lateral.

Approach: Posterolateral thoracotomy.

Steps in procedure:

(1) Posterolateral thoracotomy
(2) Incision of pleura at the upper lobar reflection and along the trachea as far as the thoracic aperture
(3) Exposure of the pulmonary veins, ligation and division
(4) Exposure of the pulmonary artery, ligation and division
(5) Exposure of the vagus nerve to the origin of the recurrent nerve
(6) Ligation and division of the azygos vein (optional)
(7) Excision of the pre- and paratracheal lymph nodes and fat, proceeding from above downward past the bifurcation so that the right main bronchus or right upper lobe bronchus is exposed
(8) Transection of the bronchus
(9) Excision of the subcarinal nodes

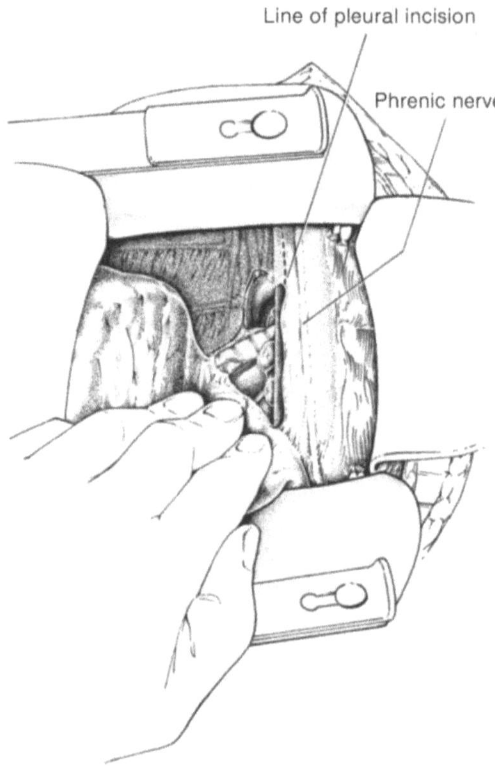

a

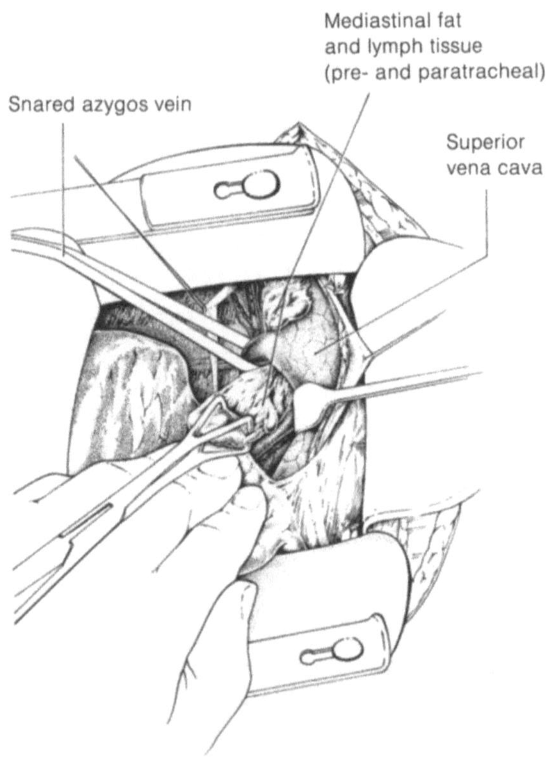

b

Fig. 5. a Pleural incision for right mediastinal lymphadenectomy. **b** Dissection of the pre- and paratracheal lymphatic and fatty tissue for lymphadenectomy. In this view the azygos vein is undivided; division of the vein facilitates exposure and allows for a more complete lymphadenectomy. **c** Status after right lymphadenectomy. The azygos vein has been divided, and the right upper lobe is preserved. **d** Closure of the mediastinum (optional)

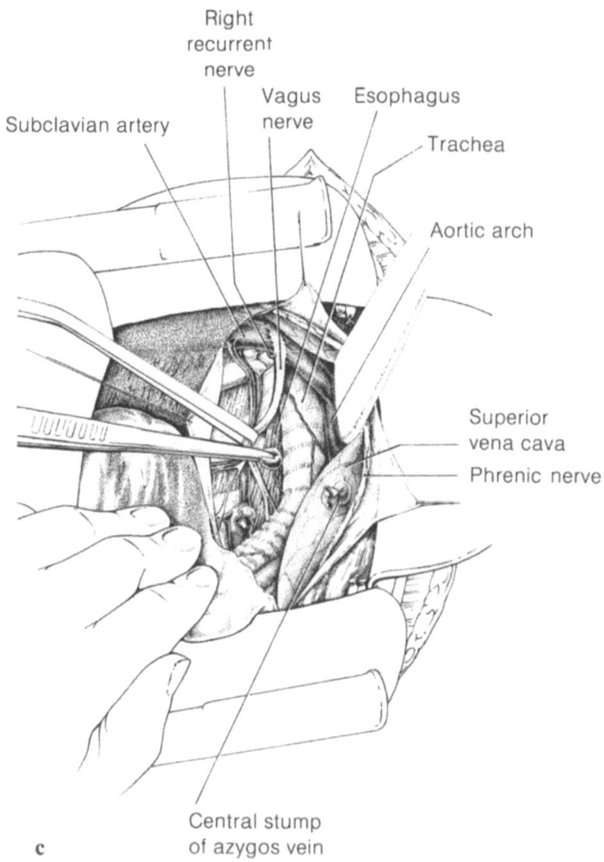

c

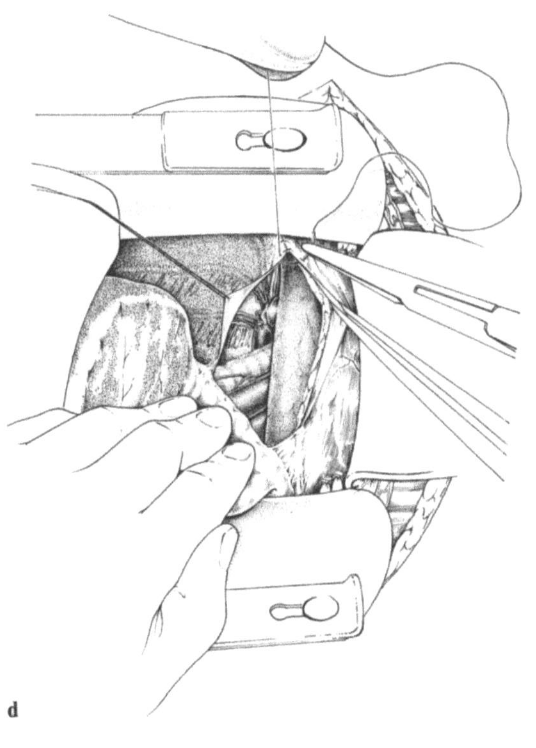

d

After thoracotomy the pleura is incised at its reflection, and the incision is extended over the trachea as far as the thoracic aperture (Fig. 5 a). The pulmonary veins are exposed, cleared, ligated and divided; the arteries are dealt with similarly. For a lower lobectomy or lower bilobectomy, the pulmonary resection is performed first; for an upper lobectomy or pneumonectomy, the lung is left in place after division of the vessels. Adequate exposure may require ligation and division of the azygos vein, in which case the proximal stump should be secured with a transfixing ligature. The vagus nerve is dissected free and snared; it is cleared to the origin of the recurrent nerve while also exposing the subclavian artery. Next the lymphatic and fatty tissue is removed from the para- and pretracheal areas, proceeding from above downward and using electrocautery to control bleeding from lymph node vessels (Fig. 5 b). The anterior and lateral walls of the trachea are completely exposed. Figure 5 c shows the appearance of the field on completion of the dissection, with the trachea, aortic arch, and vena cava exposed. The dissection is continued distally past the tracheal bifurcation. If the azygos vein is preserved, the mediastinal fat and lymphatic tissue must be extracted from beneath the vein. After the bronchus has been cleared, divided and secured, the specimen is removed, and at that time the subcarinal nodes are taken. Before closing, the surgeon palpates carefully behind the trachea and about the retrohilar esophagus for additional lymph nodes. Suture closure of the mediastinal pleura (Fig. 5 d) is optional. Chest tubes are inserted, and the wound is closed in layers.

Complications: Recurrent nerve injury. Postoperative bleeding from lymph node vessels. Chylothorax from perforation of major lymph channels.

4.3 Left Mediastinal Lymphadenectomy

Given the topographic location of the aortic arch and great mediastinal vessels, this resection may encompass only portions of the mediastinal lymphatic drainage tracts. Left thoracotomy does not afford access to the right paratracheal or superior pretracheal lymph nodes. When a pneumonectomy is performed, the lymph nodes about the bifurcation are easier to remove than during a lobectomy.

Steps in procedure:

(1) Left posterolateral thoracotomy
(2) Incision of the pleura at its reflection on the upper lobe, longitudinal incision of the pleura over the aortic arch into the upper mediastinum
(3) Pulmonary resection
(4) Exposure of the vagus nerve and recurrent nerve. Excision of lymph nodes in the aortic arch and bifurcation
(5) Excision of anterior mediastinal lymph nodes proximal to the phrenic nerve
(6) Insertion of chest tubes, wound closure in layers

The mediastinal pleura is incised from its reflection to a point past the aortic arch, the pulmonary artery is dissected free (Fig. 6 a,b), and the pulmonary resection is carried out. The vagus nerve and recurrent nerve are exposed, and the lymph nodes in the aortic arch are removed together with the subcarinal, left tracheobronchial, and paraesophageal nodes. The lymph nodes in the pulmonary ligament are also excised.

Complications: Recurrent nerve or left phrenic nerve injury, lymphatic fistula, postoperative bleeding.

All excised nodes should be described in terms of their topographic location, adhering to a standard scheme (e.g., the Naruke scheme).

5 Procedures on the Anterior Mediastinum

5.1 Parathyroidectomy in the Anterior Mediastinum

Indication: Excision of diseased parathyroid glands in the mediastinum with a negative exploration of the typical parathyroid sites and with laboratory or scintigraphic evidence of mediastinal parathyroids.

Instruments: Thoracic set.

Position: Supine.

Approach: Median sternotomy.

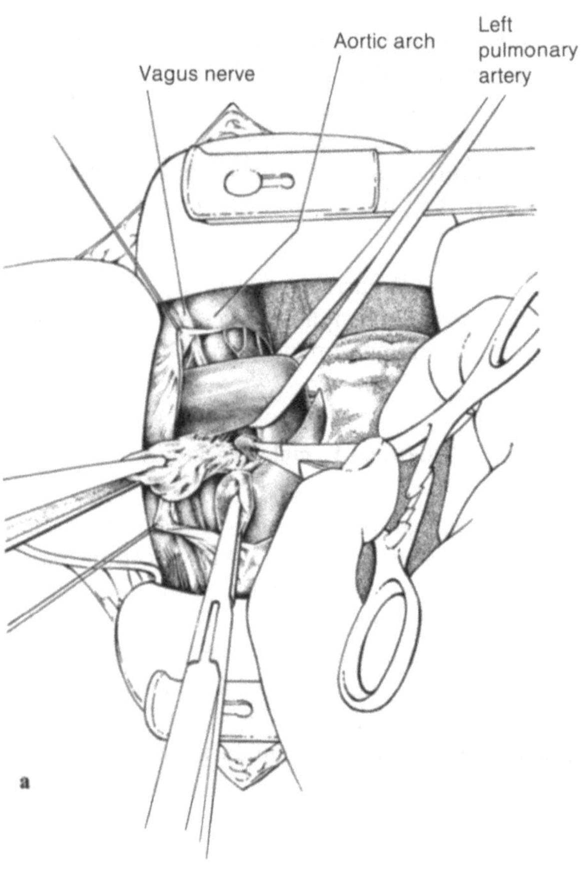

a

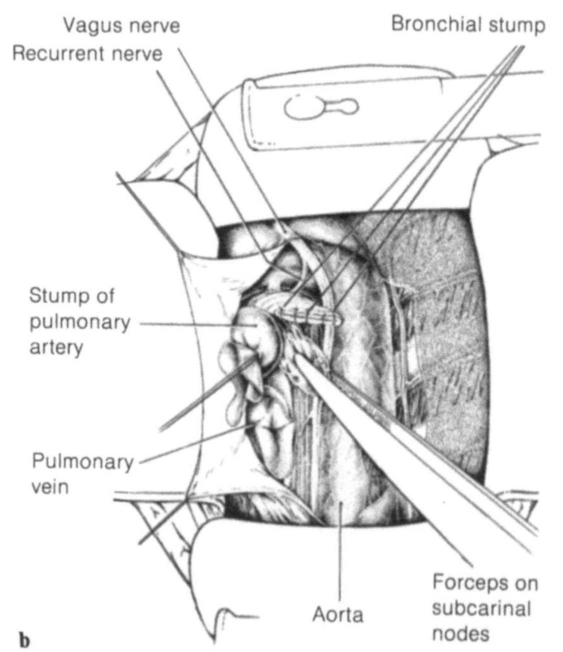

b

Fig. 6. a Left-sided lymphadenectomy: resection of the parabronchial lymph nodes and fatty tissue. **b** Lymphadenectomy for left pneumonectomy

Steps in procedure:

(1) Median sternotomy
(2) Identification and excision of the parathyroid gland with concomitant removal of the thymus and mediastinal fat
(3) Closure of the chest in layers

The thymic region is exposed through a median sternotomy. Pathologically altered parathyroid glands can usually be grossly identified. The recommended treatment is systematic removal of the prepericardial fatty tissue, taking the thymus even if an abnormal parathyroid gland cannot be visualized. A chest tube is inserted, and the wound is closed in layers.

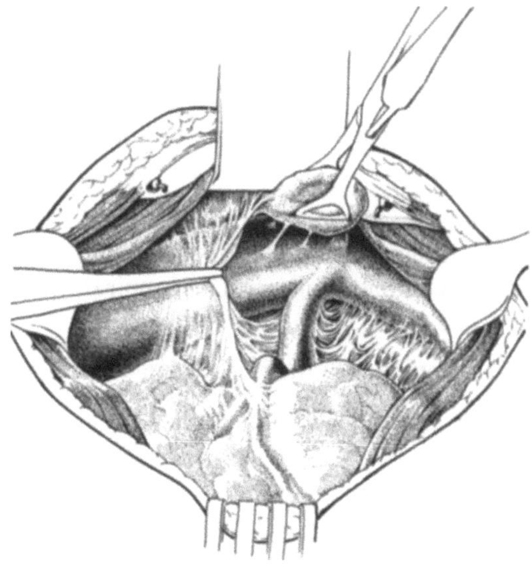

Fig. 7. Transcervical thymectomy, anterosuperior view. The manubrium is elevated anteriorly with a Roux retractor. Here a nub of thymic tissue has been separated from the thyrothymic ligament and is being pulled anteriorly with a forceps. Note the short vessels bridging from the thymic tissue to the left brachiocephalic vein

5.2 Procedures on the Thymus

Thymectomy is indicated:

- for treatment of myasthenia gravis even if the thymus appears normal,
- for thymic tumors.

5.2.1 Transcervical Thymectomy

Indication: Myasthesia gravis with a normal-appearing thymus on X-rays and CT scans.

Preoperative preparation: Empty stomach, general anesthesia. The patient should be prepared and draped for a median sternotomy, should it prove necessary.

Instruments: Small basic set; on hand: thoracic set, sternal saw.

Position: Supine with the neck extended.

Approach: Small Kocher collar incision.

Steps in procedure:

(1) Supine position with the neck extended
(2) Collar incision
(3) Midline incision of the cervical muscles
(4) Bilateral exposure of the thyrothymic ligaments
(5) Division of each ligament, which is grasped with a Pean clamp
(6) Bilateral, stepwise dissection of the thymus with traction on the clamp, which is repositioned as the dissection proceeds
(7) Wound closure in layers over a suction drain

A small Kocher collar incision is made, and the platysma is divided. The cervical muscles are split vertically to their attachment on the manubrium or sternoclavicular joint and are held laterally with Kocher retractors. The lower pole of the thyroid gland is exposed, and the thyrothymic ligament is identified on each side. The ligament on the right side is divided, seized with an Ellis clamp, and elevated (Fig. 7). The thymus is progressively dissected free, giving close attention to the small veins on its posterior surface that enter the left innominate vein. These vessels must be isolated, ligated, and divided. The thymus itself is distinguished from the surrounding fatty tissue by its firmer consistency and anatomic boundaries. Both lobes of the thymus are removed, and a suction drain is inserted.

It is possible to remove the thymus completely through a suprasternal incision, but this approach has its disadvantages. On the one hand, troublesome bleeding can result from inadvertent tearing of the left innominate vein, and a sternotomy may be necessary to secure hemostasis; on the other, there is no assurance that a total thymectomy has been accomplished. The major advantage of transcervical thymectomy is its relatively low morbidity and shorter hospital stay compared with the transsternal procedure.

5.2.2 *Transsternal Thymectomy*

Indications: Thymic tumors, thymectomy for myasthenia gravis.

Preoperative preparation: Empty stomach, special consult with anesthesiologist about potential postoperative complications such as respiratory distress.

Position: Supine with the neck extended.

Approach: Median sternotomy.

Steps in procedure:

(1) Median sternotomy (full or partial)
(2) Exposure of both thymic lobes from below upward
(3) Extirpation of the thymus
(4) Closure of the chest

A full or partial median sternotomy exposes the thymus gland anterior to the pericardium and great veins, bounded laterally by the parietal pleura. Beginning at the lower poles of the thymus and proceeding upward, the gland is progressively freed from the pericardium and elevated anteriorly by careful traction. The arterial supply is derived chiefly from small branches of the internal mammary artery and occasionally from the inferior thyroid. Typically the thymus is drained by two veins on its posterior aspect that enter the left innominate vein (Fig. 8). These vessels may be very short, so there is a significant potential for avulsion-type injury. In rare cases the thymus may be situated behind the innominate vein. The thymus is usually distinguishable from fatty tissue in the neck by its distinctive color and consistency and also by its boundaries, which become apparent when traction is placed on the gland. Some authors recommend that the thymectomy include removal of the surrounding fat as far as the pulmonary hilum, since it may contain detached thymic tissue. Care is taken to protect the phrenic nerve during removal of the fatty tissue.

In the presence of localized thymic tumors, removal of the entire gland is indicated. The transsternal approach is recommended even when X-rays show a laterally situated tumor arising from the thymus.

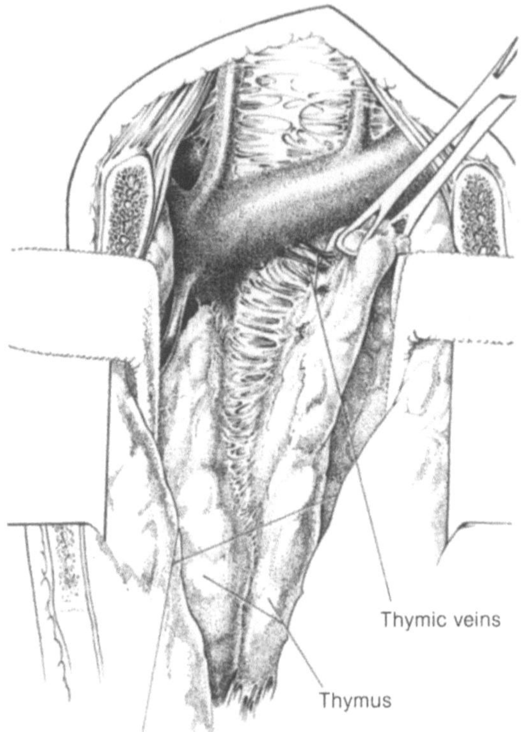

Fig. 8. Exposure of the thymus through a full sternotomy. The short thymic veins are visible

Intraoperative complications: Pleural entry, bleeding from thymic veins avulsed from the left innominate, phrenic nerve injury.

It is not uncommon for myasthenia gravis patients to require prolonged postoperative ventilatory support.

5.3 Other Lesions of the Anterior Mediastinum

Most lesions of the anterior mediastinum, including those that are paramediastinal on X-rays, originate from the thymus, the thyroid, or are congenital lesions of dysontogenic origin. If preoperative findings (X-ray tomography, CT, isotope scans) are consistent with a process originating from the thyroid, a median sternotomy is recommended if the size of the lesion is such that it can be adequately removed through that approach. Use of the lateral or anterolateral transpleural approach (e.g., for intrathoracic goiter) poses greater technical problems, especially regarding the exposure of tumor-feeding vessels. Transsternal extension may prove necessary, or a cervical approach may have to be used. Enucleation of the usually well-encapsulated tumors requires a complete exposure of the lesion and its vascular relationships (most thymic tumors occur anterior to the great veins, most thyroid nodules posterior). The left innominate vein may be ligated and divided with no adverse consequences.

It is not unusual for anterior mediastinal masses to cause significant neurovascular displacement (vagus nerve, recurrent nerve, phrenic nerve), and it is essential that anatomic orientation be maintained throughout the procedure. Before any procedure is undertaken on the anterior mediastinum, the patient's vocal cord function and phrenic nerve function should be tested to establish a baseline, and the patient should be well informed about possible complications involving those functions.

Malignant, infiltrative tumors of the anterior mediastinum are usually inoperable, and attempts at resection are problematic due to the risk of hemorrhage. Generally the scope of the resection must be limited to excisional biopsy.

5.3.1 Paratracheal Cysts

These rare lesions are usually detected on roentgenograms or CT scans. Symptoms result from tracheal compression, which may be severe.

Instruments: Small basic set (on hand: thoracic set, sternal saw).

Position: Supine with the neck extended.

Approach: Small collar incision extended on the affected side.

Steps in procedure:

(1) Collar incision
(2) Division of the platysma, release of the strap muscles and sternocleidomastoid muscle on the affected side
(3) Exposure of the anterior tracheal wall
(4) Exposure and isolation of the cyst
(5) Extirpation of the cyst
(6) Suction drainage
(7) Wound closure in layers

A small suprasternal incision (Kocher collar incision) is made and is extended on the affected side. After division of the platysma, the sternocleidomastoid muscle and pretracheal strap muscles are released, and the anterior wall of the trachea is dissected free. Usually the cysts are easy to palpate in their superior portion, and they are progressively mobilized from the trachea. Exposure of the recurrent nerve is desirable on the left side, although it may be difficult due to adhesions and scar-tissue bands. The cyst is mobilized as close to its wall as possible to avoid recurrent nerve injury. Occasionally it is necessary to open and decompress the cyst to create enough space for further dissection. If the trachea is entered during extirpation of the cyst, it is repaired with absorbable (monofilament) suture material.

After complete removal of the cyst, the trachea is checked for aerostasis by partially withdrawing the endotracheal tube. A Redon suction drain is inserted, the divided cervical muscles are reattached to the manubrium or clavicle, and the rest of the wound is closed in layers.

Complications: Left recurrent nerve palsy.

5.3.2 Transthoracic Removal of a Paratracheal Cyst

After posterolateral thoracotomy and incision of the parietal pleura, the cyst may be seen bulging into the mediastinum. The lesion is freed from surrounding tissues; large vascular connections are seldom encountered. If the trachea is entered, it is repaired with absorbable monofilament suture material.

5.3.3 Intrathoracic Goiter

Indication: Mediastinal mass that is consistent with extension of goiter based on preoperative studies and is inaccessible through a cervical approach.

Preoperative preparation: As for median sternotomy.

Instruments: Thoracic set.

Position: Supine with the neck extended.

Approach: Collar incision combined with partial or full median sternotomy.

Steps in procedure:

(1) Suprasternal collar incision, median sternotomy
(2) Exposure of thyroid
(3) Mobilization of intrathoracic part of thyroid
(4) If necessary, subtotal resection of goiter, extirpation of the mediastinal part of the thyroid
(5) Insertion of drains
(6) Wound closure in layers

A suprasternal collar incision is extended downward to the midsternum or into the epigastrium to form a T-shaped incision. After division of the platysma and upward dissection of the cutaneous-platysma flap, the cervical muscles are split on the midline, and the goiter is exposed. The incision is carried into the sternal manubrium, and a median sternotomy is performed; the sternotomy may be partial (third interspace) or full, depending on the size of the substernal extension of the goiter. The right and left innominate veins and the superior vena cava are often stretched over the mass and must be isolated. The thyroid mass may be bluntly mobilized; it does not have a vascular supply within the mediastinum. The blood supply is usually derived from the inferior thyroid artery, which is ligated and divided in standard fashion (see Strumectomy). The pedicle from the thyroid gland to the substernal mass may be extremely thin, requiring that the cervical and substernal portions of the goiter be dealt with separately. A pleural drain is inserted in the event of pleural entry. Two Redon suction drains are placed substernally, and the sternotomy is closed.

Complications: Recurrent nerve palsy (especially on the left side), injury to the great vessels, pleural entry.

5.4 Tumors of the Anterior Inferior Mediastinum

The most common mass lesions in this region are lipomas, fibromas, fibrosarcomas, and pericardial cysts, which may be approached through an anterolateral or posterolateral thoracotomy, depending on their location. The lesions are well circumscribed, and most can be enucleated without difficulty. Diaphragmatic hernias presenting as mediastinal masses are described in Chap. H.

6 Procedures on the Middle Mediastinum

Most lesions of the middle mediastinum arise from the lymphatic system, and the main role of surgery is in obtaining biopsy specimens and determining their histology. In addition, bronchogenic or enteric cysts or teratomas can develop in close relation to the hilum or trachea, and an attempt must be made to enucleate these lesions without jeopardizing nearby structures (see Chap. F).

7 Procedures on the Posterior Mediastinum

7.1 Neurogenic Tumors

Neurogenic tumors of the posterior mediastinum arise from the peripheral nerves or from the sympathetic or parasympathetic chain.

Most of these lesions occur in the paravertebral area. Whereas benign tumors such as neurinoma, neurofibroma, and ganglioneuroma can usually be enucleated without difficulty, malignant tumors such as neurosarcoma and neuroblastoma can grow invasively and often are not amenable to radical removal.

Indication: Radiologically apparent, usually asymptomatic tumor of the posterior mediastinum.

Preoperative preparation: CT evaluation of hourglass tumors, neurosurgical consult.

Instruments: Thoracic set.

Position: Lateral.

Approach: Posterolateral thoracotomy; the level depends on the site of the neoplasm.

Steps in procedure:

(1) Posterolateral thoracotomy
(2) Incision of the parietal pleura
(3) Isolation and division of intercostal vessels overlying the tumor
(4) Mobilization and extirpation of the tumor with removal of intervertebral and intraspinal extensions
(5) Insertion of drainage tube
(6) Closure of the chest

Through a posterolateral thoracotomy, the lung is retracted anteriorly, and the pleura over the tumor is incised and pushed aside. Often it is necessary at this stage to ligate intercostal vessels coursing over the tumor. The tumor is progressively freed from the vertebral column, the ribs, and the intervertebral foramina. Many tumors extend through the foramina and into the spinal canal, forming an hourglass-shaped growth with associated neurologic symptoms. In this case neurosurgical assistance is needed to accomplish a complete removal. Dissection into the foramina can provoke venous bleeding that is difficult to control.

Following removal of the neoplasm, a chest tube is inserted and the thoracotomy is closed.

Complications: Segmental motor deficits from nerve damage in the region of the lower thoracic spine. With tumors at the thoracic inlet, injury can occur to the recurrent nerve or sympathetic trunk leading to Horner's syndrome.

7.2 Other Lesions (Teratomas, Dermoid Cysts, Hydatid Cysts, Enteric Cysts, Bronchogenic Cysts)

These lesions usually cannot be assigned to a particular organ or structure, and their vascular supply is highly variable. They are exposed through a posterolateral thoracotomy and excised locally, sparing nearby structures (nerves, vessels, esophagus).

8 Procedures Involving the Lymphatic System

The most important of these procedures are performed on the thoracic duct. Systematic lymphadenectomy is discussed in Sect. 4 of this chapter.

8.1 Thoracic Duct Injury

The thoracic duct, which runs posterior to the esophagus, is susceptible to injury during surgical procedures on the esophagus and posterior mediastinum. If chylous leakage from the thoracic duct is noted intraoperatively, the stump is ligated. Attempts at reconstruction are usually futile, and the duct may be ligated without harmful effects owing to adequate collateral vessels. If the injury is recognized postoperatively from drainage of lymph through the chest tube, oral feeding should be discontinued and parenteral nutrition maintained for 10–14 days. In most cases the fistula will resolve spontaneously with fusion of the pleural layers. If the leak persists for more than 2–3 weeks, a repeat thoracotomy should be considered.

Preoperative preparation: Cream is ingested 3 h before surgery to aid intraoperative recognition of the leak.

Instruments: Thoracic set.

Position: Lateral.

Approach: Through the original thoracotomy.

Steps in procedure:

(1) Reopening of the original incision
(2) Identification and ligation of the thoracic duct stump
(3) If the stump is not found: parietal pleurectomy
(4) Insertion of two chest tubes
(5) Closure of the chest in layers

The old thoracotomy is reopened, or for a primary operation a posterolateral thoracotomy is performed on the side of the chylothorax. The pulmonary ligament is ligated and divided, and the lung is dissected free posteriorly as far as the lower lobe vein. The lung is retracted superiorly and the diaphragm inferiorly. The esophagus is exposed and snared. The thoracic duct is then identified posterior to the esophagus, isolated, and ligated.

Spontaneous chylothorax is caused in about 50% of cases by malignant disease of the posterior mediastinum leading to obstruction and spontaneous perforation of the thoracic duct. Surgical repair of the chylous leak is rarely possible. A better option is parietal pleurectomy so that the lung will fuse to the chest wall and mediastinum and seal off the fistula.

Complications: There are no specific complications relating to the surgical procedure.

8.2 Lymphocele, Lymphangioma

Localization: Usually in the left upper mediastinum.

Indication: Radiologic evidence of a mediastinal mass.

Preoperative preparation: As for thoracotomy.

Instruments: Thoracic set.

Position: Lateral.

Approach: Posterolateral thoracotomy.

Steps in procedure:

(1) Posterolateral thoracotomy
(2) Incision of the parietal pleura over the lesion
(3) Exposure and local excision of the lymphangioma
(4) Insertion of two chest tubes
(5) Closure of the thoracotomy

The mass usually can be localized by palpation and is exposed by incision of the parietal pleura. It is dissected free in stepwise fashion. Radical local excision is difficult because of the delicate walls of the lymphocele or lymphangioma. It is important to preserve structures coursing in proximity to the lesion. If continuity of the lymphatic duct cannot be restored, ligation is advised. Two chest tubes are placed, and the wound is closed in layers.

References

1. Carlens E (1959) Mediastinoscopy: a method for inspection and tissue biopsy in the superior mediastinum. Dis Chest 36:343
2. Goldberg EM, Glicksman A, Khan F, Nickson J (1970) Mediastinoscopy for assessing mediastinal spread in clinical staging of carcinoma of the lung. Cancer 25:347
3. Hata E, Ohara T, Harada M, Kimura K, Fukushima K, Kotoda K, Hasegawa T, Matsuoka R, Arai T, Kira S (1982) Superradical operation for carcinoma of the left lung through the median sternotomy. III. World Conference on Lung Cancer R 147, Tokyo
4. Thermann M, Poser H, Müller-Hermelink KH, Troidl H, Brieler S, Amend V, Schröder D (1984) Evaluation of tomography and mediastinoscopy for the detection of mediastinal lymph node metastases. The Annals of Thor Surg, Volume 37, Nr 6

H. Procedures on the Diaphragm

R. GRUNDMANN

CONTENTS

1 Anatomy

1.1 Sites of Predilection for Herniation (see 3.1.2)

1.2 Innervation of the Diaphragm

The only motor nerve of the diaphragm is the phrenic nerve. Sensory innervation is additionally supplied by the 6th through 12th intercostal nerves. Both the left and right phrenic nerve divide into branches of variable number before reaching the diaphragm. The right phrenic nerve ramifies while still within the fatty tissue of the right cardiac angle (before entering the central tendon of the diaphragm), usually lateral to the inferior vena cava. The left phrenic nerve ramifies about 3 cm from the central tendon while still within the fatty tissue of the left cardiac angle [49].

2 Incisions of the Diaphragm (Fig. 1)

The diaphragm is best exposed through a thoracotomy in the seventh or eighth intercostal space. Incisions in the diaphragm should be placed to avoid division of the phrenic nerve branches so as to minimize the extent of postoperative paralysis [46, 47]. The best technique is to incise the diaphragm parallel to the costal arch at a distance of 2–3 cm from its line of attachment [49]. This incision may be used for all operations involving

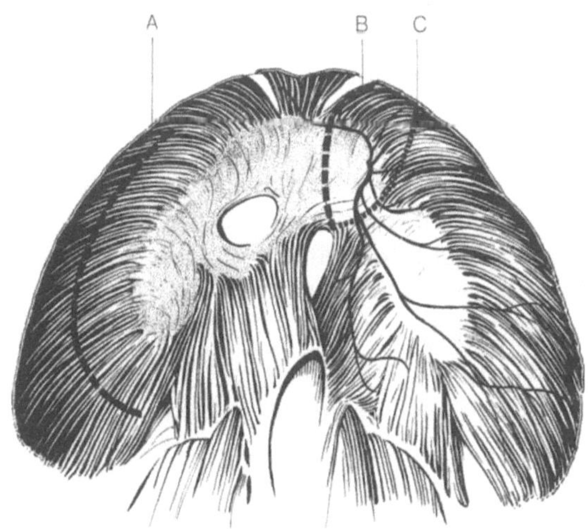

Fig. 1. Incisions of the diaphragm. *A* An incision parallel to the costal arch, 2–3 cm from the attachment of the diaphragm, is best functionally. *B* Extension of the esophageal hiatus in the sagittal plane, medial to the site of entry of the phrenic nerve. *C* Lateral radial phrenotomy. Incision of this type should be avoided

the diaphragm and disrupts only the terminal extensions of the intradiaphragmatic motor nerve branches and the terminal sensory branches of the intercostal nerves (Fig. 1, incision A).

If extension of the esophageal hiatus is required, the incision should be placed on the sagittal midline. Because both phrenic nerves descend lateral to the esophagus in the area of the hiatus, they are not vulnerable during exposure of the esophagus, nor are they injured by dissection upward into the central tendon or downward between the diaphragmatic crura. If extension of the esophageal hiatus on the sagittal plane is not sufficient, an anterior extension may be made medial to the site of entry of the phrenic nerve, as suggested by Sery et al. [71]. However, this incision severs the anterior division of the phrenic nerve and thus damages the branches that are distributed to the anteromedial portions of the diaphragm (pars sternalis and a portion of the pars costalis). This incision (Fig. 1, incision B) is less favorable, therefore, than the semicircular phrenotomy mentioned above.

Incision of the crura should be avoided, as it invariably results in nerve division. The same applies to a lateral radial incision (Fig. 1, incision C), which interrupts all the posterolateral nerve branches and largely denervates the diaphragm on the affected side. It is best to avoid radial incisions of the diaphragm whenever possible.

Instruments: Basic set, extra thoracic set.

Position and approach: These depend on the type of procedure. The supine position with an upper midline laparotomy or transverse laparotomy is indicated for a transabdominal procedure, and the lateral position with an anterolateral or posterolateral thoracotomy for the repair of muscular defects (see below).

Suture technique: Divided muscle tissue is reapproximated with a single row of 2-0 sutures.

3 Procedures

The decision to undertake a surgical procedure on the diaphragm depends to a large extent on the patient's age: The principal indications for surgery in infants are congenital hernias, prolapses, and eventrations of the diaphragm; the main indications in adults are traumatic ruptures. Resections of the diaphragm for primary tumors are infrequently performed.

3.1 Congenital Anomalies

3.1.1 Eventration of the Diaphragm

Diaphragmatic eventration is defined as a partial or complete elevation of the intact diaphragm as a result of muscular aplasia, atrophy, or paralysis on the affected side [14].

In the *congenital* form the muscular portion of the diaphragm is poorly developed *(aplasia)* so that the thoracic and abdominal cavities are separated only by pleura and peritoneum. The cause is an anomaly of embryonic development in which the small intestine reenters the abdominal cavity prematurely, prior to the ingrowth of muscle fibers into the rudimentary diaphragm.

The *paralytic (acquired)* form of eventration results from damage to the brachial plexus during obstetric manipulations or from phrenic nerve injury following birth [7].

Localization: The congenital (aplastic) form most commonly affects the right hemidiaphragm. The acquired forms affect the right and left sides with equal frequency [80].

3.1.1.1 Transperitoneal Plication of the Diaphragm [56]

Instruments: Basic set.

Position and approach: Supine, subcostal incision.

Steps in procedure:

(1) Subcostal incision
(2) Exteriorization of the eventrated diaphragm
(3) Fixation of the plicated diaphragm to the costal arch and to the posterior abdominal wall

A long forceps with serrated jaws is introduced into the abdomen through a subcostal incision, and the center of the eventrated diaphragm is grasped and exteriorized. The base of the plicated diaphragm is fixed to the costal arch with a row

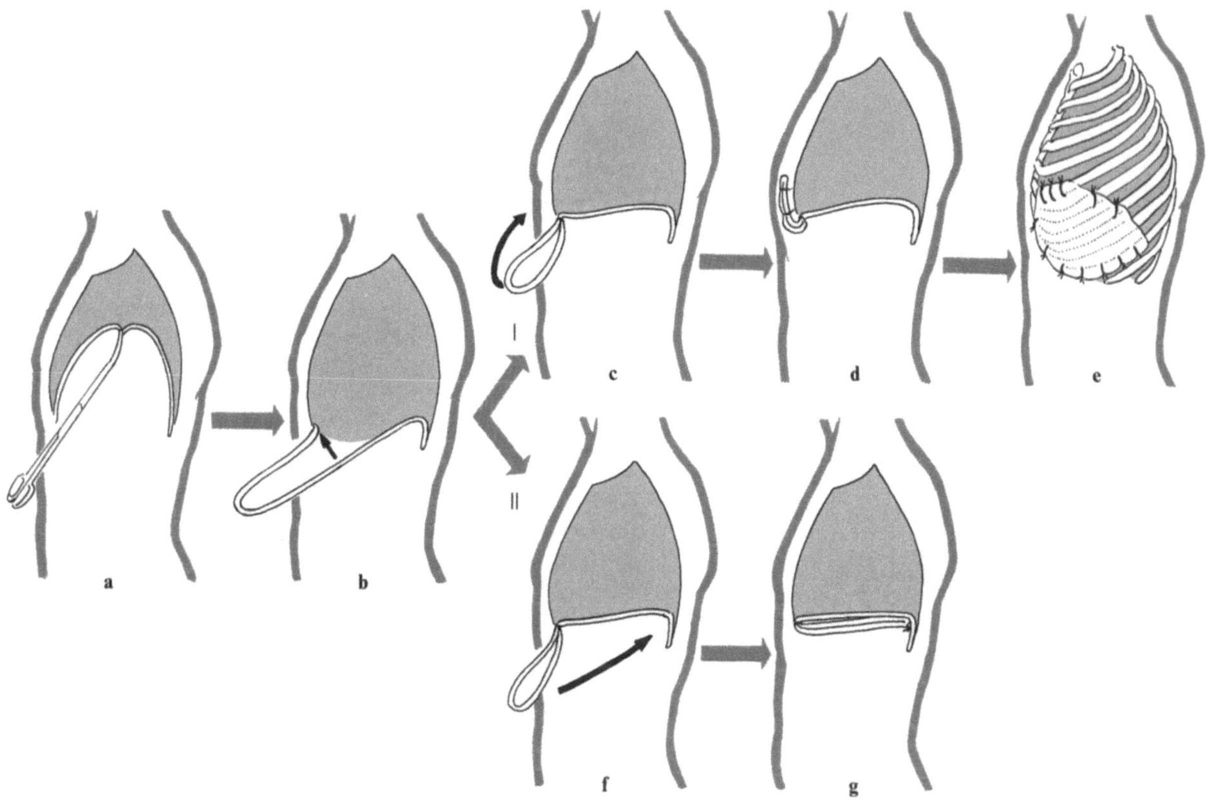

Fig. 2a–g. Transperitoneal plication of the diaphragm. The redundant diaphragm is exteriorized. It can either be tacked to the anterior chest wall with heavy pericostal sutures (I) or swung posteriorly and sutured to the attachment of the diaphragm (II)

of pericostal or perichondral sutures. The remainder may be tacked to the anterior chest wall with heavy pericostal sutures, after first mobilizing the skin of the laparotomy wound upward (Fig. 2, I), or it may be reflected posteriorly and sutured to the base of the posterior attachment of the diaphragm [32] (Fig. 2, II). The latter technique creates a three-layer plication that effectively prevents recurrence of the elevation, even when the muscle is profoundly hypoplastic.

Another means of preventing recurrence is to resect the exteriorized, attenuated portion of the diaphragm and then plicate and fix the remaining diaphragmatic tissue [62]. Resection should be avoided, however, if the phrenic nerve is not irreversibly damaged [48, 70].

3.1.1.2 Transthoracic Plication of the Diaphragm

Eventrated diaphragm can be plicated from either the abdominal or thoracic side [70]. The abdominal approach is preferred for the inspection or correction of any abdominal malformations that may coexist with the eventration [80]. The thoracic approach gives access to coexisting pulmonary malformations [14], although such malformations are far less common with congenital diaphragmatic eventration than, say, with congenital diaphragmatic hernias. The thoracic approach is technically less complex and is especially advantageous for the repair of right-sided eventrations. Left-sided eventrations and the rare bilateral forms of diaphragmatic paralysis are best approached by the abdominal route.

Instruments: Basic set, extra thoracic set.

Position and approach: Lateral position, posterolateral thoracotomy in the seventh or eighth interspace.

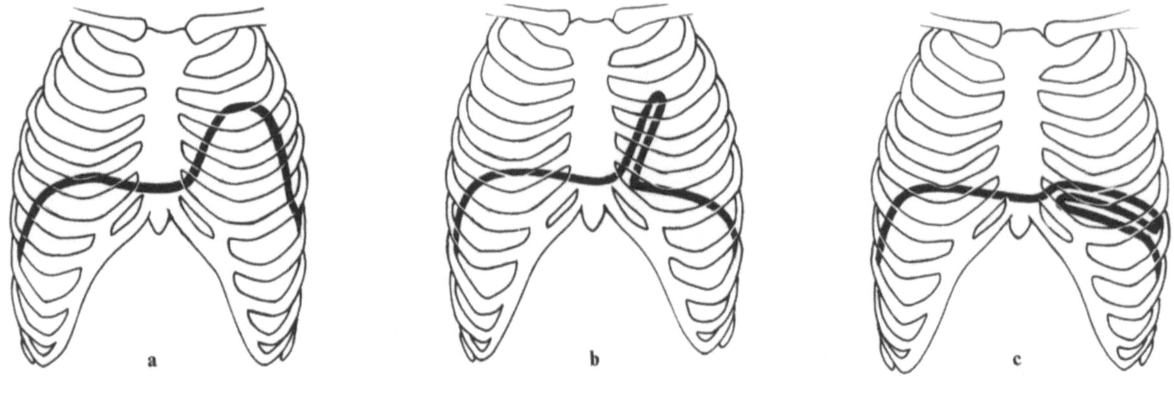

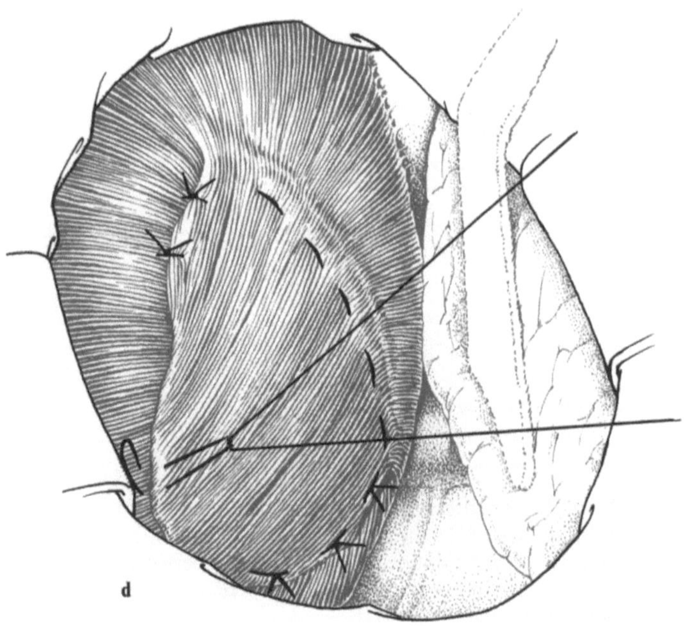

Fig. 3a–d. Transthoracic plication of the diaphragm. The redundant diaphragm is sutured at its base and fixed to the thoracic cage near the line of attachment of the diaphragm. **a** Eventration of the diaphragm; **b** redundant fold of diaphragm; **c** fixation of the fold to the thoracic cage; **d** appearance of the operative field

Steps in procedure: [77]:

(1) Posterolateral thoracotomy in the 7th or 8th interspace
(2) Diaphragm is grasped and elevated
(3) Plicated diaphragm is sutured at the base
(4) Tissue fold is sutured to the chest wall.

The eventrated diaphragm is grasped with Babcock forceps and elevated. The redundant fold of diaphragmatic tissue is sutured along its base and is then sutured to the thoracic cage in the area of attachment of the diaphragm (Fig. 3).

Another technique [44] is to place heavy stay sutures medial and lateral to the central tendon of the diaphragm and tie them in a manner that inverts the redundant tissue into the abdomen (Fig. 4) (cf. technique of Schwartz and Filler [70]). A potential disadvantage of this repair is that the plicated area of the diaphragm (i.e., the area of reinforcement) is smaller than with the other plication techniques [63].

The above procedure is acceptable only if the eventrated diaphragm can be securely plicated, and the base of the plication can be sutured without injuring the underlying viscera (especially the stomach, colon, and spleen) or catching them in the suture line. If difficulties arise or if it is necessary to explore the abdomen for coexisting anomalies, it is better to perform an open transthoracic plication (see below).

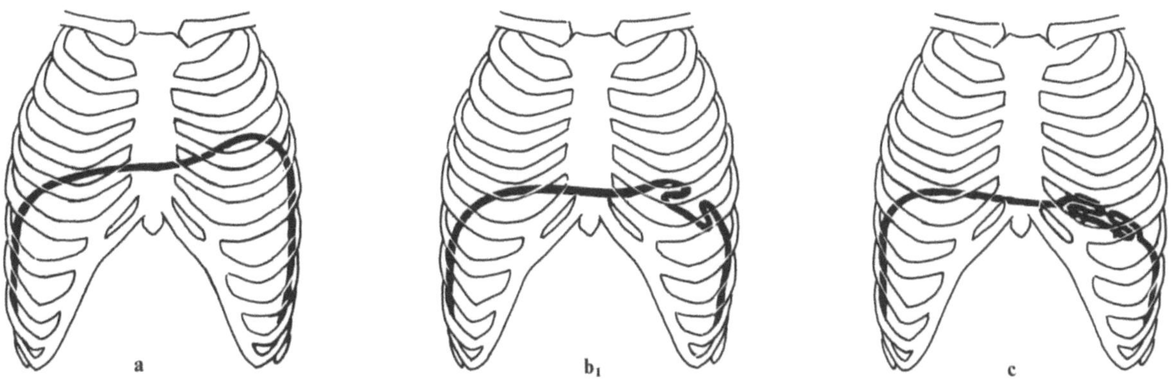

3.1.1.3 Open Plication of the Diaphragm [63]

Instruments: Basic set, extra thoracic set.

Position and approach: Lateral position, anterolateral thoracotomy in the seventh or eighth interspace.

Steps in procedure:

(1) Anterolateral thoracotomy in the 7th or 8th interspace
(2) Anteroposterior incision through the eventrated diaphragm
(3) Cut edges are overlapped, the medial overlying the lateral
(4) Layers are stitched together

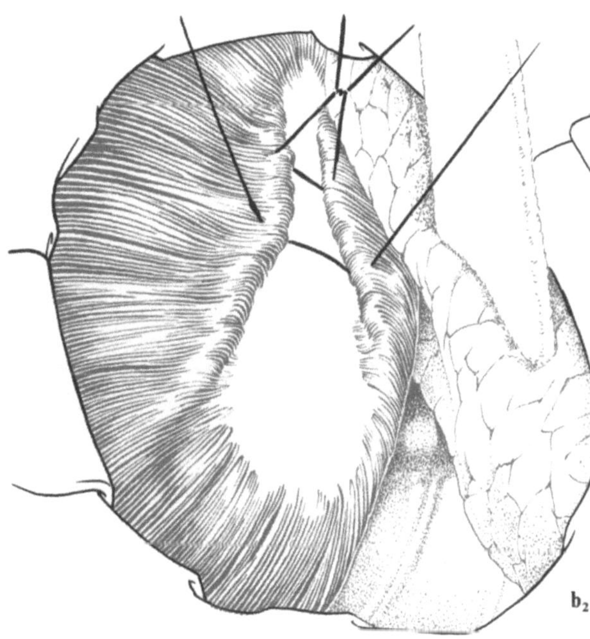

The chest is entered, and an anteroposterior incision is made through the apex of the elevated diaphragm (Fig. 5) to within 2–3 fingerwidths of the chest wall. The abdominal cavity is entered from above, and the medial portion of the diaphragm is pulled over the lateral portion with sharp forceps until the diaphragm assumes the desired, lowered contour. With a protecting hand beneath the diaphragm, the overlapping layers are stitched together with two rows of interrupted sutures. Both rows are placed before the sutures are tied.

Occasionally the aplastic diaphragm may be too weak for plication, and a reconstructive technique must be employed (see Sect. 3.4). The use of autogenous material is preferred in children due to the risk of growth disturbance (scoliosis) [7, 72], although favorable long-term results have been reported with prosthetic meshes [73].

Fig. 4a–c. Transthoracic plication of the diaphragm. The diaphragm is engaged with a heavy suture medial and lateral to its central tendinous portion, and the redundant tissue is inverted into the abdomen. **a** Eventration of the diaphragm; **b** the redundant tissue is inverted into the abdomen before the retention sutures are tied; $\mathbf{b}_1$ schematic diagram; $\mathbf{b}_2$ appearance of the operative field; **c** the completed plication

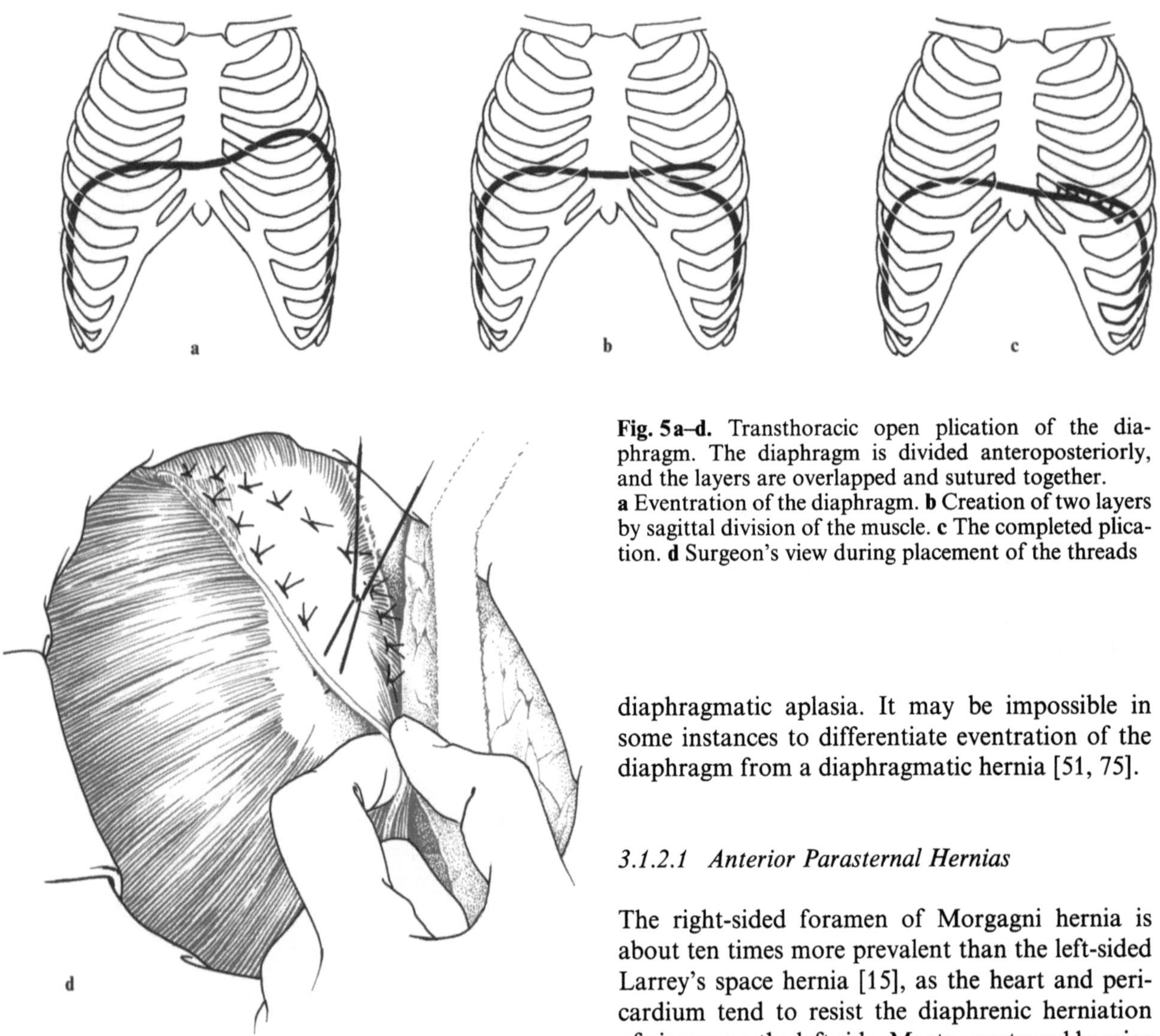

Fig. 5a–d. Transthoracic open plication of the diaphragm. The diaphragm is divided anteroposteriorly, and the layers are overlapped and sutured together.
a Eventration of the diaphragm. **b** Creation of two layers by sagittal division of the muscle. **c** The completed plication. **d** Surgeon's view during placement of the threads

3.1.2 Congenital Diaphragmatic Hernias and Aplasias

The location of these hernias is determined by preformed weak spots in the right (foramen of Morgagni) and left (Larrey's space) parasternal portions of the diaphragm and in the right and left lumbocostal areas (Bochdalek's triangle).

True diaphragmatic hernias possess a hernial sac consisting of pleuroperitoneal membrane. The majority of these lesions do not have a sac, however, and involve the protrusion of viscera through a complete defect ("diaphrenic prolapse"). The prolapse can also occur at weak points that are not preformed–usually a site of partial or complete diaphragmatic aplasia. It may be impossible in some instances to differentiate eventration of the diaphragm from a diaphragmatic hernia [51, 75].

3.1.2.1 Anterior Parasternal Hernias

The right-sided foramen of Morgagni hernia is about ten times more prevalent than the left-sided Larrey's space hernia [15], as the heart and pericardium tend to resist the diaphrenic herniation of viscera on the left side. Most parasternal hernias are acquired and are diagnosed after 40 years of age. Small parasternal hernias are asymptomatic and are discovered incidentally on chest X-rays. Large hernias that cause displacement of intrathoracic structures produce cardiopulmonary symptoms or episodes of pain due to incarceration of the herniated viscera. Surgical repair is indicated for these lesions [12, 15, 37, 66].

Instruments: Basic set.

Position and approach: Supine position, upper midline laparotomy or subcostal incision.

Either the transthoracic or transabdominal route may be used, but laparotomy is preferred for adult as well as pediatric cases [12, 32].

Procedure: This consists in exposing the hernial sac, reducing its contents, and repairing the defect with simple interrupted sutures (2-0).

3.1.2.2 Posterolateral (Bochdalek) Hernias

Posterolateral hernias are most commonly detected in children and are extremely rare in adults [57]. In infants the condition has a very grave prognosis [43]. The high mortality is due in part to the frequent coexistence of pulmonary hypoplasia [16, 19, 28, 29, 55] and to the high pulmonary vascular resistance in these children [74]. Survival has been improved by administering a vasodilator and lowering the vascular resistance in the pulmonary circuit [74].

The majority of these hernias occur on the left side. Left-sided hernias are associated with more serious respiratory problems than right-sided hernias, because the right-sided defect is usually covered by the liver [9].

Instruments: Basic set.

Position and approach: Supine position, subcostal incision on the affected side or upper transverse laparotomy [51].

Generally the transabdominal approach is preferred. It affords an opportunity to deal with associated gastrointestinal anomalies and also satisfies the frequent need for creation of a ventral hernia to provide space for the reduced viscera [9, 25]. The transthoracic route is acceptable for the very rare right-sided Bochdalek hernias [16] and for the occasional hernias diagnosed in mature patients [57]. The advantage of the thoracic approach is that it provides a clearer view of the lesion.

Procedure: The herniated viscera are reduced from the thorax, and the diaphragmatic defect is repaired by direct suture. If the defect is very large and it is feared that intraperitoneal pressure will be raised excessively, a ventral hernia can be created [51, 75]. This is done by simply closing the skin over the viscera while leaving the muscular and fascial layers open.

Occasionally the defect is so large that it cannot be completely closed by direct suture. In these cases a patch of plastic mesh may be used to obliterate the defect in adults [13] (see also 3.4). In children it is preferable to cover the defect with a vascularized tissue flap.

3.1.2.3 Repair of a Diaphragmatic Defect with a Pedicled Muscle Flap [69]

Instruments: Basic set.

Position and approach: See Sect. 3.1.2.2.

Steps in procedure:

(1) Subcostal incision, division of the transversus abdominis muscle inferiorly
(2) Mobilization of the diaphragmatic remnant and transversus abdominis muscle from the costal arch to the midaxillary line
(3) Posterior transfer of the muscle flap to obliterate the defect

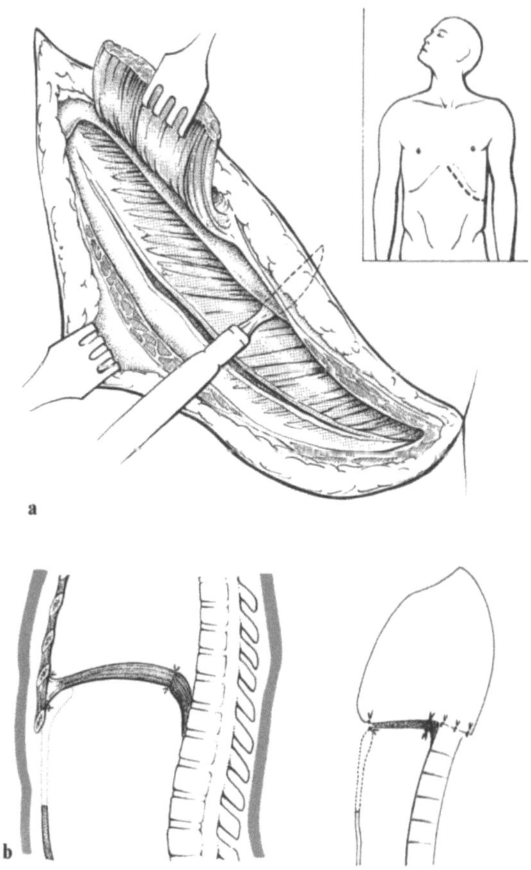

Fig. 6a, b. Repair of a diaphragmatic defect with a pedicled muscle flap. The diaphragmatic remnant and transversus abdominis muscle are separated from the posterior surface of the ribs to the midaxillary line and swung posteriorly. Insert: line of incision. **a** Separation of the transversus abdominis muscle from the posterior surface of the ribs. **b** Lateral view of the transposed muscle flap

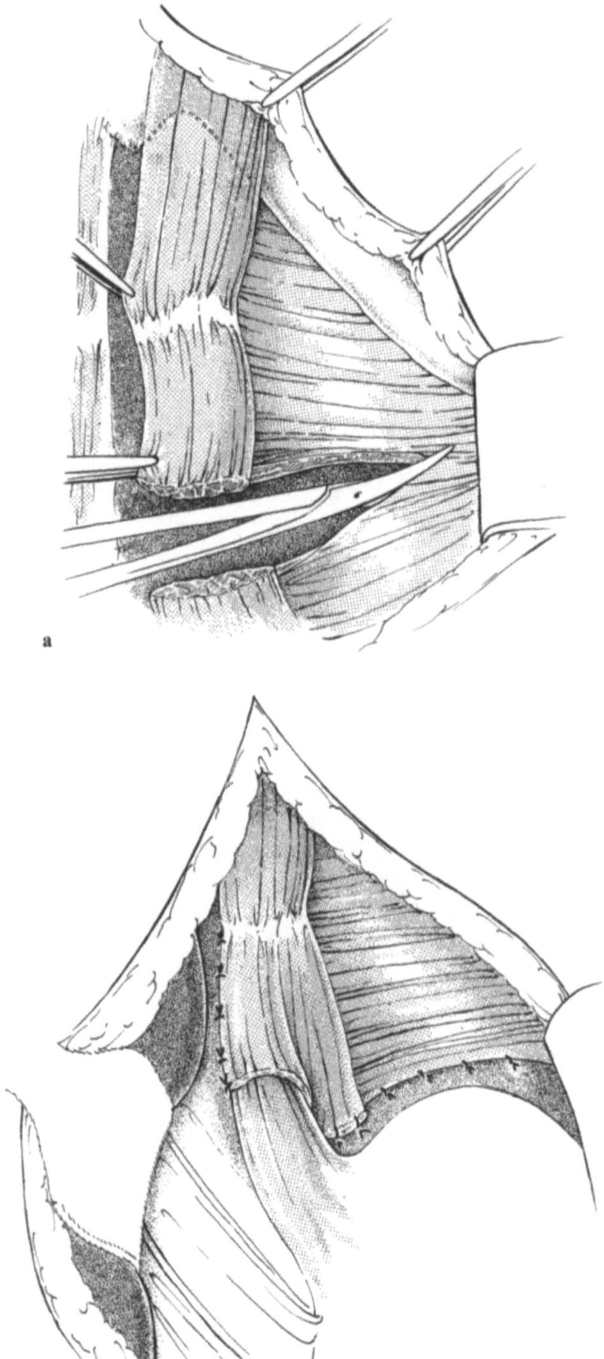

Fig. 7 a, b. Repair of a diaphragmatic defect by the Rosenkrantz technique. A laterally based flap is developed from the abdominal wall muscles of the left or right upper quadrant (*a*) and transposed over the defect.
b Appearance of the flap after it has been sutured into the defect

Operative technique: The technique is based on the fact that the transversus abdominis muscle and the anterior and lateral portions of the diaphragm are intimately blended in the area of their common costal attachment. The diaphragmatic remnant and the transversus abdominis muscle are sharply dissected from the costal margin, keeping the knife blade directed toward the ribs and carrying the dissection back to the midaxillary line or slightly beyond it (Fig. 6).

If the abdomen has already been opened by a subcostal incision for reduction of the hernia, this incision will have divided the transversus abdominis inferiorly, resulting in a laterally based muscle flap that can be swung posteriorly and sutured to the posterior chest wall with interrupted pericostal sutures.

Rosenkrantz and Cotton [65] propose a similar technique in which a flap, also laterally based, is developed from the abdominal muscles of the left or right upper quadrant (transversus abdominis and rectus abdominis muscles) and transposed into the diaphragmatic defect (Fig. 7).

3.1.3 Accessory Diaphragm (Fig. 8)

Accessory diaphragm [26, 50, 67] is a rare anomaly in which the intrathoracic cavity (usually the right) is partly or completely subdivided into two compartments by a fibromuscular septum that communicates with the diaphragm [31]. Because the septum generally is in the area of the interlobar fissure, it is apt to be mistaken on X-rays for inflammatory or neoplastic interlobar disease or an atelectatic middle lobe. Most cases are asymptomatic, although respiratory complaints are occasionally seen, especially if lobar atelectasis supervenes. Surgical resection is advised in symptomatic cases.

Procedure: Removal of the anomalous membrane is most commonly performed through a right posterolateral thoracotomy in the seventh interspace [30].

3.2 Traumatic Rupture of the Diaphragm

Rupture of the diaphragm due to blunt abdominal trauma is a relatively rare injury and is correspondingly difficult to diagnosis [10]. Many ruptures of this type remain undetected for years. Di-

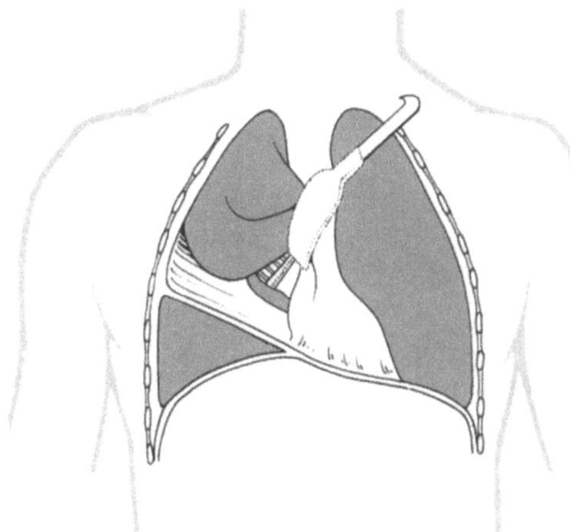

Fig. 8. Accessory diaphragm. The right intrathoracic space is divided into compartments by a fibromuscular septum that communicates with the diaphragm

agnosis formerly relied on biplane chest films, contrast instillation through a nasogastric tube, pneumoperitoneum by gas injection [34], and hepatic scintigraphy for right-sided ruptures [5]. In recent years CT has contributed greatly to the diagnosis of diaphragmatic ruptures [4], but it is still possible to miss these injuries even at laparotomy [36]. This has led authors to speculate about "two-stage" ruptures, although it is unclear whether the ruptures were actually preceded by an incomplete tear, or whether diagnosis was simply delayed [53].

The majority of diaphragmatic ruptures occur on the left side. However, the frequency of right-sided ruptures increases with the accuracy of the diagnostic evaluation [42], and it appears that up to 40% of all ruptures may involve the right hemidiaphragm [79]. Typically, the ruptures extend radially from the posterolateral quadrant of the diaphragm.

Timing of repair: If no associated injuries are present, immediate (acute) repair is not essential. Excellent results have been reported in cases where surgery was delayed for up to two months after the injury [8]. Even so, the danger of incarceration provides a rationale for undertaking surgical repair as soon as the rupture is diagnosed.

Instruments: Basic set, extra thoracic set (in some cases).

Position: Supine for laparotomy, lateral for posterolateral thoracotomy.

Approach: Laparotomy is generally preferred over thoracotomy in the acute phase [58], as it permits the detection and treatment of coexisting intrabdominal injuries. This is true even for right-sided ruptures, which are not as accessible as left-sided injuries, although some authors favor a transthoracic approach in these cases [17]. Right-sided ruptures may occasionally necessitate a combined transthoracic and transabdominal repair [42].

Posterolateral thoracotomy [76] is the incision of choice for traumatic hernias of long standing. It gives excellent exposure and also facilitates the separation of adhesions, which may be very extensive in old ruptures [6].

Procedure: In the great majority of cases, the rupture can be repaired with a single suture line (2-0 material). Very extensive ruptures, especially on the right side, may require closure with a graft of Marlex mesh [18].

3.2.1 Pericardiophrenic Hernias

Pericardiophrenic hernia is a rare posttraumatic [1, 52] or congenital condition [39] in which a communication exists between the cavities of the peritoneum and pericardium. Intraabdominal hemorrhage occurs when there is associated cardiac injury [3].

Procedure: Repair by the transabdominal route (upper midline laparotomy) is recommended so that the abdomen can be inspected for associated injuries.

3.3 Primary Tumors of the Diaphragm

Primary diaphragmatic tumors are more often benign than malignant, although both types are rare [78, 84]. The most important benign tumors are lipomas, mesothelial cysts, neurofibromas, and angiofibromas. The principal malignant tumor is fibrosarcoma.

Position and approach: Lateral position, posterolateral thoracotomy. A combined thoracoabdominal approach may be necessary for tumors expanding into both the chest and abdominal cavity [68].

Operative technique: The removal of smaller, benign tumors leaves a defect that usually can be closed by direct suture. With tumors close to the chest wall, primary closure can be effected by reapproximating the diaphragm to the rib cage.

The removal of malignant tumors always necessitates reconstruction of the diaphragm. Various techniques are available for this (see Sect. 3.4), but in cancer patients who have a relatively limited life expectancy, one should not hesitate to opt for the simplest solution and use a prosthetic mesh (e.g., Marlex) for repair of the defect [78]. In operations for right hemidiaphragmatic malignancies, closure of the thoracic outlet can be accomplished by fixation of the liver to the anterior chest wall [27, 54]. However, the advantage of technical simplicity with this method must be weighted against the risk of herniation.

3.4 Replacement of the Diaphragm

The great majority of diaphragmatic defects, regardless of their etiology, are amenable to repair by direct suture. However, there are two types of situation in which replacement of the diaphragm should be considered: 1) children with congenital aplasias and hypoplasias of the diaphragm, and 2) adults undergoing removal of diaphragmatic malignancies.

While autologous materials such as pedicled muscle flap (see 3.1.2.3) are preferred for diaphragm reconstructions in children, patients with limited life expectancy are good candidates for the technically simpler prosthetic replacements. Prosthetic materials in the form of plastic meshes are also suitable for younger patients; growth disturbance has not proved to be a problem with these materials [73]. At present the prosthetic material of choice is Marlex mesh [33, 38], although the risk of infection is theoretically greater than with homologous biologic material such as stored dura [64, 81, 82] or pericardium [20]. A potential advantage of dura or pericardium over Marlex, dacron, or nylon meshes [2] is their greater flexibility. Another basic requirement of reconstructive materials is that they incite little or no inflammatory response in surrounding tissues. It remains unclear which type of material is superior in this regard [20].

Autologous cutis grafts [21] are even more biologically favorable than the foregoing materials, and their elasticity makes them excellently suited for diaphragmatic replacement, especially in adults [60].

In selected cases it is possible to replace the left hemidiaphragm (e.g., after resection of a pleural mesothelioma) with a pedicled flap mobilized from the pericardium (Fig. 9). Studies by Hahnloser and Geroulanos [27] have shown this to be an excellent replacement material, and the resulting cardiac displacement did not lead to problems of venous inflow stasis.

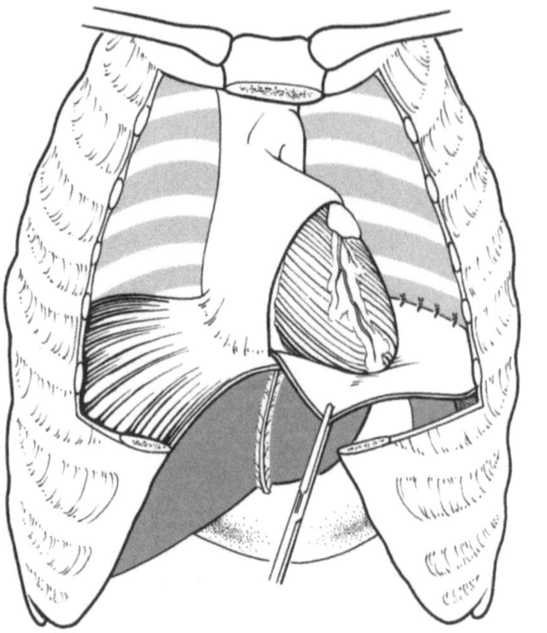

Fig. 9. Replacement of the left hemidiaphragm by a pedicled pericardial flap (here after a pleuropneumonectomy with resection of the diaphragm)

3.5 Use of the Diaphragm for Reconstructive Procedures in the Esophagus and Tracheobronchial Tree

Flaps of diaphragmatic tissue can be used for the repair of defects in the esophagus and tracheobronchial tree. This is an especially useful technique when overt or latent infection makes it difficult to effect closure by direct suture alone. Success relies on an adequate blood supply to the flap, which will otherwise succomb to scarring and contracture. Various *indications* have been described, including esophageal perforations (iatrogenic or in Boerhave's syndrome), large wall defects created by the removal of leiomyomas [59] or other tumors, tracheobronchial fistulas, and traumatic defects (especially posterior) in the tracheal wall [83].

Operative technique: Care is taken when mobilizing the muscle flap to preserve the nerve supply to the rest of the diaphragm. The flap itself should not have a nerve supply so that it will not contract with the rest of the muscle. Basically two types of flap are used: flap grafts consisting of a long strip of diaphragm with a vascular and muscular pedicle, and pedicle grafts that are based on the mammary vessels.

3.5.1 *Flap Grafts*

These flaps are taken from the posterior musculotendinous region of the diaphragm about the hiatus, using radial incisions (Figs. 10, 11). The muscular base of the flap remains in continuity with the diaphragm, and the flap is nourished by the inferior diaphragmatic vessels. Flaps of this kind can be reflected as far upward as the aortic arch. When the flap is mobilized, care is taken to avoid entering the peritoneal cavity if at all possible; this is easier on the right side than on the left. The donor defect is closed with simple interrupted sutures (2-0 material).

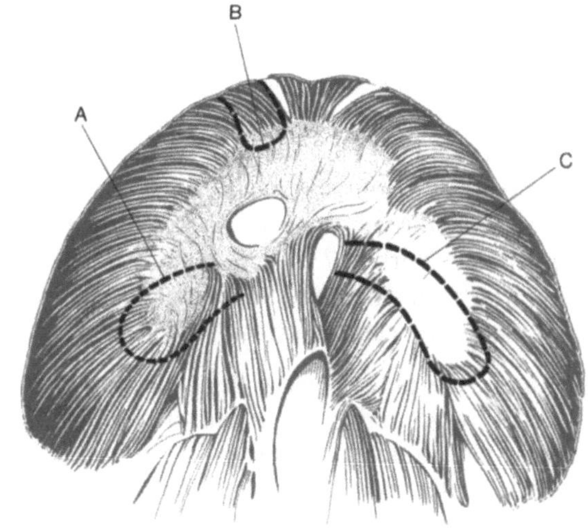

Fig. 10. Use of the diaphragm for repairing defects in the esophagus or tracheobronchial tree. *A, B, C* Incisions used to mobilize the pedicled flaps

3.5.2 *Pedicle Grafts*

These are taken from the anterior border of the diaphragm close to its sternal attachment. They are vascularized by branches of the internal mammary artery.

Approach: Median sternotomy.

Operative technique: The mammary vessels are exposed, and the vascular pedicle is traced to the diaphragm, where a suitable piece of muscle is cut from the anterior border. The pedicled flap can be transposed a considerable distance–into the cervical region if necessary–after first ligating the epigastric vessels.

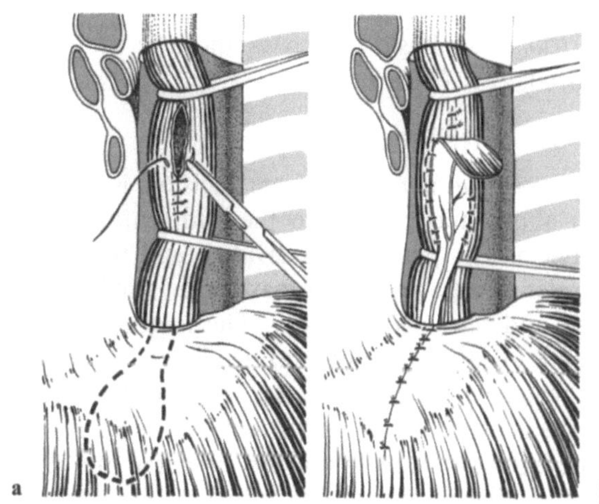

Fig. 11 a, b. Repair of an esophageal defect with a diaphragmatic flap. **a** Closure of the defect, and the incision used to create the flap. **b** The flap is elevated onto the defect and sewn into place

3.6 Diaphragm Pacing

Electrical stimulation of the diaphragm by an implanted pacemaker [22, 24, 45] may be considered a) in quadriplegic patients with spinal cord lesions above the C6 level [24], b) in patients with central alveolar hypoventilation depressing the respiratory response to hypoxia and hypercapnia (with a near-normal ventilatory capacity), c) in children with congenital hypoventilation syndrome [61] who have hypoventilation during sleep and lack of respiratory response to hypercapnia [35]. (Patient selection in these cases depends on the severity of the syndrome: patients requiring continuous ventilation are probably not good candidates for phrenic nerve stimulation [40].) d) The implantation of diaphragm pacemakers has also been described in patients with chronic obstructive pulmonary disease [23].

The success of diaphragm pacing depends upon two factors: a functionally intact connection between the phrenic nerve and diaphragm, and a stable chest wall. Generally the two hemidiaphragms are paced *alternately* for 12 hours each [11, 41]. At least this is the recommended schedule for adult quadriplegics who require full-time ventilatory support and have normal phrenic nerves. (This mode requires bilateral pacemaker implantation; see below.) In adults and especially in children who have less than normal phrenic nerve function, activation of *one* hemidiaphragm is not sufficient, and only *simultaneous bilateral* pacing will suffice. These patients will continue to require supplementary mechanical ventilation because of diaphragm fatigue, which limits electrical stimulation of the diaphragm to a maximum of 16 h in any 24-h period.

Principle of diaphragm pacing: The pacing system (manufactured by Avery Laboratories, Farmingdale, New York 11735) consists of an external transmitter with antenna, a subcutaneous receiver, and a platinum neural electrode (Fig. 12).

Approach: The phrenic nerve electrode may be implanted through either a cervical or thoracic approach. The thoracic approach is preferred, despite its greater risk, because it tends to be more effective (the cervical region contains accessory branches of the phrenic nerve that may not be stimulated with the rest of the nerve).

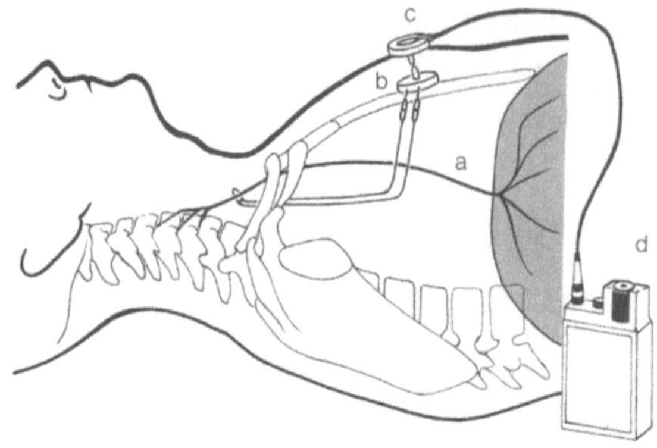

Fig. 12. Diaphragm pacing. *a* phrenic nerve; *b* receiver; *c* antenna; *d* external transmitter

3.6.1 Cervical Approach

Instruments: Basic set; extra thoracic set as required.

Position: Supine.

Operative technique: A 5-cm incision is made 2 cm above and parallel to the midportion of the clavicle. The platysma is divided, and the lateral border of the sternocleidomastoid muscle is identified and retracted medially. The internal jugular vein is exposed and displaced medially. The anterior scalene muscle is dissected free, and the phrenic nerve is exposed and undertunneled with a clamp. The electrode is pulled under the nerve and fixed to the adjacent tissue. The receiver is inserted into a subcutaneous pocket fashioned in the chest wall, and finally the electrode wire is passed to the receiver through a subcutaneous tunnel.

3.6.2 Thoracic Approach

Instruments: Basic set; extra thoracic set as required.

Position: Supine.

Approach: Anterolateral thoracotomy in the third or fourth interspace.

Operative technique: The chest is entered, the lung is retracted laterally, and the phrenic nerve is dissected free 5–10 cm above the heart (stimulation at that level will not precipitate cardiac arrhythmia). As in the cervical approach, a tunnel is made under the nerve, and the electrode is pulled through and fixed to the adjacent tissue. The electrode wire is passed through the third or fourth interspace into a subcutaneous pocket in the anterior chest wall, where it is connected to the receiver.

References

1. Adamthwaite DN, Snyders DC, Mirwis J (1983) Traumatic pericardiophrenic hernia: a report of 3 cases. Br J Surg 70:117–119
2. Adler RH, Firme CN (1957) The use of nylon prostheses for diaphragmatic defects. Surg Gynecol Obstet 104:669–674
3. Anders A, Breyer HG, Waldschmidt J (1981) Linksseitige Ventrikelruptur mit Perikard-Diaphragma-Verletzung. Chirurg 52:654–657
4. Arendrup HC, Jensen BS (1982) Traumatic rupture of the diaphragm. Surg Gynecol Obstet 154:526–530
5. Ball T, McCrory R, Smith JO, Clements JL (1982) Traumatic diaphragmatic hernia: errors in diagnosis. AJR 138:633–637
6. Baudrexl A (1979) Beitrag zur Problematik der veralteten Zwerchfellruptur. Zbl Chirurgie 104:704–712
7. Bowen TE, Zajtchuk R, Albus RA (1982) Diaphragmatic paralysis managed by diaphragmatic replacement. Ann Thorac Surg 33:184–188
8. Brearley S, Tubbs N (1981) Rupture of the diaphragm in blunt injuries of the trunk. Injury 12:480–484
9. Campell DN, Lilly JR (1982) The clinical spectrum of right Bochdalek's hernia. Arch Surg 117:341–344
10. Christophi C (1983) Diagnosis of traumatic diaphragmatic hernia: Analysis of 63 cases. World J Surg 7:277–280
11. Collier PS, Wakeling LM (1982) Diaphragmatic pacing. A new procedure for high spinal cord lesions. Physiotherapy 68:47

12. Comer TP, Clagett OT (1966) Surgical treatment of hernia of the foramen of Morgagni. J Thorac Cardiovas Surg 52:461–468
13. Cuschieri RJ, Wilson WA (1981) Incarcerated Bochdalek hernia presenting as acute pancreatitis. Br J Surg 68:669
14. Döhler R, Heinemann G (1979) Angeborene Zwerchfell-Eventration. Fortschr Med 40:1769–1771
15. Düx A (1982) Zwerchfellhernien und -Prolapse. Radiologe 22:7–21
16. Ehrlich FE, Salzberg AM (1978) Pathophysiology and management of congenital posterolateral diaphragmatic hernias. Am Surg 44:26–30
17. Estrera AS, Platt MR, Mills LJ (1979) Traumatic injuries of the diaphragm. Chest 75:306–313
18. Estrera AS, Platt MR, Mills LJ, Urschel HC (1980) Rupture of the right hemidiaphragm with liver herniation: report of a case with extension of a tear of previously undiagnosed ruptured right hemidiaphragm. J Trauma 20:174–176
19. Fitzgerald RJ (1977) Congenital diaphragmatic hernia: a study of mortality factors. Ir J Med Sci 146:280–284
20. Gallo JI, Artinano E, Val F, Duran CG (1982) Glutaraldehydepreserved heterologous pericardium for the repair of diaphragmatic defects. J Thorac Cardiovasc Surg 83:905–908
21. Geever ED, Merendino KA (1952) The repair of diaphragmatic defects with cutis grafts. An experimental study. Surg Gynecol Obstet 95:308–316
22. Glenn WWL (1978) Diaphragm pacing: Present status. PACE 1:357–370
23. Glenn WWL, Gee JBL, Schachter EN (1978) Diaphragm pacing. Application to a patient with chronic obstructive pulmonary disease. J Thorac Cardiovasc Surg 75:273–281
24. Glenn WWL, Hogan JF, Phelps ML (1980) Ventilatory support of the quadriplegic patient with respiratory paralysis by diaphragm pacing. Surg Clin N Am 60:1055–1078
25. Grmoljez PF, Lewis JE (1976) Congenital diaphragmatic hernia: Bochdalek Type. Am J Surg 132:744–746
26. Haeberlin P (1945) Eine seltene Zwerchfellmißbildung (partielle einseitige Doppelbildung). Schweiz Med Wochenschr 75:510–511
27. Hahnloser P, Geroulanos S (1976) Der Zwerchfellersatz mit Perikard bei Radikaloperation des Pleuramesothelioms. Thoraxchirurgie 24:1–5
28. Harrington J, Raphaely RC, Downes JJ (1982) Relationship of alveolar-arterial oxygen tension difference in diaphragmatic hernia of the newborn. Anesthesiology 56:473–476
29. Harrison MR, Jester JA, Ross NA (1980) Correction of congenital diaphragmatic hernia in utero. I. The model: Intrathoracic balloon produces fatal pulmonary hypoplasia. Surgery 88:174–182
30. Hart JC, Cohen IT, Ballantine TVN, Varrano LF (1981) Accessory diaphragm in an infant. J Pediatr Surg 16:947–949
31. Hartmann CA, Lange S (1982) Das akzessorische Diaphragma. Fortschr Röntgenstr 137:103–106
32. Hecker WCh (1975) C. Zwerchfellhernien und Relaxationen. In: Zenker R, Berchtold R, Hamelmann H (Hrsg) Die Eingriffe in der Bauchhöhle, 3. völlig neubearbeitete Auflage, Bd VII/Teil 1, Springer, Berlin Heidelberg New York, S 812–825
33. Hubbard SG, Todd EP, Carter W, Zeok J, Dillon ML, Luce E (1979) Repair of chest wall defects with prosthetic material. Ann Thorac Surg 27:440–444
34. Hussain SA (1980) Delayed Rupture of the diaphragm following blunt trauma. Int Surg 65:269–270
35. Ilbawi MN, Hunt CE, DeLeon SY, Idriss FS (1980) Diaphragm pacing in infants and children: report of a simplified technique and review of experience. Ann Thorac Surg 31:61–65
36. Jensen BS, Arendrup HC (1981) Rupture of diaphragm. Acta Chir Scand 147:729–730
37. Kumar KL, Forse MA (1982) Herniation through the Foramen of Morgagni presenting as cardiomegaly. South Med J 75:894
38. Lacey SR, Goldthorn JF, Kosloske AM (1983) Repair of agenesis of hemidiaphragm by prosthetic materials. Surg Gynecol Obstet 156:310–312
39. Larrieu AJ, Wiener I, Alexander R, Wolma FJ (1980) Pericardiodiaphragmatic hernia. Am J Surg 139:436–440
40. Liu HM, Loew JM, Hunt CE (1978) Congenital central hypoventilation syndrome: A pathologic study of the neuromuscular system. Neurology 28:1013–1019
41. Lozewicz S, Potter DR, Costello JF, Moyle JB, MacCabe JJ (1981) Diaphragm pacing in ventilatory failure. Br Med J 283:1015–1016
42. Luiting MG, Den Otter G (1982) Rupture of the diaphragm due to blunt trauma. Neth J Surg 34:13–17
43. Manthei U, Vaucher Y, Crowe CP (1983) Congenital diaphragmatic hernia: immediate preoperative and postoperative oxygen gradients identify patients requiring prolonged respiratory support. Surgery 93:83–87
44. Marcos JJ, Grover FL, Trinkle JK (1974) Paralyzed diaphragm – Effect of plication on respiratory mechanics. J Surg Res 16:523–526
45. McMichan JC, Piepgras DG, Gracey DR, Marsh HM, Sittipong R (1979) Electrophrenic respiration. Report of six cases. Mayo Clin Proc 54:662–668
46. Merendino KA, Johnson RJ, Skinner HH, Maguire RX (1956) The intradiaphragmatic distribution of the phrenic nerve with particular reference to the placement of diaphragmatic incisions and controlled segmental paralysis. Surgery 39:189–198
47. Merendino KA (1964) The intradiaphragmatic distribution of the phrenic nerve. Surgical significance. Surg Clin N Amer 44:1217–1226
48. Michelson E (1961) Eventration of the diaphragm. Surgery 49:410–422
49. Middendorp UG (1964) Zur Frage der Zwerchfellincisionen. Helv chir Acta 31:220–227
50. Minnis JF, Reingold M (1963) Accessory diaphragm. Report of a case. Dis chest 44:554–558
51. Mishalany HG, Nakada K., Woolley MM (1979) Congenital diaphragmatic hernias. Arch Surg 114:1118–1123
52. Morrison JA, Mullens JE (1978) Traumatic intrapericardial rupture of the diaphragm. J Trauma 18:744–745

53. Müller-Färber J, Katthagen BD (1981) Die Zwerchfellruptur nach stumpfer Gewalteinwirkung. Unfallchirurgie 7:147–155
54. Neville WE, Clowes GHA (1954) Congenital absence of hemidiaphragm and use of a lobe of liver in its surgical correction. Arch Surg 69:282–290
55. Nielsen OH, Jørgensen AF (1978) Congenital posterolateral diaphragmatic hernia. Factors affecting survival. Z Kinderchir 24:201–215
56. Nissen R (1956) Transperitoneale Zwerchfellraffung bei Lähmungshochstand und Relaxation. Thoraxchirurgie 4:222–225
57. Osebold WR, Soper RT (1976) Congenital posterolateral diaphragmatic hernia past infancy. Am J Surg 131:748–754
58. Payne JH, Yellin AE (1982) Traumatic diaphragmatic hernia. Arch Surg 117:18–24
59. Petrovsky BV (1961) The use of diaphragm grafts for plastic operations in thoracic surgery. J Thorac Cardiovasc Surg 41:348–355
60. Piza-Katzer H, Appel WH, Kotz R, Wagner O (1983) Funktionsgerechte Wiederherstellung eines kombinierten Bauch-, Thoraxwand- und Zwerchfelldefektes mit Corium nach Sternum-Tumorresektion. Chirurg 54:157–160
61. Radecki LL, Tomatis LA (1976) Continuous bilateral electrophrenic pacing in an infant with total diaphragmatic paralysis. J Pediatr 88:969–971
62. Ramakrishnan MS (1981) Eventration of diaphragm. Ann Acad Med Singapore 10:409–412
63. Reitter H, Konrad R (1959) Die transthorakale offene Zwerchfelldoppelung zur Beseitigung einer Relaxation. Chirurg 30:172–177
64. Rodgers BM, Maher JW, Talbert JL (1981) The use of preserved human dura for closure of abdominal wall and diaphragmatic defects. Ann Surg 193:606–611
65. Rosenkrantz JG, Cotton EK (1964) Replacement of left hemidiaphragm by a pedicled abdominal muscular flap. J Thorac Cardiovasc Surg 48:912–920
66. Saha SP, Mayo P, Long GA (1982) Surgical treatment of anterior diaphragmatic hernia. South Med J 75:280–281
67. Sappington TB, Daniel RA (1951) Accessory diaphragm. A case report. J Thorac Surg 21:212–216
68. Sbokos CG, Salama FD, Powell V, McMillan IKR (1977) Primary fibrosarcoma of the diaphragm. Br J Dis Chest 71:49–52
69. Schwaiger M (1955) Zur Operation der echten und falschen Zwerchfellhernien. Langenbecks Arch Klin Chir 282:366–375
70. Schwartz MZ, Filler RM (1978) Plication of the diaphragm for symptomatic phrenic nerve paralysis. J Pediatr Surg 13:259–263
71. Serý Z, Králík J, Hiklová D, Malinská J (1956) Beitrag zur Technik der schonenden Zwerchfellincision bei abdomino-thorakalen Operationen. Thoraxchirurgie 4:125–135
72. Shaffer JO (1964) Prothesis for agenesis of the diaphragm. JAMA 188:1000–1002
73. Shaffer JO (1981) Treatment of agenesis of the diaphragm and esophageal crura. West J Med 134:361–363
74. Shochat SJ, Naeye RL, Ford WDA, Whitman V, Maisels MJ (1979) Congenital diaphragmatic hernia. Ann Surg 190:332–341
75. Snyder WH, Greaney EM (1965) Congenital diaphragmatic hernia; 77 consecutive cases. Surgery 57:576–588
76. Spelsberg F, Pichlmaier H, Junginger Th (1972) Die traumatische Zwerchfellruptur. Chir Praxis 16:33–40
77. Symbas PN, Hatcher CR, Waldo W (1977) Diaphragmatic eventration in infancy and childhood. Ann Thorac Surg 24:113–119
78. Tanaka F, Sawada K, Ishida I, Seki Y, Ohmori Y, Kuwahara T, Maruyama K, Sagara T (1982) Prosthetic replacement of entire left hemidiaphragm in malignant fibrous histocytoma of the diaphragm. J Thorac Cardiovasc Surg 83:278–284
79. Waldschmidt ML, Laws HL (1980) Injuries of the diaphragm. J Trauma 20:587–592
80. Wayne ER, Campbell JB, Burrington JD, Davis WS (1974) Eventration of the diaphragm. J Pediatr Surg 9:643–651
81. Wernitsch W, Kümmerle F (1973) Der plastische Verschluß von Zwerchfelldefekten. Akt Traumatologie 3:129–134
82. Wernitsch W, Stötzer M, Herbst H, Schrank H, Kessler E (1977) Experimentelle, licht- und elektronenmikroskopische Untersuchungen zum Verschluß von Zwerchfelldefekten mit lyophilisierter Dura. Akt Traumatologie 7:57–64
83. Westaby S, Shepherd MP, Nohl-Oser HC (1982) The use of diaphragmatic pedicle grafts for reconstructive procedures in the esophagus and tracheobronchial tree. Ann Thorac Surg 33:486–490
84. Wiener MF, Chou WH (1965) Primary tumors of the diaphragm. Arch Surg 90:143–152

I. Procedures on the Esophagus

H. PICHLMAIER and J. M. MÜLLER

1 Techniques of Esophageal Suture and Anastomosis

CONTENTS

1.1 Anatomy of the Esophagus

1.1.1 Structure of the Esophageal Wall

The laminar structure of the esophageal wall (Fig. 1) follows the same general pattern as the rest of the alimentary tract [21, 27]. In the thoracic part of the esophagus, the entire right side and the upper and lower portions of the left side receive a serous covering from the mediastinal pleura. The abdominal part of the esophagus is covered anteriorly by peritoneum. Interposed between the serosa and underlying muscular coat is the adventitia, a loose layer of connective tissue which is a downward continuation of the pharyngeal fascia and which gives the esophagus its mobility in the neck and posterior mediastinum. The pleural serous coat is lost when the esophagus is surgically exposed. The underlying adventitia should be preserved, as it is a semipermeable membrane with

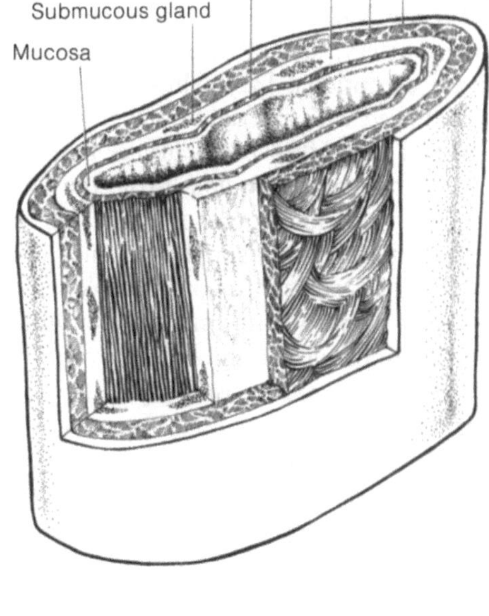

Fig. 1. Structure of the wall of the esophagus (modified from Lanz and Wachsmuth [21])

the capacity for rapid adhesion, although it does not match the quality of the intestinal serosa in that regard. The muscularis, or muscular coat of the esophagus, consists of an interwoven mass of apolar helical fibers (Fig. 2). The bundles of muscle fibers course obliquely upward and downward in both clockwise and counterclockwise fashion and may wind round the esophagus in a nearly circular pattern [31]. The submucosa is permeated by numerous mucous glands, its collagenous fiber architecture paralleling that of the muscular layer [17]. The collagenous fibers of the submucosal layer, together with the muscularis mucosae, form the actual suture bed of the esophagus; its capacity to hold a suture line is entirely comparable to other portions of the alimentary tract. The muscularis itself is inadequate for placing a suture line. The esophagus retracts markedly when divided owing to its myoelasticity, and this loss of length must be taken into account when a substitute is prepared. The mucosa presents a three-layered structure, the inner lining consisting of a multilaminar, nonkeratinizing squamous epithelium. The mucosa and submucosa possess a longitudinal fold that augments the distensibility of the organ ("stretch reserve" [8]).

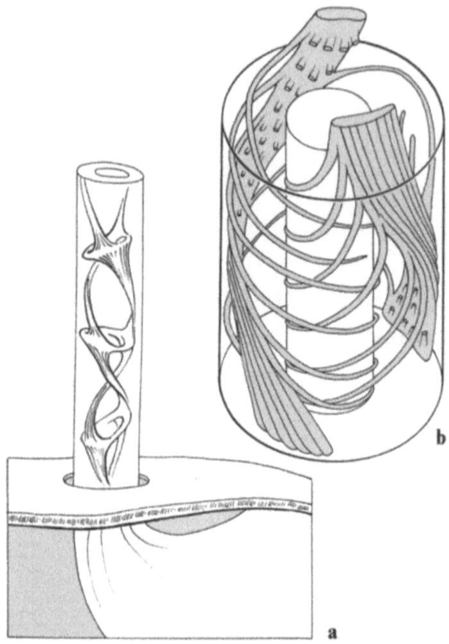

Fig. 2a, b. The muscular architecture of the esophagus (modified from Stelzner [31])

1.1.2 Blood Supply

In 90% of cases, the upper segment of the esophagus from the esophagopharyngeal junction to the thoracic inlet is supplied by constant, large branches from the paired inferior thyroid arteries (Fig. 3). Esophageal branches from the ascending pharyngeal artery, subclavian artery, and vertebral artery are exceptional [33]. Thus, the esophagus is well endowed with arterial vessels in its cervical portion, and blood-flow problems are rare following anastomoses in that region. From the thoracic inlet to the superior border of the pulmonary veins, the arterial blood supply becomes less copious [34] and is subject to considerable variation (Fig. 4 a,b). Two to four small-caliber branches pass to the esophagus from one or two bronchial arteries, usually on the left side [5]. In about 20% of cases lateral branches of the fifth or sixth right intercostal arteries are distributed to the esophagus. As many as two esophageal arteries proper may arise from the descending aorta at the level of the eighth to tenth thoracic vertebra. They pass distally in the posterior mediastinum to the posterior wall of the esophagus, divide into an ascend-

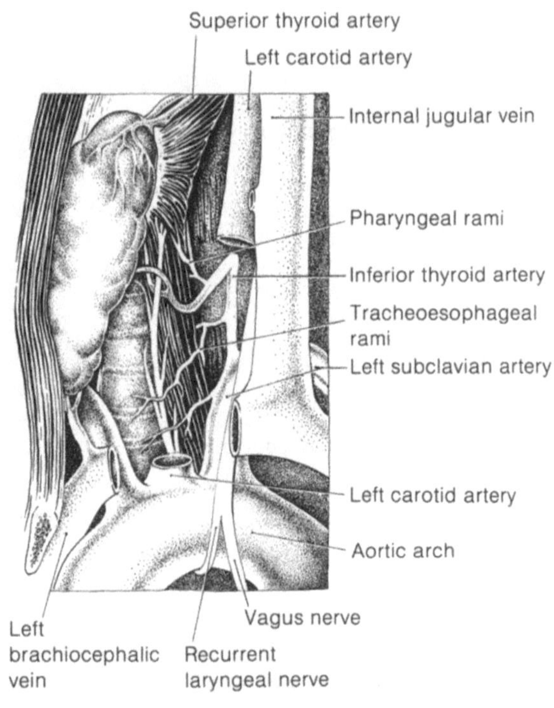

Fig. 3. The arterial supply of the cervical esophagus

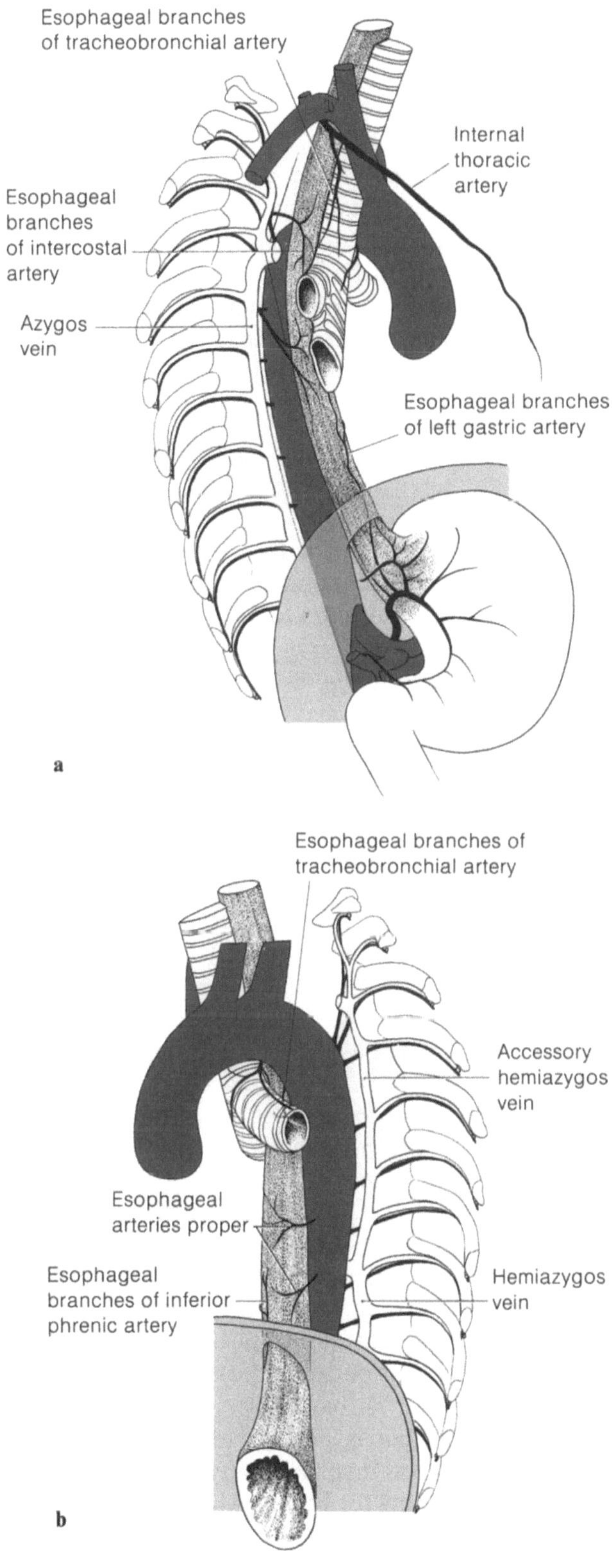

Fig. 4a, b. Vascular supply of the thoracoabdominal esophagus. **a** View from the left side; **b** view from the right side

ing and descending ramus, and frequently communicate with the esophageal branches of the bronchial arteries [23]. The abdominal esophagus is supplied by two to six branches from the left gastric artery, which ascend through the hiatus to supply the lower thoracic esophagus as well. The distal esophagus receives branches from the left inferior phrenic artery in about half of cases, and rarely from the right phrenic artery. When the left gastric artery is ligated, Stelzner and Kunath [30] advise placing an esophageal anastomosis immediately distal to the azygos vein, since this portion of the esophagus is outside the distribution of the left gastric artery. We can confirm the value of this tactic in diseases (e.g., adenocarcinoma of the esophagocardial junction) that require a combined thoracoabdominal approach. But if the disease permits the anastomosis to be performed through the abdominal route, we consider the risks of the two-cavity operation to be greater than the potential danger of anastomotic disruption due to deficient blood flow in the distal esophagus. The fact that the intrathoracic esophagus is supplied largely by end-arteries [34] is advantageous in terms of blunt dissection (see Sect. 6.7). If the esophageal branches of the left gastric and inferior thyroid arteries have been ligated, the intrathoracic esophageal arteries may be divided without preliminary ligation. Their muscular walls will cause them to retract and close off when cut [20], and bleeding should cease spontaneously within a few minutes even without compression.

The venous return from the arborizing submucous networks of the cervical esophagus is into the inferior thyroid vein. The proximal and middle thirds of the esophagus are drained by the azygos vein and hemiazygos vein, while the lower thoracic and abdominal portions are drained by the coronary vein [23].

1.1.3 Lymphatic Drainage

There are two intricate lymphatic plexuses in the esophagus, one arising from the mucosa and the other from the muscularis [20, 25]. The capillaries of the mucosal plexus are arranged longitudinally over the full length of the esophagus and have variable connections with the the capillaries of the muscular layer. Their collecting trunks lie in the submucosa. Some of them drain directly into the adjacent periesophageal lymph nodes, while others run for variable distances in the submucosa before penetrating the muscularis to drain into a lymph node. The absence of segmental collecting sites explains why lymph node metastases from esophageal carcinoma can spread over the entire viscus, regardless of the location of the primary tumor [3].

1.2 Basic Technical Aspects of Esophageal Suturing and Anastomosis

A meticulous suturing technique is essential for the undisturbed healing of an esophagotomy or esophagoenterostomy. Because the esophagus lacks a serous coat, a careless suturing technique or traumatic handling of the tissues can have particularly adverse consequences. The principles of an adequate lumen, water- and airtight closure without tension, and preservation of blood supply apply to the esophagus just as they do to other portions of the gastrointestinal tract.

We routinely test the integrity of every esophageal suture line or anastomosis during the operation. We temporarily occlude the lumen distal to the anatomosis by means of a finger or sponge stick. We then insert a tube into the area of the anastomosis and inject a methylene blue solution (0.5 ml/100 ml NaCl 0.9%) under moderate pressure until the anastomotic site balloons outward slightly. The suture line is then carefully inspected for fluid leakage. Any defects are immediately oversewn.

A tension-free anastomosis relies on adequate mobilization of the esophageal substitute. We additionally anchor the substitute in the posterior mediastinum with several sutures to protect the anastomosis from tension.

Blood flow disturbances in the area of the anastomosis can be largely avoided by skeletonizing the esophagus sparingly and by suitable preparation of the substitute organ. Intraluminal decompression is provided by a transnasal tube, which is advanced through the anastomosis under vision until its tip is about a hand's width distal to the anastomosis. We leave the tube in place until the second or third postoperative day. It is uncertain, however, whether the advantages of this decompression and removal of gastrointestinal secretions outweigh the disadvantages of the tube, such as interference with respiration, the risk of pressure necrosis, reflux, and (as studies of the removed tube have shown) the creation of a permanent conduit for bacterial growth [28].

1.3 Techniques of Esophageal Suturing and Anastomosis

1.3.1 Manual versus Mechanical Suture Techniques

Mechanical sutures of the gastrointestinal tract represent a fundamental departure from traditional manual techniques, of which no fewer than 250 variations have been described. It may be assumed that, other conditions being equal, the mechanical techniques are superior to manual suturing. There are several reasons for this [16]:

- the perpendicularity of the sutures relative to the wound surfaces, which, combined with the thin material of the staples, causes minimal tissue trauma;
- the uniform pressure of the staples (B-shaped when closed), which do not devitalize the tissue and permit blood vessels to pass through;
- uniform stress distribution across the staple line; minimal tissue trauma, since all the staples are inserted at one time; and
- the speed with which anastomoses can be performed, reducing the likelihood of contamination and sepsis.

A potential disadvantage of mechanical sutures is they necessarily produce an inversion or eversion of the wound margins. Studies by Herzog [14] have shown that an anatomic (end-on) coaptation of the wound layers is essential for rapid, primary healing of the bowel wall. However, previous clinical results of mechanical suturing in the gastrointestinal tract [9, 15, 16, 18, 29] show that the principle of the end-on closure is of minor significance compared with the pure technical quality of the suture, and that it may assume importance only in cases where a perfect manual suture has been performed.

We personally use the EEA stapling instrument for esophagoenteric anastomoses whenever technically possible. It must be emphasized, however, that mechanical suture techniques do not release the surgeon from the basic rules of anastomotic surgery. Tissue that is poorly perfused, traumatized, inflamed, or involved by tumor will have just as little prospect for healing when stapled than when sutured manually. Only surgeons who are already well versed in manual suturing techniques should attempt to use a stapling device. By the same token, the stapling instrument will not enable surgeons to do what they otherwise could not do

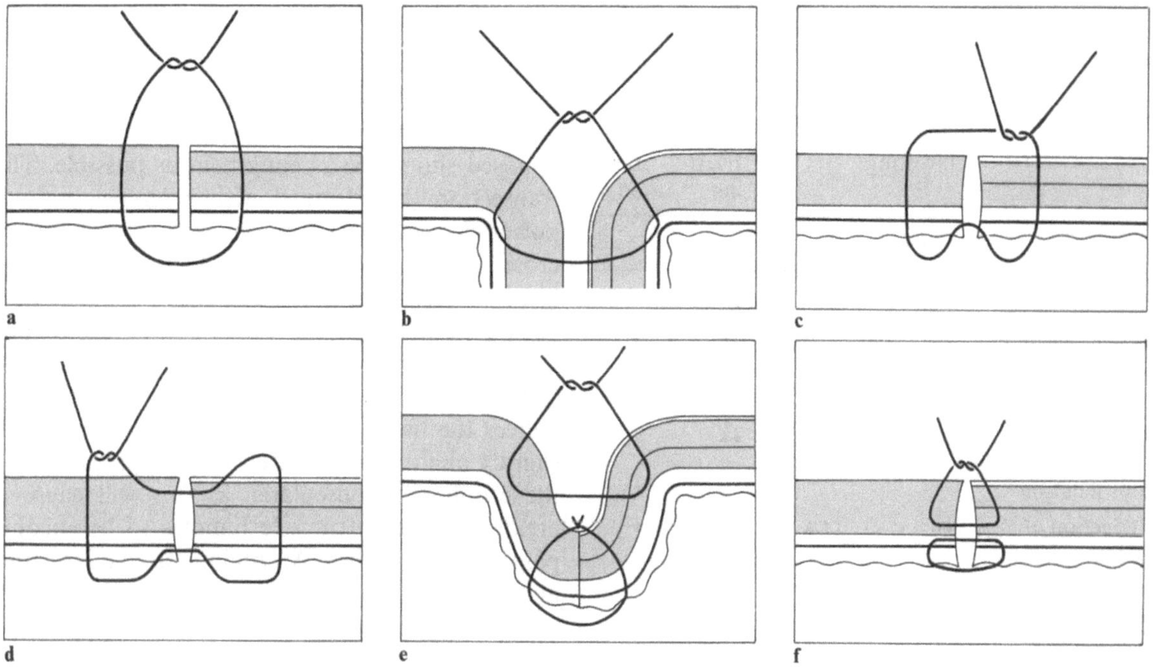

Fig. 5a–f. Suture techniques: **a** Albert suture (all coats, single layer); **b** Lembert suture (single layer, inverting); **c** Gambee suture (single layer, all coats, end-on); **d** Herzog suture (single layer, all coats, end-on); **e** Albert-Lambert suture (two layers, strongly inverting); **f** modified Wölfler suture (inner continuous mucosal suture, outer seromuscular suture)

manually. We tend to favor a less broad approach to the use of stapling instruments than some other authors [36]. Except where the GIA instrument is needed for simultaneous division and closure of gastrointestinal structures, all maneuvers can be performed manually with a high degree of precision, and we do not feel that the time saved with mechanical sutures outweighs their markedly higher costs.

1.3.2 Manual Sutures

1.3.2.1 Suture Materials

Wound healing depends not just on the suture technique but also on the tissue compatibility of the suture material, the amount of material used, and the trauma associated with its use [24].

For esophageal procedures we use only absorbable synthetic suture material swaged on an atraumatic needle. We suture the mucosa and submucosa with 4-0 poly-p-dioxanon monofilament, and the muscularis with 4-0 braided polyglycolic acid or polyglactin. We perform ligations with polyglactin threads of size 2-0 to 0, depending on the diameter of the vessel.

1.3.2.2 Suture Techniques

Of the basic types of suture shown in Fig. 5 –everting, inverting, and end-on– the everting suture has proved to be the least satisfactory (Table 1).

The end-on technique, described by Gambee [11] for the accurate coaptation of wound layers, has been modified by Herzog [13] and subjected to extensive experimental testing. It leads to primary consolidation of the wound, permits rapid bridging of the anastomosis by blood vessels, and avoids the stricturing effect of an inverting suture. It is technically more difficult than an inverting suture and must be performed with great care to ensure a watertight closure. The advantage of stricture prevention is assured only if the suture is made in a single layer. So far there has been only limited clinical experience with the end-on technique in esophageal surgery. One of the oldest techniques, the inverting Lembert suture, is still widely used. It leads to secondary wound healing

Table 1. Clinical and experimental rating of various manual suture techniques (after Pichlmaier and Junginger [25])

Criteria	Rating			
	Inverting		Everting	End-on
	1-layer	2-layer		
Burst strength	○	○	▲	
Tensile strength	◆○	○○○	▲▲	◆
Histologic consolidation	○○	○○	▲	
Microangiographic consolidation	◆	○○	▲▲	◆
Reduction of lumen	◆□	○□▲	○□	◆
Inflammatory response	◆	○		
Local complications	+◆◆◆○+□+□	○○○□□	▲	+◆
Suturing time	◆	○		
Mortality	+○○+□+□	+○○+□+□		+◆

+ = clinical results, ◆ = good, ○ = fair, ▲ = poor, □ = no difference

and therefore is more apt to incite scar formation and scar contraction than the end-on technique. Combining the Lembert suture with a second, deeper layer of through-and-through sutures (Albert-Lembert) or even with a third seromuscular suture layer [32] does not improve the strength of the anastomosis, increases the luminal reduction and inflammatory response of the tissue, and restricts blood flow in the anastomitic area. We routinely employ a two-layer suture line in the esophagus, following the technique of Akiyama [2], which is drawn from the technique described by Wölfer in 1881. We agree with Herzog [13] that like structures should be approximated to each other. However, we feel that this applies most critically to the submucosa, which serves as the actual suture bed and determines the strength of the anastomosis. The muscularis suture, we believe, serves an approximating function only. Given the structural disparity between the esophagus and the rest of the gastrointestinal tract and the lack of a serous coat on the esophagus, the single-layer end-on suture cannot ensure apposition of the submucosal layers and promotes pressure necrosis of the muscle, which is included in the suture line to augment its strength.

The technical details are the same whether an inverting or end-on suture is employed. For an accurate anastomosis, the lumina that are to be apposed should be as congruent as possible. The transection is performed with a scalpel or low-power electrocautery to minimize wound edge necrosis. Bleeding vessels on the cut surfaces are isolated with a small forceps and selectively coagulated; "mass cautery" is avoided. For a mucosa-submucosal suture, the needle is inserted toward the center of the lumen, imagined to be circular, and pierces the tissue at right angles to its surface. A slightly oblique needle insertion is appropriate for the esophageal muscularis, as this will cause a greater number of muscle bundles to be encompassed by the suture. An oblique needle insertion may be used in the esophageal substitute to correst minor luminal discrepancies. The round half-circle needle is passed through the tissue on a line that follows the needle shape. For some time we have used a heavier suture in the muscularis in an effort to reduce the pressure on the encompassed muscle bundles. The sutures are spaced 4–5 mm apart so that the necrotic areas that form around every needle track do not overlap [24].

When a braided suture material is used, an accurately placed square knot should be sufficient. With monofilament material, we add a third knot whose threads are directed opposite to the second knot. Under no circumstances should a "granny" type of knot be tied for the sake of speed or simplicity. Neither can the security of this knot be increased by making multiple knots. This will result only in a hillock of suture material that, if large enough, can produce a significant foreign body effect [25].

1.3.2.3 Anastomotic Technique

In terms of technique, it does not matter whether an anastomosis is constructed between the esophagus and the stomach, small intestine, or colon. The substitute is apposed to the esophagus such that both structures overlap by about 1–2 cm. At this point the lumina of both organs are still occluded. About 1 cm oral to the esophageal stump, which is occluded with a clamp or staple line, a corner suture is placed through the muscularis of the lateral esophageal wall. The suture is placed slightly obliquely so that it will encompass several muscle bundles at once. At a corresponding site on the substitute, the same suture is passed through the seromuscular layer and tied. The thread is cut about a hand's width from the knot and is grasped with a clamp. Starting from this corner suture, a row of simple interrupted suture is placed along what will be the posterior portion of the anastomosis (Fig. 6 a). The sutures are spaced at 4- to 5-mm intervals. When each suture is placed, it is tied immediately and cut 2–4 mm above the knot, depending on the material. One thread of the final suture is cut a hand's width from the knot and seized with a clamp; it serves as the second corner suture. Because the anastomotic suture line is actually held by the submucosa in both the esophagus and the transplant, the first row of sutures serves merely to approximate the segments. Thus, to avoid necrosis of the muscularis, the initial threads are not tied very tightly. Next an opening is made into the esophagus (Fig. 6 b) 2–3 mm from the posterior suture line using a scalpel or electrocautery. Tags of mucosa within the lumen of the stoma are removed by suction, and the mucosa is cleaned with dissecting patties soaked in antiseptic solution. At that point the amputation of the esophageal stump may be completed. The substitute is also opened 2–3 mm from the suture line and similarly cleansed. Bleeding points on the cut edge are selectively cauterized. At the level of one of the corner threads the esophageal mucosa is grasped with a forceps and pulled forward slightly, and a monofilament suture on an atraumatic needle is inserted into the lumen, at right angles to the tissue plane. The mucosa of the substitute is similarly grasped and pulled forward, and the needle is passed from within the lumen outward. The suture is tied, making certain that the submucosal layers of both structures are apposed.

The end of the thread opposite the needle is left uncut so that it can be used to hold the mucosae forward as the anastomosis is performed. Next the needle is inserted back into the lumen, and a continuous suture line is placed on the posterior side of the anastomosis (Fig. 6 c), making certain

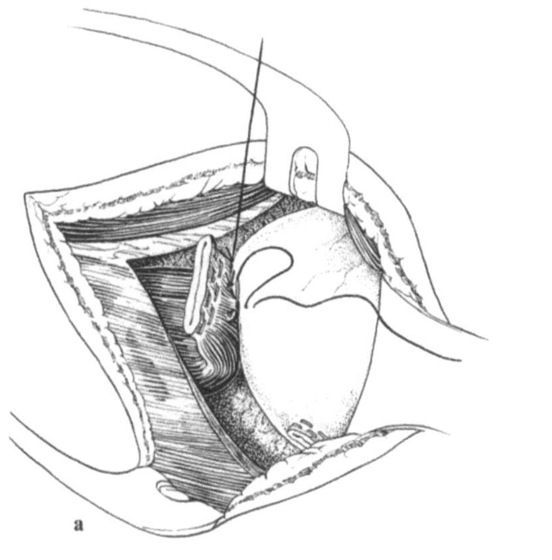

a

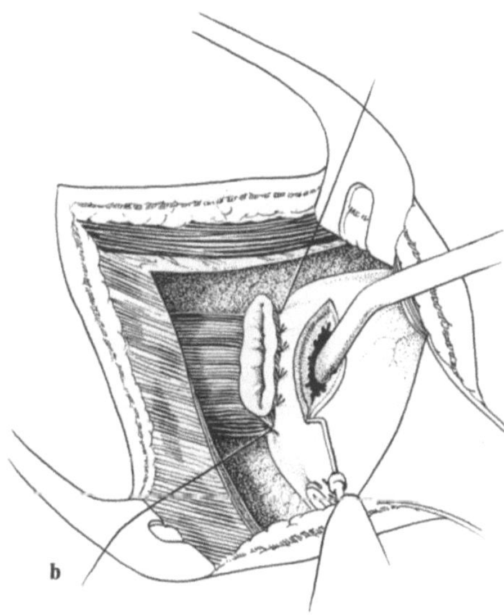

b

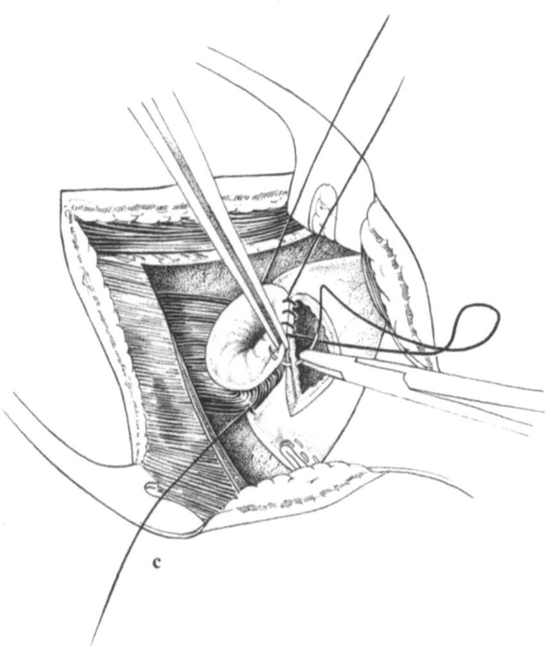

c

Fig. 6a–g. Technique of esophagogastrostomy in the cervical region (following subtotal esophagectomy and elevation of the stomach). **a** Posterior row of interrupted seromuscular sutures. **b** The staple line is excised, the stomach is opened at the appropriate site, and its contents are aspirated. **c** Continuous mucosa-to-mucosa suture completes the posterior part of the anastomosis. **d–g** see p. 232

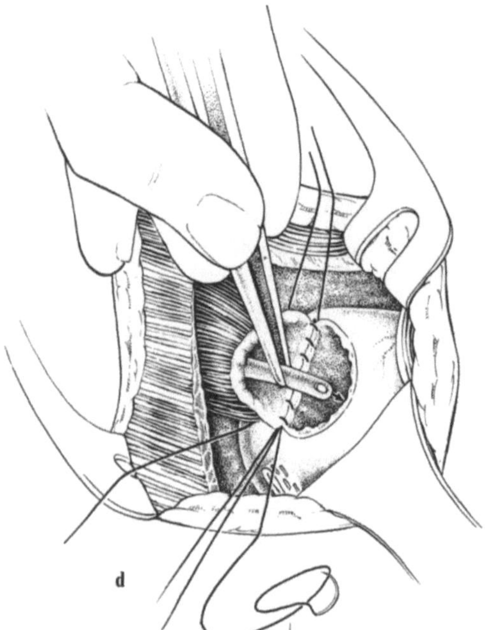

d

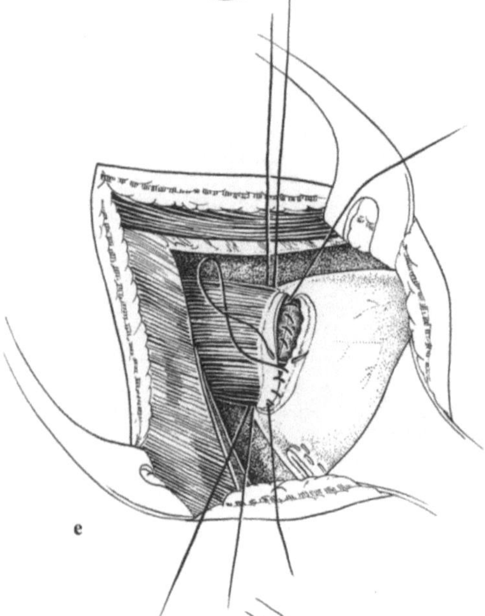

e

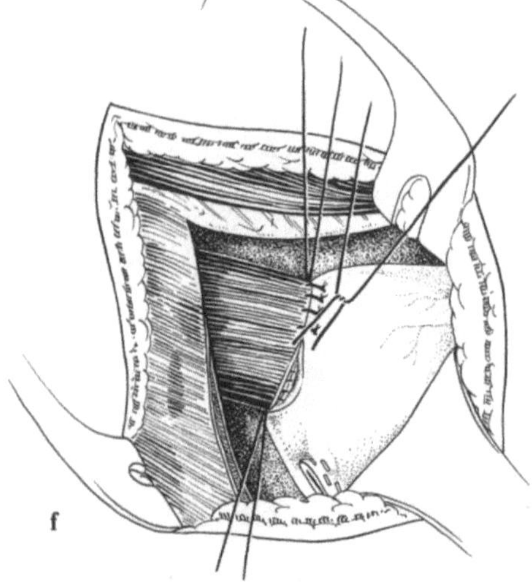

f

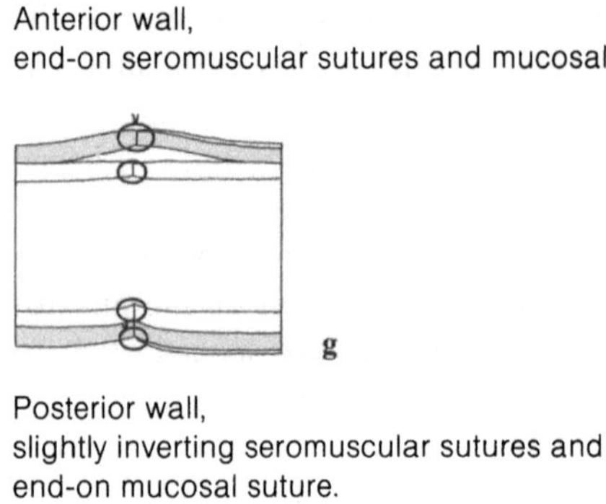

Fig. 6. d Nasogastric tube is passed into the esophageal substitute. **e** Continuous mucosa-to-mucosa suture forms the anterior first row. **f** Interrupted seromuscular sutures complete the anterior side. **g** Longitudinal section through the anastomosis

that submucosa apposes to submucosa. When the opposite corner thread is reached, the suture line may be directly continued onto the anterior side of the anastomosis. However, to avoid stricture formation during subsequent tightening of the running suture, we usually bring the needle out of the lumen, apply a holding stitch, and unite the running suture to it. Once the posterior wall has been completed, a nasogastric tube is advanced to the site of the anastomosis, grasped with a forceps, and passed on into the transplant for a distance of about 10 cm (Fig. 6 d). There it is secured nasally with a strip of adhesive tape to provide decompression of the esophageal substitute during the initial days after surgery.

The atraumatic needle is inserted back into the lumen, and the running mucosa-submucosal stitch is continued to complete the anterior part of the anastomosis (Fig. 6 e). The last stitch is brought out of the lumen and tied to the end that was left uncut initially. When this suture line (which we regard as definitive) has been completed, it is covered by loosely approximating the esophageal muscularis to the seromuscular layer of the substitute with slightly inverting or end-on interrupted sutures (Fig. 6 f,g).

Fig. 7. a EEA stapling instrument for circular anastomoses, supplied with disposable cartridges for different anastomostic diameters. **b** GIA stapling instrument for concurrent enterotomy and closure. **c** TA-55 Premium stapling instrument with disposable cartridges for definitive enterotomy closure (other sizes: TA-30, TA-90, and cartridges with different staple heights) ▷

1.3.3 Mechanical Sutures

1.3.3.1 Stapling Instruments and their Applications

Stapling instruments (Fig. 7 a–c) can be used in a variety of ways for repairs or anastomoses of the esophagus itself, for mobilizing an organ that is to be anastomosed to the esophagus, for subsequent restoration of alimentary continuity, for construction of a substitute gastric reservoir, and for the closure of enterostomies. We do not feel that every possible application is appropriate. In Table 2 we have italicized the indications that we consider to be relevant.

All stapling instruments operate by the same basic principle. The EEA and TA instruments employ compression, and the GIA a pusher mecha-

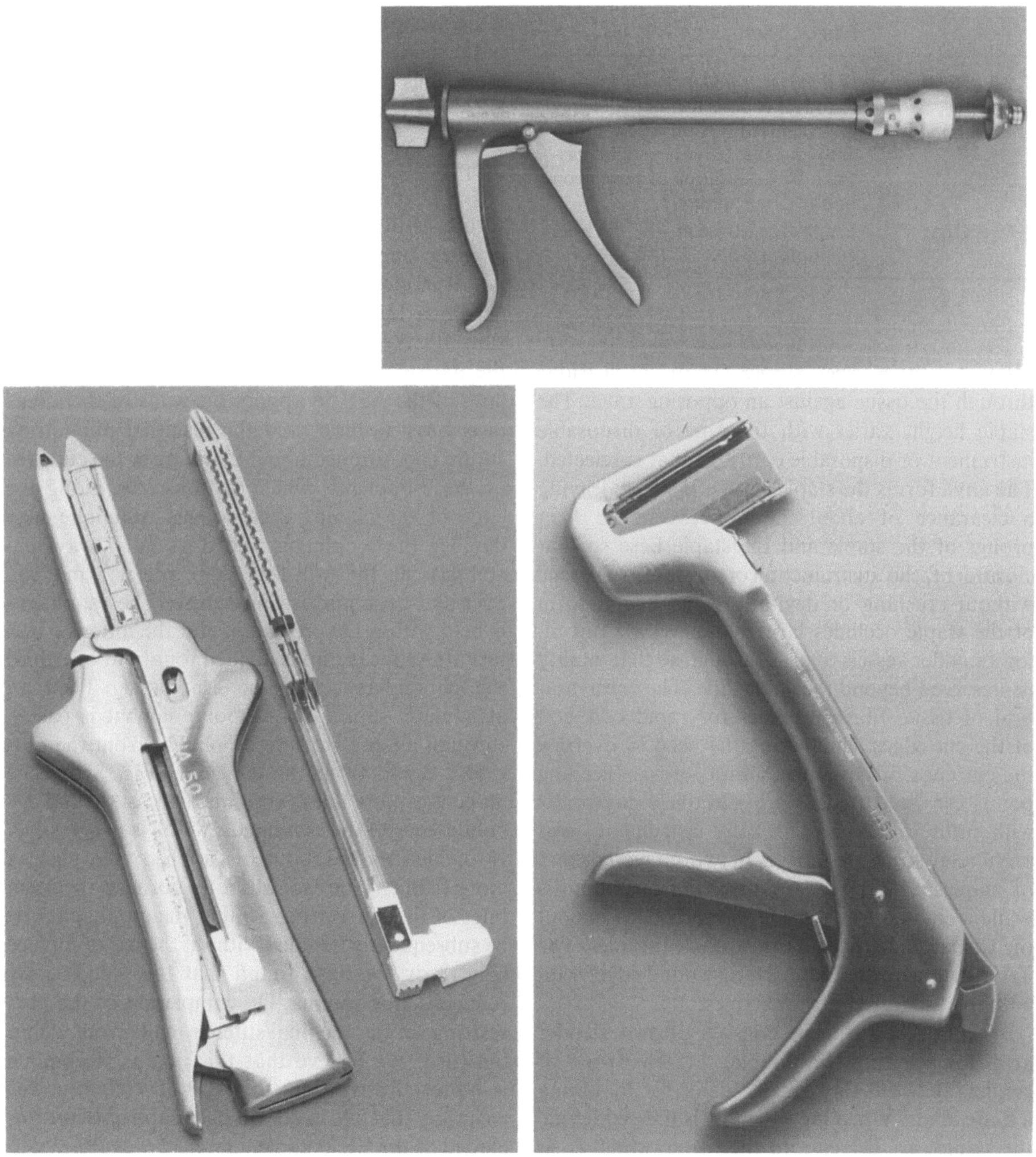

a b c

Table 2. Possible applications of stapling instruments in esophageal surgery

Instrument type	Application
EEA, DEEA, CDEEA	*Esophagoenteral* or enteroenteral end-to-end or side-to-side anastomosis. Van Kemmel dissection anastomosis
GIA-50 Premium	*Enterotomy with simultaneous closure. Construction of substitute gastric pouch* (jejunojejunostomy). Construction of antiperistaltic or isoperistaltic gastric tube. Collis gastroplasty [7] Finney pyloroplasty [10]
TA-30/55/90 Premium DTA-30/55/90	*Definite enterotomy closure* Removal of diverticulum, Collis gastroplasty [7]. Construction of antiperistaltic or isoperistaltic gastric tube Restoration of bowel continuity (triangulation)
TA + GIA	Esophagogastrostomy by the triangulation principle

nism, to drive steel staples from a cartridge through the tissue against an opposing anvil. The staple height varies with the type of disposable instrument or disposable cartridge that is selected. The anvil forms the staples into a B shape, leaving a clearance of about 2 mm between the bent prongs of the staple and the staple base so that closure of the instrument compresses the tissue without crushing or devitalizing it. The B form of the staple occludes large blood vessels but allows smaller vessels to pass through so that vitality is preserved beyond the staple line. The extravasation of tissue fibrin provides for rapid cohesion of the cut edges, eliminating the need to oversew the cut ends or cover them with serosa. Bleeding points on the cut edges are selectively controlled with suture ligatures. The EEA instrument, used on tubular structures, drives in two staggered rows of staples to produce an inverting anastomosis while a circular knife inside the cartridge cuts out the tissue inside the innermost ring of staples. The TA instrument closes and everts wound edges with a double staggered row of staples.

The GIA instrument consists of two slender arms for inserting two double, staggered rows of staples. Between the arms is a slot for mounting a knife blade. When the assembly is pressed home, the staples are driven into the tissue, which is simultaneously divided between the two arms. The instruments currently marketed are extremely reliable when properly used. However, beginners are urged to read the manufacturer's instructions carefully before proceeding, and even to practice closures and anastomoses on anatomic specimens or a bicycle inner tube.

1.3.3.2 Esophagoenterostomy with the EEA Instrument

Below we shall describe the technique for an esophagogastrostomy using the EEA instrument. The basic details are the same as for anastomosing the esophagus to the small intestine or colon with the EEA, DEEA, or CDEEA instrument.

The esophagus is grasped at the level of the proposed resection with a pursestring clamp (ASP 50) or Dixon clamp for placement of a pursestring suture. If the ASP 50 is used, it should be locked in place only once to avoid esophageal damage. A 2-0 monofilament suture swaged on a straight needle at both ends is passed through the guides slots on the ASP 50 (Fig. 8 a), which open on the narrow sides of the instrument. The rakelike jaws of the ASP 50 appose the walls of the viscus in a wavy fashion, and the resulting pursestring suture is positioned about 2 mm from the cut edge of the esophagus, which is transected along the edge of the clamp. Because this technique may damage the esophagus and does not always encompass all the wall layers, we prefer a manual, over-and-over pursestring suture. The esophagus is held with a Dixon clamp, and the anterior wall just above the clamp is divided for about one-third the circumference of the esophagus. Then an atraumatic suture of 2-0 monofilament is passed through all coats of the esophagus from the outside 2–3 mm from the cut edge (Fig. 8 b). The all-coats suture line is continued about the full circumference of the esophagus, which is progressively divided as the suture is applied. We place a monofilament thread at both corners, between bites of the pursestring, so that the esophagus can be subsequently handled without the use of forceps (Fig. 8 c). We have found that this significantly reduces tissue trauma. On completion of the pursestring suture, the final stitch is made from within outward. We believe that this manual technique is more effective than the ASP 50 technique for ensuring that all coats of the esophagus are included in the EEA staple lines.

The method of inserting the EEA instrument depends on the level at which the anastomosis is to be performed. For anastomoses of the lower and middle esophagus, the instrument may be introduced through the abdomen or thorax. For anastomoses of the upper thoracic or cervical esophagus, insertion of the straight EEA instrument tends to be difficult, and it is better to use the curved disposable instrument (CDEEA), which can be introduced by either the transthoracic or transoral route.

A pursestring suture about 1 cm in diameter is placed at the top of the gastric fundus. A gastrostomy opening is made between two holding sutures in the anterior wall of the stomach, about 10 cm below the intended site of the anastomosis, using the electrocautery. The cartridge end of the EEA instrument, with the anvil removed, is inserted into the stomach through the gastrostomy (Fig. 8 d) until the central rod is at the center of the pursestring suture. The fundus is opened at that site with the electrocautery, and the central rod is passed through. The pursestring suture is tightened snugly around the rod, and the threads are tied (four knots maximum) and cut close to the knot so that their ends will not get in the way of the circular blade. Now the anvil is screwed onto the central rod (Fig. 8 e) until the upper edge of the knurled screw engages against the top of the rod. The wing nut at the handle end of the instrument is turned in counterclockwise fashion until maximum separation of the anvil and cartridge is achieved. Now the instrument is pushed upward so that the cut end of the esophagus can be slipped over the anvil (Fig. 8 f).

The preplaced holding sutures are exceedingly helpful during this stage. Trauma to the esophagus is minimized by using a small cartridge size; we prefer the 25-mm cartridge, or in exceptional cases the CDEEA 21. In all cases the luminal diameter should be measured using the supplied gauge. The pursestring suture in the esophagus is tightened, tied, and cut close to the knot. The holding sutures are removed. Now the anvil and cartridge are brought together by turning the wing nut at the end of the instrument in a clockwise direction (Fig. 8g). The view window on the shaft of the instrument will indicate when the segments have been apposed (some leeway is allowed for individual differences). The mark on the shaft should touch the mark in the view window; they need not overlap completely. The instrument is rotated in both directions so that the entire circumference of the planned anastomosis can be inspected. Once it is certain that both segments are perfectly apposed and there is no intervening foreign material, the safety catch is released, and the handle is squeezed firmly until it is fully closed. Resistance will be felt and a crunching sound heard as the tissue is cut and the staples are driven home. The end point of the cutting and suturing step is indicated by additional markings in the view window (Fig. 8 h). The cartridge and anvil are separated by three half turns of the wing nut in the counterclockwise direction. The instrument is then rotated 180° clockwise or counterclockwise, and additional, gentle twisting movements are made as the instrument is disengaged from the anastomosis and withdrawn through the gastrostomy. The anvil is detached, and both excised tissue cylinders are removed. We position the specimens on the operating table as they were in the instrument; that way if the specimens are incomplete, the site of the defect in the anastomosis can be recognized. If both tissue cylinders are complete, we additionally test the anastomosis by injecting methylene blue dye. The gastrostomy may be closed manually or with the TA instrument (Fig. 8 i).

The transoral approach is technically very similar to the transgastric, although it has been found that passage of the instrument into the cervical esophagus is usually difficult and can cause significant mucosal injury. Therefore we prefer a manual anastomosis of the cervical esophagus in most cases. But if stapling is decided upon, the instrument with anvil attached is passed transorally into the esophagus under laryngoscopic control. A short rubber tube mounted on the anvil screw can facilitate the insertion. When the cut edge is reached, the instrument is opened. The preplaced pursestring suture in the esophagus is tightened and tied around the central rod. The wall of the stomach is opened at the center of a pursestring suture, the anvil is advanced through the incision, and the second suture is tightened. Then the stapler is closed, fired, and removed as previously described.

The above technique can also be used after fundectomy to create an anastomosis between the esophagus and the anterior or posterior wall of the body of the stomach. The fundectomy may be performed with the GIA instrument, or the stomach may be transected between a clamp and a TA staple line. It is not necessary to oversew or invaginate the staple lines, although small bleeding points in the anastomosis should be ligated or coa-

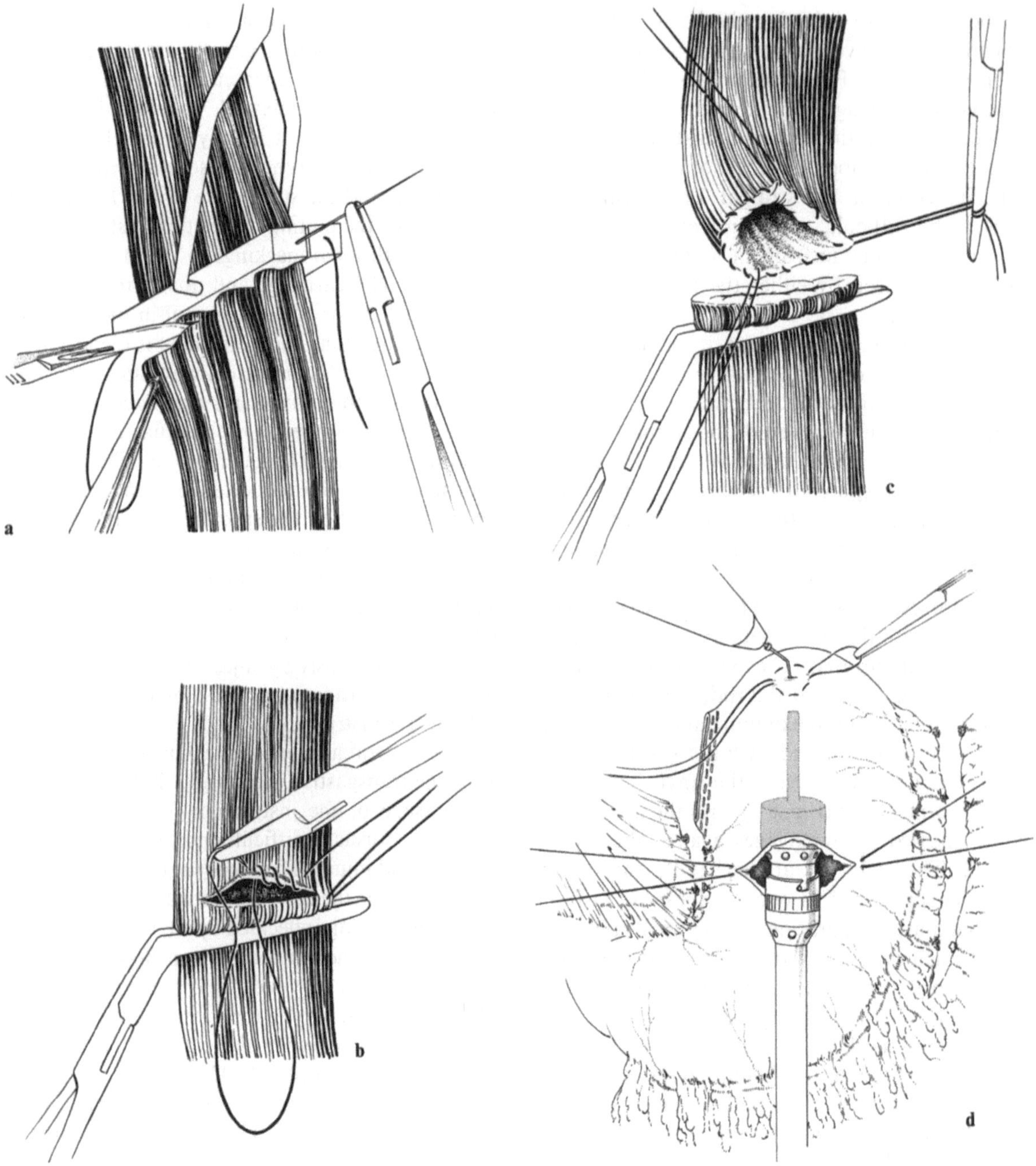

Fig. 8a–i. Technique of esophagogastrostomy with the EEA stapling instrument. **a** Placement of the pursestring suture with the ASP-50. **b** Manual placement of the pursestring suture, with progressive transection of the esophagus. **c** The proximal end of the esophagus is controlled with holding sutures. **d** The EEA instrument is inserted through a transverse gastrotomy. The stomach is opened within a pursestring suture at the intended anastomotic site on the fundus. **e** The anvil is attached. **f** Anvil is inserted into the esophagus. **g** The segments are approximated, and the stapler is fired. **h** Longitudinal section through the stapled anastomosis (all-layer, two staggered rows of staples). **i** Gastrostomy is closed with the TA-55 stapler

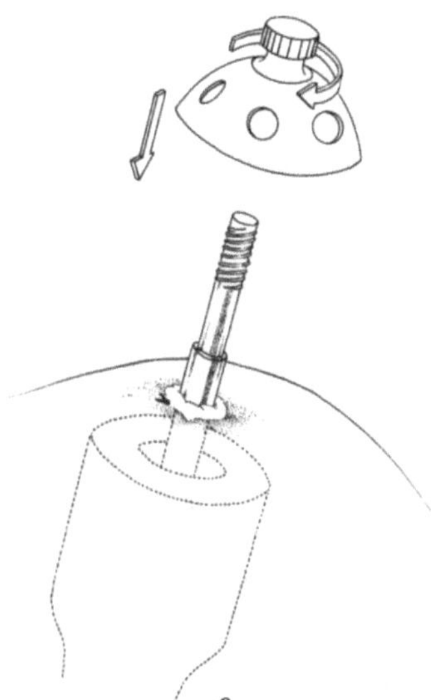

e

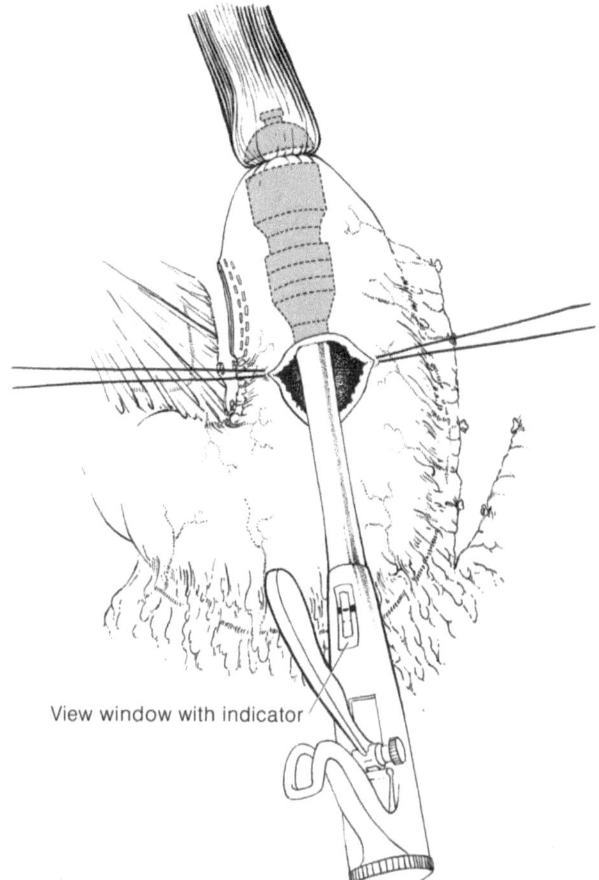

g

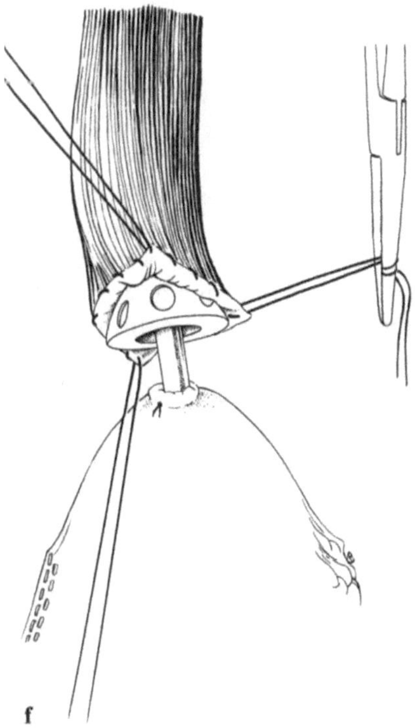

f

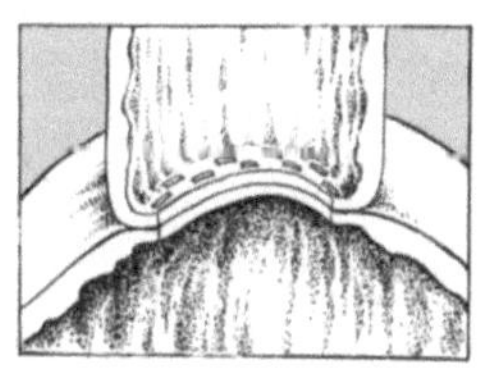

h

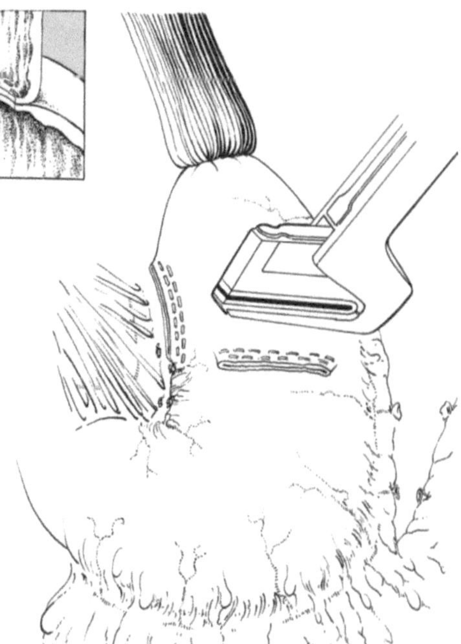

i

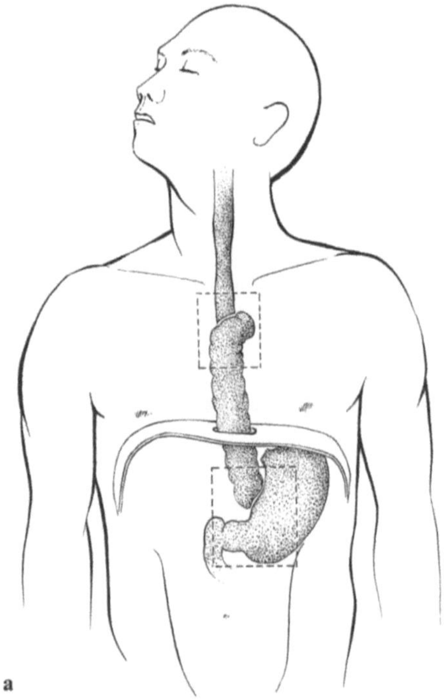

a

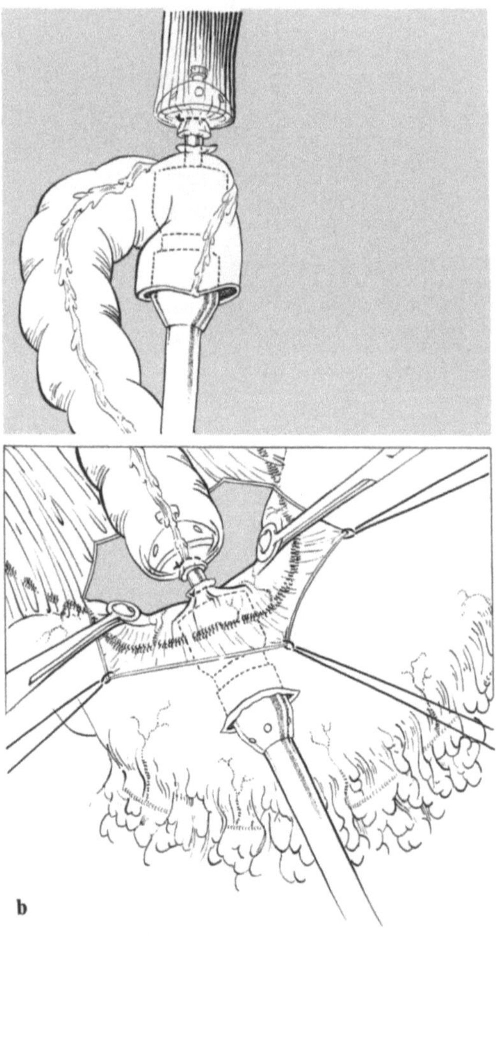

b

Fig. 9a, b. Colon reconstruction of the esophagus. End-to-side anastomoses are made between the esophagus and colon (**a**) and between the colon and body of the stomach (**b**) with the EEA stapling instrument

gulated. One should be careful about using electrocautery close to staples, as the current can heat the metal staples, which in turn can cause thermal necrosis of tissue. When colon is used as the esophageal substitute, the EEA instrument can be used to anastomose the colon to the esophagus (Fig. 9 a) as well as to the stomach (Fig. 9 b). We prefer to join the esophagus to the colon in end-to-side fashion, since an end-to-end anastomosis with the EEA instrument cannot adequately compensate for the unequal lumina. The device may be inserted into the colon segment through its proximal end or through a separate colotomy made in the area of the taenia libera. In either case the TA instrument can be used to close the colotomy after the EEA instrument is withdrawn.

The technique of esophagojejunostomy corresponds to that described for esophagocolostomy, except that there is no definite preference in this case for an end-to-end or end-to-side anastomosis.

Triangulation techniques involving use of the GIA and TA instruments have been described for esophagoenterostomies [6, 29], but we do not feel that they have practical significance.

1.3.3.3 Other Applications of the Stapling Instruments

All anastomoses or enterostomy closures involved in a gastric reconstruction or Roux-type esophagojejunostomy (Fig. 10) can be performed with stapling instruments. Following gastrectomy, the duodenal stump can be closed with the TA or GIA instrument. The jejunum is divided 20–40 cm behind the ligament of Treitz with the GIA instrument. The distal loop of jejunum is brought up in front of or behind the colon and anastomosed to the esophagus with the EEA device. For construction of a gastric reservoir, two loops of jejunum are apposed side to side and held in position proximally and distally with traction sutures. The two loops of bowel are opened transversely between the traction sutures, and the GIA instrument is inserted into each limb to construct a side-to-side jejunojejunostomy. The jejunotomies are closed transversely with the TA stapler.

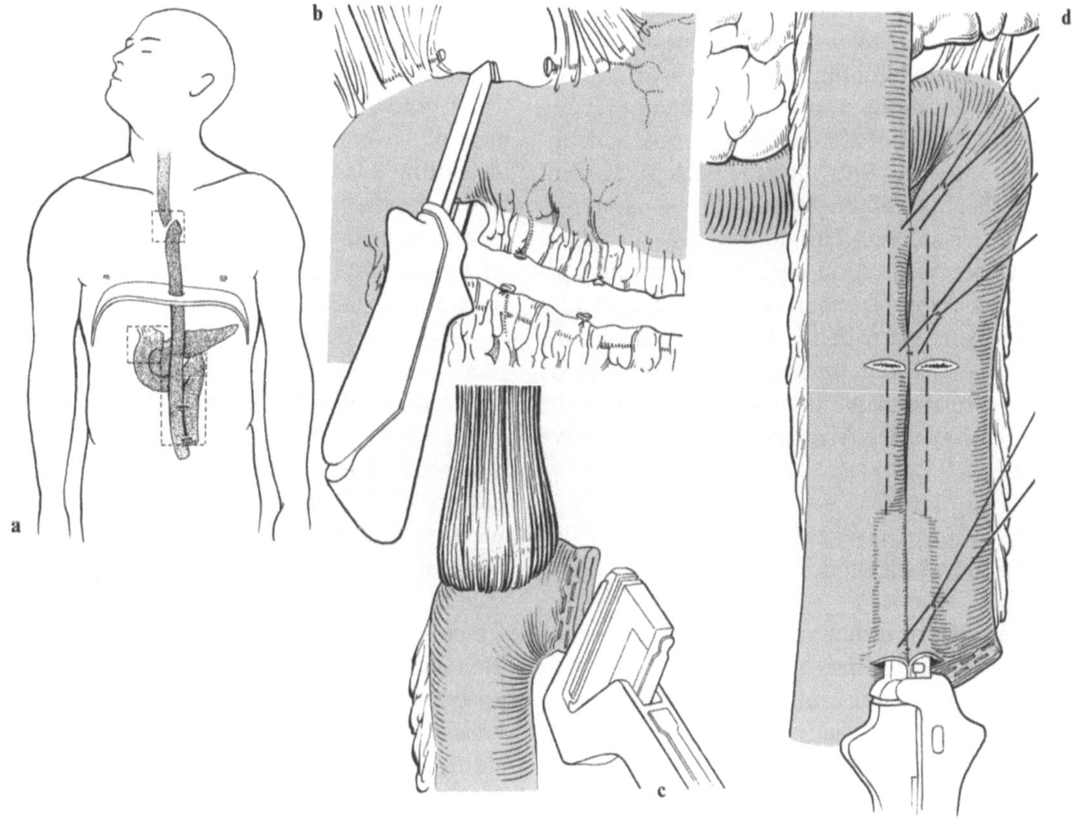

Fig. 10a–d. Gastric reconstruction performed entirely with stapling instruments. **a** General view, **b** transection of the stomach and closure of the duodenum with the GIA instrument, **c** end-to-side anastomosis between the esophagus and mobilized jejunum with the EEA instrument and closure of the jejunal stump with the TA-55, **d** construction of a substitute gastric reservior by side-to-side jejunojejunostomy with the GIA instrument. The remaining jejunotomies can be closed with the TA-55 or TA-90

There is no question that mechanical suturing with the TA or GIA instrument saves much time in constructing an antiperistaltic or isoperistaltic gastric tube for esophageal replacement. In patients with a short esophagus, the GIA instrument can be applied next to the cardioesophageal junction to construct a Collis gastroplasty [7]. In principle the TA stapler can be used for the closure and removal of esophageal diverticula, but we favor a manual suture in these cases due to limitations of space.

Potential applications of the stapling instruments that relate indirectly to esophageal surgery include the reapproximation of severed bowel segments by the triangulation principle ("functional end-to-end anastomosis" [29, 36]) and various types of pyloroplasty (Finney [10], Heineke-Mikulicz [22]) to promote gastric emptying.

1.3.3.4 Potential Complications with Stapling Instruments

Most stapler-related complications are due to technical errors in the use of the instruments. With the EEA instrument, failure to tie the pursestring suture tightly enough can place the edge of the tissue within the path of the cutting blade or staple line. The faulty anastomosis is evidenced by the failure to obtain intact discs of full-thickness tissue. The esophagus can become damaged by the insertion of a cartridge that is too large for the lumen or by rough withdrawal of the anvil after the stapler has been fired. If the anvil is not fully seated onto the central rod or if there is extraneous suture material in the area of the anastomosis, the circular knife will not be able to divide the tissue cleanly. Mechanical failure of the stapling instruments is also a possibility, although their simple design makes this unlikely. The B shape of the staples is designed to preserve the blood supply, but anastomotic bleeding can occur if an arterial vessel is caught in the staple line. With an everting suture, the source of the bleeding is easily identified and controlled. But when the EEA instrument is used, the interior portion of the anastomosis cannot be visualized. The double row of staples provides some protection against hemorrhage, although this is by no means certain. In inverting anastomoses made with the GIA instrument, the surgeon should always look inside the anastomosis to make sure the staple lines are dry. This is the only effective safeguard against postoperative bleeding.

1.4 Mechanical Ligation

Blood vessels are mechanically ligated by means of V-shaped metal clips (hemoclips) applied with special forceps. In the simplest model the clip is manually loaded into the tip of the instrument before it is applied. Clip-applying forceps with cartridges containing 15 to 30 clips allow multiple closures to be performed without reloading. The efficacy of the mechanical closure is equivalent to that of a manual ligature.

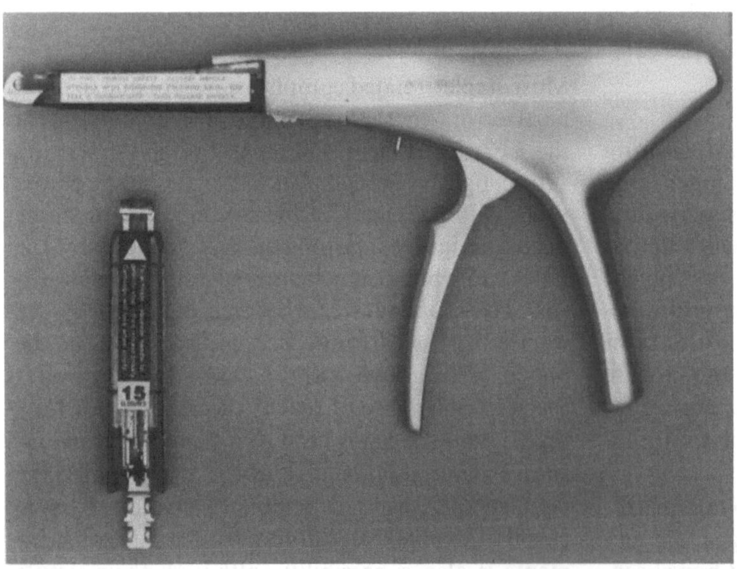

Fig. 11. LDS-2 instrument for the simultaneous ligation and division of tissue

The LDS instrument (Fig. 11) ligates and divides tissues or vessels in a single step. The vessel is picked up in the hook-shaped tip of the instrument, and the handle is squeezed to compress a pair of U-shaped staples into a semilunar curve. A cutting blade follows, severing the tissue between the clips. The greatest time saving is realized when the instrument is used to divide a large area of vascularized tissue (e.g., detaching the greater omentum from the stomach).

1.5 Use of Adhesives on the Esophagus

Synthetic adhesives with an alkyl-2-cyanoacrylate base or the biologic "fibrin glue" made by polymerizing a concentrated fibrinogen solution with a mixture of thrombin, calcium, and aprotinin are still in the experimental stage as a solitary means for closing gastrointestinal incisions or reinforcing anastomoses [12, 19]. We do not consider them adequate for the repair of suture line leaks [26], which we manage by the placement of additional sutures.

1.6 Techniques for Reinforcing Repairs and Anastomoses

A meticulous, atraumatic suturing technique combined with adequate preparation of the esophageal substitute and atraumatic dissection of the free end of the esophagus continue to offer the best assurance of uncomplicated anastomotic healing. Even so, there are situations in which it is advantageous to reinforce the suture line by covering it with adjacent tissue or protecting it from tension. This may be done routinely for esophagoenterostomies, or it may be indicated when the removal of a benign tumor leaves a sizable defect in the muscularis, or when it is necessary to repair an esophageal perforation in an infected area.

The easiest way to remove tension from an esophagoenterostomy is to fix the transplanted organ to the pleura or to structures of the posterior mediastinum. The suture line should be covered with tissue that adheres rapidly and has a rich blood supply separate from that of the area being covered. It should be emphasized that none of the methods described below can prevent the disruption of a poorly constructed anastomosis.

1.6.1 Pedicled Omental Flap

A pedicled flap of greater omentum can be elevated to virtually any site on the esophagus [4, 9]. The omentum satisfies the above criteria for most situations, except in gastric tube reconstructions of the esophagus, in which case the omentum is supplied by the same system that perfuses the stomach, the right gastroepiploic artery. Thus a reduction of flow in this artery will produce similar effects in the stomach and omentum. A particular advantage of the greater omentum as a pedicled flap is its rich lymphatic network with "windows" that permit the absorption of macromolecules. This provides a biologic cleansing mechanism that is highly beneficial when the flap is applied to tissue that is necrotic or infected. The immune complex of the omentum, composed of lymphoid cells and histiocytes, is of additional value in the control of infection [1].

Operative technique: The greater omentum is exposed through the same approach used for mobilizing the esophageal substitute, or through an upper midline laparotomy. The omentum is freed of adhesions with the abdominal wall and bowel, reflected upward, and detached from the transverse colon. Its vascular supply is inspected by transillumination. The right gastroepiploic artery is usually very well developed. It gives rise to the right and middle epiploic arteries and unites in the left third of the greater curvature with the left gastroepiploic artery, from which the left epiploic artery arises. The epiploic arteries interanastomose through Haller's arcades. Detached from the transverse colon, the greater omentum is brought up into the chest through the hiatus or through a separate incision in the diaphragm. If it is not long enough to reach the intended site, it may be based on one of the two gastroepiploic arcades. If the right gastroepiploic artery serves as the pedicle, the left gastroepiploic artery is divided just below its origin from the splenic artery. The omentum is detached from the stomach as far as the origin of the right gastroepiploic artery, at about the level of the pylorus, so that the vascular arch of the gastroepiploic artery is preserved on the omental side. Additional length can be gained [4] by incising the omentum between the right and middle epiploic arteries and incising it again parallel to Haller's arcade. If the flap is to be supplied by the left gastroepiploic artery, the omentum may be mobilized distal to the right gastroepiploic artery so that it retains both its right- and left-sided connections with the stomach. The portion of the omentum that is advanced into the chest or neck may be tacked over the area to be covered with simple interrupted sutures or wrapped around it, depending on the degree of mobilization of the esophagus.

1.6.2 Pedicled Pleural Flap

The mediastinal pleura is very rarely suitable for coverage of an esophageal suture line, which is accomplished more effectively with a rotation flap of parietal pleura (Fig. 12). Conditions for creating a adequately vascularized flap are less favorable on the left side than on the right due to the presence of the aorta. A pleural flap of sufficient size, based close to the esophagus, is cut out with a scissors. Starting at one corner, the flap is carefully mobilized, reflected over the esophageal suture line, and secured there with several interrupted sutures. Larger flaps have a more precarious blood supply and therefore should be mobilized along with intercostal muscles pedicled on their nutrient vessels. This is more easily accomplished with individual strips of pleura and muscle than with a single, large flap. The pleura is incised along the center line between two adjacent ribs and freed from the posterior aspect of the ribs with a periosteal elevator as far as the attachment of the intercostal musculature. The musculature along the superior, avascular border of one rib

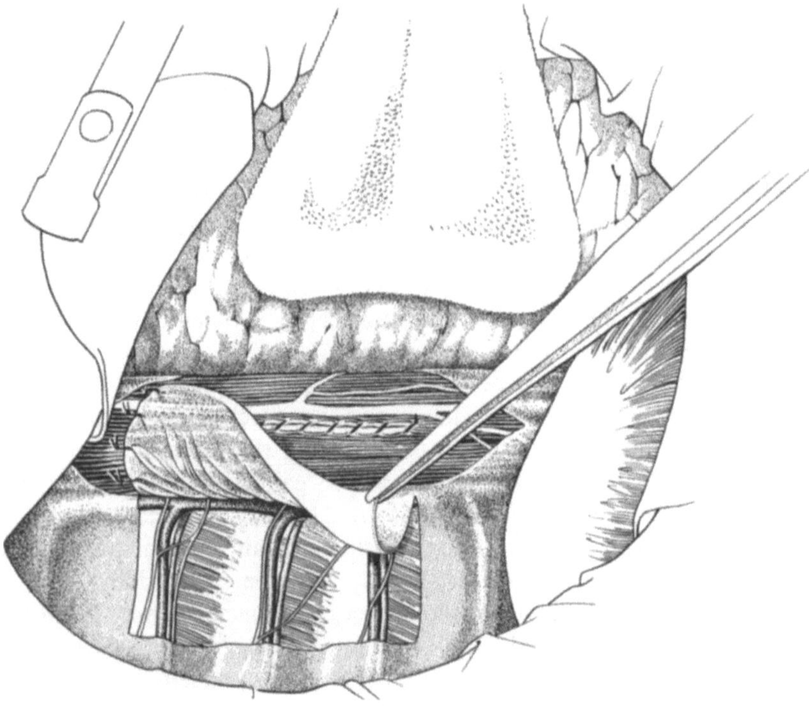

Fig. 12. Coverage of the suture line in the esophagus with a pleural flap

is divided with a scalpel. The intercostal vessels at the inferior border of the higher rib must be carefully preserved, as they will provide the pedicle for the musculopleural flap. The vessels at the edge of the flap are exposed, divided between small clamps, and ligated. From there the flap is dissected toward its base near the esophagus. Proximal branches from the intercostal arteries are coagulated or ligated. The artery coursing at the level of the costovertebral joints must be preserved. The musculopleural flap is wrapped around the esophagus and fixed with several interrupted sutures. It may be necessary to develop multiple flaps, depending on the area to be covered.

1.6.3 Lung Flap

The use of lung tissue for the coverage of esophageal defects was originally described by Nissen [23]. Today this method is considered to be obsolete.

1.6.4 Reinforcing a Suture Line Close to the Diaphragm

The most effective way to protect a suture line in the abdominal or lower thoracic esophagus is by means of a fundoplication or semifundoplication procedure (see Sect. 11). Fundoplication is indicated for an intrathoracic suture line to prevent reflux through the intrathoracic cardia. A diaphragmatic flap is less acceptable for suture line coverage, since development of the flap frequently leads to phrenic nerve injury.

1.6.5 Invagination of the Anastomosis

The simplest way to protect an anastomosis is by invagination (Fig. 13). It employs the same principle as the (now obsolete) three-layer esophagoenterostomy described by Sweet [32]. The only difference is that the third row of sutures is placed farther from the anastomotic suture line, and fewer sutures are placed to maintain the invagination. This is believed to prevent the blood flow disturbances frequently seen with the classic three-layer anastomosis and the resulting proneness to

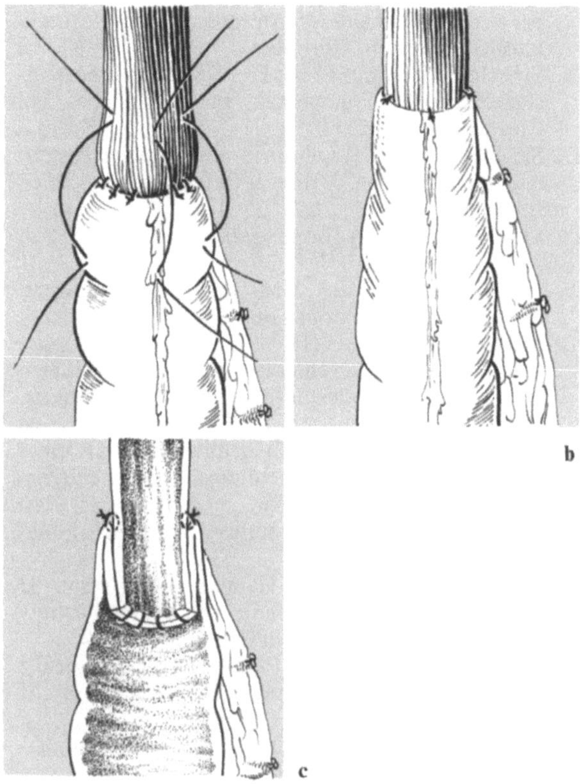

Fig. 13a–c. Anastomotic reinforcement by invagination. **a** Several sutures are placed 1.5–2 cm from the anastomosis. **b** The sutures are tied, imbricating the transplant (colon) over the anastomosis. **c** Longitudinal section through the invaginated anastomosis

stricture formation. Comparative, prospective data are needed to determine whether the newer technique reduces the incidence of anastomic leak. Methods available for the coverage of end-to-side anastomoses depend on the organ used for reconstruction and are discussed in Sect. 7.

1.7 End-to-End versus End-to-Side Anastomosis of the Esophagus

It is our view that the end-to-end and end-to-side techniques are equivalent in their ability to produce an effective, functional esophageal anastomosis. For statistical reasons alone, we must reject retrospective attempts to demonstrate the superiority of one method over the other [6]. Arguments that have been advanced in favor of end-to-side anastomoses, such as better blood flow to the esophageal substitute and better opportunities for reinforcing the suture line or establishing luminal congruity, are unconvincing. With proper selection and mobilization of the esophageal substitute, there should be no blood flow problems with either the end-to-end or end-to-side technique. If additional protection of the anastomosis by coverage with the transplanted organ is felt to be indicated (we consider this unnecessary with proper anastomotic technique), this can be done by invagination in an end-to-end anastomosis and by overlapping or plication in an end-to-side anastomosis, regardless of the organ used for the reconstruction (see Sect. 7). In both cases sufficient material must be available in the transplanted organ. The end-to-side anastomosis carries the risk of creating a blind pouch conducive to bacterial growth, but this should not occur if proper technique is used.

The lumina of the esophagus and transplant are usually congruent when the small intestine is used as the substitute. When the stomach is used, luminal equality is established in the same way for both types of anastomosis. For an end-to-end esophagocolostomy, the lumina are made equal by longitudinal incision of the esophagus.

References

1. Abbes MJ, Richelme H, Demard F (1974) The greater omentum in repair of complications following surgery and radiotherapy for certain cancers. Internat Surg 59:81
2. Akiyama H (1973) Esophageal anastomosis. Arch Surg 107:512
3. Akiyama H (1980) Surgery for carcinoma of the esophagus. Curr Probl Surg 17:1
4. Alday ES, Goldsmith HS (1972) Surgical technique for omental lengthening based on arterial anatomy. Surg Gyn Obstet 135:103
5. Caudwell EW, Sieckert RG, Lininger RE, Anson BJ (1948) The bronchial arteries: An anatomic study of 150 human cadavers. Surg Gyn Obstet 86:395
6. Chassin JL (1978) Esophagogastrectomy: Data favoring end-to-side anastomosis. Ann Surg 188:22
7. Collis JL (1957) An operation for hiatus hernia with short esophagus. Journ Thorac Cardiovasc Surg 34:768
8. Eichfuss HP, Schreiber HW (1981) Anastomosentechnik am Ösophagus. In: Häring R (Hrsg) Chirurgie des Ösophaguskarzinoms. Edition Medizin Weinheim, Deerfield, Burg
9. Fekete F, Breil P, Ronsse H, Tossen JC, Langonnet F (1981) EEA[R] stapler and omental graft in esophagogastrectomy. Experience with 30 intrathoracic anastomoses for cancer. Ann Surg 193:825
10. Finney JMT (1902) A new method of pyloroplasty. Bull Johns Hopkins Hosp 13:155

11. Gambee LP (1951) A single-layer open intestinal anastomosis applicable to the small as well as to the large intestine. World J Surg 59:1
12. Heiss WH (1971) Technik und Resultate der Gewebsklebung. Bull Soc Int Chir 6:549
13. Herzog B (1974) Die Darmnaht. Hiter, Bern
14. Herzog B (1972) Hat die Lembert'sche Theorie heute noch ihre Gültigkeit in der Darmchirurgie? Langenbecks Arch. Chir Suppl Forum 281
15. Hollender LT, Blanchot P, Meyer C, DaSilva E, Costa JM (1981) Erfahrungen mit der Anwendung von Nahtapparaten in der Magen-Darmchirurgie. Zbl Chirurgie 106:74
16. Junginger Th, Walgenbach S, Pichlmaier H (1983) Die zirkuläre Klammeranastomose (EEA) nach Gastrektomie. Chirurg 54:161
17. Kaufmann I (1971) Das Bauprinzip der Muscularis mucosa. Acta anat Basel 80:305
18. Kivelitz H, Ulrich B, Mahmud H (1980) Zur Chirurgie des Speiseröhrencarcinoms. Chirurg 51:717
19. Kort J (1971) Klebstoffe in der Chirurgie. Schattauer, Stuttgart
20. Kunath U (1980) Die stumpfe Dissektion der Speiseröhre. Chirurg 51:296
21. Lanz v.T., Wachsmuth W (1955) Praktische Anatomie, Bd I/12. Springer, Berlin Göttingen Heidelberg
22. Mikulicz J (1888) Zur operativen Behandlung des stenosierenden Magengeschwürs. Arch Klin Chir 37:79
23. Nissen R (1954) Operation am Ösophagus. Thieme, Stuttgart
24. Nockemann PT (1975) Die chirurgische Naht. Thieme, Stuttgart
25. Pichlmaier H, Junginger Th (1977) Nahttechniken bei gastrointestinalen Anastomosen. Chir.-gastroenterol. Symposium, Göttingen
26. Scheele J, Herzog J, Mühe E (1978) Anastomosensicherung am Verdauungstrakt mit Fibrinkleber. Zbl Chirurgie 103:1325
27. Sieglbauer F (1963) Lehrbuch der normalen Anatomie des Menschen. Urban & Schwarzenberg, Wien Innsbruck
28. Skinner DB (1980) Esophageal reconstruction. Am Journ Surg 139:810
29. Steichen FM, Ravitch MM (1973) Mechanical sutures in surgery. Br Journ Surg 60:191
30. Stelzner F, Kunath U (1977) Ergebnisse bei ösophagointestinalen Anastomosen und Untersuchungen der Durchblutung des dafür mobilisierten Magens. Chirurg 48:651
31. Stelzner F, Lierse W (1972) Strukturen des Ösophagus im Hinblick auf Beobachtungen beim operativen Eingriff. Zbl Chir 26a:1857
32. Sweet R (1950) Thoracic surgery. Saunders, Philadelphia London
33. Swigart VL, Siekert RG, Hambley WC, Anson BJ (1950) The esophageal arteries. An anatomic study of 150 specimens. Surg Gyn Obstet 90:234
34. Szabò EE, Karàcsonyi S, Paraky Z (1961) Über die Blutversorgung des Ösophagus und die chirurgische Bedeutung derselben. Zbl Chirurgie 86:619
35. Terracol J, Sweet RH (1958) Diseases of the esophagus. Saunders, Philadelphia
36. United States Surgical Corporation (1980) Stapling techniques. General surgery, 2nd edn

2 Esophagotomy and Esophagostomy

CONTENTS

2.1 Esophagotomy

This procedure is indicated for the extraction of foreign bodies lodged in the esophagus or for the excision of benign tumors (see Sect. 8) or constricting rings [25] or webs [8, 27] that are not amenable to endoscopic removal, division, or dilatation.

2.1.1 Cervical Esophagotomy

Preoperative preparation: All procedures on the cervical esophagus carry a risk of recurrent laryngeal nerve injury with vocal cord paralysis. Hence the vocal cords should be inspected for recurrent nerve integrity with the laryngoscope before and after surgery.

Instruments: Basic set.

Position and approach: Supine with the upper body slightly elevated and the arms adducted. The head is extended and turned toward the opposite side. The incision (Fig. 14 a–d) is made either along the anterior border of the sternocleidomastoid muscle from the mandible to the sternoclavicular joint, or on a transverse cervical skin crease just above the jugular fossa (unilateral Kocher collar incision), extending 1–2 cm past the anterior border of the sternocleidomastoid muscle on the side of the approach and also past the midline. This transverse incision parallel to the skin lines gives a better cosmetic result [4], although the exposure of the cervical esophagus is more limited. The side that is elected depends on the portion of the esophagus that is involved. Given the physiologic rotation of the stomach, the left-sided approach is advantageous in that the cervical esophagus bows slightly toward the left, and the recurrent nerve coursing between the esophagus and trachea is less vulnerable than in the right-sided approach.

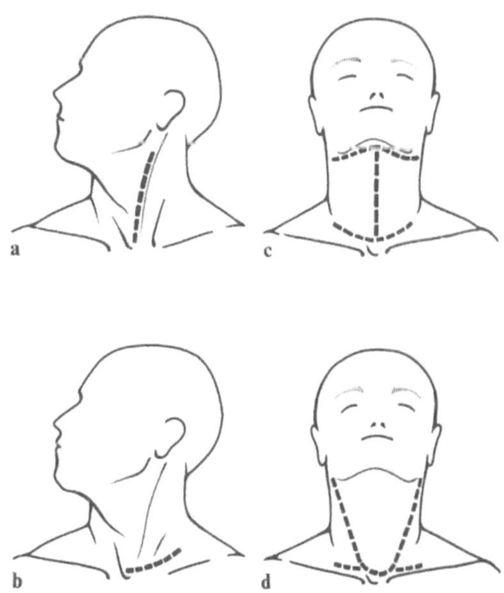

Fig. 14a–d. Approaches to the cervical esophagus: skin incisions. **a** Longitudinal incision along the anterior border of the sternocleidomastoid muscle. **b** Unilateral Kocher collar incision. **c** Trapdoor incision. **d** Extended Kocher collar incision with supraclavicular extensions

Steps in procedure:

(1) Skin incision along the anterior border of the sternocleidomastoid muscle or unilateral collar incision
(2) Exposure of the strap muscles and sternocleidomastoid
(3) Medial retraction of the thyroid gland with division of the thyroid veins
(4) Ligation of the inferior and/or superior thyroid artery
(5) Partial or circumferential exposure of the esophagus
(6) Incision of the esophagus
(7) Removal of the lesion
(8) Closure of the esophagus in two layers
(9) Drain insertion
(10) Wound closure in layers

Operative technique: The skin is incised with a scalpel, and the wound margins are retracted. The superficial fascia and platysma are divided with the electrocautery. The subcutaneous cervical veins are identified and divided. The dissection is carried sharply toward the anterior side of the vertebral column using a scissors or scalpel, preserving the anatomic structures (Fig. 15). The middle cervical fascia is incised at the anterior border of the sternocleidomastoid muscle, and the omohyoid muscle is mobilized and either retracted superiorly or divided in its tendinous midportion.

The strap muscles overlying the lobe of the thyroid gland are retracted medially with a Roux retractor or divided transversely. The sternocleidomastoid muscle and neurovascular bundle are retracted laterally, taking care that the retractor pressure does not restrict carotid blood flow. The superior thyroid artery is seen entering the upper lobe of the thyroid from above; that vessel and its accompanying veins are ligated only if they interfere with exposure of the esophageal-hypopharyngeal junction. The ligature is placed close to the capsule to avoid superior pharyngeal nerve injury. The connective tissue at the posterior border of the thyroid gland is bluntly mobilized, and the lateral thyroid veins are severed close to the gland. The lobe of the thyroid gland can be displaced farther medially at this time (Fig. 16 a). The inferior thyroid artery is visible at the distal end of the gland, entering from the lateral side. The recurrent laryngeal nerve usually courses between the branches of that artery in proximity to the gland; to avoid injuring the nerve, the inferior thyroid artery should be traced to its origin from the thyrocervical trunk and divided there (Fig. 16 b). Because of the highly variable course of the recurrent laryngeal nerve (Fig. 16 c [12]), we use a magnifying loupe and two fine dissecting patties to identify the nerve and follow its course. We have found this to be the best way of avoiding injury.

Fig. 15. Approaches to the cervical esophagus. *a* Anterior approach, *b* lateral (standard) approach, *c* posterior approach

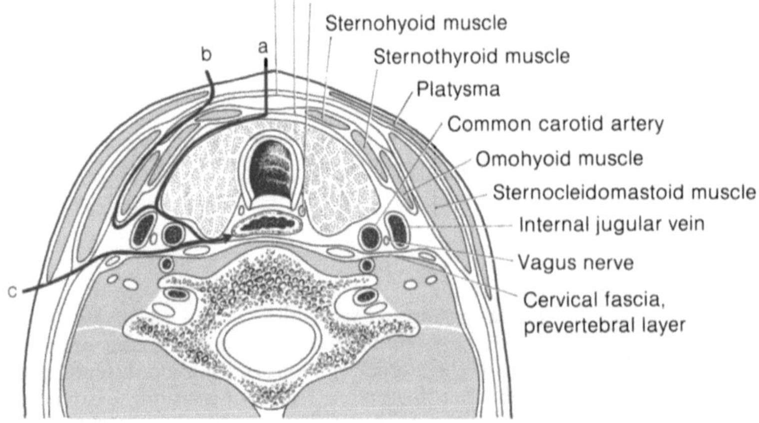

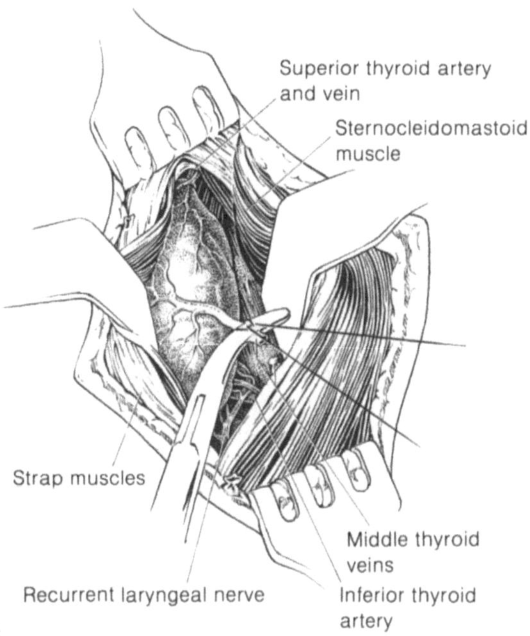

a

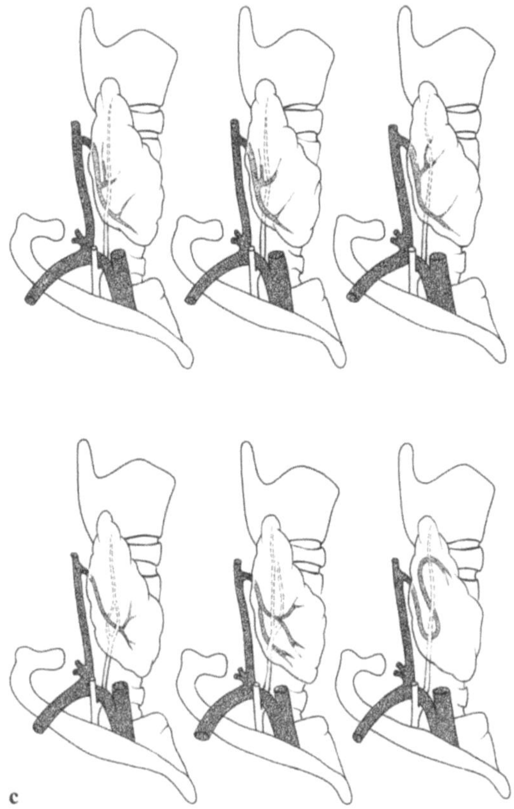
c

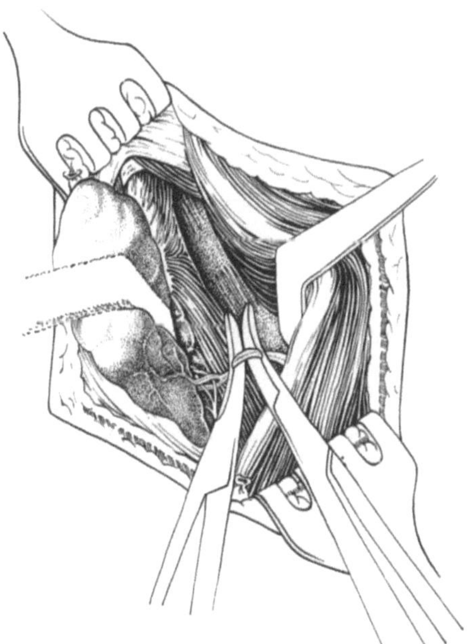
b

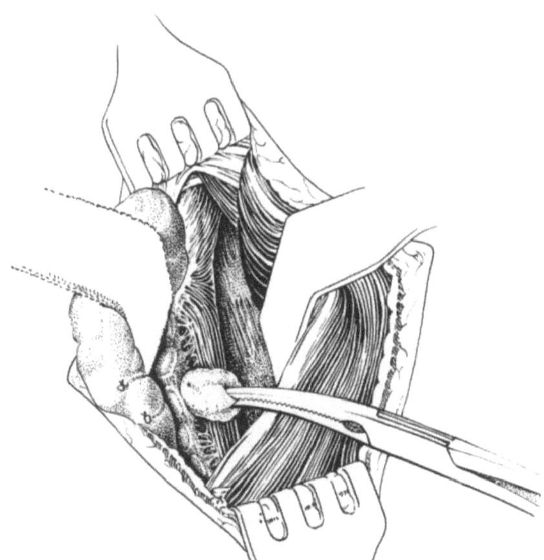
d

Fig. 16a–d. Exposure of the cervical esophagus through a unilateral Kocher collar incision (viewed from the left side). **a** Ligation of the lateral thyroid veins. **b** Ligation of the inferior thyroid artery. **c** Variations in the course of the recurrent laryngeal nerve (modified from Lanz and Wachsmuth [12]). **d** Dissection of the trachea from the anterior wall of the esophagus

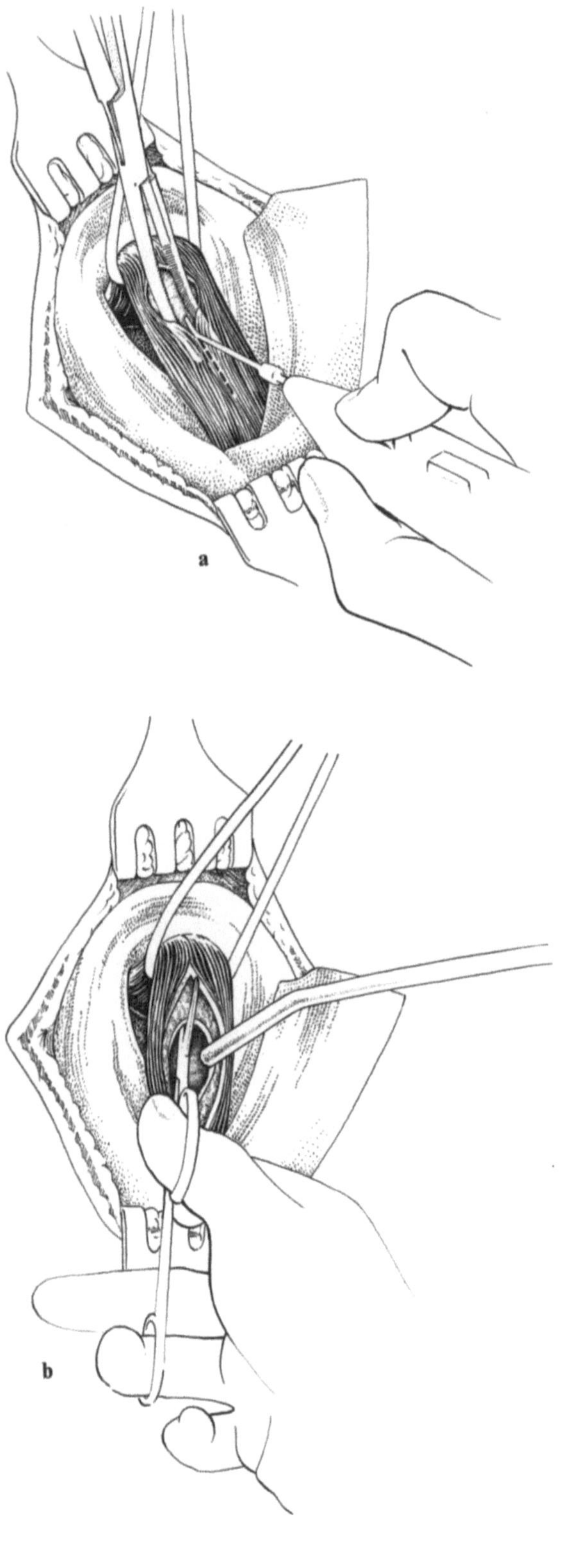

Fig. 17a, b. Opening the cervical esophagus. **a** Vertical incision of the muscular layer. **b** Incision of the mucosa and aspiration of esophageal contents

The esophagus is exposed between the trachea and vertebral column and is freed from the prevertebral fascia. Circumferential mobilization of the esophagus is usually unnecessary for the extraction of a foreign body. But if it is considered necessary to dissect the posterior tracheal wall from the esophagus, care must be taken not to injure the membranous portion of the trachea (Fig. 16 d). For orientation at this stage, the superior end of the esophagus can be identified by palpation of the cricoid plate; the mouth of the esophagus is level with its lower third. Before the lumen of the esophagus is entered, the surrounding area should be packed off with antiseptic-soaked gauze to protect the cervical soft tissues from contamination by spilled esophageal contents. The esophagus is opened by making a vertical incision through the muscularis at the designated site, which if necessary may be confirmed by intraoperative endoscopy (Fig. 17 a). The underlying submucosa and mucosa will bulge up somewhat between the incised edges of the muscle. To facilitate subsequent closure, the muscular edges are pushed back several millimeters with a dissecting patty before incising the mucosa with a scissors or scalpel while aspirating the luminal contents (Fig. 17 b). The wound margins are held widely open with small, atraumatic forceps to afford good exposure for removal of the foreign body or tumor.

We close the esophagotomy longitudinally in two layers (see Sect. 1). Transverse closure has been recommended to prevent stricturing but is unnecessary with a normal esophageal wall. The mucosa is closed with a continuous watertight suture (Fig. 18 a), and a second layer of interrupted sutures is placed to reapproximate the muscularis loosely over the mucosa (Fig. 18 b). The wound is closed in layers over a Penrose drain. Cosmesis is an important concern in the cervical area. To achieve a tension-free skin closure, we first suture the platysma. The skin wound is closed with intracutaneous or vertical mattress sutures of fine monofilament material. When interrupted sutures are used, every second thread is removed on the second postoperative day, and the remaining sutures are removed on day four. Since there is no epithelial ingrowth into the needle tracks by that time, there should be no visible puncture marks. The patient is fed through a preplaced nasogastric tube or parenterally until X-rays confirm the integrity of the suture line. At that time the patient is gradually returned to a normal diet.

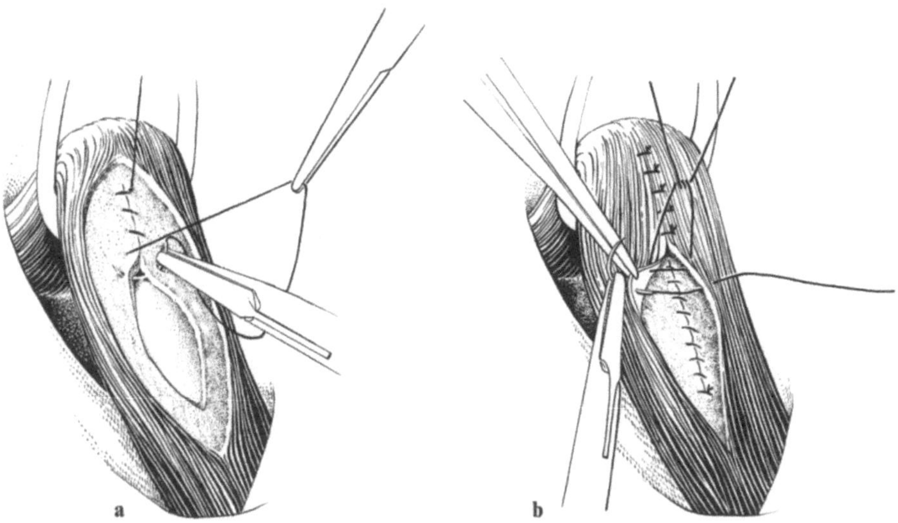

Fig. 18a, b. Closure of the esophagotomy. **a** Continuous mucosal suture. Large-gauge stomach tube is passed into the esophagus to prevent stricturing. **b** Muscular coat is approximated over the mucosal suture line with simple interrupted sutures

2.1.2 Thoracic Esophagotomy

Preoperative preparation: See Chap. C.

Instruments: Basic set, extra thoracic set.

Position and approach: Posterolateral thoracotomy (see Chap. B); the position of the incision depends on the level of the disease and the affected side. For lesions close to the aortic arch, a right-sided approach gives better exposure and makes it easier to mobilize the esophagus.

Steps in procedure:

(1) Posterolateral thoracotomy according to the level of the lesion and the side involved
(2) Anterior retraction of the lung
(3) Incision of the mediastinal pleura (sparing the vagus nerve) and dissection of the pleura from the esophagus
(4) Mobilization and snaring of the esophagus
(5) Incision of the esophagus
(6) Removal of the lesion
(7) Closure of the esophagus in two layers
(8) Closure of the mediastinal pleura
(9) Chest tube insertion
(10) Closure of the thoracotomy in layers

Operative technique: The chest is entered (see Chap. B) and the lung retracted anteriorly with a broad spatula. The mediastinal pleura covering the esophagus is picked up with a forceps and incised for a length of 1–2 cm with a scissors (Fig. 19 a). The incision is then extended superiorly and inferiorly with the scissors, whose jaws are opened only slightly for this maneuver. In a right-sided approach the pleural incision is extended upward past the crossing of the azygos vein to make the vessel somewhat more mobile. The esophagus can then be mobilized below the vein. It may occasionally be necessary to divide the azygos vein, although it must be considered that the vein is a major collateral vessel between the superior and inferior vena cava, and its disruption can have adverse consequences in the event of a subsequent pelvic vein thrombosis or in rare instances where the inferior vena cava is aplastic. After the pleura has been incised, each edge is grasped with a forceps and freed from the esophagus by blunt patty dissection (Fig. 19 b). The vagus nerve is picked up on a small nerve hook or snared with a tape and is freed from its connective tissue attachments with the esophagus. Larger connecting branches between the two main trunks should be spared if at all possible. In a simple esophagotomy, as performed for the extraction of a foreign body, it is unnecessary to free the esophagus circumferentially. However, benign neoplasms with a broad area of attachment may require that the esophagus be rotated for better exposure, making it necessary to free the esophagus completely from its bed. We do this by bluntly dissecting around the esophagus with the thumb and forefinger (Fig. 19 c) to clear its attachments with the opposite pleura. This is

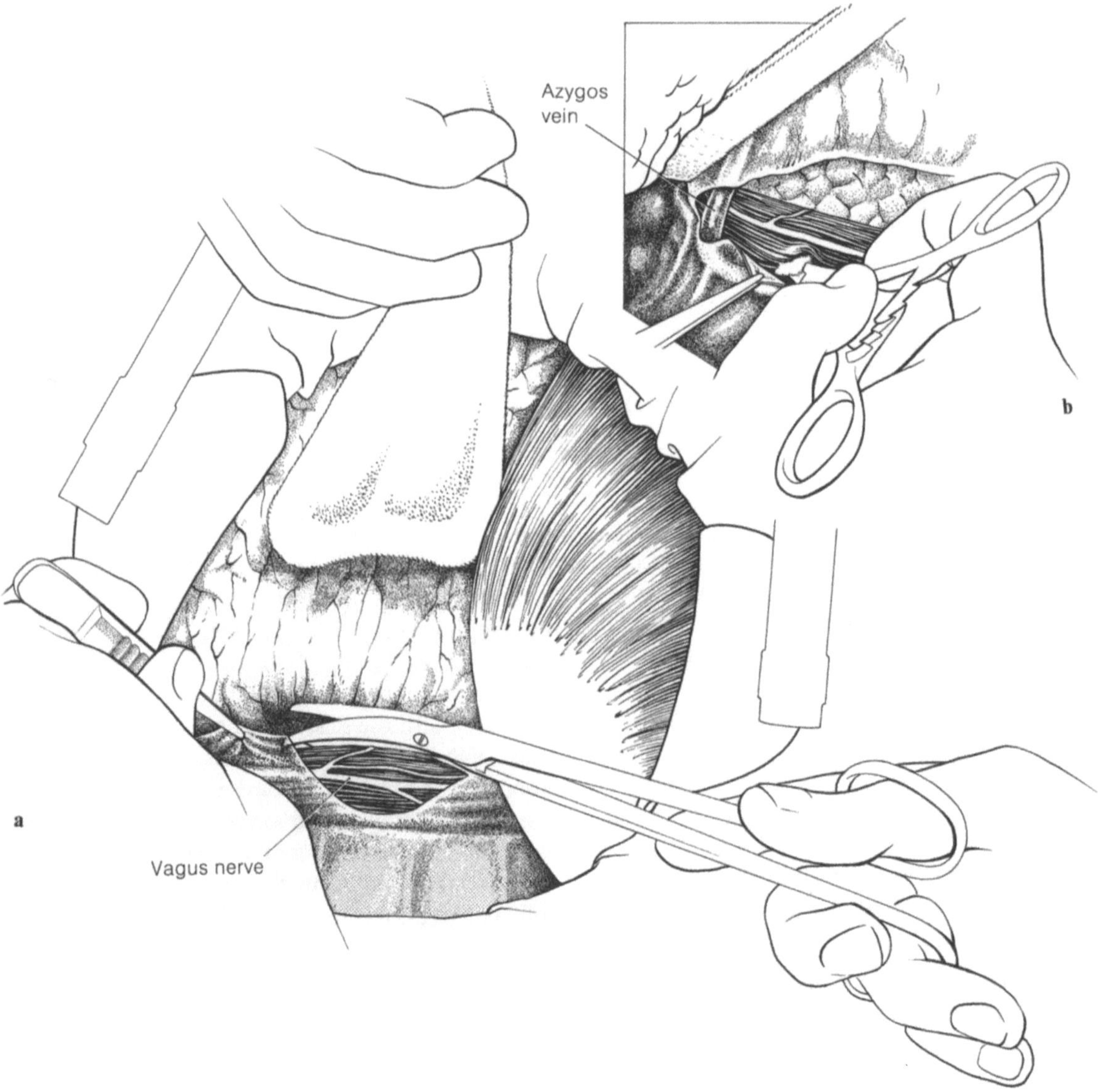

Fig. 19a–d. Exposure of the thoracic esophagus through a right-sided approach. **a** The mediastinal pleura is incised longitudinally over the esophagus, carefully sparing the vagus nerve. **b** The pleura is freed from the esophagus, sparing the azygos vein. **c** The esophagus is encircled and freed from the contralateral pleura. **d** Vessels entering the esophagus posteriorly are cauterized

continued until the thumb and forefinger completely encircle the esophagus and are touching. The vagus nerve branch on that side is palpable as a cordlike structure; it is left on the esophageal wall. After the esophagus has been cleared by finger dissection, it is encircled with a Guyon clamp and snared with a rubber tape. The esophagus is elevated from its bed by traction on the snare. Blood vessels entering the esophagus posteriorly are made taut by this maneuver; larger vessels are ligated, smaller ones are cauterized (Fig. 19 d). If the contralateral pleura is entered during mobilization of the esophagus, it is repaired with a continuous suture while the end-expiratory pressure is raised slightly to +2 or +3 cm H_2O to prevent the entry of air, tissue fluid, or blood. Because the lung cannot collapse under the positive ventilatory pressure, it usually is unnecessary to place a contralateral drain at the end of the operation. However, after every thoracic procedure we

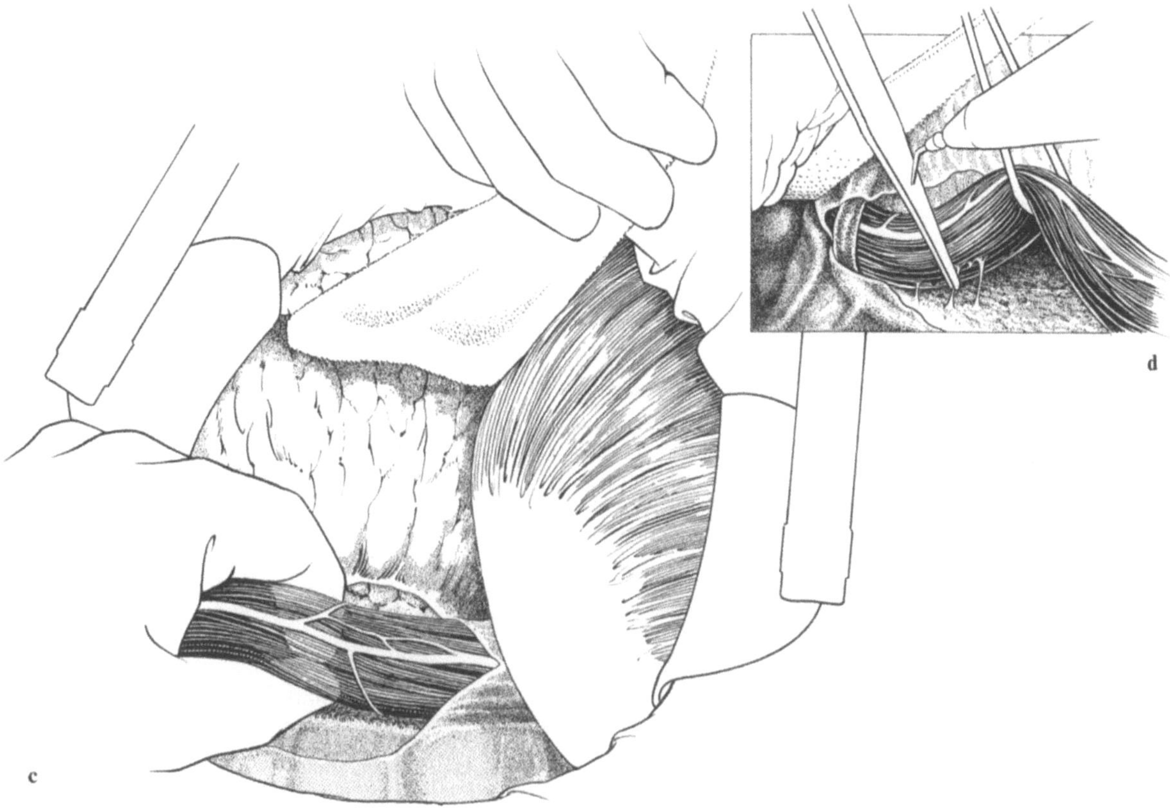

d

c

monitor pulmonary expansion radiologically in the operating suite before the patient is extubated. Incision and closure of the esophagus are described in 2.1.1. There is disagreement concerning the need to close the pleura over the esophagotomy. We close it whenever possible with a continuous suture to restore anatomic relations and avoid extensive adhesions (Fig. 20). Skinner et al. [28] point out that disruption of the suture line under a closed pleura would promote the spread of inflammation in the posterior mediastinum, where it would be more difficult to control. When the pleura is left open, they maintain, the secretions can drain through the chest tube, and infection is easier to control.

At the end of the operation the pleural cavity needs to be drained. A finger inside the chest marks the lowest intercostal space on the midaxillary line, and the skin over the fingertip is incised with a scalpel. A long clamp is introduced from the outside through the intercostal musculature and pleura at the upper border of the rib. The distal end of the drainage tube is grasped, brought out through the incision, and connected to an underwater seal. The proximal end of the drain is positioned just below the esophagotomy. The drain is secured to the skin, and the lung is inflated with positive pressure to eliminate areas of atelectasis. Finally the thoracotomy is closed in layers (see Chap. C).

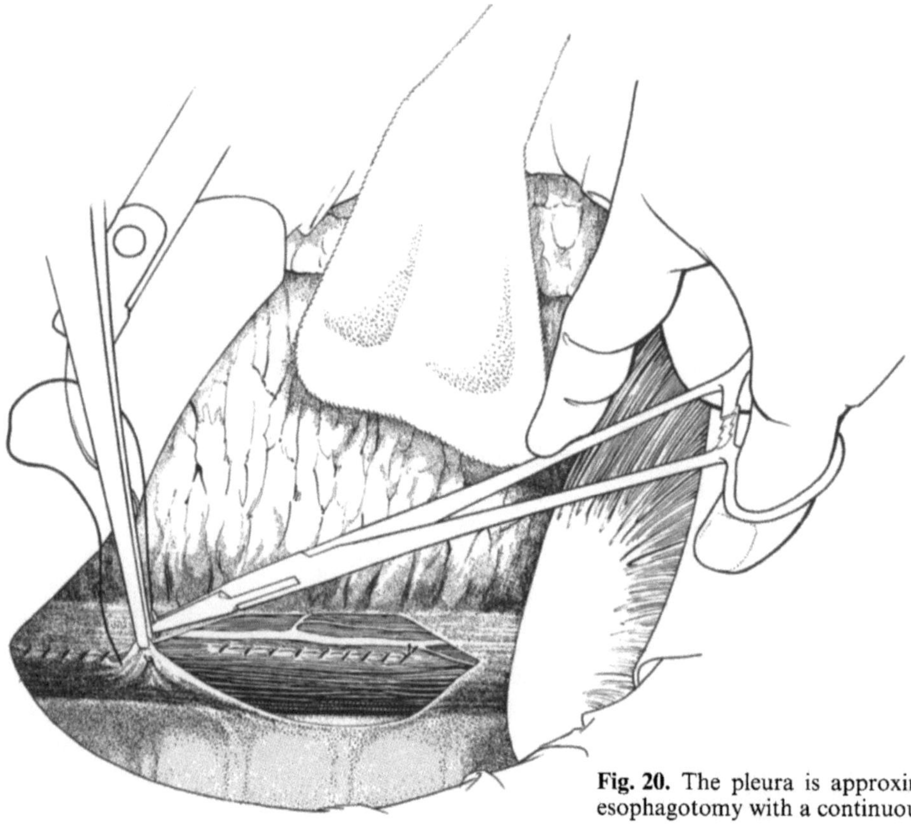

Fig. 20. The pleura is approximated over the thoracic esophagotomy with a continuous suture

2.2 Esophagostomy

2.2.1 Lateral Cervical Esophagostomy

This procedure may be used to establish a portal for tube feeding after surgical procedures on the oropharynx, or it can provide for drainage of oroesophageal secretions in dysphagic patients. A double-barreled cervical esophagostomy can be used in conjunction with a feeding gastrostomy [15] to temporarily defunctionalize the esophagus. In patients who require prolonged tube feedings, cervical esophagostomy is superior to a nasogastric tube in that it eliminates irritation of the nose and throat and the danger of aspirating mucous secretions [32]. Another advantage from the patient's standpoint is the ease of concealing a cervical esophagostomy tube beneath the collar or a scarf. This cannot be done with a nasogastric tube, which is far more conspicuous. The surgical procedure and its aftermath (e.g., care of the stoma) are more easily tolerated than a gastrostomy.

2.2.1.1 Simple Lateral Esophagostomy

Preoperative preparation: See 2.1.1.

Instruments: Basic set, esophagoscope, feeding tube.

Position and approach: The procedure corresponds to that for a cervical esophagotomy (see 2.1.1). The length of the incision depends on the application of the stoma. If only one tube is to be inserted, a 2- to 3-cm incision will suffice.

Operative technique: The esophagus is exposed as described in 2.1.1. With a very small incision, identification of the esophagus is aided by inserting an esophagoscope and pressing its tip against the lateral wall of the esophagus. In a darkened operating room, the light beam of the scope is easily seen through the cervical soft tissues (Fig. 21 a). When the lateral wall of the esophagus has been visualized through the scope, and the insertion of only one tube is planned, a stab incision is made

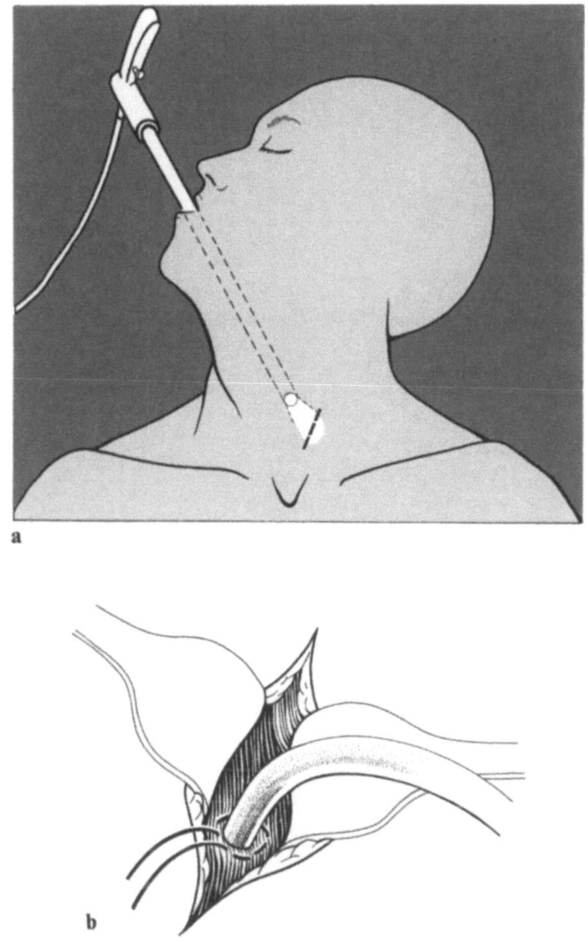

Fig. 21a, b. Simple lateral esophagostomy. **a** With a very short incision, an endoscope beam is useful for locating the esophageal wall. **b** A tube is passed into the cervical esophagus for feeding and to aspirate gastric contents. The pursestring suture is optional

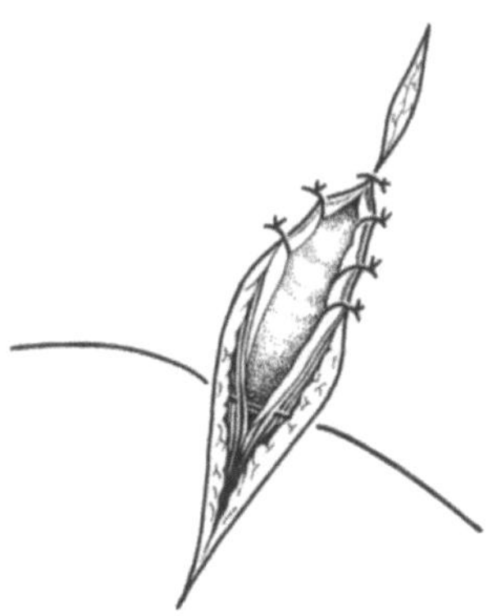

Fig. 22. Esophagostomy for feeding and/or partial defunctionalization of the esophagus (salivary drainage)

at the appropriate site in the esophageal wall, and the tube is introduced and passed into the stomach under endoscopic guidance. If the esophageal wall fits snugly about the tube, a pursestring suture is unnecessary (Fig. 21 b). The wound is closed without a drain, as the tube will provide adequate drainage of secretions. Generally a drainage tract will be well established after one week, and at that time the tube may be changed as required. If the tube is no longer needed, it may be removed without having to close the defect surgically. The fistula should close spontaneously within a few days.

If a larger stoma is needed to provide for simultaneous drainage of saliva, a 2- to 3-cm longitudinal incision is made in the esophagus, and its wall is sutured to the skin with interrupted all-coats sutures (Fig. 22). The two sutures at the upper and lower limits of the esophagotomy must encompass the esophageal wall as well as both margins of the skin wound. The remainder of the skin incision is closed.

2.2.1.2 Percutaneous Tube Esophagostomy

We prefer a modification of the technique used by Graham and Royster [7] in adults and by Talbert and Haller [30] in children. Its advantage is that the initial puncture of the esophagus is made with a thin steel needle. Should the needle enter an artery or vein, the bleeding is easily controlled by compression.

Preoperative preparation: No special preparation.

Instruments: Scalpel, peel-away introducer (Fig. 23 a), feeding tube, esophagoscope.

Position and approach: Supine with the upper body slightly elevated and the head extended and turned to the right side. The puncture site is two fingerwidths above the jugular fossa at the anterior border of the sternocleidomastoid muscle, preferably on the left side.

Operative technique: With the operating room darkened, the rigid esophagoscope is passed perorally into the esophagus. The tip of the scope is easily located by the light spot visible through the cervical soft tissues. The tip is advanced to the proposed site of needle insertion and elevates the lateral esophageal wall in the direction of that site. The carotid pulse is palpated to make sure the needle is inserted well medial to it. The steel needle is introduced from above downward into the esophageal wall, guided by the light spot, while constant aspiration is applied (Fig. 23 b). Entry of the needle tip into the lumen is confirmed by direct observation through the esophagoscope. A flexible guide wire is inserted through the needle into the esophagus, and the needle is withdrawn (Fig. 23 c). About a 1/2-cm incision is made in the skin over the guide wire with the scalpel, and the dilator with peel-away introducer is threaded over the wire into the esophagus (Fig. 23 d). The dilator and steel

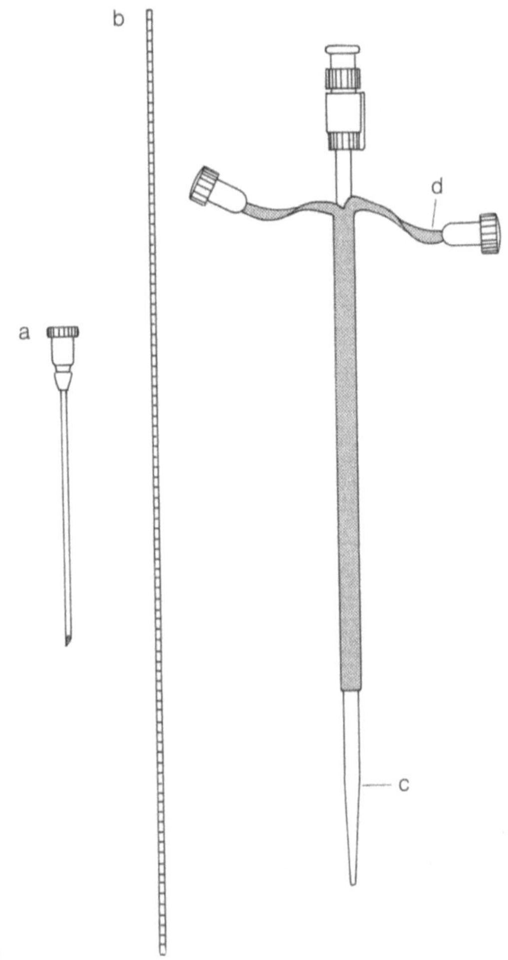

a

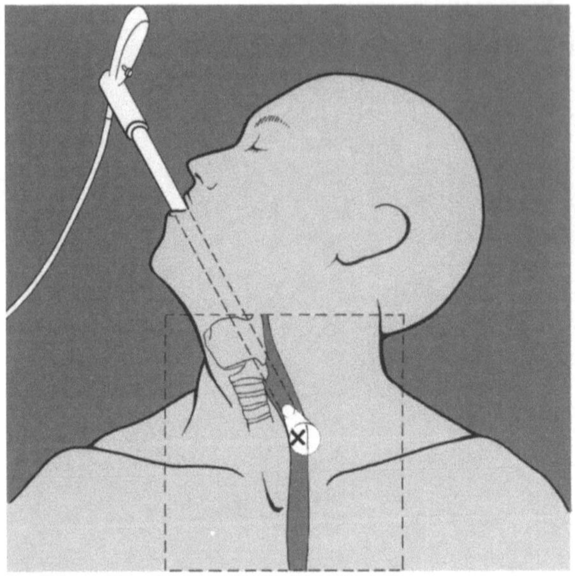

b

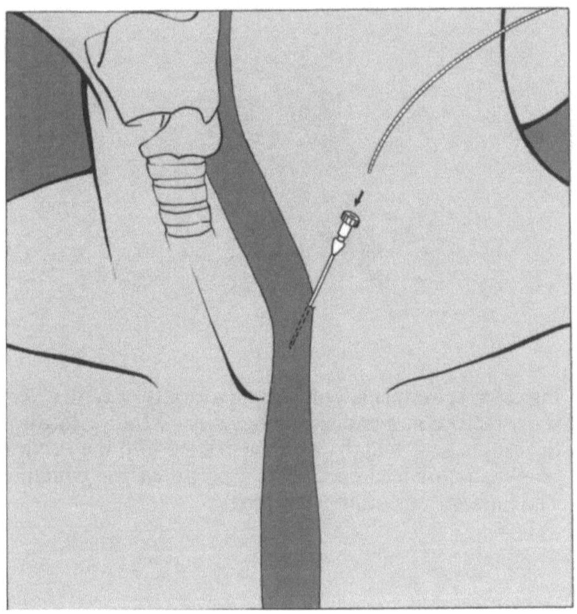

c

Fig. 23a–e. Percutaneous tube esophagostomy. **a** Instruments: *a* Needle, *b* guidewire, *c* dilator, *d* peel-away introducer. **b** An endoscope is used to help locate the puncture site. **c** The needle is passed into the esophagus under endoscopic guidance, and the guidewire is inserted. **d** The dilator with peel-away introducer is threaded over the wire into the esophagus. **e** The peel-away introducer is removed, and the feeding tube is inserted

wire are removed, and the feeding tube is inserted into the esophagus through the peel-away introducer and passed on into the stomach. As the ends of the peel-away introducer are pulled apart, the introducer splits into halves and slips easily from the wound (Fig. 23 e). The feeding tube is fixed to the neck with a stay suture of nonabsorbable material.

This procedure, used in conjunction with thin oligopeptide nutrient solutions, is excellent for patients who are severely malnourished or have lost lengthy portions of the bowel. The solution, packaged in a plastic bag, is easily carried in a pocket or vest along with an infusion pump without significantly limiting the patient's mobility.

2.2.1.3 Double-Barreled Lateral Cervical Esophagostomy

The advantage of this method over transection of the esophagus or the separate construction of two stomata

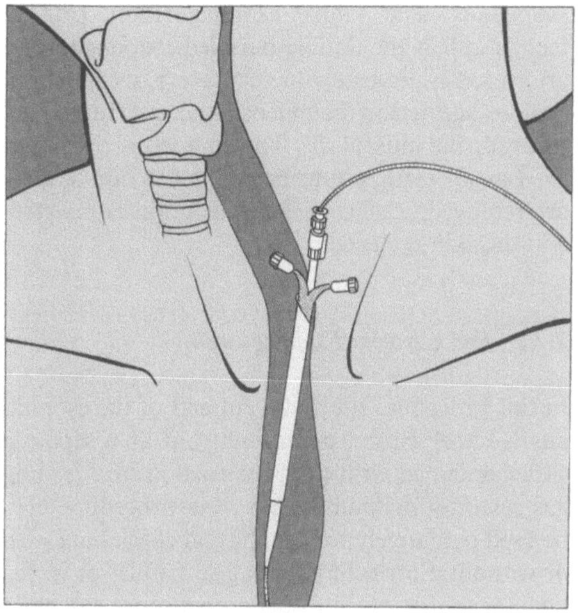

d

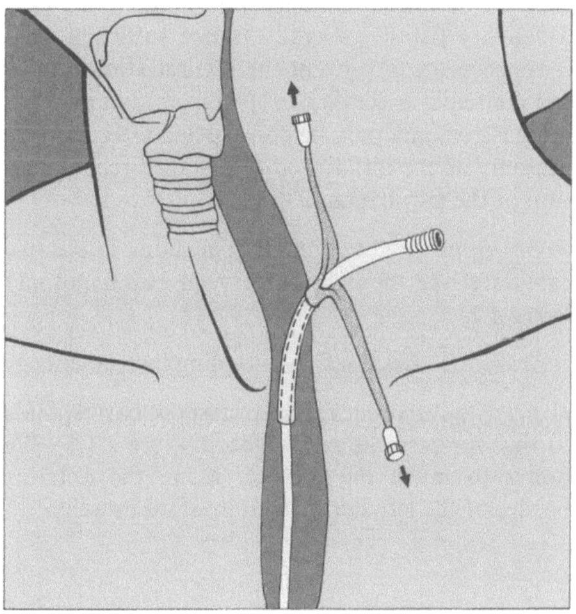

e

is that one wall of the esophagus is left intact [15], facilitating reanastomosis.

Preoperative preparation: See 2.1.1.

Instruments: Basic set.

Position and approach: See 2.1.1.

Operative technique: The esophagus is exposed from the hypopharynx to the thoracic inlet as described for cervical esophagotomy (see 2.1.1) and is snared with a Penrose drain. If the entire circumference of the esophagus cannot be brought to the level of the skin, the mobilization is continued bluntly into the posterior mediastinum to gain additional length. A loop of esophagus is delivered into the skin wound by traction on the Penrose drain. The skin directly below the drain is closed (Fig. 24a) with two interrupted sutures. This bridge of skin serves a supporting and dividing function analogous to the plastic rod in a double-barreled colostomy. The esophagus over the skin bridge is opened longitudinally with a 3- to 4-cm incision, and the wall is sutured to the margins of the skin incision with interrupted all-coats sutures (Fig. 24 b). This creates a double-barreled stoma that permits the attachment of an extracorporeal bypass tube (see 2.4) while effectively defunctionalizing the thoracic esophagus.

Fig. 24a, b. Double-barreled lateral cervical esophagostomy. **a** A narrow skin bridge is created below the exteriorized loop of esophagus. **b** The esophageal wall is fixed to the skin margins with all-coats sutures

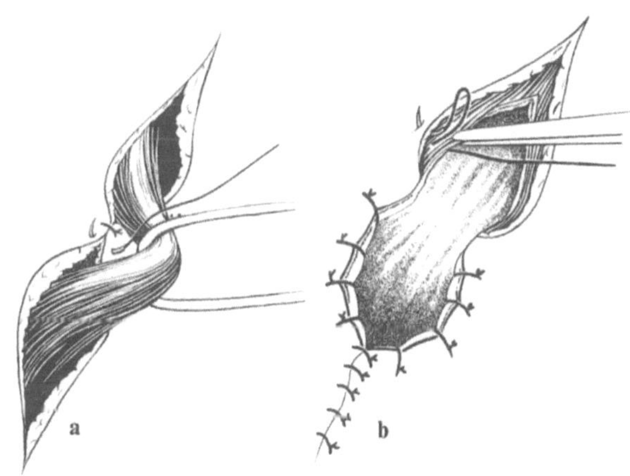

2.2.1.4 *Closure of a Lateral Esophagostomy*

Open or percutaneous tube esophagostomies do not require surgical closure, as the fistula left by removal of the tube will close spontaneously. But if a stoma has been constructed by suturing a portion of the esophageal wall to the skin, surgical closure is necessary.

Preoperative preparation: No special preparation.

Instruments: Basic set, red stomach tube (Ch 32).

Position and approach: The patient is positioned as for a cervical esophagotomy (see 2.1.1). The incision is made in the old scar.

Operative technique: The scar is excised, and the stoma is circumscribed leaving a rim of skin about 1 mm wide (Fig. 25 a). The esophagus is mobilized only enough to enable a tension-free closure. The side walls of the stoma are pulled apart with a pair of laterally placed traction sutures. The cutaneous rim may be left in place to serve as a second suture bed. The stomach tube is advanced beyond the esophagotomy to prevent narrowing of the esophagus. The simple esophagostomy (Fig. 25 b,c) as well as the double-barreled esophagostomy are closed transversely in two layers, using a continuous suture for the mucosa and interrupted sutures for the muscularis. The cutaneous rim is utilized as an extra suture bed. The traction sutures are removed, a silicone Penrose drain is inserted, and the skin is closed.

2.2.2 *End Cervical Esophagostomy*

In this procedure the distal cut end of the esophagus is either closed or brought out at a separate site. Combined with the construction of a feeding gastrostomy or jejunostomy, the procedure may be used palliatively for esophageal carcinoma with or without a bronchioesophageal fistula, or in patients who are too ill to undergo a more extensive thoracic or abdominal operation. In the latter case a salivary fistula generally is not sufficient, and it is necessary to prevent the regurgitation of gastric contents. A cervical esophagostomy and feeding gastrostomy may be constructed after esophagectomy as the initial step of a staged reconstruction of the esophagus [23].

Preoperative preparation: Preparations in elective cases are like those for a cervical esophagotomy (see 2.1.1).

Instruments: Basic set, TA stapling instrument.

Position and approach: The procedure corresponds to that for cervical esophagotomy (see 2.1.1). We prefer to make the incision along the anterior border of the left sternocleidomastoid muscle.

Fig. 25a–c. Closure of a lateral esophagostomy. **a** The stoma is circumferentially excised, leaving a narrow rim of skin. A large-gauge stomach tube functions as a stent to prevent narrowing of the esophagus during the closure. **b** Transverse closure of the stoma in two layers. **c** (Detail of 25 b) The muscularis is approximated with simple interrupted sutures over the continuous mucosal suture. The rim of skin left on the stoma provides an additional suture bed

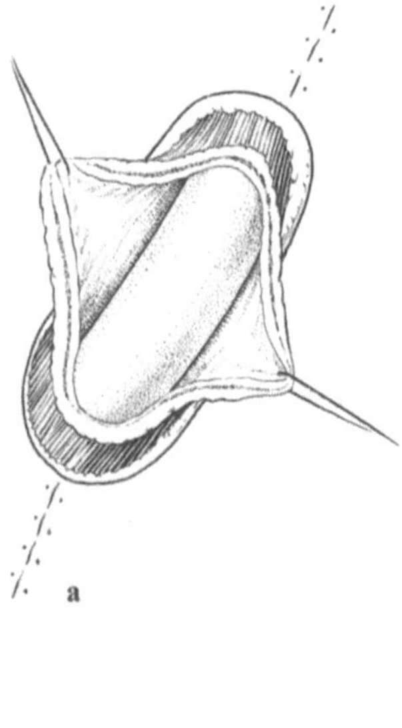

a

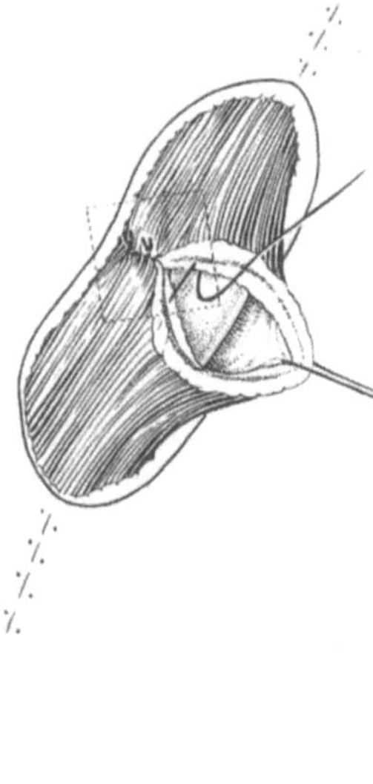

b

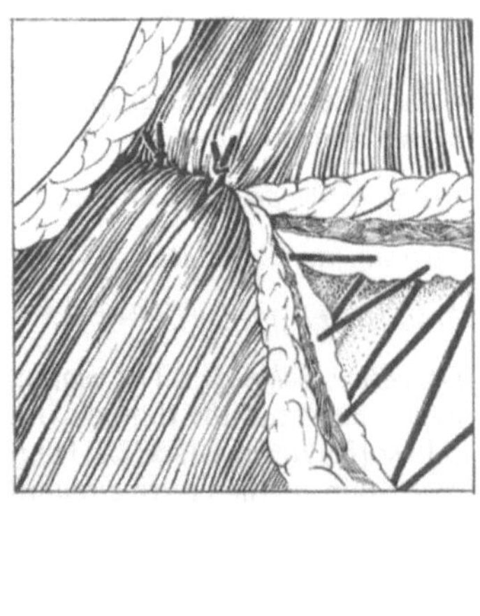

c

Steps in procedure:

Steps 1 through 5 are as described in Sect. 2.1.1.

(6) Snaring of the esophagus
(7) Placement of two guide sutures on each side
(8) Closure of the esophagus close to the thoracic inlet with the TA stapler
(9) Incision of the anterior esophageal wall, cleaning of the lumen
(10) Division of the posterior wall (watch for mucosal bleeding)
(11) Fixation of the proximal cut end to the skin wound with all-coats interrupted sutures
(12) Closure of the remaining skin wound

Operative technique: The cervical esophagus is exposed, freed circumferentially, and snared with a soft Penrose drain as in a cervical esophagotomy (see 2.1.1). A loop of esophagus is delivered into the skin wound by traction on the drain; at this point the esophagus may require additional mobilization by blunt dissection in the posterior mediastinum. All-coats guide sutures are placed on each side of the esophagus above and below the proposed site of the transection. The cervical soft tissues around the esophagus are packed off with gauze soaked in antiseptic. If the distal stump is to be closed, this is done most easily with the TA stapler (Fig. 26 a). With traction on the guide sutures, the anterior wall of the esophagus is incised with the electrocautery about 2 mm proximal to the staple line. Residual mucus and saliva are aspirated, and the lumen is cleaned with dissecting patties soaked in antiseptic (Fig. 26 b). Only then is the posterior wall of the esophagus divided. The distal stump is pulled forward on its guide sutures to check for hemostasis and completeness of the staple line. Inversion of the staple line with sutures is both difficult and unnecessary [29].

Alternatively, the esophageal stump may be closed manually using a two-layer technique in which the continuous mucosal suture is buried with a row of inverting muscularis sutures.

There is some concern about closing the distal stump if a complete distal obstruction of the lower esophagus exists or is anticipated. It is feared that gas or secretions will accumulate between the closed end and the distal obstruction, causing a pressure buildup that may blow out the closure

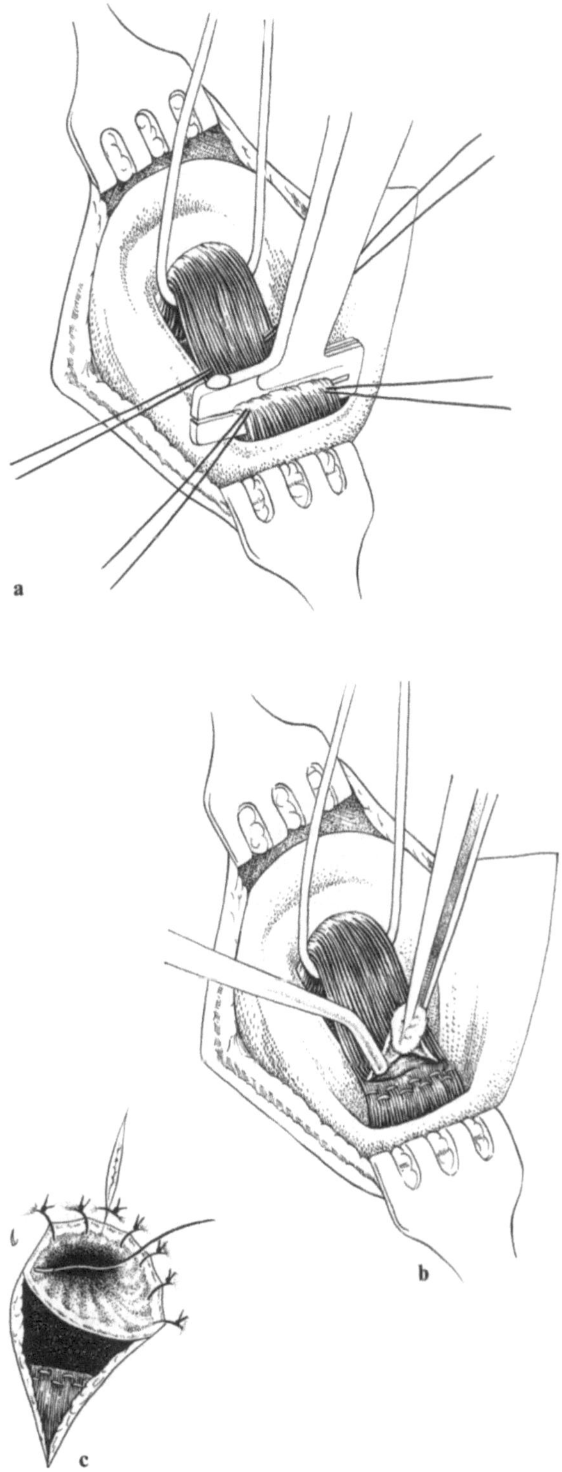

Fig. 26a–c. Construction of an end cervical esophagostomy. **a** The esophagus is closed distal to the planned stoma with the TA stapler. **b** The esophagus is opened proximal to the staple line, suctioned, and its lumen cleaned with dissecting patties soaked in antiseptic. **c** The proximal end of the esophagus is sutured into the skin wound

or esophageal wall [22], resulting in a life-threatening mediastinitis. This complication can be avoided by suturing the distal end to the lower margin of the skin wound to form a mucous fistula. However, this cannot always be done due to longitudinal tension on the esophagus or a deficiency of material. The placement of the end cervical esophagostomy depends on the type of procedure that is planned thereafter. If reanastomosis to the esophagus or esophageal substitute is planned, we suture the cervical stoma into the skin wound (Fig. 26 c). The proximal segment should be as straight as possible to aid salivary drainage. The esophageal wall is attached to the margins of the skin wound with all-coats interrupted sutures, and the rest of the skin wound is closed. If the stoma is permanent, placing it lateral to the skin incision on the flat surface of the sternocleidomastoid muscle [24] will permit a collection bag or extracorporeal tube to be attached to it with less difficulty (see 2.4) than placement at any other site. The skin is grasped two to three fingerwidths above the clavicular insertion of the sternocleidomastoid muscle with a sharp forceps, and a circular opening about 2 cm in diameter is made with a scalpel. The subcutaneous fat and platysma are resected with the electrocautery down to the level of the sternocleidomastoid muscle, which is split in the direction of its fibers with a closed scissors over an opposing fingertip held below the muscle. This opening is bluntly extended. A long clamp is introduced to grasp the guide sutures on the esophageal stump and deliver the stump through the muscle and skin incision without twisting it. The esophageal wall is sutured to the skin using the technique described above, and the cervicotomy is closed over a Penrose drain with interrupted sutures. A stoma placed in the skin wound should be covered for two to three days with compresses, and a collection bag is not attached until there is adequate cohesion of the wound edges. When the stoma is placed separate from the skin wound, a bag may be glued to it right away.

2.2.3 Thoracic Esophagostomy

Thoracic esophagostomy with a T-tube as described by Thorek [31] for the treatment of severe inflammatory esophageal stricture is reserved for highly selected cases. It may be tried as a last resort in patients with a longstanding, refractory esophageal perforation to seal off the defect and decompress the lumen [1, 26]. The operative technique is described in I.13.

2.3 Nutrition Following Defunctionalization of the Esophagus

2.3.1 Selection of Procedure

Patients who have undergone surgery that excludes the esophagus from the alimentary tract must be nourished either parenterally or enterally through a feeding fistula. Parenteral nutrition has the advantage of greater efficiency. Even in severely malnourished cancer patients, it can usually establish an anabolic state and correct nutritional deficit regardless of whether adjuvant measures such as chemotherapy or radiotherapy are required [18]. The abdomen is not entered. This can be advantageous when esophageal reconstruction is planned, although it precludes effective, orthograde cleansing of the large bowel as a prelude to colon replacement of the esophagus. With the catheter techniques and nutrient solutions currently available, it is possible to maintain prolonged intravenous nutritional support in both the hospital and home settings [19]. However, the high material costs and the exigencies of caring for the infusion system limit use of this method to cases where resumption of oral feedings is anticipated within a few weeks. Conventional feeding fistulas as well as needle gastrostomy or jejunostomy [14] necessitate laparotomy. The technique that is best in terms of nutritional physiology and is least disturbing to the stomach and bowel [9] involves the continuous infusion of an oligopeptide solution by a portable pump through a needle jejunostomy, but again the costs are high. An apparently good technique for mananaging patients with a malignant stricture that is nonresectable and prevents the placement of an endoesophageal tube involves the use of an extracorporeal bypass tube connecting a cervical stoma with a gastrostomy (see 2.4). The patient is still able to eat normally, and this is considered a major psychological benefit. Our standard procedure for reconstructing the esophagus after a carcinoma resection is to perform a esophagogastrostomy in the same sitting, thereby eliminating the problem of a feeding fistula. If this cannot be done for anatomic reasons (e.g., a prior gastric resection) or if the esophageal reconstruction is performed for benign disease, we utilize the colon or jejunum so that a gastrostomy will not interfere with further procedures [23]. We no longer recognize any indications for a conventional jejunostomy.

2.3.2 *Parenteral Nutrution*

In-hospital parenteral nutrition is administered through a central venous catheter that is inserted into the superior vena cava via the internal jugular vein or subclavian vein. The infusion solutions and infusion schedule follow standard recommendations for the preoperative and postoperative period (see Chap. C). If the patient is to be discharged home during the interval between defunctionalization and reconstruction of the esophagus, we implant [11] a Silastic catheter (Fig. 27 a) of the type described by Broviac et al. [3].

Preoperative preparation: No special preparation.

Instruments: Broviac Silastic catheter, peel-away introducer, image intensifier, scalpel, long clamp.

Position and approach: Supine with the arms adducted. The head of the operating table is tilted downward to improve venous filling. We prefer the subclavian vein for access, inserting the needle at the inferior border of the midpoint of the clavicle.

Fig. 27 a–d. Placement of a Broviac catheter for home parenteral nutrition. **a** The Broviac catheter: *a* intravascular segment, *b* Dacron cuff, *c* extravascular segment with connector. **b** The subclavian vein is punctured below the left clavicle. **c** The Broviac catheter is passed through a subcutaneous tunnel formed in the anterior chest wall. A guidewire has been previously inserted through the puncture needle into the superior vena cava. **d** The intravascular segment of the Broviac catheter is inserted into the superior vena cava through the peel-away introducer

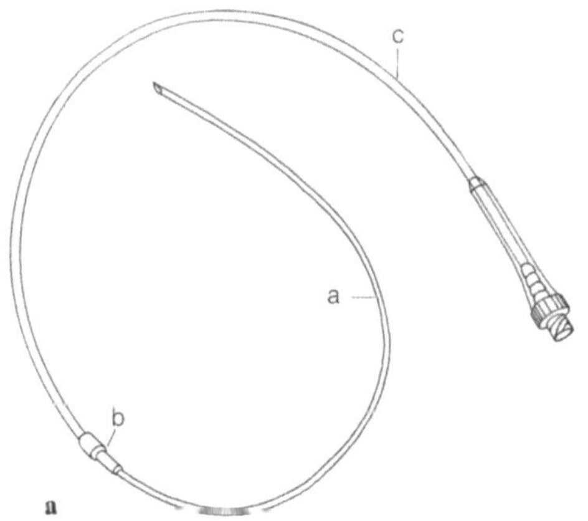

a

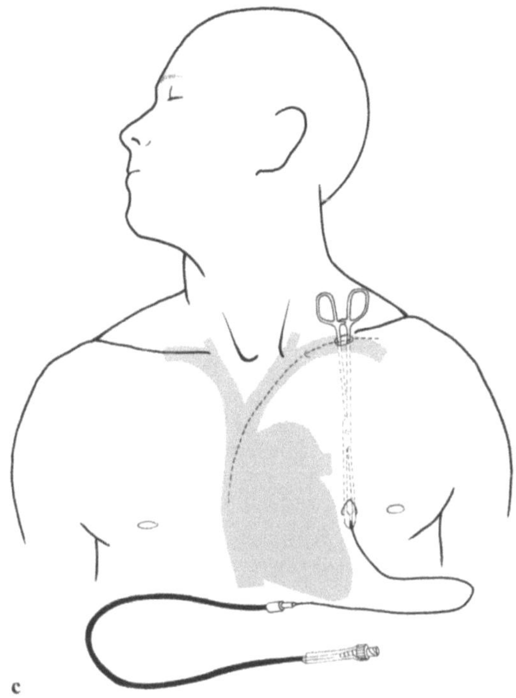

c

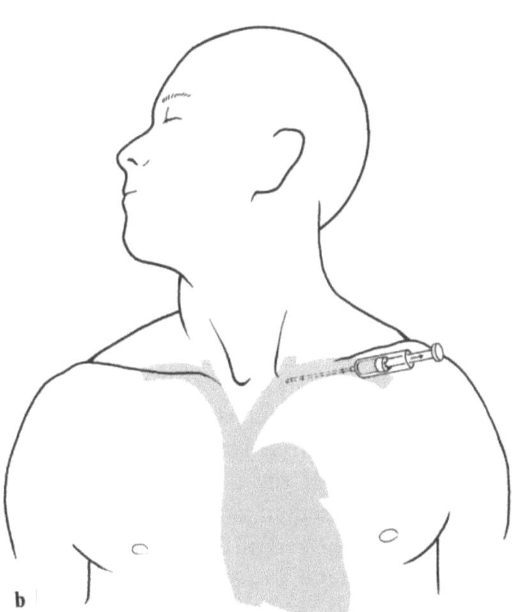

b

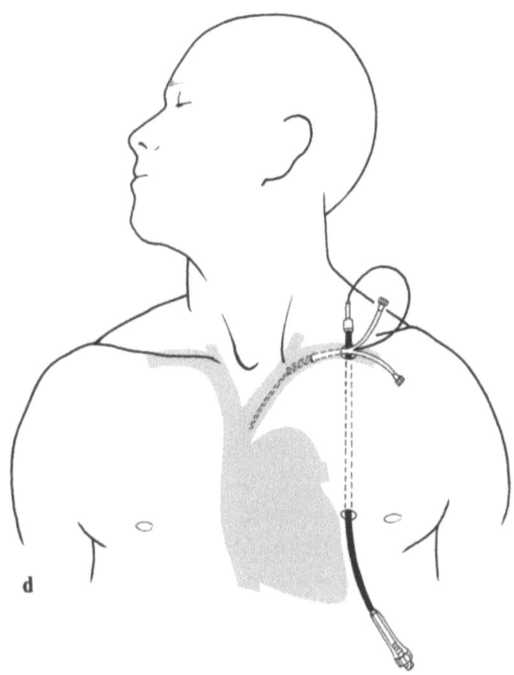

d

Technique: After the needle has pierced the skin, it is advanced along the inferior border of the clavicle toward the jugular fossa while the plunger is raised (Fig. 27 b). The aspiration of dark red blood signifies puncture of the vein. Under image intensifier control, a guide wire is passed through the needle and into the superior vena cava. The needle is removed, and about a 1-cm scalpal incision is made in the skin at the insertion site. A second incision of equal length is made between the sternum and nipple, and a long clamp is used to create a subcutaneous tunnel between the two incisions (Fig. 27 c). The venous catheter is drawn up through the tunnel until its Dacron cuff appears in the proximal opening. At that point the venous dilator in a peel-away introducer is threaded over the guide wire into the superior vena cava, and the patient is asked to perform a Valsalva maneuver. The guide wire with dilator is removed, and the intravascular segment of the Broviac catheter is inserted into the superior vena cava through the peel-away introducer (Fig. 27 d). Finally the ends of the introducer are pulled apart to split the introducer tube and extract it from the wound. Placement of the catheter tip is checked with the image intensifier and adjusted if necessary so that the tip lies just above the right atrium.

Both skin incisions are closed with simple interrupted sutures, and the catheter is secured to the skin exit site with an additional suture. On the day after catheter placement, patients are enrolled in a teaching program for home parenteral nutrition [17]. They are instructed in the techniques that will be used in caring for the catheter infusion system. After about 10 days they are able to care for themselves and can continue their nutrition at home.

2.3.3 Gastrostomy

The major difference between the various gastrostomies is in the type of connection that is established between the wall of the stomach and the skin. In the mucosa-line gastrostomy of Glassmann [6] and Deucher [5], a channel is fashioned from the gastric wall and brought out on the skin. Nutrient fluids are administered through a tube (Ch 20) that is temporarily inserted for the gastrostomy feedings. Since the tract is lined entirely by mucosa, there is no danger that it will become narrowed or obliterated when the tube is removed. Between feedings the stoma is covered with a small pad and sealed with a plastic sheet. In the Witzel [33] and Kader [10] gastrostomies, the connection between the stomach and skin is formed by a tube or Foley catheter. The fistula will close spontaneously when the tube is removed, so the tube should not be withdrawn between feedings. The Kader gastrostomy [10] is technically simple to construct. We prefer it in cases where only a temporary gastrostomy is required. Recently we abandoned use of the Witzel technique [33], described in volume VII/1 of this series.

2.3.3.1 *Kader Gastrostomy* [10]

Preoperative preparation: No special preparation.

Instruments: Basic set, Foley or de Pezzer catheter (Ch 20–24).

Position and approach: Supine position, 5-cm transrectus or upper midline laparotomy below the left costal arch.

Steps in procedure:

(1) Transrectus or upper midline abdominal incision (5 cm)
(2) Delivery of the anterior gastric wall into the wound
(3) Placement of two concentric pursestring sutures
(4) Incision of the gastric wall at the center of the sutures
(5) Insertion of a the Pezzer catheter into the gastrostomy through a separate skin incision
(6) Pursestring sutures are tightened, ends are brought out through the abdominal wall
(7) Pursestring sutures are tied over a pledget, the laparotomy is closed

Technique: Following laparotomy, a site of entry for the gastrostomy tube is selected on the wall of the stomach at the junction of the body and fundus. That site is grasped with an Ellis clamp and pulled into the wound. Two concentric pursestring sutures of nonabsorbable monofilament material (inside diameter 5–6 mm) are placed around the entrance site with their free ends on opposite sides (Fig. 28 a). A pair of temporary pullout sutures are placed opposite the thread ends. Traction is placed on the sutures to aid incision of the gastric wall with the electrocautery and lessen the danger of cutting the pursestring sutures (Fig. 28 b). The gastric contents are aspirated, mucosal bleeding points are carefully controlled, and the Foley or the Pezzer catheter is inserted into the stomach. The pursestring sutures are immediately tightened after removal of the traction threads. The ends of the pursestring sutures are not cut, but are used to fix the stomach to the abdominal wall. The end of the catheter is brought out through a lateral incision separate from the laparotomy wound (Fig. 28 c). The ends of both pursestring sutures are passed through the abdom-

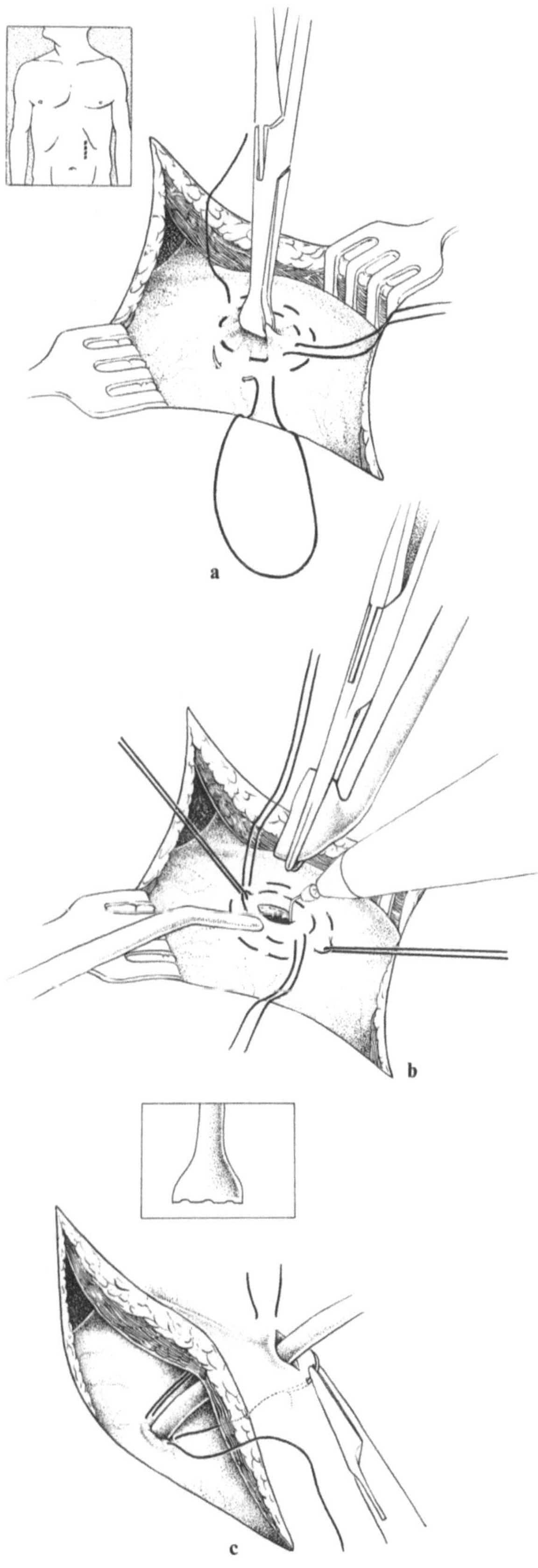

a

b

c

Fig. 28 a–c. Construction of a Kader gastrostomy [10]. **a** High transrectus laparotomy. The anterior gastric wall is grasped with an Ellis forceps, and two concentric pursestring sutures are applied. **b** The stomach is opened within the pursestring sutures, which are made tense by traction sutures. **c** A cut de Pezzer catheter is introduced (insert) into the stomach through a separate skin incision. The catheter is secured with the pursestring sutures, and the gastrostomy site is fixed with the ends of the sutures to the anterior abdominal wall

inal wall on large needles and tied over small pledgets. If the Foley or the Pezzer catheter is additionally secured to the skin under slight tension with a suture or adhesive tape, the gastric wall will fuse to the peritoneum and form a watertight seal. The laparotomy incision is closed. The catheter will serve to decompress and drain the stomach until peristalsis resumes. It can then be used as a portal for feeding.

The untied threads within the abdomen may be removed in eight to ten days. If the catheter is left in place for at least ten days before it is changed, there is no need to fear retraction of the stomach wall with leakage of gastric juice into the peritoneal cavity. A constant, slight tension on the Foley or the Pezzer catheter will ensure that contact is maintained between the stomach and peritoneum and also will prevent maceration of the skin by constant leakage of gastric juice between the tube and gastrostomy.

2.3.3.2 Gastrostomy of Glassmann [6] *and Deucher* [5]

Preoperative preparation: No special preparation.

Instruments: Basic set, catheter (Ch 16 to 20).

Position and approach: Supine position; 10-cm upper abdominal transrectus incision below the left costal arch.

Technique: After incision of the abdomen, the anterior wall of the stomach is grasped with an Ellis clamp and pulled into a cone-shaped pouch whose length approximately equals the thickness of the abdominal wall. Deucher [5] fashions the gastric pouch with two concentric pursestring sutures, and Glassmann [6] with three concentric sutures (inside diameter 2 cm) spaced about 1 cm apart (nonabsorbable monofilament material) (Fig. 29 a). These sutures are tightened until the lumen of the pouch is constricted but can still accommodate a Ch 16–20 catheter. When the pursestring sutures are placed, care is taken to pass the needle beneath all visible arteries and veins of the gastric wall to ensure that the pouch will not become necrotic and slough. In Glass-

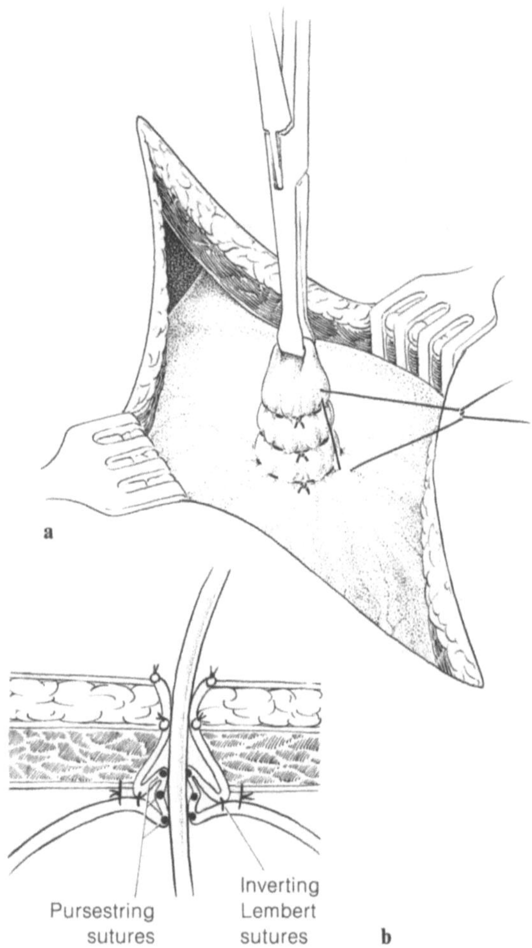

Fig. 29 a, b. Glassmann's gastrostomy [6]. **a** A gastric pouch is formed by means of three concentric pursestring sutures. Inverting sutures are then placed to transform the pouch into a valve. **b** Cross-section through the completed valve

mann's technique [6], Lembert sutures are placed in the gastric wall below the three pursestring sutures and into the wall of the newly formed "diverticulum" above the pursestring sutures. When the Lembert sutures are tied, a circular valve is formed at the base of the gastric pouch (Fig. 29 b). Deucher [5] sutures the "diverticulum" to the skin right away. The first row of interrupted sutures engages the peritoneum, the posterior rectus sheath, and the stomach at the level of the lowest pursestring suture. The second suture line fixes the anterior rectus sheath to the greatest diameter of the gastric pouch. The outermost row of sutures unites the skin and stomach wall so that the tip of the gastric pouch is exposed over an area about 1 cm wide.

After 48 h the tip of the pouch is opened with an electrocautery, the catheter is passed into the stomach, and feeding can be commenced.

2.3.3.3 Needle Gastrostomy or Jejunostomy

Preoperative preparation: No special preparation.

Instruments: Basic set, Jejunocath set (Fig. 30 a).

Position and approach: Supine position. The gastrostomy is performed through an upper paramedian laparotomy, the jejunostomy through a midline laparotomy that starts several centimeters above the umbilicus, curves around the left side of the umbilicus, and terminates a few centimeters below it.

Steps in procedure:

(1) Midline laparotomy extended around the left side of the umbilicus
(2) Delivery of the proximal jejunum into the incision
(3) Placement of a pursestring suture on the antimesenteric bowel wall
(4) Insertion of a split needle between the seromuscular layer and mucosa (5 cm)
(5) Penetration of the mucosa
(6) Insertion of the feeding catheter, removal of the split needle
(7) Pursestring suture is tied, catheter is secured by a second seromuscular suture
(8) Fixation of the bowel wall to the anterior peritoneum
(9) Closure of the laparotomy in layers

Technique: After incision of the abdomen, an Ellis clamp is used to grasp the stomach wall close to the junction of the body and fundus or the antimesenteric wall of the small bowel just behind the ligament of Treitz and deliver it into the wound. A pursestring suture is placed, and the split needle is inserted at its center, passing through the seromuscular layer but keeping above the mucosa. A blunt stylet is introduced through the needle and projects slightly beyond its tip; this stylet protects the mucosa from injury as the needle is tunneled between the seromuscular layer and mucosa for about 5 cm (Fig. 30 b). The stylet is withdrawn, and the sharp needle is advanced through the mucosa. Then the catheter is passed through the needle into the lumen of the jejunum. At that point the catheter is flushed with 10 ml of physiologic saline solution to confirm that it has entered the lumen. The steel needle is withdrawn and split

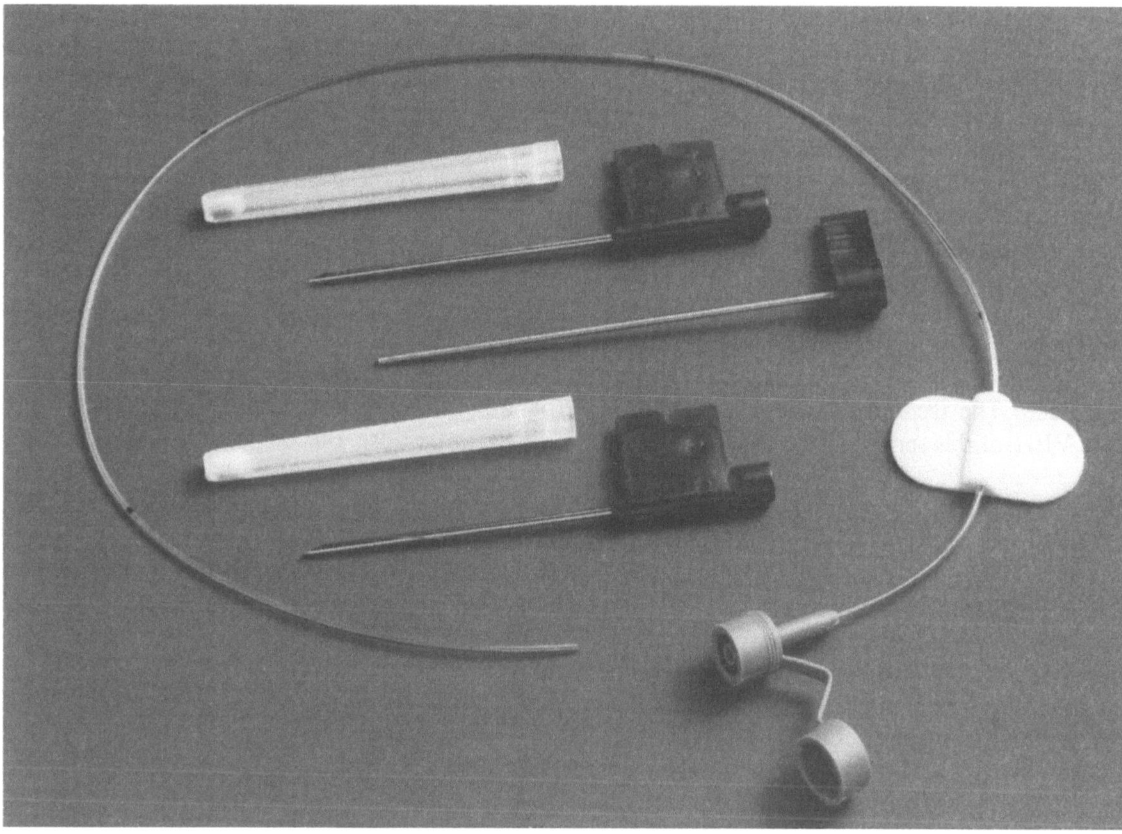

a

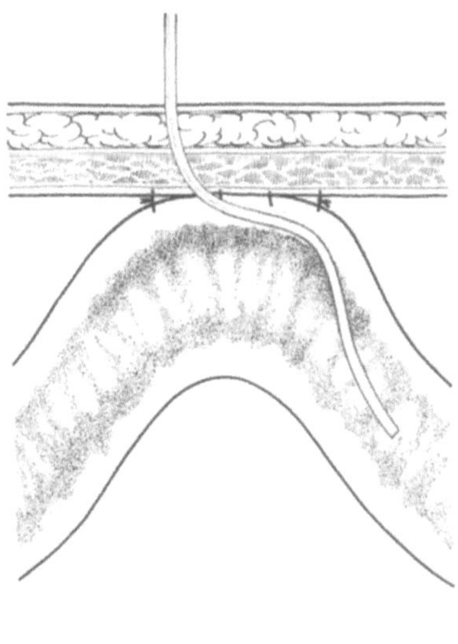

b

Fig. 30 a, b. Needle gastrostomy or jejunostomy. **a** Jejunocath set: 1. split needles, 2. trocar, 3. jejunostomy catheter with means for fixation. **b** Cross-section through the needle jejunostomy. The long intramural course of the feeding tube prevents the escape of intestinal secretions

apart as it is removed. The pursestring suture is tightened and tied so that the gastric or jejunal wall envelops the catheter snugly. The catheter is further secured with a second seromuscular suture placed 1–2 cm from the pursestring suture. Both these sutures, possibly augmented by one or two additional sutures, serve to fix the gastric or bowel wall to the peritoneum of the anterior abdominal wall after the catheter has been brought out through an incision separate from the original laparotomy. The skin wound is closed, and the catheter is additionally secured by one or two cutaneous sutures.

The disadvantages of this method are that only thin nutrient solutions may be administered, and the catheter cannot be changed because of its intramural placement. An advantage is that intestinal secretions cannot escape to the skin along the catheter, nor can they leak into the peritoneal cavity.

2.3.4 Conventional Jejunostomy

The jejunostomy can be constructed in the fashion of a Witzel [33] or Kader gastrostomy [10] or by using an isolated loop of jejunum as described by Maydl [13]. For the past few years, we have had no occasion to perform a conventional jejunostomy in our patients. It might be appropriate in the case of an extensive cardia carcinoma where there is concern about tumor ingrowth into a gastrostomy, or as a means of avoiding gastrostomy prior to a staged esophageal reconstruction using the stomach. The technique is described fully in volume VII/1 of this series.

2.4 Extracorporeal Bypass Tube

The major advantage of an extracorporeal tube connecting a cervical esophagostomy with a gastrostomy [2, 21] is that it permits feeding by the oral route. For psychological reasons, it is best not to impose dietary restrictions; adequate nutrition is ensured by feeding concentrated solutions directly into the gastrostomy. In the simplest type of extracorporeal esophageal replacement, a colostomy bag is glued over the cervical stoma, and the distal end of the bag is connected to the gastrostomy tube [32]. The colostomy bag must be securely attached to the cervical stoma, which must be carefully constructed, and the bag should be attached to the gastrostomy tube in a manner that prevents secretions from collecting around the tube opening. This can be done by wrapping tape tightly around the lower end of the bag and the upper end of the tube to create a funnel-shaped orifice.

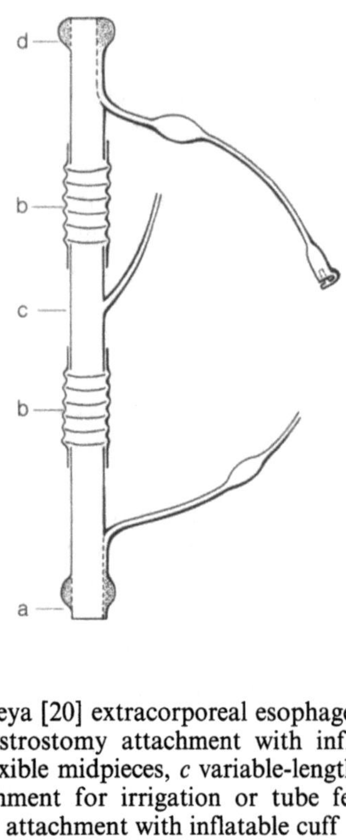

Fig. 31. The Nabeya [20] extracorporeal esophageal bypass tube. *a* Gastrostomy attachment with inflatable rubber cuff, *b* flexible midpieces, *c* variable-length midpiece with attachment for irrigation or tube feeding, *d* esophagostomy attachment with inflatable cuff

Nabeya [20] has developed an excellent design for an extracorporeal esophageal bypass tube (Fig. 31). Because the device consists of several parts, it can be individually adapted. The ends that connect to the esophagostomy and gastrostomy have inflatable cuffs to prevent leakage of saliva and gastric fluids. A T-shaped tube in the midportion of the prosthesis permits nutrient concentrates to be infused without having to remove the prosthesis.

References

1. Abbott OA, Mansour KA, Logan WD (1970) Atraumatic so-called "spontaneous rupture of the esophagus". J Thorac Cardiovasc Surg 59:67–83
2. Akiyama H (1980) Surgery for carcinoma of the esophagus. Curr Probl Surg 17:1
3. Broviac JW, Cole JJ, Scribner BH (1973) Silicone rubber atrial catheter for prolonged parenteral alimentation. Surg Gynec Obstet 136:602
4. Denecke HJ (1973) Plastische und rekonstruktive Chirurgie des Halses (Teil II). Handbuch der plastischen Chirurgie, Bd. 2. De Gruyter, Berlin New York
5. Deucher A (1967) Allgemeine und spezielle chirurgische Operationslehre Bd. VI/1 2. Aufl. Springer, Berlin Heidelberg New York
6. Glassmann JA (1939) A new aseptic double-valved tubogastrostomy. Surg Gynecol Obstet 68:789
7. Graham WP, Royster HP (1967) Simplified cervical esophagostomy for long term extraoral feeding Surg Gynec Obstet 125:127–129
8. Goyal RK, Bauer JL, Spiro HM (1971) The nature and location of lower esophageal ring. N Engl J Med 248:1175
9. Heberer M, Brandl M (1982) Sondenernährung chirurgischer Patienten. Klinische Ernährung 10:110
10. Kader B (1896) Zur Technik der Gastrostomie. Zbl Chirurgie 23:665
11. Keller HW, Müller JM, Pichlmaier H (1983) „Peel-away-introducer" – Eine Technik der Implantation von zentralen Venenkathetern für die Langzeit-parenterale Ernährung. Infusionstherapie 10:79
12. Lanz v T, Wachsmuth W (1955) Praktische Anatomie, Bd I/12. Springer, Berlin Göttingen Heidelberg

13. Maydl K (1898) Über Jejunostomie. Mitt Grenzgeb Med Chir 3:532
14. Mc Donald HA (1954) Intrajejunal drip in gastric surgery. Lancet 1:1007
15. Menguy R (1971) Near-total exclusion by cervical esophagostomy and tube gastrostomy in the management of massive esophageal perforation. Ann Surg 173:613
16. Müller JM, Pichlmaier H (in Vorber) Die gestochene zervikale Katheterfistel zur Sondenernährung. Ernährung
17. Müller JM (1982) Die parenterale Ernährung zu Hause – Ein Handbuch für Patienten – Travenol Eigenverlag
18. Müller JM, Brenner U, Dienst C, Pichlmaier H (1982) Praeoperative parenteral feeding in patients with gastrointestinal carcinoma. Lancet 1:68
19. Müller JM, Keller H, Vleeschauwer B, Schmitz M (1982) Die parenterale Ernährung von ambulanten Patienten. Klinische Ernährung 10:153
20. Nabeya K (1977) Radical operation for esophageal cancer. Ishigaku Publishers Inc, Tokyo
21. Nakayama K, Nakayama M, Kinoshita Y (1974) Erfahrungen bei der Behandlung des Ösophaguskarzinoms im oberen und mittleren thorakalen Drittel. Zentralb f Chirurgie 99:1352
22. Ong GB (1975) Unresectable oesophagus carcinoma. Ann Roy Coll Surg 56:3
23. Pichlmaier H, Müller JM, Wintzer G (1978) Ösophagusersatz. Chirurg 49:65
24. Rush BJ, Lazuaro EJ, Vaughan LH (1970) Cervical esophagostomy – a neglected operation. Arch Surg 101:145
25. Schatzki R, Gary JE (1956) The lower esophageal ring. Amer J Roentgol 75:246
26. Schroeder L, Bock JU (1978) Zur chirurgischen Problematik iatrogener Ösophagusperforationen. Langenbecks Arch Chir 346:201
27. Shamma MH, Benedict EB (1958) Esophageal web: A report of 58 cases and an attempt at classification. N Engl J Med 259:378
28. Skinner DB, Little AG, DeMeester TR (1980) Management of esophageal perforation. Am Journ Surg 139:760
29. Steichen FM, Ravitch MM (1980) Mechanical sutures in esophageal surgery. Ann Surg 191:373
30. Talbert JL, Haller JA (1965) Temporary tube pharyngostomy in the staged repair of congenital tracheoesophageal fistula. Surgery 58:738
31. Thorek P (1951) Surgical treatment of stenosis due to eosophagitis: Formation of temporary external fistula over T-tube. JAMA 147:640
32. Ware L, Garrett WS, Pickrell K (1967) Cervical esophagostomy: A simplified technic. Ann Surg 165:142
33. Witzel O (1891) Zur Technik der Magenfistelanlegung. Zbl Chir 18:601

3 Bougienage of the Esophagus

In collaboration with G. BUESS

CONTENTS

Rapid technical advances have made peroral esophageal dilatation safer, more effective, and far easier for patients to tolerate. With increasing frequency, bougienage can obviate the need for the operative treatment of esophageal strictures in patients who are poor surgical risks. Post-therapeutic strictures have increased markedly in recent years and have become an important indication for conservative dilatation therapy. These lesions include:

- strictures secondary to the sclerotherapy of esophageal varices;
- anastomotic strictures, especially after the reconstruction of esophagectomies and gastrectomies;
- rare cicatricial strictures of the lower esophagus after SPV.

Neoplastic strictures of the esophagus and gastric inlet have also become a major area of interest in dilatation therapy. Many lesions of this kind are no longer amenable to a curative operation. An attempt can be made to control dysphagia by performing bougienage at intervals, but most cases are managed by initial dilatation of the stricture with appropriate monitoring (see 3.3.1 and 3.3.2) followed by the placement of an endoesophageal tube under combined endoscopic and radiologic control.

3.1 Preparations for Bougienage

The stomach must be empty to prevent aspiration during the procedure.

3.1.1 Sedation and Anesthesia

The necessity and degree of analgesia depend on the nature of the stricture as well as on the patient's tolerance for pain and especially for the method that is used. With the Eder-Puestow system, the need for instrument changes and the potentially traumatizing surface of the instrument used to pass the dilator make the procedure difficult to tolerate. This led Manegold [5] to recommend that the Eder-Puestow system be used only under general inhalation anesthesia, although we have used it successfully under diazepam sedation (5–10 mg i.v.). Use of the newer stepped dilators obviates the need for instrument changes, and the surface of the instrument is nontraumatizing. In 500 dilatations performed to date we have not found it necessary to use general anesthesia, and some of our patients did not even require sedation.

3.1.2 Timing the Steps of the Dilatation

The initial dilation of a very tight stricture should be conducted in several steps. We space the sessions several days apart, dilating the stricture in increments of approximately 4 mm. Thus, for a high-grade stricture with a residual lumen of 4 mm, it takes about 12 days to dilate the esophagus to 16 mm. Any further dilations after that time are for the control of restricturing. We schedule a repeat dilation whenever the patient reports incipient dysphagia for solid food. At that time the stricture will still permit the passage of a small-caliber gastroscope, and we dilate to the maximum diameter of 16 mm in one sitting. The intervals between dilatations range from three weeks to three months, depending on the tendency toward restricturing.

3.1.3 Determining the Necessary Extent of the Dilatation

When a short segment of the esophagus is strictured, a patient with good masticatory function will begin to experience dysphagia when the lumen narrows to about 10 mm. Bougies up to 45 Ch (i.e., about 15 mm in diameter) are most commonly used, although dilation to 60 Ch has been reported in the Angloamerican literature. Maximum dilatation with the stepped endoscopic dilator is to 16 mm.

3.2 Postdilatation Monitoring

As in any other surgical procedure, the risk of perforation depends not just on the properties of the instrument but also on the personal experience and diligence of the operator. Because a perforation cannot be confidently excluded on the basis of clinical signs, additional monitoring is needed. After dilatation with the Eder-Puestow system, swallowing ability should always be assessed by giving the patient a water-soluble X-ray contrast medium. When using a method that is endoscopically controlled, we limit our monitoring to that control and give water-soluble contrast medium only after the initial dilatation. If endoscopy shows evidence of a perforation, this should be checked by placing the patient in a head-down posture and testing for contrast leakage, perhaps with the simultaneous administration of buscopan.

3.3 Systems for Bougienage

3.3.1 Guidewire Systems Adapted for Use with a Flexible Endoscope and Radiologic Monitoring

In these methods the stricture is visualized through a flexible endoscope, and the flexible tip of a guidewire is passed into the stricture under vision. Once the wire has traversed the proximal part of the stricture, its tip cannot be visualized, and the rest of the procedure can no longer be monitored endoscopically; it must be conducted under fluoroscopic control. Close monitoring is needed to avoid kinking or looping of the guidewire, which is a common source of complications.

3.3.1.1 The Eder-Puestow System [6]

Preparation: See 3.1.

Instruments: The metal olive dilator is introduced over a long steel wire with an atraumatically shaped metal spring at its tip (Fig. 32). The spring is 1.5 mm in diameter and will fit through the biopsy channel of a standard endoscope. The metal olives have a polished surface that glides easily through the esophagus and come in 13 sizes ranging from 7 to 15 mm in diameter. The guide rod is a semiflexible metal spring that permits straight insertion of the dilator, but its spiral surface can traumatize tissues. The distal end of the guide rod consists of a short tapered spring. The components of the system are interconnected by screw threads (Fig. 32).

Position: Facilities must be available for conducting endoscopy and fluoroscopy concurrently. The dilatation may be performed in the endoscopic unit when a portable C-arm fluoroscope is available. The endoscope is then introduced with the patient positioned on his left side. When an X-ray table is used, the patient is positioned supine. In that case particular care must be taken to prevent aspiration.

Steps in procedure:

(1) Endoscopic evaluation of the esophagus
(2) Insertion of a guidewire under combined endoscopic and radiologic control
(3) Removal of the endoscope and dilatation of the stricture with metal olives of increasing size passed over the indwelling guide rod under continuous radiologic control
(4) Endoscopic inspection of the dilated area

Technique: The stricture is visualized with an endoscope. If the lesion can be negotiated with small-caliber instruments, the guidewire is passed into the stomach under endoscopic control. If the lesion is impassable, the guidewire is advanced into

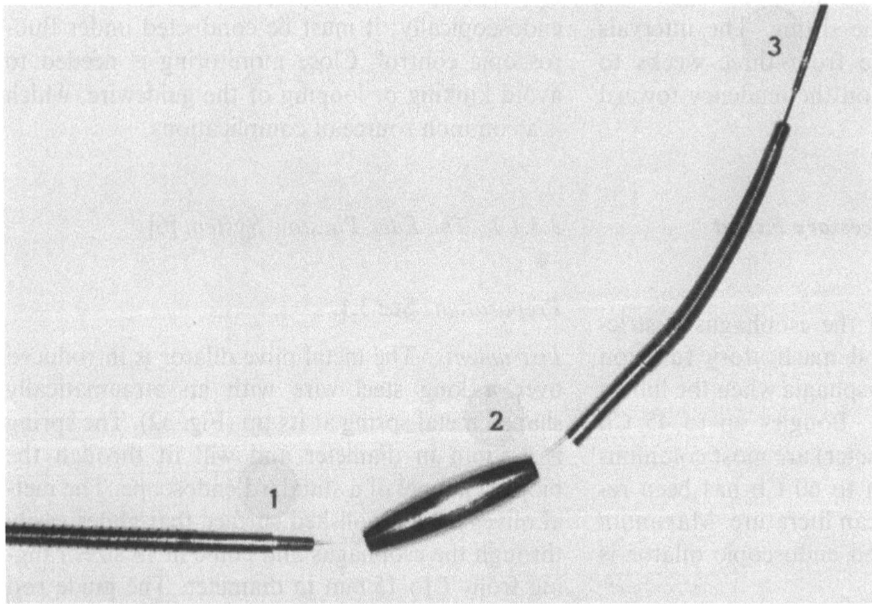

Fig. 32. Dilating portion of the Eder-Puestow system: *1* end of the guide rod, *2* metal olive dilator, *3* distal end of the guide rod and (at far right) the tip of the guidewire

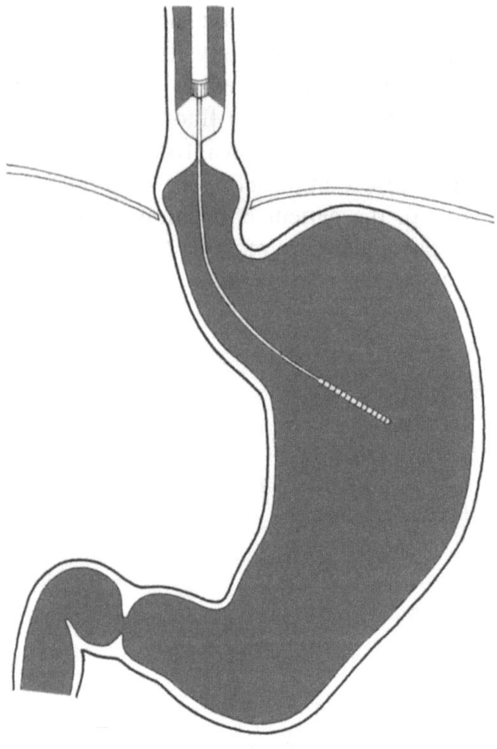

Fig. 33. The stricture is visualized through the endoscope, and the guidewire is passed into it. The advance of the guidewire beyond that point is monitored radiologically

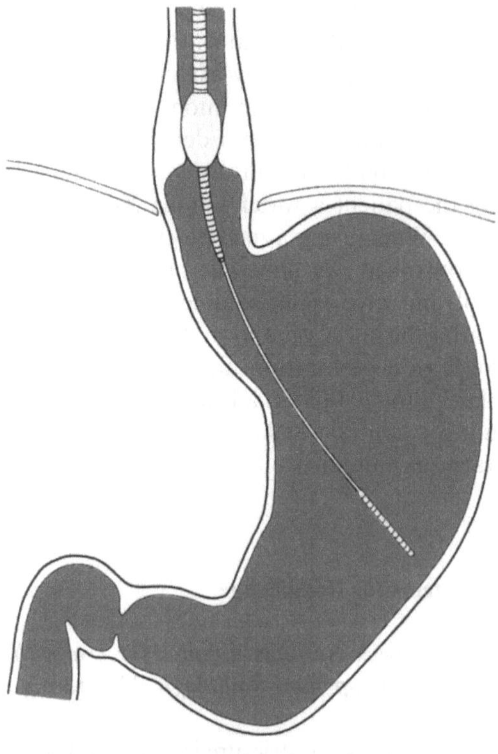

Fig. 34. The stricture is dilated with olives of increasing size under radiologic control

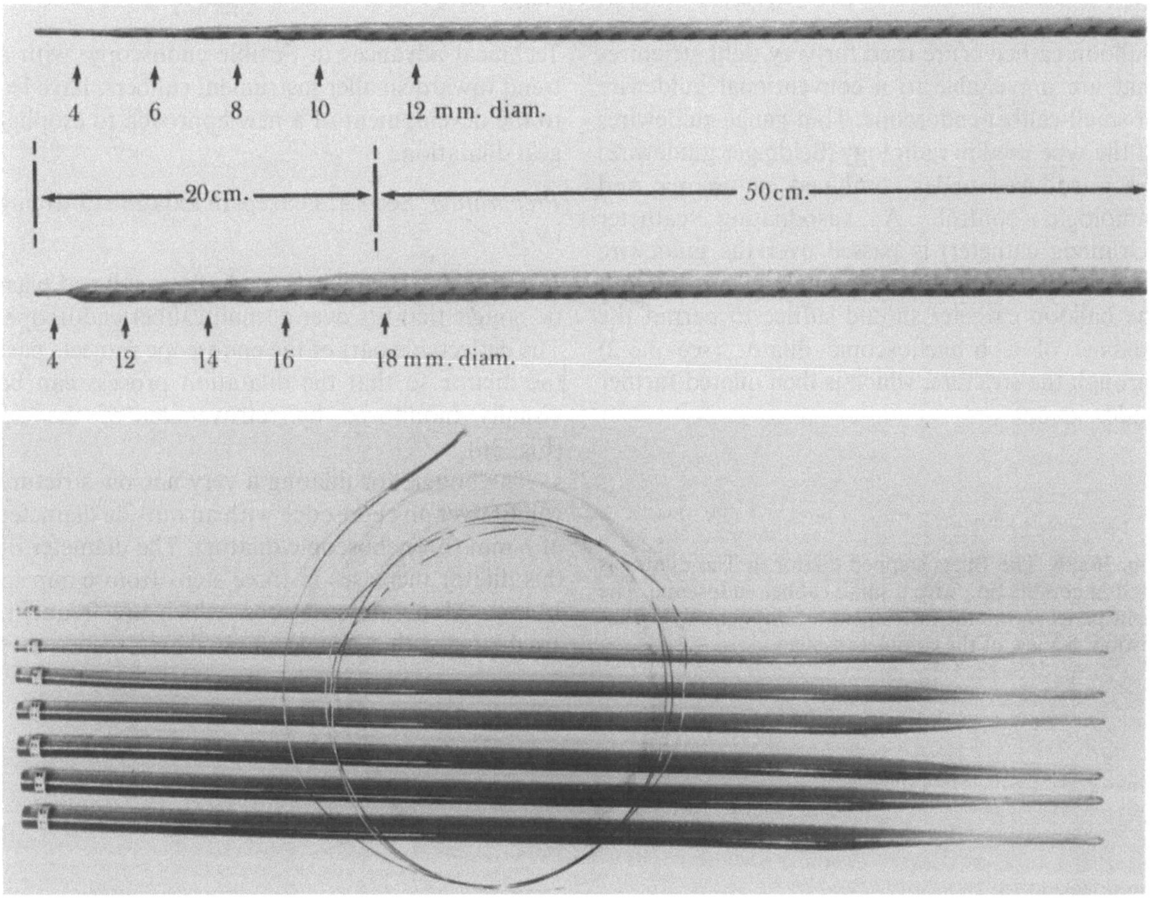

a
b

Fig. 35a, b. The Celestin and Savary plastic dilators and guidewires. **a** The Celestin stepped dilator, **b** the Savary system

the stricture under endoscopic vision, and further insertion of the instrument is monitored radiologically (Fig. 33). Once the tip of the guidewire has reached the gastric outlet, the endoscope may be withdrawn. The guidewire must be held firmly in place at this time so that it will not ride upward past the stricture. Dilatation is begun with the smallest dilator that is accepted. As the olive is introduced perorally on its flexible carrier, care is taken not to injure the teeth, lips, or corners of the mouth. This is done most effectively by using a bite ring of the type used in endoscopy or by guiding the instrument through the oral cavity with two fingers. Once the dilator enters the upper esophagus, its progress is monitored radiologically (Fig. 34). An assistant, braced against the operator's shoulder, holds the guidewire steady to keep it from displacing as the dilator is advanced. The dilatation is completed when the desired olive diameter is reached.

3.3.1.2 The Celestin and Savary Systems

Celestin [4] uses two plastic dilators whose diameters increase in steps from the leading end to the main shaft. The first dilator covers the range of 4–12 mm, the second 4–18 mm, each in 5 increments (Fig. 35). Advantages are the atraumatic surface of the instrument and fewer instrument changes. The dilators are passed over a guidewire introduced through an endoscope under radiologic control. The system of Savary [7] is similar to the Eder-Puestow system (see 3.3.1.1): dilators of increasing size are passed into the esophagus over a wire guide. Frequent instrument changes are necessary, but the procedure is less traumatizing owing to the atraumatic surface of the bougies (Fig. 35).

3.3.1.3 Balloon Catheter Systems

Balloon catheters are used for very tight strictures that are impassable to a conventional guidewire or small-caliber endoscope. Thin-gauge guidewires of the type used in radiology (Seldinger guidewire) are introduced under combined endoscopic and radiologic control. A vasodilating catheter (Grüntzig catheter) is passed over the guidewire under radiologic control. A single dilatation with the balloon catheter should suffice to permit the passage of a bronchoscopic dilator (see 3.3.2) through the stricture, which is then dilated further under vision.

Fig. 36a, b. The Buess stepped dilator. **a** The dilator is used in conjunction with a small-caliber endoscope. The right panel shows the instrument assembly ready for insertion. **b** View of the complete system

3.3.2 ***The Buess System*** [1–3]

Technical advances in flexible endoscopy, with a trend toward smaller instrument calibers, have led to the development of a new approach to esophageal dilatation.

Preparation: See 3.1. Diazepam sedation (5–10 mg i.v.).

Instruments: The dilator is a hollow, stepped plastic bougie that fits over a small-caliber endoscope. The deflectable part of the endoscope projects past the dilator so that the dilatation process can be visually monitored by retroversion of the tip (Fig. 36).

The bougie for dilating a very narrow stricture will fit over an endoscope with an outside diameter of 6 mm (bronchoscopic dilator). The diameter of this dilator increases in three steps from 6 mm to 14 mm. Moderate strictures, which are frequent, are dilated with a bougie whose diameter increases

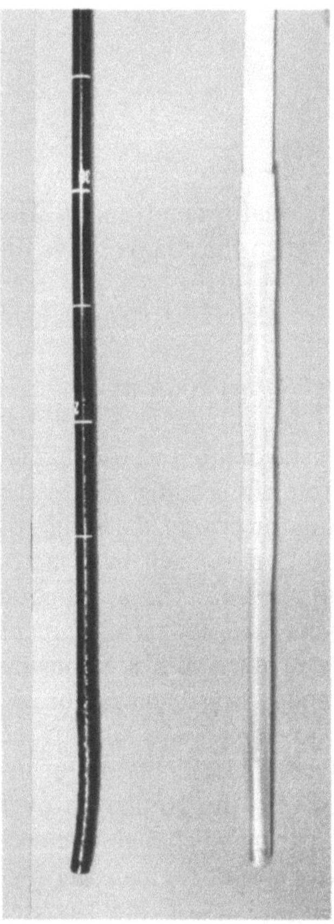
a

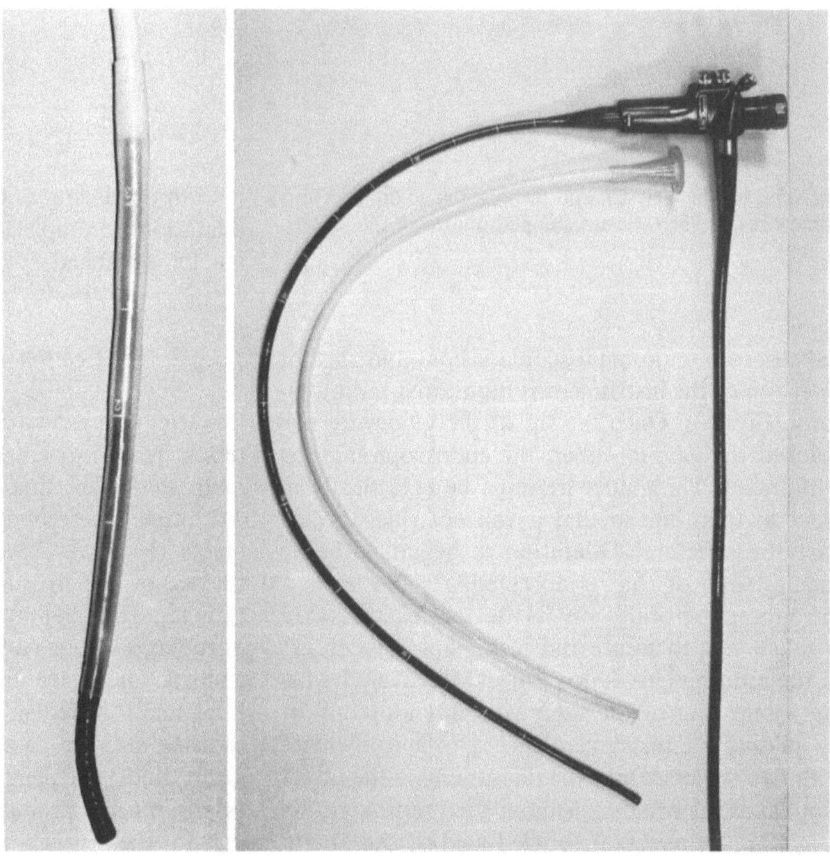
b

in 4 steps from 9 mm distally to 16 mm at the shaft. This device can be used in conjunction with most pediatric endoscopes.

Position: Left lateral.

Steps in procedure:

(1) Insertion of the endoscope-dilator assembly into the esophagus
(2) Passage of the assembly through the stricture under endoscopic control
(3) Dilatation by simple distal advancement of the dilator assembly
(4) Endoscopic evaluation of the stricture during withdrawal of the scope

Technique: The procedure is similar to that for standard endoscopy of the upper gastrointestinal tract.

With the patient on his left side, the dilator-endoscope assembly is introduced perorally under the protection of a bite ring, and the upper esophagus is evaluated. The endoscope is advanced to the stricture under vision. Air insufflation is helpful in delineating tortuosities, even in long strictures, which are negotiated by carefully advancing the instrument under vision and deflecting its tip. This technique eliminates the danger of perforation (Fig. 37). After the deflectable part of the endoscope has passed through the stricture, the actual dilatation process is begun. The lumen of the hollow viscus is observed continuously as the dilator is advanced. At this stage the operator must guide the instrument himself so that he can assess the resistance to dilation and control the advance of the bougie. With suitably equipped endoscopes, the dilatation process can be directly monitored by the retroversion maneuver (Fig. 38). On completion of the dilatation, the hollow viscus and the dilated area are evaluated as the instrument is withdrawn. Both of the stepped dilators are designed to eliminate the need for instrument changes during a single session. The atraumatic instrument surface and lack of radiation exposure are additional factors that minimize patient discomfort. Sedation may not even be required. In the rare cases where strictures are too tight to admit a small-caliber endoscope, we begin the dilatation with a balloon catheter passed over a Seldinger guidewire (see 3.3.1.3). Invariably, we are able to pass the endoscopic bougie after this initial dilatation.

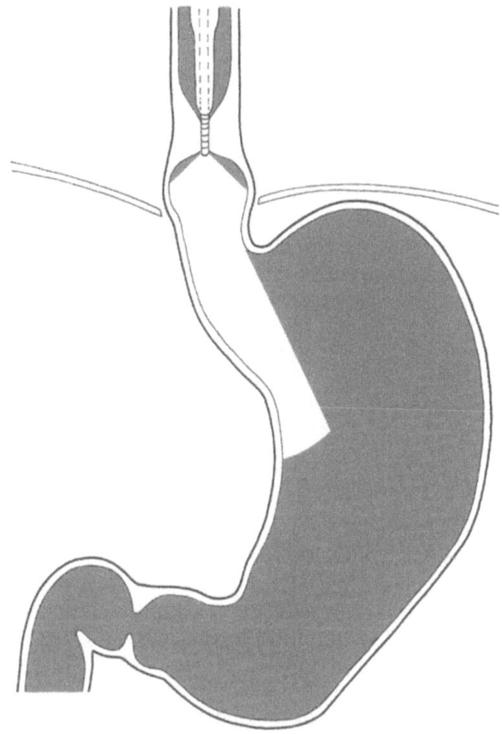

Fig. 37. Bougienage with the endoscopic stepped dilator: The deflectable tip of the endoscope negotiates the stricture

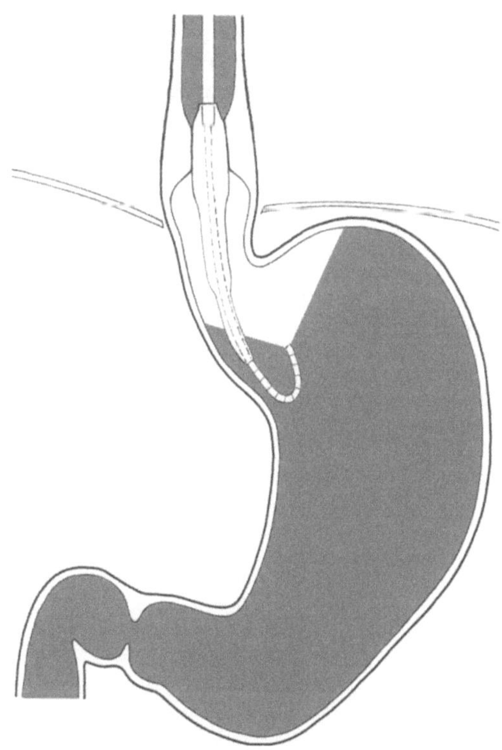

Fig. 38. The stricture is dilated simply by advancing the assembly. The dilatation can be monitored by retroversion of the endoscope tip

3.3.3 Bougienage Using a Rigid Endoscope

Long before the introduction of flexible endoscopy, rigid endoscopes were used to visualize esophageal strictures, guide the insertion of Chevalier-Jackson type bougies, and dilate the stricture under endoscopic vision, to the degree permitted by the inside diameter of the rigid scope. Generally these techniques cannot be tolerated without general anesthesia, so they have been largely abandoned in favor of systems adapted for use with flexible endoscopes. However, strictures involving the upper esophagus are difficult to visualize with a fiberoptic endoscope, and use of a rigid endoscope in conjunction with the Chevalier-Jackson dilator or Eder-Puestow system can be an effective solution in these cases.

3.3.4 Blind Dilatation

3.3.4.1 Plastic and Rubber Dilators

Instruments: In contrast to the bougienage systems described thus far, dilatation with conventional plastic and rubber bougies is not subject to external control by an operator. The dilators are introduced while the patient is seated, and the patient is told to swallow. Since the path of the instrument tip cannot be directly visualized, only minimal pressure may be applied to push it through the esophagus. If the stricture is severe or if there is angulation or pocketing, the contours of the lesion can be visualized radiologically by administering a water-soluble contrast medium. This allows for safer insertion of the dilator under fluoroscopic control. We feel today that blind bougienage is appropriate only for the self-dilation of recurring stenoses that require frequent retreatments.

3.3.4.2 Dilators with Mercury-Filled Tips

The mercury-filled tip enables the leading end of the dilator to conform better to the shape of the passageway, and the heavier tip is believed to make the dilatation less traumatizing. Today the applications of these dilators are limited to the same types of cases that are managed with rubber bougies.

References

1. Buess G, Thon J, Hutterer F (1983) A multiple-diameter bougie fitted over a small-caliber fiberscope. Endoscopy 15
2. Buess G, Keller HW (1983) Therapie schwerer Schluckstörungen nach proximal gastrischer Vagotomie. Chirurg 54
3. Buess G, Thon J, Eitenmüller J, Schellong H, Hildebrand E, Hutterer F (1983) The endoscopic multiple-diameter bougie – clinical results after one year of application. Endoscopy 15:337
4. Celestin LR, Campbell WB (1981) A new and safe system for oesophageal dilation. Lancet 1:74
5. Manegold BC (1982) Diagnostik und Differentialtherapie der benignen Ösophagusstenosen. Internist 23:257
6. Puestow KL (1955) Conservative treatment of stenosing diseases of esophagus. Postgrad Med 18:6
7. Savary M, Miller G (1977) Der Oesophagus: Lehrbuch und endoskopischer Atlas. Solothurn: Gaumann

4 Plastic Procedures for the Repair of Esophageal Strictures

CONTENTS

4.1 Indications

Plastic procedures are indicated for the repair of severe, fixed, benign esophageal strictures no more than 8 cm in length that are nondilatable or not adequately dilatable by bougienage. It should be emphasized, however, that endoscopic or open transgastric dilatation under vision, possibly combined with an antireflux procedure, will be successful in the majority of patients. It should also be noted that segmental resection of the esophagus and reconstruction with interposed bowel can be performed for strictures at any level and offers an alternative to the procedures described below. For long strictures and strictures caused by systemic diseases such as scleroderma, we prefer primary resection and replacement with small intestine or colon.

4.2 Plastic Repair of Cervical Esophageal Strictures

4.2.1 Repair by Longitudinal Incision and Transverse Closure

Very short strictures can be widened by incising the affected area longitudinally and closing it transversely as in the Heineke-Mikulicz pyloroplasty [13]. The procedure is applicable at any level of the esophagus, although, if used at all, it should be limited to the cervical portion. This is because it is very rarely possible to achieve a tension-free closure of the esophagotomy. While suture line leak in the cervical esophagus usually can be managed without difficulty, and fistulas developing in that area tend to close spontaneously, an intraabdominal or intrathoracic leak is a potentially life-threatening complication.

Preoperative preparation: Prophylactic antibiotics (see Chap. C).

Instruments: Basic set, stomach tube (Ch 32).

Incision: Along the anterior border of the sternocleidomastoid muscle, or the unilateral Kocher collar incision (see 2.1.1).

Operative technique: The esophagus is exposed and snared (see 2.1.1). It can be mobilized further, and some additional length gained, by blunt dissection past the thoracic inlet. The strictured area is identified. If the location of the stricture is uncertain, the stomach tube may be advanced to the stricture or the lesion localized with a flexible esophagogastroscope. The affected area is incised longitudinally between two traction sutures (Fig. 39 a). The sutures are pulled taut so that the extent of the stricture can be determined. If it is found that the stricture is longer than 1 cm, the original plan for transverse closure should be abandoned, and one of the procedures described below should be employed. If the length of the stricture does not exceed 1 cm, the incision is extended for 1–2 cm above and below the lesion. Then the stomach tube is advanced down past the level of the incision to prevent narrowing while the sutures are placed. The transverse closure is performed with two rows of simple interrupted sutures (Fig. 39 b).

The integrity of the closure is tested by instillation of methylene blue solution. A Penrose drain is placed at the site of the esophagotomy, and the wound is closed in layers.

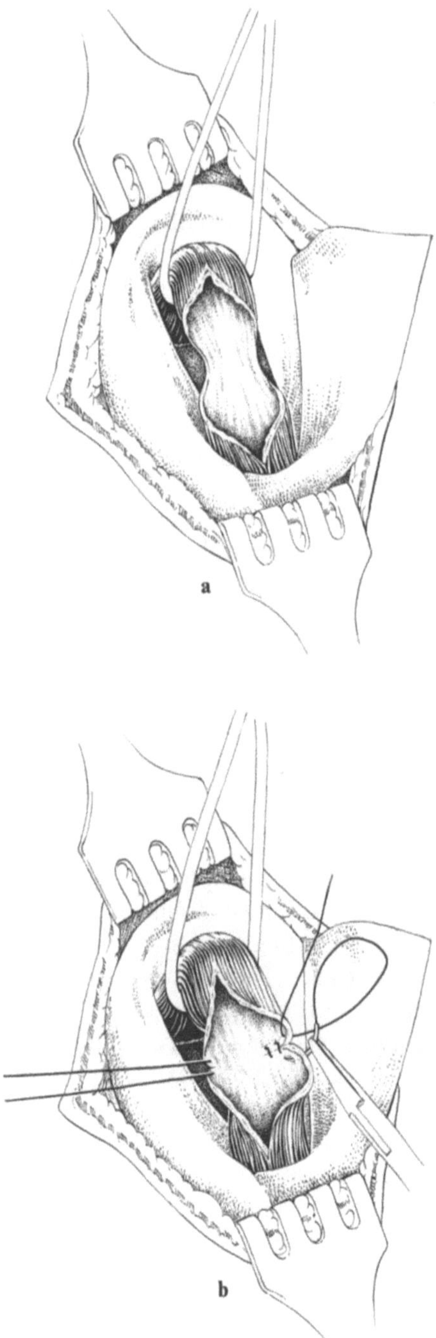

Fig. 39 a, b. Plastic repair of an esophageal stricture. **a** The stricture is opened longitudinally. **b** The incision is closed transversely. The initial sutures for widening the posterior wall of the esophagus are placed from inside the lumen

4.2.2 Free Jejunal Patch [16]

Seidenberg [19] in 1957 was the first to replace the resected cervical esophagus with a free, tubular segment of transplanted jejunum. Due to problems with thrombosis of the arterial or venous limb of the graft, few surgeons in later years were successful with the free transplantation of segments of the stomach [8], jejunum [15, 17, 18], or colon [2, 14] for reconstruction of the cervical esophagus. With advances in microvascular surgery, free jejunal transfer in particular has assumed major importance for cervical esophageal replacement in the last 10 years, and it appears to be supplanting older techniques such as the antethoracic skin tube [1, 6, 12, 24].

Some years ago we came to believe that benign strictures of the cervical and upper thoracic esophagus could be managed by a lesser procedure than segmental esophagectomy and replacement with a free transplant. This prompted us, in 1970, to widen a strictured cervical esophagus by the transfer of a free jejunal patch [16]. This procedure offers the significant advantages of preserving esophageal continuity and avoiding vagotomy. Since the vascular supply of the esophagus is not disturbed, the danger of suture line leak is less with the jejunal patch than with an interposed intestinal tube.

Preoperative preparation: Prophylactic antibiotics, intestinal lavage (see Chap. C).

Instruments: Basic set, microsurgical set, operating microscope or optical loupe, stomach tube (Ch 32), cooled Collins' solution (optional).

Position and approach: The esophagus is exposed through an incision along the anterior border of the sternocleidomastoid muscle (see 2.1.1). The graft is obtained through a left paramedian midabdominal incision 6–8 cm long.

Operative technique: A two-team approach is recommended to shorten the operating time. While one team removes the graft, the other team exposes the esophagus.

The jejunal patch is obtained by opening the abdomen and identifying the jejunum at the ligament of Treitz. A large branch of the superior mesenteric artery is consistently found at the first or second loop of jejunum and will serve as the vascular pedicle for the graft. The vascular supply of the jejunum is inspected by transillumination until about a 4- to 6-cm long segment of bowel is identi-

Steps in procedure:

(1) Identification of a suitable jejunal segment using transillumination
(2) Dissection of the vascular pedicle
(3) Removal of the jejunal segment with the GIA instrument and division of the vascular pedicle an adequate distance from the bowel
(4) Reanastomosis of the jejunum and closure of the mesenteric incision
(5) Exposure of the esophagus in the neck (see 2.1.1)
(6) Dissection of the donor vessels
(7) Longitudinal incision of the esophageal stricture
(8) Adaptation of the jejunal patch and its pedicle
(9) Vascular anastomoses
(10) Attachment of the patch graft with two layers of sutures
(11) Drain insertion

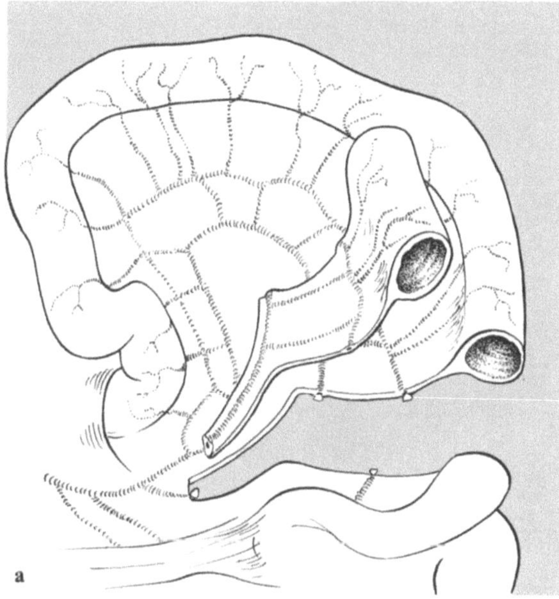

a

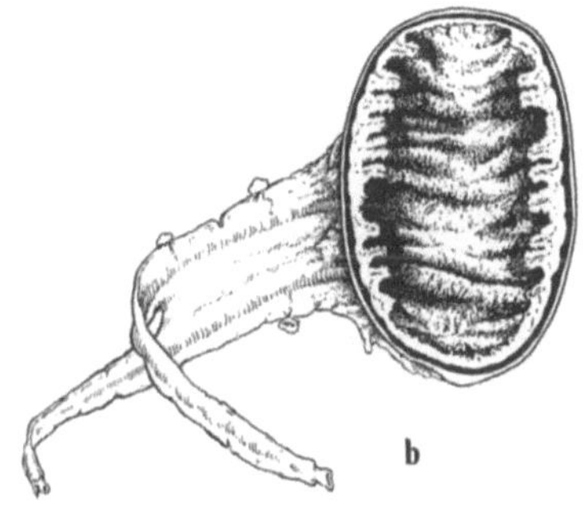

b

Fig. 40a, b. Free jejunal patch for widening the strictured cervical esophagus. **a** A jejunal segment with a satisfactory vascular supply is removed. **b** The patch ready for grafting to the esophagus

fied whose marginal arcade is supplied by an artery of substantial size and is drained by an adequate accompanying vein (Fig. 40 a). The mesentery is incised with a scalpel about 0.5 cm from the nutrient vessels on each side, carrying the incision close to the bowel wall; the arcades are divided between ligatures. The adjacent bowel wall is dissected free from the mesentery, and the jejunal segment is mobilized by trasecting the jejunum in line with the mesenteric incisions using the GIA instrument. The vascular pedicle is followed toward the mesenteric artery and is isolated just above its junction with the parent vessel. The artery and vein of the vascular pedicle are openly divided and the central stumps ligated. While intestinal continuity is restored by end-to-end anastomosis and the mesenteric incision and abdomen are closed, the patch is prepared for transplantation. Both rows of GIA staples are cut from the graft, and the segment is opened on its antimesenteric side (Fig. 40 b). The mucosa is cleaned with cooled Ringer's solution containing a dissolved antibiotic. The artery may be flushed with cooled Collins' solution, though this is not essential. Even without cold perfusion and storage, the bowel segment will tolerate ischemia for up to 3 h at room temperature.

During or after removal of the graft, the cervical esophagus is exposed while carefully preserving the artery and vein that will serve as donor vessels (see 2.1.1). The artery of the graft may be anastomosed end-to-end to the superior or inferior thyroid artery, lingular artery or maxillary artery, or side-to-end to the external carotid. Because we prefer to perform end-to-end anastomoses between arteries having like diameters and wall thicknesses, and the inferior thyroid artery is a major supplier of the cervical esophagus, we generally use the superior thyroid artery as the donor, although the choice will ultimately depend on anatomic factors. The selected vessel is snared with a small rubber tape, and a segment 1–2 cm long is dissected free (Fig. 41 a). The peripheral part

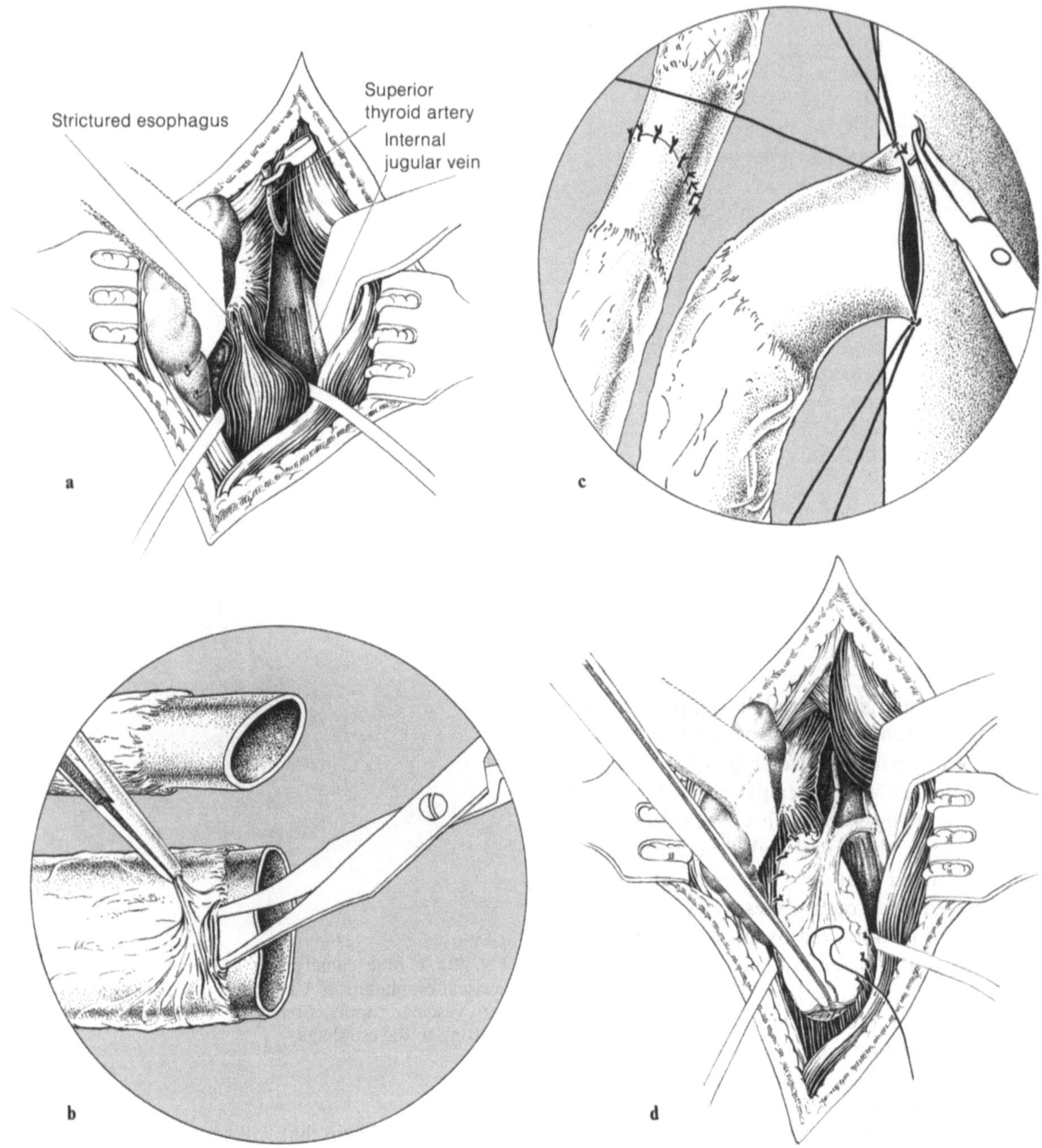

Fig. 41 a–d. Free jejunal patch for widening the strictured cervical esophagus. **a** Preparation of the strictured esophagus for receiving the graft. The superior thyroid artery is isolated for anastomosis to the patch. Note the high-grade stricture just distal to the pharynx (view from the left side). **b** The adventitia is removed from the vessels under the operating microscope or optical loupe. **c** The artery of the jejunal patch is anastomosed end-to-end to the superior thyroid artery, and the vein of the patch is anastomosed end-to-side to the internal jugular. The anastomoses are performed with simple interrupted sutures using the operating microscope or loupe. **d** The patch is sewn in place with an inner, continuous mucosal suture line and an outer row of interrupted seromuscular stitches of the vessel is ligated, the central stump is occluded with a small vascular clamp, and the artery is divided. The vein of the graft may be anastomosed end-to-end to the superior thyroid vein or facial vein, or end-to-side to the internal jugular vein.

The esophageal stricture is opened longitudinally, making sure that the incision extends 1–2 cm into normal esophagus above and below the lesion. The lumen is cleaned with dissecting patties soaked in antiseptic. The length of the incision is measured, and the patch is cut to a corresponding elliptical shape with the vascular pedicle at its center. Then the patch is placed over the defect, and its vascular pedicle is approximated to the donor vessels so that the pedicle is straight but tension-free.

The sequence of the vascular anastomoses is probably of no consequence. We prefer to start with the vein. Using an optical loupe or operating microscope with 16X magnification, the adventitia is removed sparingly (0.5 mm) from the end of the vessel (Fig. 41 b). Eight to 10 interrupted sutures of 9-0 nylon or 7-0 Poly-P-Dioxanon (PDS) should be enough to unite the vessels securely (Fig. 41 c). The number of sutures can be decreased by using fibrin glue, which will also lessen the risk of anastomotic stricture. When the anastomoses have been completed, the clamps are released at once to reestablish flow. Marked pulsations of the artery and bleeding from the margins of the patch confirm adequate perfusion. At this time the stomach tube is passed down through the opened stricture and into the distal esophagus. It will serve to keep the esophagus dilated while the patch is sewn into place. The patch is sutured to the margins of the esophagotomy using a two-layer technique (see 1.3.2.2 and 1.3.2.3) (Fig. 41 d). The patch should be attached tightly enough to prevent the formation of a blind sac. The integrity of the suture line is checked by instillation of methylene blue. With watertightness confirmed, the wound is closed in layers over a soft Penrose drain.

4.3 Plastic Repair of Thoracoabdominal Esophageal Strictures

4.3.1 Selection of Procedure

The choice of procedure depends on the level of the stricture. Lesions of the upper to midthoracic third can be managed by the free transfer of a jejunal patch. Lesions of the middle and lower thoracic third can be repaired by the transfer of a pedicled jejunal or antral patch. Strictures close to the diaphragm can be widened with a fundic patch, or a wide communication can be established between the stomach and the portion of the esophagus above the stricture. However, we feel that these operations promote esophagogastric reflux, even when combined with an antireflux procedure, and so we prefer to construct the esophagogastrostomy with interposed small bowel.

4.3.2 Free Jejunal Patch

The techniques for removing, revascularizing, and suturing the graft are described in 4.2.2. The graft artery may be anastomosed to an intercostal artery located close to the strictured area. An end-to-side anastomosis to the aorta is also possible. For this the aorta is partially occluded with a Satinski clamp. A punch of the type used in cardiac surgery for aortocoronary venous bypass is utilized to create a lumen matching the caliber of the recipient artery, and the anastomosis is performed. The vein of the graft may be anastomosed end-to-end to an intercostal vein or, preferably, end-to-side to the azygos or hemiazygos vein.

4.3.3 Pedicled Jejunal Patch

The pedicled jejunal patch based on a branch of the superior mesenteric artery can occasionally be transferred as far as the cervical esophagus or its upper thoracic third [10]. Generally, however, the range of the transfer extends no farther than the middle and distal thoracic thirds.

Preoperative preparation: Prophylactic antibiotics, intestinal lavage (see Chap. C).

Instruments: Basic set, stomach tube (Ch 32).

Position and approach: Upper midline laparotomy. The patient is repositioned for a right- or left-sided posterolateral thoracotomy according to the level of the stricture.

Steps in procedure:

(1) Identification of a suitable jejunal segment using transillumination
(2) Dissection of the vascular pedicle
(3) Mobilization of the jejunal segment with the GIA instrument
(4) Reanastomosis of the jejunum and closure of the mesenteric incision
(5) Retrocolic and retrogastric advance of the pedicled jejunal segment
(6) Closure of the abdomen
(7) Thoracotomy according to the side and level of the stricture
(8) Delivery of the pedicled jejunal segment into the chest through a phrenotomy
(9) Exposure and incision of the esophageal stricture
(10) Adaptation of the patch
(11) Attachment of the patch
(12) Drain insertion

Operative technique: The abdomen is incised, and the first loop of the jejunum is identified at the ligament of Treitz. Its vascular pattern is evaluated by transillumination (Fig. 42 a). If the superior mesenteric artery ramifies into small, individual branches (see 7.4.2), it is unlikely that a viable graft can be obtained. But if the superior mesenteric divides into a few large jejunal arteries that form well-developed marginal arcades, the outlook is generally favorable. The first branch of the superior mesenteric artery is identified at its origin just below the duodenojejunal flexure. It usually runs parallel to the first coil of the jejunum. Its course is followed until its marginal arcades unite with those of the second branch. If it appears that the vascular pedicle will have sufficient length to reach the esophageal stricture, the mesentery on both sides of the pedicle is inspected by transillumination. Branches arising from the mesentery distal to the marginal arcade are isolated with small clamps and divided. The dissection is continued as far as the origin of the superior mesenteric artery. The sites of bowel transection are designated according to the proposed length of the patch. The jejunum is skeletonized at those sites, and the segment is mobilized using the GIA instrument.

Once the jejunal segment has been isolated, it may be found that portions of the adjacent bowel are no longer adequately perfused due to the previous vascular dissections. These areas must be resected before bowel continuity is reestablished by an end-to-end anastomosis. The mesenteric incision is closed with interrupted sutures. Then the omental bursa is opened, adhesions between the posterior gastric wall and peritoneum are cleared, and the pedicled jejunal segment is brought up through an incision in the transverse mesocolon and lesser omentum, passing behind the transverse colon and stomach. Care is taken to avoid twisting of the vascular pedicle. To avoid internal herniation, the mesocolic incision is narrowed with a suture that catches the fringe of mesentery remaining on the vascular pedicle (Fig. 42 b).

The transplant may be passed into the chest through the esophageal hiatus or through a separate radial incision in the diaphragm. We prefer a separate incision, as this avoids disruption of the hiatus that might cause reflux problems. The oral end of the transplant is engaged with a heavy traction suture tied to a sponge. The sponge, with suture attached, is passed up through the phrenotomy and will be used later to pull the patch into the chest. Then the abdomen is closed, and the patient is repositioned for thoracotomy.

The chest is entered, and the lung is retracted anterosuperiorly. The phrenotomy is identified, and the transplant is pulled into the thorax using the preplaced traction suture, carefully avoiding trauma to the vascular pedicle. The pedicle may be secured at the diaphragm by stitching its mesenteric rim loosely to the edges of the phrenotomy. The mediastinal pleura over the esophageal stricture is widely opened longitudinally, and the anterolateral wall of the esophagus is freed of connective tissue, sparing the underlying vagus nerve

Fig. 42a–d. Pedicled jejunal patch for widening the strictured thoracic esophagus. A jejunal segment with a vascular pedicle of adequate length and caliber is mobilized. Adjacent bowel (**a** broken line) should be resected if underperfused. **b** The pedicled jejunal segment is brought up behind the colon and stomach. A traction suture tied to a dissecting patty marks the oral end of the segment (isoperistaltic interposition) and is used to pull the segment into the chest. **c** The stricture is opened longitudinally, and the patch is cut to definitive size. **d** The patch is sewn into place with an inner, continuous mucosal suture line followed by an outer row of interrupted seromuscular sutures ▷

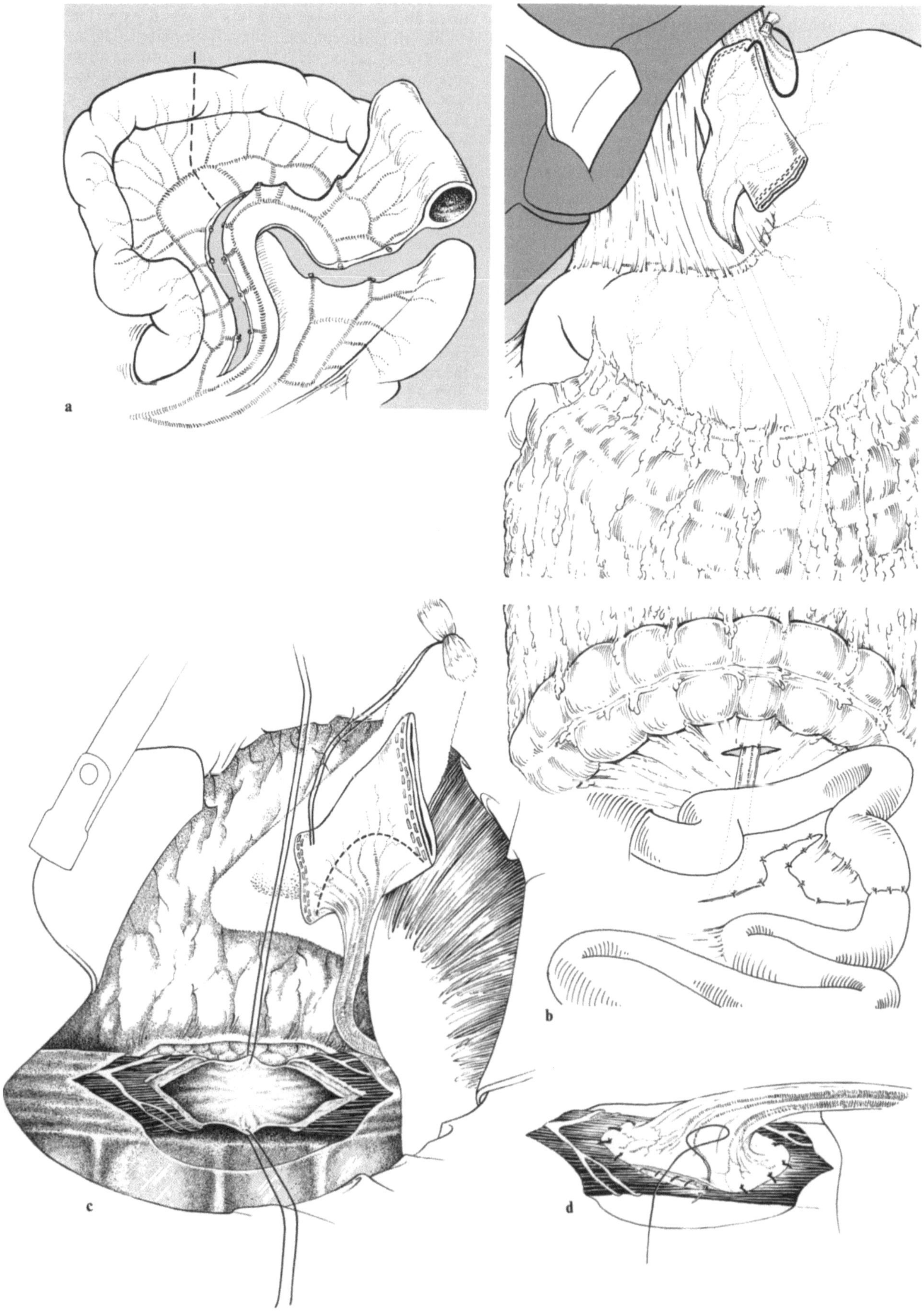
a
b
c
d

branch. We try to mobilize the stricture no more than is absolutely necessary. The stricture is opened longitudinally between two traction sutures. This incision should extend 1–2 cm into normal esophagus above and below the stricture. At this point the necessary size of the patch can be determined (Fig. 42 c). The staple lines on the jejunal segment (still closed at both ends) are removed, and the intestinal tube is opened on its antimesenteric side. Its mucosa is by wiped clean with antiseptic solution. The patch is cut to the shape of an ellipse long enough to cover the defect, with the vascular pedicle at its center. Bleeding points on the cut surface of the bowel are selectively cauterized. Then the orogastric tube is advanced through the opened stricture into the stomach, and the patch is sutured in isoperistaltic position over the indwelling tube (Fig. 42d) using a two-layer technique (see 1.3.2.2). The patch should be sutured without tension, but it should be flush with the esophageal wall so that a cul-de-sac is not formed.

The orogastric tube is replaced with a small-caliber nasogastric tube, and the integrity of the suture line is tested with methylene blue solution. If sufficient material is present, the mediastinal pleura may be loosely reapproximated over the patch. Finally a chest tube is inserted, the lung is inflated, and the thoracotomy is closed in layers.

4.3.4 Pedicled Antral Patch [9]

The advantage of using an antral patch to widen the strictured esophagus lies in the resistance of the antral mucosa to gastric acid. Thus the patch may even be placed at the esophagogastric junction without danger of peptic ulceration. It is reported that serum gastrin levels are not increased after the operation [9].

Preoperative preparation: Prophylactic antibiotics (see Chap. C).

Instruments: Basic set, stomach tube (Ch 32), sterile pH probe, pentagastrin.

Position and approach: Upper midline laparotomy for a stricture at the esophagogastric junction, thoracoabdominal incision in the bed of the seventh left rib for a higher stricture.

Operative technique: A pentagastrin infusion (6 µg/kg b.w./h) is commenced at the start of the operation to ensure maximum parietal cell stimulation.

The abdomen or chest is entered, and the strictured portion of the esophagus is exposed and snared (see 2.1.2). The length of the stricture is estimated so that the necessary size of the patch can be ascertained. Then the stomach is opened about 8 cm proximal to the pylorus.

Fig. 43a–c. Pedicled antral patch for widening the strictured abdominal esophagus. **a** The antral patch, based on the left gastroepiploic artery, is mobilized. The lesser omentum is incised close to the cardia, forming an aperture through which the patch can be brought up to the stricture behind the stomach. **b** The patch is sewn into place to widen the stricture; the antral defect is closed with interrupted inverting sutures. **c** Following the antral patch esophagoplasty, fundoplication is done to prevent reflux. The vascular pedicle passes outside the gastric wrap ▷

A sterile pH probe is used to establish the distal limit of the parietal cell area so that a portion of the antrum free from acid-secreting mucosa can be selected for the patch. The size of the antral patch is determined, and the right gastroepiploic artery is divided at its distal end. Then a pedicle is formed from the part of the gastroepiploic arcade supplying the pedicle, making certain that it is long enough to reach the stricture without tension. The oval-shaped antral patch is excised from the greater curvature (Fig. 43 a), and the defect is closed transversely to preserve the gastric lumen. The posterior gastric wall is freed of peritoneal adhesions, and the lesser omentum is divided close to the cardia. The antral patch is passed behind the stomach to the site of the stricture, taking care not to twist its vascular pedicle. If the stricture is intrathoracic, the patch may be passed into the chest through the bluntly enlarged hiatus after division of the esophagophrenic membrane. Then the esophageal stricture is opened longitudinally, and a specimen is taken for frozen section biopsy to exclude carcinoma. The large-bore orogastric tube is advanced past the stricture into the stomach to serve as a stent, whereupon the patch is cut to final size and sutured into position using a two-layer technique (see 1.3.2.2) (Fig. 43 b). Hugh [9] routinely performs a fundoplication (see 11.5) around the distal end of the patch, making certain that the pedicle is left free (Fig. 43 c). We consider a semifundoplication to be more appropriate for this situation (see 11.6) and at least functionally equivalent to a complete fundoplication.

4.3.5 Fundic Patch [4, 22]

The first description of this procedure [21] left the impression that it was sufficient to incise the strictured esophagus longitudinally and then cover the defect with a fold of gastric fundus. An essential part of the procedure, the creation of an esophagogastric valve, was not described in detail. This led to a number of failures [20, 25], due mostly to reflux. Later Thal [22] and Hatafuku [3] published new descriptions of the procedure and added a semifundoplication.

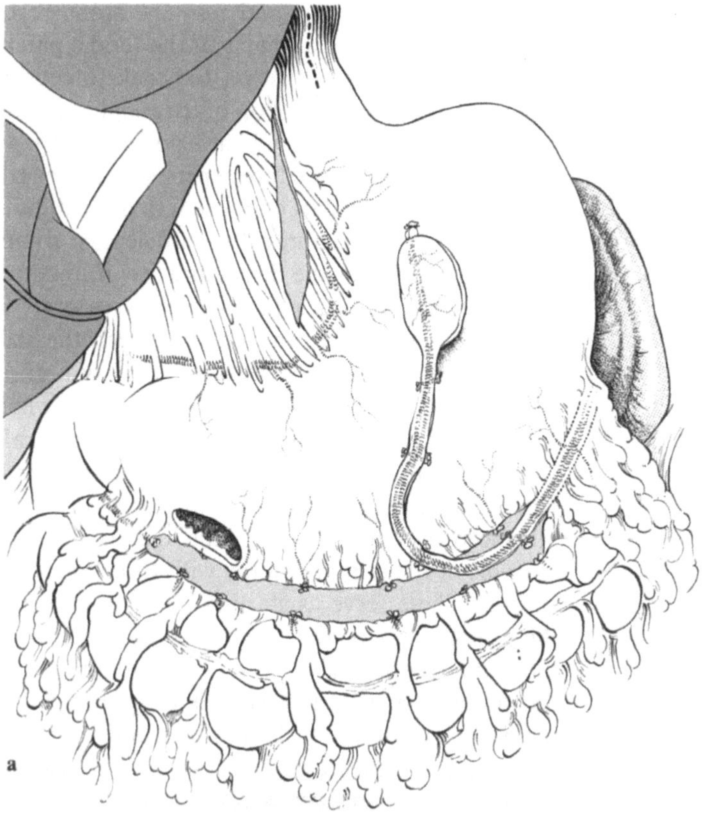

a

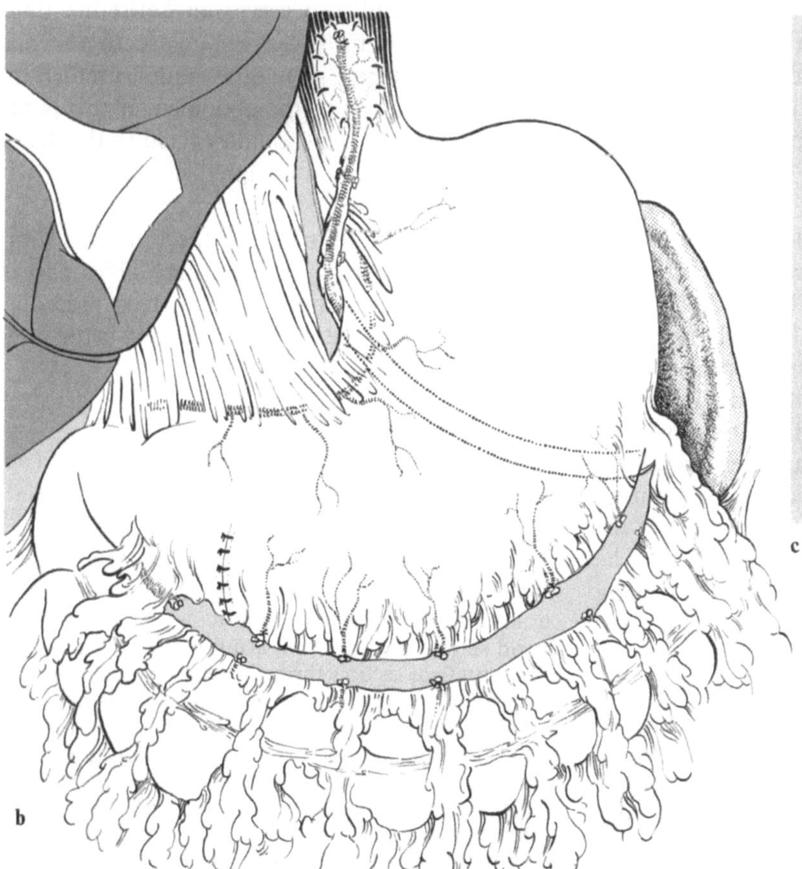

b

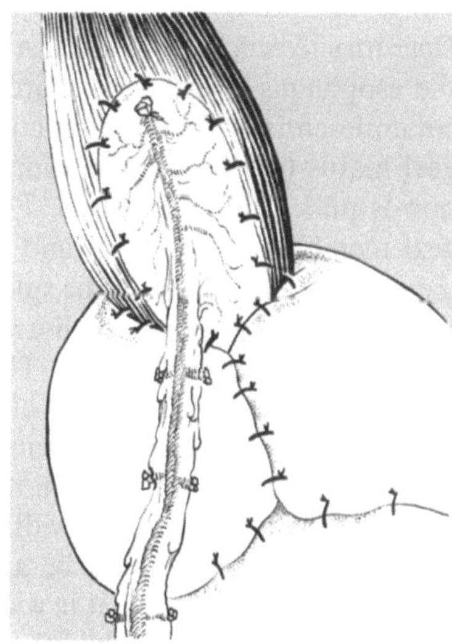

c

Preoperative preparation: Prophylactic antibiotics (see Chap. C).

Instruments: Basic set, extra thoracic set, stomach tube (Ch 32), dermatome.

Position and approach: Left posterolateral thoracotomy, possibly with division of the eighth rib, or upper midline abdominal incision extending around the left side of the umbilicus, depending on the level of the stricture.

Steps in procedure:

(1) Exposure of the stricture
(2) Longitudinal incision of the stricture
(3) Widening of the posterior esophageal wall
(4) Construction of an esophagogastric valve
(5) Removal of split-thickness skin graft
(6) Placement of the skin graft over the fundic fold that will cover the esophageal defect
(7) Fixation of the fundic fold over the esophageal defect
(8) Semifundoplication
(9) Drainage

Operative technique: For a transthoracic procedure the esophagus is exposed, snared, and mobilized circumferentially from the stricture to the esophageal hiatus (see 2.1.2). The esophagogastric junction is pulled into the hiatus. The phrenoesophageal membrane is divided, and the diaphragm is incised in the direction of the splenic compartment until the fundus can be delivered into the chest through the enlarged hiatus. The fundus can be mobilized further by division of the short gastric arteries. The esophageal stricture is opened longitudinally between two traction threads. When the threads are pulled taut, the width of the posterior wall of the esophagus can be appreciated. If the wall appears too narrow, it is widened by suturing the cut edges of the esophagus transversely at the narrowest point of the stricture (Fig. 44 a). The esophagogastric valve is constructed by placing three sutures that unite the distal edge of the esophagotomy with the fundus–two placed near the corners of the incision, and one placed centrally (Fig. 44 b). When tied, the sutures imbricate the fundus over the lower part of the esophagotomy, creating an esophagogastric valve that projects into the lumen of the stomach (Fig. 44 c). The valve is additionally secured with several interrupted sutures. A large-bore tube is passed through the esophagus and into the stomach to serve as a stent for placement of the fundic patch. The fundus is grasped with a Babcock forceps at a point that will meet the top of the esophagotomy when the flap is advanced into position (Fig. 44 d). The rest of the procedure depends on the length of the stricture and thus on the length of the fundic patch. For stort strictures it is sufficient to rotate the fundic fold over the defect and sew it in place. For long strictures a split-thickness skin graft is taken from the thigh and cut to match the size of the fundic patch. The surface of the skin graft is sutured to the serosa of the fundus so that, when the patch is in place, the inner surface of the graft will appose to the esophageal lumen and will provide a granulating surface. The fundic fold is now advanced over the stomach tube and fixed to the margins of the esophagotomy with three retention sutures. These serve as starting points for closing the lateral sides of the patch with continuous or interrupted sutures (Fig. 44 e). The remaining fundus on both sides of the patch is wrapped around the esophagus in the fashion of a semifundoplication (see 11.6) and secured with several interrupted sutures. This maneuver covers the sutures of the fundic patch and also serves an antireflux function. If the stricture was very close to the diaphragm, an attempt should be made to return the semifundoplication to the abdomen. If this is not possible, the stomach should be fixed to the hiatus or phrenotomy with interrupted sutures.

Strictures of the abdominal esophagus are best exposed transabdominally, as the fundus is more easily mobilized from that approach. This part of the procedure is identical to the steps preceding a fundoplication (see 11.5), and the rest is the same

Fig. 44a–f. Fundic patch for widening the strictured abdominal or lower thoracic esophagus (view from the left side). **a** The stricture is opened longitudinally, and the posterior wall of the esophagus is widened with transverse sutures placed at the narrowest part of the lesion. **b** Construction of the esophagogastric valve. The two corner threads encompass more tissue than the central thread so that the valve will acquire a semilunar shape. **c** Longitudinal section through the esophagus and stomach after construction of the esophagogastric valve. **d** A fold of fundus is created, and the side of the fold facing the esophageal lumen is covered with split-thickness skin. Three retention sutures fix the fundic patch to the esophagus. **e** Definitive fixation with a continuous suture line placed between the retention sutures. **f** A fundoplication is performed to cover the patch sutures and prevent reflux ▷

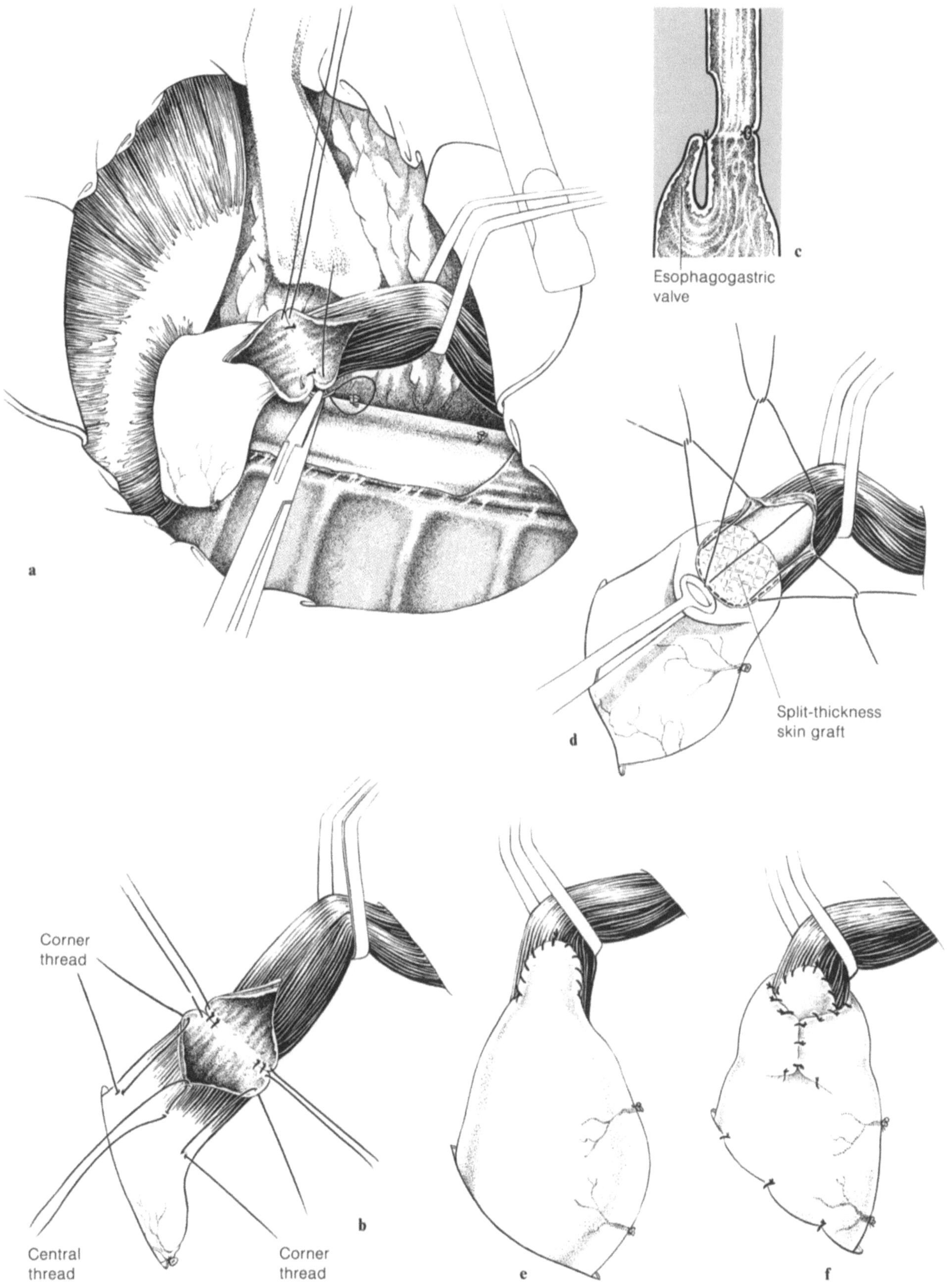
a
Esophagogastric
valve
c
Split-thickness
skin graft
d
Corner
thread
Central
thread
Corner
thread
b
e
f

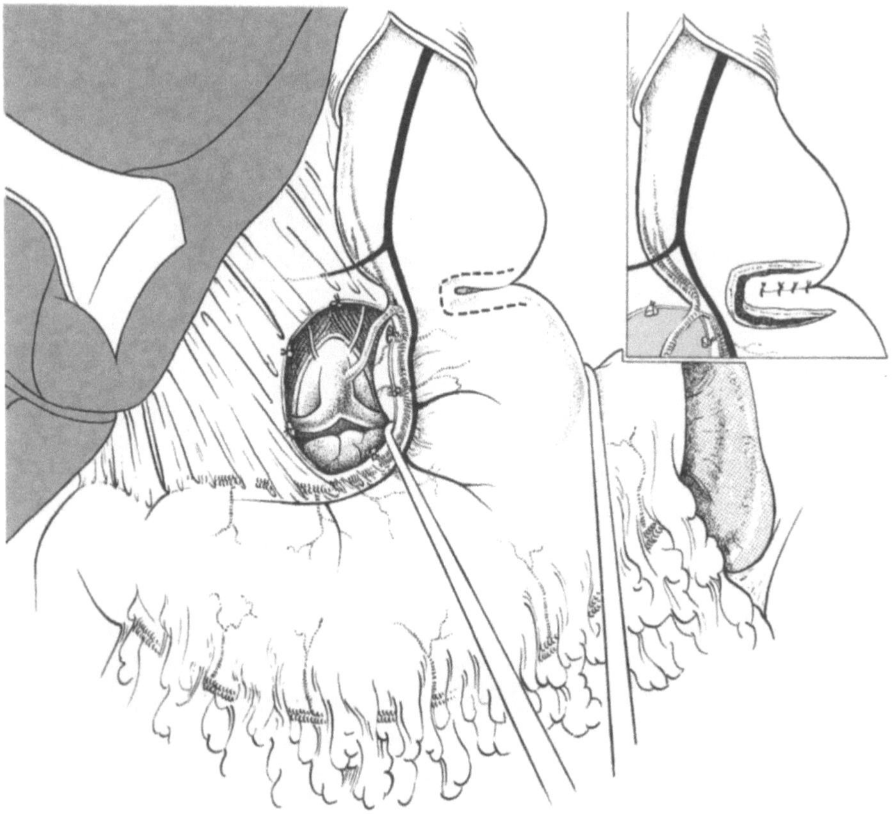

Fig. 45. Esophagogastrostomy for widening the strictured abdominal esophagus. The dilated esophagus above the stricture is approximated to the gastric fundus and fixed to it with interrupted seromuscular sutures. The esophagus and fundus are opened, and mucosal sutures are placed to create a wide communication between the esophagus and stomach. The anterior part of the anastomosis is likewise constructed in two layers

as described above. Both the abdominal and thoracic procedures can be modified by performing a complete fundoplication instead of a semifundoplication [11, 24]. After the patch is sewn into place, a cuff of gastric fundus is wrapped around the esophagus, and both folds are united with three or four interrupted sutures. The wrap is additionally fixed to the stomach with several sutures to prevent telescoping (Fig. 44 f).

4.3.6 Esophagogastrostomy

The abdominal [7] or thoracic [3, 5] esophagogastrostomy consists of a side-to-side anastomosis between the dilated esophagus above the stricture and the gastric fundus so that a broad communication is established between the esophagus and stomach (Fig. 45). There is a significant potential for gastroesophageal reflux in this procedure, even when it is combined with fundoplication. Because of this, and because of the effective alternatives that are available, we no longer perform esophagogastrostomy for the treatment of esophageal stricture.

References

1. Ancona E (1981) Gastrointestinal microsurgery: Colonic and jejunal autotransplants for cervical esophagoplasty. Internat Surg 66:39
2. Chrysospathis P (1966) The contribution of vascular surgery to esophageal replacement. Brit J Surg 53: 122
3. Frey EK (1938) Die cardioplastische Ösophago-Gastrostomie. Zbl Chir 65:2
4. Hatafuku T, Maki T, Thal AP (1972) Fundic patch operation in the treatment of advanced achalasia of the esophagus. Surg Gynecol Obstet 143:617
5. Henschen C (1936) Transpleurale Ösophagus-Gastroanastomose. Langenbecks Arch klin Chir 186:20

6. Hester TR, McConnel FMS, Nahal F, Jurkiewicz MJ, Brown RG (1980) Reconstruction of cervical esophagus, hypopharynx and oral cavity using free jejunal transfer. Am Journ Surg 140:487
7. Heyrovsky H (1913) Kasuistik und Therapie der isopathischen Dilatation der Speiseröhre. Arch Klin Chir 100:703
8. Hiebert CA, Cummings SO (1961) Successful replacement of the cervical esophagus by transplantation and revascularisation of a free graft of gastric antrum. Ann Surg 154:103
9. Hugh TB, Lusby RJ, Coleman MJ (1979) Antral patch esophagoplasty. A new procedure for acid-peptic esophageal stricture. Am Journ Surg 137:222
10. Kasai M, Abols SI, Makino K, Yoshida S, Taguchi Y (1965) Reconstruction of the cervical esophagus by a pedicled jejunal graft. Surg Gynec Obstet 121:102
11. Maher JW, Hocking MP, Woodward ER (1981) Long-term follow up of the combined fundic patch fundoplication for treatment of longitudinal peptic strictures of the esophagus. Ann Surg 194:69
12. McKee DM, Peters CR (1978) Reconstruction of the hypopharynx and cervical esophagus with microvascular jejunal transplant. Clin Plast Surg 5:305
13. Mikulicz J (1888) Zur operativen Behandlung des stenosierenden Magengeschwürs. Klin Chir 37:39
14. Nakayama K, Yamamoto K, Tamiya T (1964) Experience with free autografts of the bowel with a new venous anastomosis apparatus. Surgery 55:796
15. Peters CR, McKee DM, Berry BW (1971) Pharyngoesophageal reconstruction with revascularized jejunal transplants. Amer J Surg 121:678
16. Pichlmaier H, Spelsberg F, Grundmann R (1971) Autologer Speiseröhrenersatz. Chirurg 9:398
17. Popow WI, Filin WI (1961) Die freie Transplantation des Darms zur Rekonstruction der Speiseröhre. Zbl Chirurgie 31:1745
18. Roberts RE, Douglas FM (1961) Replacement of cervical esophagus and hypopharynx by revascularized free jejunal autograft. N Engl J Med 264:342
19. Seidenberg B, Rosenak SS, Hurwitt ES, Som ML (1959) Immediate reconstruction of the cervical esophagus by a revascularized isolated jejunal segment. Ann Surg 149:162
20. Skinner DB, DeMeester TH (1976) Gastroesophageal reflux. Curr Probl Surg 13:52
21. Thal AP, Hatafuku T, Kurzman R (1965) New operation for distal esophageal stricture. Arch Surg 90:464
22. Thal AP (1968) A unified approach to surgical problems of the esophagogastric junction. Ann Surg 168:542
23. Thomas HF, Clarke JM, Ragl JE, Woodward ER (1972) Results of the combined fundic patch-fundoplication in the treatment of reflux esophagitis with stricture. Surg Gynecol Obstet 135:241
24. Ti-Sheng C, Oi-Ling H, Wang-Wei (1980) Reconstruction of esophageal defects with microsurgically revascularized jejunal segments: A report of 13 cases. J Microsurg 2:83
25. Wise WS, Rivarola CH, Williams GD (1970) Experience with the Thal gastroesophagoplasty. Ann Thorac Surg 10:213

5 Endoesophageal Tubes

In collaboration with G. Buess

CONTENTS

5.1 Tumor Extent and Dysphagia

Carcinoma of the esophagus tends to grow longitudinally in its early stages. By the time dysphagic symptoms appear, it is common for two-thirds of the circumference to be involved. The further progression of disease leads to circumferential stricturing with dysphagia for solid foods when the lumen reaches 10 mm, and dysphagia for strained foods when the lumen reaches 5 mm. Longitudinal tumor extension additionally impairs peristaltic propulsion. A desparate situation arises when the patient becomes unable to swallow liquids. Saliva cannot be swallowed during sleep, and spontaneous aspiration results.

5.2 Evolution of Intubation Methods

The development of rigid esophagoscopy by Mikulicz [6] laid the groundwork for dilatation and intubation of the esophagus under partial endoscopic control. However, the small tube sizes and high risk of perforation during rigid endoscopic insertion limited the applications of this method, which was unlikely to be successful in cardia carcinoma with angulation in the area of the neoplasm. The surgical (pull-through) method of tube insertion was able to overcome angulations of this type and also avoid perforation below the tumor by the leading end of the tube. However, local and systemic complications of the laparotomy were common in patients with advanced disease. Finally the introduction of intubation methods using flexible endoscopes made it possible to avoid the high complication rates associated with surgical insertion. Intubation under endoscopic control alone is associated with a much shorter hospital stay and significantly lower costs. Some years ago we abandoned pull-through methods of esophageal intubation, and we no longer construct a Witzel fistula in patients with a malignant stricture.

5.3 Indications for Esophageal Intubation

Since intubation does not have a curative or tumor-reducing effect in esophageal carcinoma, it should first be determined whether surgical resection or irradiation might be curative or yield a better palliative result. As a rule, intubation is indicated only if the patient is no longer able to swallow strained foods, and the stricture does not permit the passage of an endoscope 10–12 mm in diameter.

5.3.1 Squamous Cell Carcinoma

The treatment of choice for nonresectable squamous cell carcinoma of the esophagus is irradiation. We have consistently observed palliation of dysphagia following radiotherapy. This effect last for an average of six months before restricturing occurs, and dilatation and intubation become necessary. If the patient is too sick to tolerate radiotherapy, intubation may be done primarily, although this has been associated with a higher rate of local complications in our patients. Contrary to earlier opinion, intubation is appropriate for carcinomas of the middle and upper third of the esophagus, provided there is a space of at least two fingerwidths between the proximal limit of the tumor and the esophageal inlet to accommodate the upper flange of the tube. With infiltration or compression of the bronchial system, there is a danger of critical stenosis of the airways during dilatation and intubation. Under these conditions, and for carcinomas situated high in the neck, the construction of a Witzel fistula is an acceptable option. However, we prefer laser coagulation in these cases as a means of reopening the obstructed esophagus.

5.3.2 Squamous Cell Carcinoma with a Tracheoesophageal Fistula

This is a serious condition that demands surgical intervention. Emergency intubation can provide significant palliation for a relative stricture in the area of the tumor. The upper flange will seat securely in these cases, and the tube will provide a satisfactory channel for food ingestion while sealing off the fistula.

5.3.3 Adenocarcinoma of the Cardia

Intubation is almost always possible in these cases, even with complete obstruction of the cardia. Radiotherapy is of no real benefit, so primary endoscopic tube insertion is appropriate for tumors that are not resectable.

5.3.4 Malignant Lesions of Adjacent Structures

Mediastinal lesions as well as advanced central bronchogenic carcinomas can narrow the esophagus as a result of infiltration or compression. Intubation generally affords palliation in these cases, although extreme care must be taken to avoid compression of the major airways during placement of the tube.

5.4 Selection of an Intubation Method

Dilatation of the neoplastic stricture is necessary prior to the insertion of an endoesophageal tube. Techniques of bougienage have improved greatly in recent years (see Sect. 3), and today it is possible to perform all dilatations under controlled conditions. Intubation methods that rely on endoscopic or combined endoscopic-radiologic guidance are superior to the pull-through methods, which today should be considered obsolete.

We recommend endoscopic dilatation of the stricture with the Buess stepped dilator, followed by the insertion of an Atkinson tube using the Nottingham tube introducer. At our center we are already working with prototypes of a new silicone tube manufactured by the Koss Company, which is claimed to be superior in design and material to devices currently on the market. This tube is inserted over the endoscope following endoscopic dilatation of the stricture. A Witzel fistula should be constructed only in cases where endoscopic tube insertion is not possible (see 5.3.1).

5.5 Tube Designs

New developments have led to improved tube durability and a more stable retention after endoscopic placement. Tubes made of latex and tubes that lack means to prevent proximal displacement should not be used.

5.5.1 Silicone Tubes

Atkinson tube. This tube (Fig. 46 a) was developed for endoscopic insertion. The material (silicone) is very soft but highly durable. The upper flange is relatively soft and is easily folded. The distal end of the tube has a shoulder to prevent upward migration. The tube expands the luminal diameter to about 18 mm during insertion. The Atkinson system (Fig. 47) is recommended for introduction of this tube (see Table 1 for tube dimensions).

Buess tube. When problems with shape and material were encountered with the latex tubes as well as with the Atkinson tube, we felt it necessary to develop a new tube design (Fig. 46 g,h). Our tube is made of highly durable silicone and has a transverse oval flange that occupies minimal space–a particular advantage in the proximal third of the

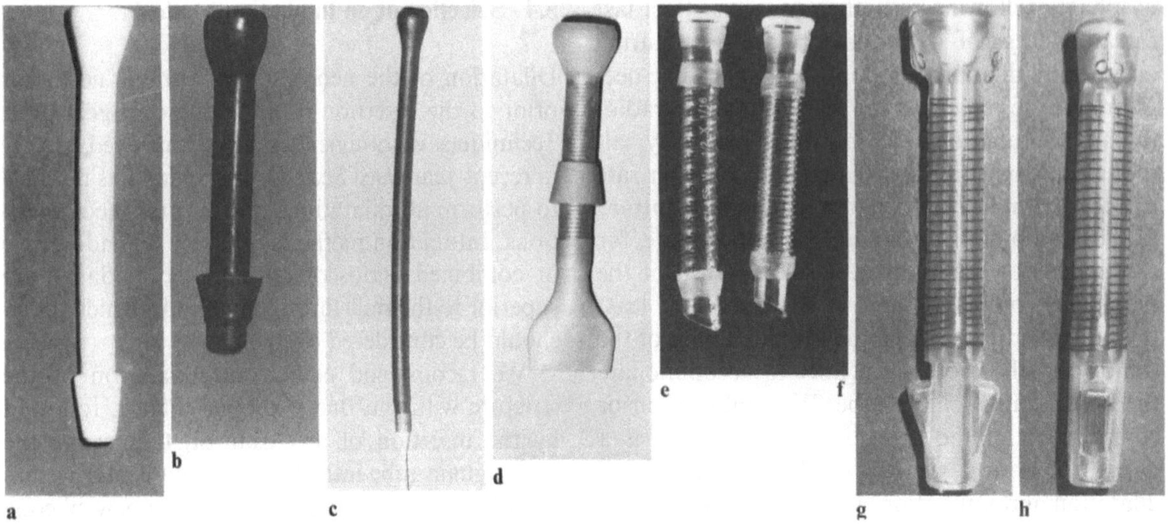

Fig. 46 a–h. Endoesophageal tube designs. **a** Atkinson tube for endoscopic insertion. **b** Celestin tube for endoscopic insertion. **c** Celestin tube for pull-through insertion (with pilot extension). **d** Häring tube for pull-through insertion (with distal flange and valve). **e,f** Tytgat tubes for endoscopic insertion. **g,h** Buess tubes for endoscopic insertion

esophagus. Integrated metal hooks make it easy to adjust the position of the tube with an endoscope. The shaft is reinforced with a metal coil, and the distal end has a pair of fold-out shoulder tabs that retract during insertion and prevent upward displacement once the tube is in position. The shape of the upper flange can be modified to deal with esophagotracheal fistulas. A transverse oval pusher rod is used to insert the tube over an endoscope. The distal tabs do not increase the luminal diameter during insertion (maximum diameter 16 mm).

5.5.2 *Celestin Tube*

For endoscopic insertion. The material (latex) has good elasticity but relatively poor tolerance to long-term placement. The upper flange of the tube is very firm and cannot be infolded; the distal end has a latex apron to prevent expulsion (Fig. 46 b). These components expand the lumen to a full 20 mm during insertion (see Table 1 for tube dimensions).

For pull-through insertion. This tube is supplied in lengths of 16 and 28.5 cm (Fig. 46 c) and is cut to the appropriate length. It comes with a pilot extension to guide the tube into the stricture. Signs of breakdown have been observed with long-term placement, and the plastic coils liberated from the tube can lead to serious complications.

Table 1. Endoesophageal tube dimensions

	Inside diameter (mm)	Outside diameter (mm)	Wall thickness (mm)	Length (cm)
Atkinson et al. [1] (Fig. 47a)	11	15	2	13.7 18.5
Celestin et al. [3] (Fig. 47b)	12	15	1.5	34
Häring [5] (Fig. 47d)	13	15	2	9 12 18
Buess et al. [2] (Fig. 47g, h)	12	16	2	11 14 17

5.5.3 *Häring Tube*

For pull-through insertion. The tube material (silicone latex) is highly elastic, and bleb formation can occur inside the lumen following endoscopic insertion. Hence the manufacturer cautions against that technique. The upper flange is very soft and easily indented; the shaft is reinforced by a metal coil. After surgical insertion, a distal flange is fitted over the end of the tube. A rubber valve can additionally be placed on the tube to prevent reflux (Fig. 46 d) (see Table 1 for tube dimensions).

5.5.4 The Tytgat Custom-Prepared Tube [7]

This prosthesis is made from Tygon tubing and is custom-prepared in a special workshop for a given tumor length. The process is so costly, however, that it is accessible only to a few centers. Two examples of the Tytgat tube are shown in Figs. 46 e, f.

5.6 Intubation under Endoscopic and Radiologic Control

Steps in procedure:

(1) Dilatation of the tumor stricture under general anesthesia using endoscopic or combined endoscopic-fluoroscopic control (see Sect. 3)
(2) Insertion of a guidewire under endoscopic and radiologic control
(3) Determination of the tumor length
(4) Selection of a suitable tube, which is mounted on the Nottingham introducer
(5) Tube insertion under radiologic guidance
(6) Endoscopic and radiologic confirmation of tube placement

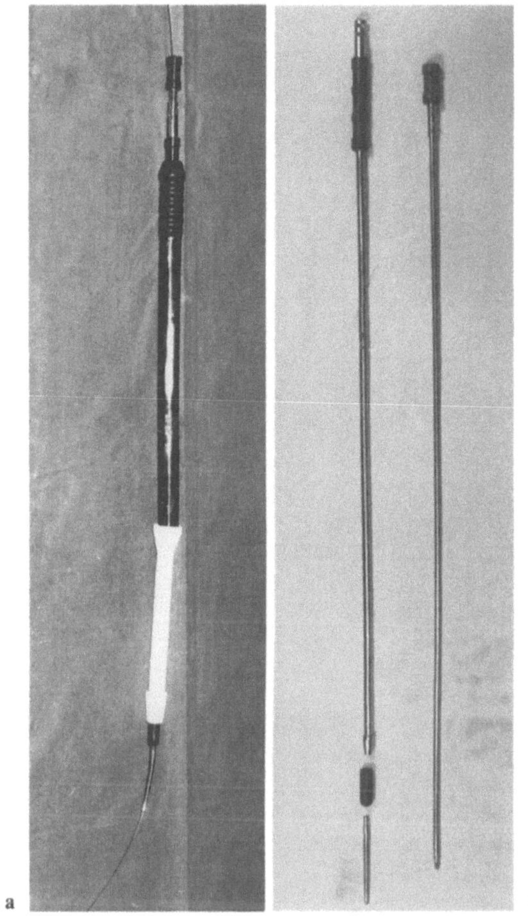

Fig. 47 a, b. The Nottingham tube introducer (Atkinson et al. [1]). **a** The fully assembled system with the Atkinson endoesophageal tube. **b** The components of the system

5.6.1 Intubation with the Nottingham Tube Introducer

5.6.1.1 Instrumentation

The tube introducer designed by Atkinson et al. [1] (Fig. 47, 48) grips the distal end of the tube from the inside by means of an expander mechanism. The tube is passed into the stricture along a guidewire under radiologic control.

The guidewire is like that used in the Eder-Puestow system. The introducer itself has a flexible tip and consists of two stainless steel spiral tubes, one of which can be slid over the other by activating a bayonet mechanism on the handle (Fig. 47). The inner tube has a tapered leader in front of an expanding plastic cup, which receives the olive-shaped end of the outer tube. Pushing the outer tube home expands the cup, which grips the tip of the prosthesis firmly from within (Fig. 48). A pusher tube (see Fig. 47) is fitted over the introducer behind the prosthesis and serves to hold it in place when the introducer is released.

5.6.1.2 Preparation and Intubation Technique

Besides the apparatus listed above, a small-caliber endoscope is needed as well as a stomach tube and gastrografin solution. The entire procedure is performed under general anesthesia on an X-ray table with the patient supine. After dilatation of the malignant stricture under appropriate control (see Sect. 3), the area of the tumor is evaluated endoscopically. The extent of the tumor and its proximal limit are determined, and the guidewire

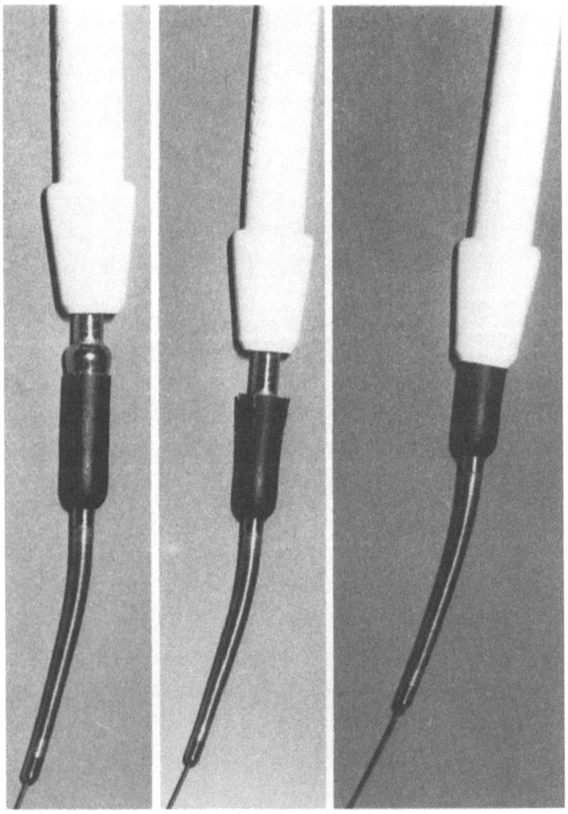

Fig. 48. The Nottingham tube introducer. Principle of the Atkinson system: The expanded plastic cup grips the end of the tube from the inside

is passed. An endoesophageal tube of appropriate length is selected or is cut to the required length. The silicone Atkinson tube is best suited for this insertion technique. It is mounted on the introducer and locked in place by means of the expanding distal cup (Fig. 48). Gliding parts are lubricated beforehand (e.g., with silicone spray) to lower resistance during intubation. Ordinarily we do not use the black pusher tube (Fig. 47); we feel that it is too rigid. The introducer/tube assembly is introduced perorally over the guidewire, taking care to avoid injury to the anterior teeth. The fingers direct the passage of the instrument through the pharynx, again making certain that the spiral metallic surface does not injure the tissues.

The first significant resistance may be felt at the level of the upper esophageal sphincter. Fluoroscopic guidance should be commenced at this level so that displacement of the guidewire or angulation can be promptly recognized. The next resistance is felt as the distal end of the introducer enters the stricture. Often an abrupt movement is felt as the tube slips through the stricture, and this can be visualized with fluoroscopy (Fig. 49). A considerable pulsion force may have to be applied at this time. We halt the insertion about 5 cm above the intended position of the upper flange and introduce a small-caliber endoscope parallel to the introducer assembly (Fig. 50). In that way we can establish the level of the proximal edge of the tube, which should be 3–5 cm from the superior edge of the neoplasm, depending on the type of tube used. At this point we also observe the behavior of the upper flange as it enters the stricture. A soft flange may become indented to the point of blockage, in which case the flange may be withdrawn slightly and allowed to reexpand, or the tube may be replaced by a model with a firmer flange. Once the flange has reached the desired position, the introducer is released, and the flange is held in position with the endoscope as the introducer is withdrawn with a gentle rotating motion under close radiologic control. The endoscope can now be used to inspect the lumen

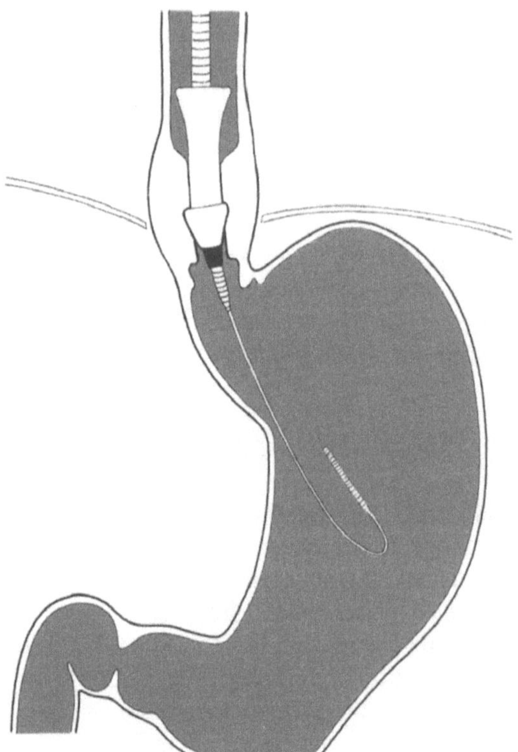

Fig. 49. The tip of the tube is passed into the stricture with the Nottingham introducer

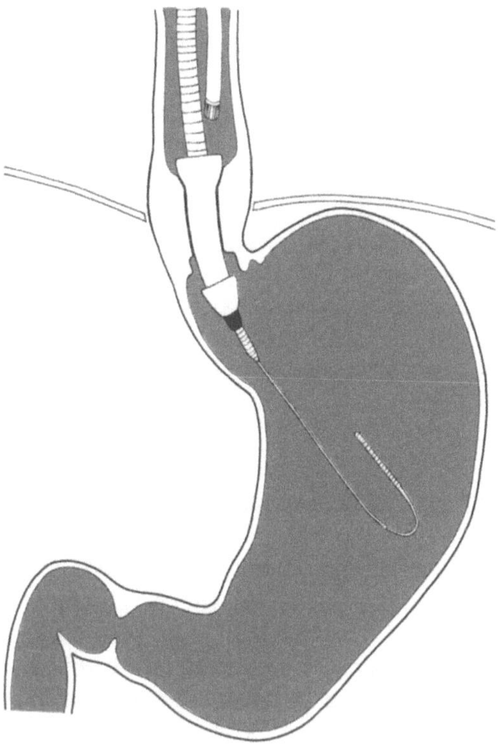

Fig. 50. The position of the tube is monitored endoscopically

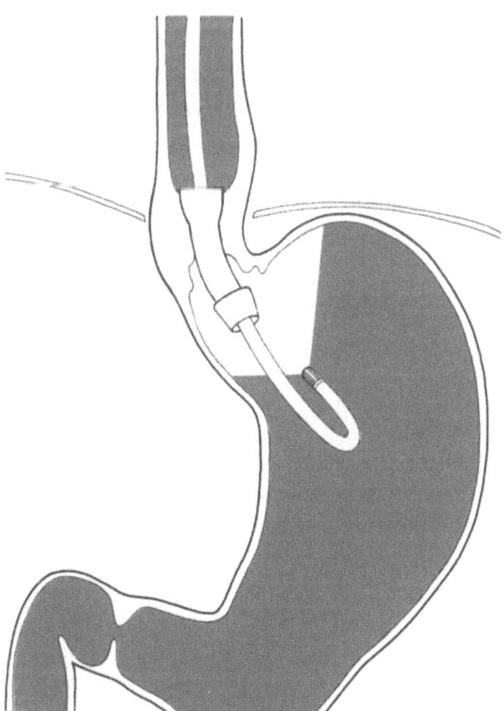

Fig. 51. After removal of the introducer, the distal end of the tube is inspected by retroversion of the endoscope tip

of the tube. The distal end of the tube is additionally evaluated, and its patency confirmed, by retroversion of the endscope tip (Fig. 51).

After removing the scope, we pass a stomach tube into the esophagus and inject a water-soluble contrast medium to exclude perforation and to document the position of the tube.

5.6.2 Tube Insertion over the Endoscope

In this technique the endoesophageal tube is fitted over a correspondingly small-caliber endoscope and inserted with the aid of a pusher tube.

Fig. 52a, b. The system of Celestin et al. [3] for endoscopic tube insertion. **a** Overall view and **b** close-up view of the connection between the pusher tube and endoscophageal tube

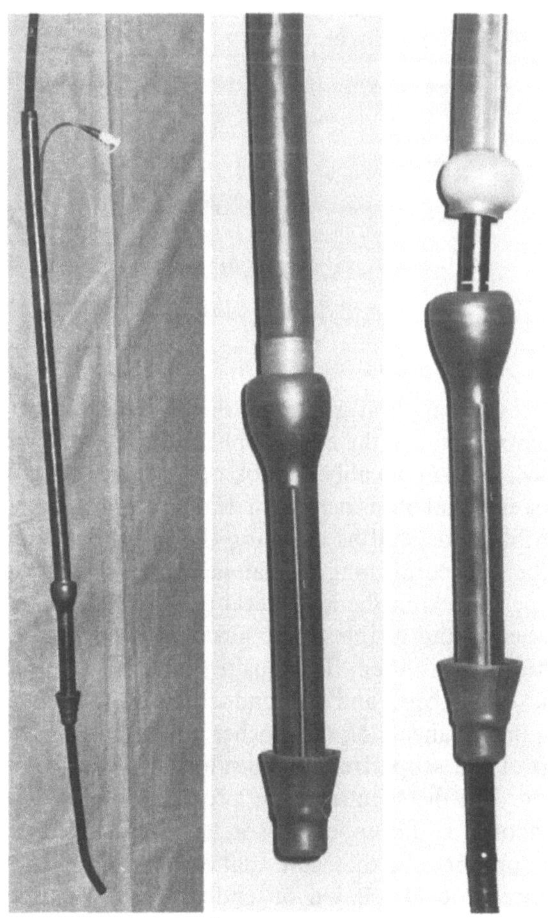

a b

5.6.2.1 The Celestin System

The pusher tube is made of latex and is reinforced by a plastic coil. The leading end of the pusher tube fits into the upper flange of the Celestin tube (Fig. 52) and engages against the top of the shaft. The pusher tube carries a balloon at its tip which, when inflated, enables the prosthetic tube to be withdrawn (Fig. 52). The pusher system of Celestin et al. [3] is often too soft to apply the pulsion force necessary to insert the tube.

5.6.2.2 The Tytgat System

A plastic tube is fitted over the endoscope for insertion of the endoesophageal tube. The principle is similar to the technique of Celestin et al. [3].

5.6.2.3 Preparation and Technique of Endoscopic Tube Insertion

Steps in procedure:

(1) Dilatation with the endoscopic stepped dilator and determination of tube length (see Sect. 3)
(2) Preparation of the endoesophageal tube/pusher/endoscope assembly, passage of the endoscope through the stricture, and insertion of the prosthesis with the pusher tube
(3) Endoscopic check of tube position

Necessary apparatus, besides the dilatation instruments, includes the endoesophageal tube, pulsion tube, and small-caliber endoscope. Fluoroscopy is not essential but is helpful in dealing with insertion problems as well as checking the position of the tube and confirming its patency. The intubation is performed in the left lateral position in sedated patients, and in the supine position when general anesthesia is used. The pusher tube is slid over the endoscope, and the endoesophageal tube is mounted ahead of the pusher tube, leaving the tip of the scope free for monitoring by retroversion. The distance from the proximal limit of the stricture to the upper incisor teeth is marked on the pusher tube to ensure that the tube is not advanced too far. Based on endoscopic evaluation of the tumor stricture, an endoesophageal tube of appropriate length is selected, making sure that the upper flange is sufficiently firm to negotiate a site of relative narrowing that may exist above the stricture. The whole assembly is now introduced into the esophagus under endoscopic guidance and advanced to the intended site. Correct placement of the upper flange and distal end of the tube is confirmed endoscopically, whereupon the endoscope is withdrawn to the upper flange while the tube is held steady with the pusher tube. When correct placement has been confirmed, the scope and the pusher tube are removed, and finally the position of the endoesophageal tube is checked radiologically.

5.7 Surgical Tube Insertion

For the surgical placement of an endoesophageal tube, the stricture is first dilated using a blind technique so that a stomach tube or pilot extension can pass through it. Complications are almost certain to arise when blind dilatation is attempted in a filiform stricture. Moreover, postoperative healing problems frequently occur with the gastrostomy that is performed for pull-through of the tube. Length of hospitalization and in-hospital mortality are markedly higher with surgical insertion techniques. We feel that the pull-through method is justified only if the patient cannot be transferred to a facility where endoscopic insertion is available.

5.7.1 Technique of Pull-Through Insertion

Preoperative preparation: Prophylactic antibiotics.

Instruments: Basic set, endoesophageal tube, pilot extension.

Position: Supine.

The stomach is exposed through a small, paramedian upper abdominal incision, and the gastrotomy is made in the midportion of the anterior gastric wall.

A stomach tube is passed orally and advanced to the stricture (Fig. 53). A guide stylet can be inserted into the tube to aid its passage through the neoplasm. The Celestin tube is supplied with a tapered pilot extension which is passed in the manner of a stomach tube and attaches flush to the distal end of the Celestin tube. The end of the stomach tube or extension is brought out through the gastrostomy and is used to pull the

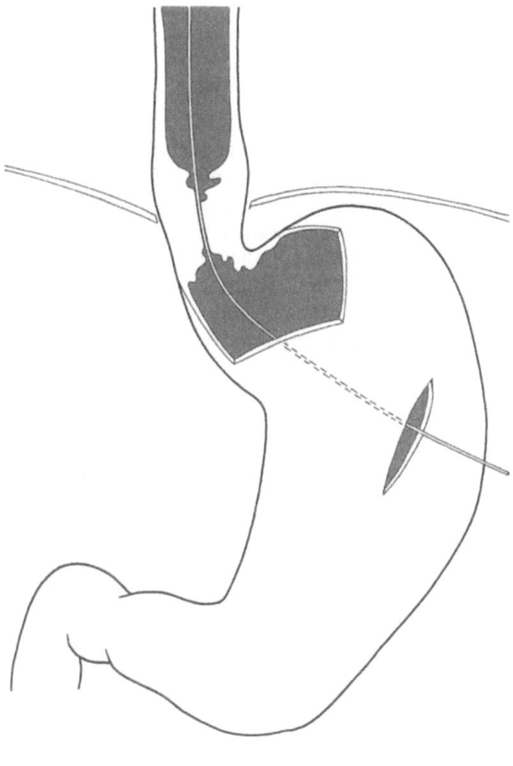

Fig. 53. Surgical tube insertion: The orogastric tube is brought out through the gastrotomy incision

prosthesis into position (Fig. 54). The tube is passed into the upper esophagus under laryngoscopic control, and continuous traction is applied to pull the prosthesis through the stricture, which becomes dilated (Fig. 54). A distal flange is attached to the leading end of the Häring tube to prevent upward migration (Fig. 55). A thin rubber antireflux cuff can also be fitted over the tube.

5.8 Nutrition after Intubation

On the day after placement of the tube, deglutiation is evaluated fluoroscopically by having the patient swallow a water-soluble contrast medium. The examiner confirms that the tube is correctly positioned, looks for signs of perforation, and makes certain that the patency of the tube is not compromised by faulty placement or by indentation of the upper flange. If the contrast medium does not pass freely into the stomach, the tube position should be adjusted. If this is unsuccessful, we replace the tube with a more suitable model. When proper tube function is confirmed, we begin oral feedings with tea and progress to solid foods.

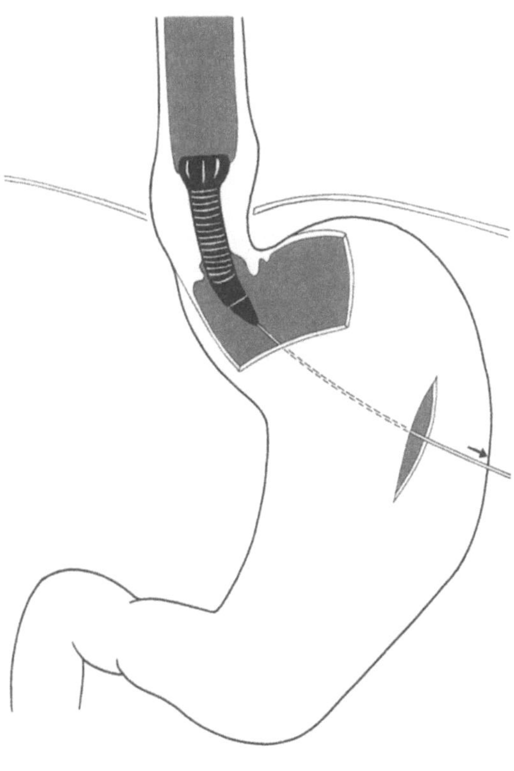

Fig. 54. The prosthetic tube is pulled into the neoplastic stricture by traction on the orogastric tube

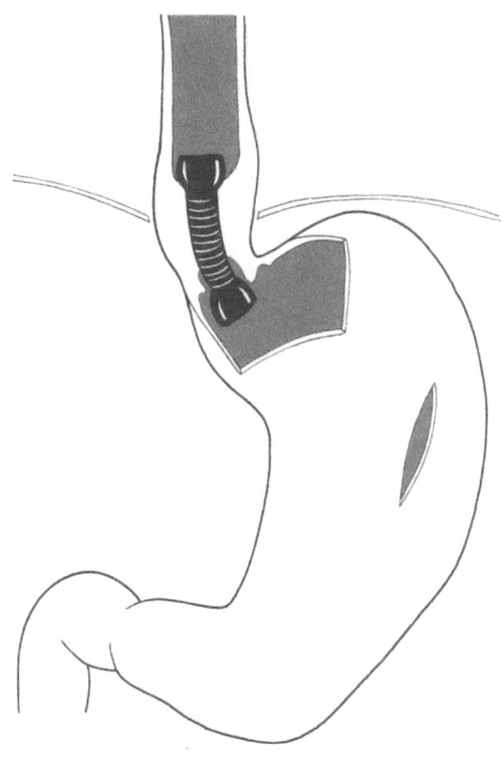

Fig. 55. A distal counterflange is fitted over the end of the tube through the gastrotomy

An important factor besides tube function is the quality of mastication. The patient with a normal or properly restored dentition should have no difficulty consuming a normal diet. We instruct the patient to chew food carefully, to avoid tough meats and foods that cannot be finely masticated, to sit while eating, and to wash food down with frequent drinks.

Swallowing difficulties. If the patient experiences dysphagia, he should first try to restore passage by drinking more liquids. If difficulties persist for more than a few hours, the patient should present at the hospital for evaluation.

Other potential problems. While some tubes are placed far enough proximally that their distal end is above the cardia, most tubes will traverse the cardia, creating a free communication between the stomach and esophagus and removing the physiologic barrier to gastroesophageal reflux. Nevertheless, only a minority of patients complain of acid reflux. Heartburn is mainly experienced in recumbency and can be relieved by elevating the upper body during sleep. An antacid should be prescribed if complaints persist.

References

1. Atkinson M, Ferguson R, Parker GC (1978) Tube introducer and modified Celestin tube for use in palliative intubation of esophagogastric neoplasms at fiberoptic endoscopy. Gut 19:669–671
2. Buess G, Lorenz B, Eitenmüller J, Steinbrich W (1982) Problems of dissolution after long-term placement of a Celestin esophageal tube. Endosc 14:182
3. Celestin LR, Etienne J, Raimbert Ph, Fallouh H, Sultan R (1980) Traitement endoscopique des sténoses oesophagiennes par prothèse de Celestin. Nouv Press Méd 30:2155–2157
4. Den Hartog Jager FCA, Bartelsman JFWM,Tytgat GNJ (1979) Palliative treatment of obstructing esophagogastric malignancy by endoscopic positioning of a plastic prothesis. Gastroent 77:1008–1014
5. Häring R (1964) Eine neue Ösophagusendoprothese als Palliativmaßnahme beim inoperablen Ösophagus- und Kardiacarcinom. Chirurg 35:549–551
6. Mikulicz J (1881) Über Gastroskopie und Ösophagoskopie. Zentralbl Chir 8:43
7. Tytgat GN, den Hartog Jager FCA (1982) Ergebnisse der endoskopischen Implantation von Überbrückungstuben. Dt Ärztebl 5:49–63

6 Esophageal Resections

CONTENTS

6.1 Extent of the Resection

The extent of the esophageal resection depends on the underlying disease. Anatomic factors such as blood supply are a secondary concern. For benign disease, part or all of the cervical, thoracic, or abdominal portions of the esophagus may be resected and replaced by appropriate reconstructive measures (see Sect. 7). For malignant disease, a segmental resection of the esophagus is rarely adequate [25]. Removal of the cervical esophagus or abdominal esophagus with gastrectomy is appropriate only in a high-risk patient with a very small carcinoma confined to the mucosa of the cervical esophagus or with an adenocarcinoma of the stomach that extends to the esophagogastric junction. As a rule, carcinomas situated above the aortic arch require extirpation of the entire esophagus along with regional lymph nodes [3, 15, 39]. With carcinoma of the cervical esophagus or hypopharynx, the procedure is extended to include partial pharyngectomy, laryngectomy, partial or complete thyroidectomy, and excision of the cervical lymph nodes [28, 30, 49]. For carcinomas at or below the aortic arch, the limits of the resection extend from the cervical esophagus to the esophagogastric junction [3, 34, 38]. Because these cancers are commonly associated with lymph node metastases along the lesser curvature of the stomach, it is recommended that the lesser curve be resected as far as the third proximal branch of the left gastric artery to ensure removal of positive nodes [3]. Partial esophagectomy combined with total or partial gastrectomy is appropriate only for adenocarcinoma of the cardia or small squamous cell cancers of the abdominal esophagus. In these cases the esophagus is resected at the level of the bifurcation or azygos vein, maintaining a clearance of 6 cm from the visible and palpable superior edge of the tumor [16, 43, 48].

6.2 Sequence of the Procedure

In a one-stage operation for benign disease, the esophageal substitute is mobilized through an abdominal or thoracic approach, the diseased esophagus is resected, and finally alimentary continuity is restored. In a two-stage operation it is customary to perform the esophageal resection and construct an esophagostomy and feeding fistula in the first sitting, and then reestablish continuity in a second sitting. Alternatively, the stomach or bowel may be transposed before the esophagus is resected.

With esophageal carcinoma, we feel that the patient's limited life expectancy requires that resection and reconstruction be performed in one stage, rather than two or three, even after a putatively curative resection. The three-stage operation [22, 35] is associated with better late results owing to patient selection, but it deprives patients of natural swallowing for some months, even with use of an extracorporeal bypass tube (see 2.4), and delays the resumption of a normal life. We initially preferred the two-stage procedure [44], anticipating that it would reduce hospital deaths. However, we found that the resection, and not the reconstruction, was the critical factor in determining patient outcomes. At present, then, we see no reason to separate the two procedures unless unfavorable anatomic conditions (e.g., due to previous surgery) so complicate the resection or reconstruction that the risk to the patient becomes excessive.

With carcinoma of the cervical or abdominal esophagus, exploration of the tumor precedes resection and replacement of the esophagus in the same or a second sitting. With carcinoma of the thoracic esophagus, there is lack of agreement on whether resectability should first be determined through a thoracotomy and the procedure continued if the lesion appears resectable, or whether a laparotomy should be performed first to exclude intraabdominal lymph node involvement. Here it should be recalled that intraabdominal lymph node involvement from intrathoracic esophageal carcinoma is considered to represent distant metastasis in the TNM classification [57]. Given the poor long-term results of surgical resection for esophageal carcinoma [14], we consider this debate to be irrelevant. If we disregard the results of Japanese and Chinese authors, whose clinical material is not comparable to that of Western authors with respect to case numbers or selection, we find that the resection of esophageal carcinoma is palliative in approximately 90% of cases. Modern radiologic techniques such as CT provide an accurate means of confirming or excluding distant metastases and, to a degree, evaluating for lymph node involvement and spread to adjacent organs [10, 43]. When these techniques are applied in conjunction with contrast studies of the esophagus, which give information on tumor extent, the esophageal axis above and below the tumor, local tumor spread, lymph node involvement, and distant metastasis [4, 5], it is possible to determine the resectability of a carcinoma with a high degree of confidence. Generally, then, the decision for resection can be made prior to operation, and the surgical procedure is dictated essentially by considerations of operative technique.

In the standard procedure – resection of the esophagus with subsequent reconstruction by stomach during a single anesthesia session – we begin with the abdominal incision, prepare the esophageal substitute, and mobilize the distal esophagus in the posterior mediastinum. The patient is then repositioned for a right thoracotomy, and the esophageal resection is carried out. With carcinoma below the aortic arch, the anastomosis can be performed at the level of the pleural apex, or the chest may be closed, the patient repositioned, and the substitute brought up subcutaneously or retrosternally to the neck, where it is united to the cervical esophagus. In terms of complete tumor removal, it is immaterial whether the anastomosis (e.g., with the EEA instrument) is placed transpleurally at the level of the thoracic inlet or directly in the neck. The intrathoracic anastomosis offers the advantage of shorter operating time, but a leak in this area poses an acutely life-threatening situation. Additional exposure of the esophagus in the neck lengthens operating time, but leakage in that area can usually be managed satisfactorily. Exposure of the cervical esophagus is imperative for supraaortic carcinoma, which requires that the esophageal substitute be anastomosed directly to the pharynx (e.g., pharyngogastrostomy).

If the thoracic phase were performed first in a single-stage operation, it would be necessary either to use a thoracoabdominal incision or perform a phrenotomy, which we prefer to avoid because of the associated compromise of diaphragmatic function. An intrathoracic anastomosis would require that the patient be moved from the lateral position to the supine position for intraabdominal mobilization of the esophageal substitute, then back to the thoracotomy position again for the anastomosis. This can be avoided by performing the anastomosis in the neck, but either option results in prolonged operating time. For resection and reconstruction in two sittings, we begin with the thoracotomy, transect the esophagus at the stomach, and construct a cervical stoma following the esophageal resection. The gastrostomy is then performed through a small laparotomy 5 cm in length. We see no justification for an extensive exploratory laparotomy at the start of the operation. Since a permanent cure is rarely achieved, involvement of the intraabdominal lymph nodes is not an absolute contraindication to resection. An extensive laparotomy needlessly prolongs the operation, and the resulting adhesions compound the difficulty of a subsequent abdominal procedure.

6.3 Selection of the Approach

Resection of the cervical esophagus can be performed through a right or left cervicotomy incision along the anterior border of the sternocleidomastoid muscle or through a unilateral collar incision. An extended resection that includes the larynx, parts of the pharynx, the thyroid, and the cervical lymph nodes can be performed through a trapdoor incision or an extended collar incision that is carried along the sternocleidomastoid muscle to the mastoid on each side (see 6.4.2, Fig. 56).

Resections of the thoracic esophagus can be accomplished through a right or left thoracotomy (see Chap. B) or bluntly through a cervicoabdominal approach. We do not see these methods as competing with each other, but rather as mutually complementary. The advantage of the right-sided approach [31, 55] is that it gives relatively unobstructed access for esophagectomy. Some cases will require division of the azygos vein; usually this will not result in significant late sequelae. Thus we consider the right-sided approach to be standard for resections of the thoracic esophagus. In the left approach [18, 54], the esophagus must be carefully mobilized below the aortic arch and then pulled upward from behind the arch. While this procedure is not inordinately difficult, it is more technically demanding and time consuming than the right-sided approach.

A resection confined to the distal intrathoracic portion of the esophagus [37] is more easily accomplished through a left thoracotomy [61]. If the incision must be extended into the abdomen, the right lobe of the liver will not be an obstacle. It is possible, however, to resect the esophagus and proximal stomach entirely through a right or left thoracic incision and follow up with a esophagogastrostomy to restore continuity [7, 15].

Esophagectomy without thoracotomy [1, 12, 56] is the method of choice for long, benign strictures that cannot be adequately dilated and for carcinomas of the abdominal or cervical esophagus in which the primary tumor and its lymphatic drainage can be exposed directly but total esophagectomy is needed to effect a radical removal or facilitate reconstruction. Omission of thoracotomy in these cases significantly reduces the risk of operation.

The abdominal esophagus can be resected through a midline or left paramedian laparotomy or through a left subcostal incision. In each approach the esophagus can be well mobilized in the posterior mediastinum through the hiatus, allowing it to be pulled several centimeters distally and the anastomosis performed with the EEA instrument. The anastomosis will retract into the chest when tension on the esophagus is released.

6.4 Resection of the Cervical Esophagus

6.4.1 Indications

Few indications exist for resection of the cervical esophagus alone [11]. It may be considered in elderly patients in poor general health who have a small carcinoma between the cricopharyngeal muscle and thoracic inlet. Benign strictures and broad-based benign tumors of the cervical esophagus rarely require a segmental resection. Nondilatable strictures can be widened by a plastic procedure (see 4.2). If resection of a broad-based benign tumor creates a wall defect so large that the mobilized esophagus cannot be closed transversely, coverage with a free intestinal patch should be considered (see 4.2.2).

The standard procedure for carcinomas that have infiltrated the cricopharyngeal muscle or extend from that muscle to within 3 cm of the thoracic inlet consists of partial pharyngectomy, laryngectomy with tracheostomy, resection of the cervical esophagus, resection of one thyroid lobe or total thyroidectomy, and excision of the cervical lymph nodes [21, 28, 49, 52]. Continuity is restored by the transfer of a free segment of jejunum or colon [36, 46]. An alternative is to add blunt removal of the thoracic esophagus followed by intrathoracic or retrosternal elevation of the stomach [30, 40, 47, 50]. This procedure is less technically demanding than a free intestinal graft with microvascular anastomosis, and we consider it less hazardous.

We no longer favor esophageal reconstruction with skin grafts [6, 59, 60] due to the limited survival time of the cancer patients and the long duration of the reconstruction, which usually must be performed in multiple stages. In patients with benign disease and good life expectancy, the unphysiologic surface loads on the skin tube predispose it to malignant change. If the carcinoma extends close to the thoracic inlet, total esophagectomy is always indicated, and continuity is restored by pharyngogastric anastomosis (see 7.3) or colon interposition (see 7.4) [3, 29, 39].

Because of the magnitude of the procedure and the associated postoperative morbidity and mortality, we are cautious about recommending these operations except in young patients who are found on exploration to have a carcinoma limited to the esophagus. We prefer radiotherapy. It is generally agreed that the resection of cervical esophageal carcinoma is contraindicated by infiltration of the prevertebral fascia, invasion of the trachea, infiltration of the neurovascular bundle (especially the carotid vessels), and the detection of multiple lymph node metastases with fixation to surrounding structures. The involvement of individual lymph nodes and tracheal infiltration to within 3 cm of the thoracic inlet are considered relative contraindications, since the cervical lymph nodes are removed at operation in any case, and resection of the manubrium can be added to ensure a safe margin. It is very common, however, to elect radiotherapy alone for the management of these cases.

6.4.2 Technique of the Simple and Extended Resection of the Cervical Esophagus

The procedure for a simple transverse resection of the cervical esophagus and its extension to include removal of the cervical viscera are begun in identical fashion and so will be described jointly. In carcinoma patients, both procedures begin with an exploration from the side of the neck toward which the tumor is spreading. Injury to major neurovascular structures is avoided. If the tumor is judged to be nonresectable, the procedure can be abandoned without significant postoperative sequelae. If resectability is confirmed, the rest of the procedure depends on whether a simple or extended resection is proposed.

Preoperative preparation: Antiseptic preparation of the pharynx, removal of teeth involved by caries or periodontal infection; prophylactic antibiotics (see Chap. C); intestinal lavage as required.

Instruments: Basic set, extra thoracic set, microsurgical set, EEA, GIA, TA.

Position and approach: See 2.1.1. Incision along the anterior border of the right or left sternocleidomastoid muscle for a simple transverse resection (Fig. 56 a). Exposure at the thoracic inlet can be improved by curving the distal end of the incision medially a thumb's width above the clavicle, resulting in a hockeystick-shaped incision. For the extended resection, the incision is carried in U-shaped fashion from the mastoid on one side along the sternocleidomastoid muscles to the mastoid on the opposite side. It may be supplemented by supraclavicular incisions to facilitate the lymph node dissection (Fig. 56 b), or trapdoor incisions may be made primarily (Fig. 56 c). If the operation is preceded by a diagnostic lymph node biopsy, the surgeon performing the biopsy should make allowance for the placement of subsequent incisions.

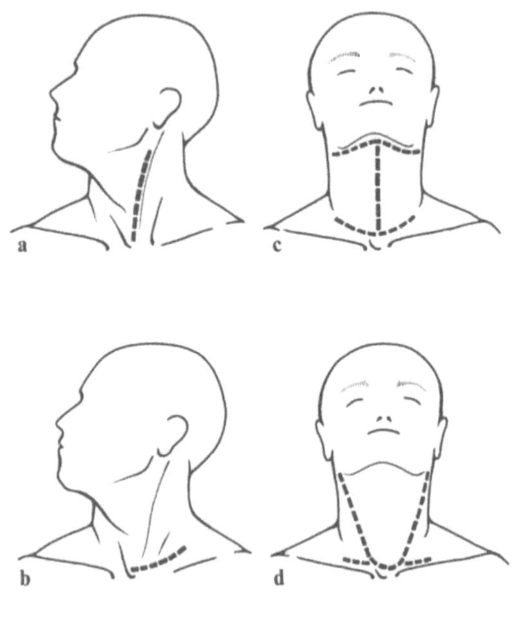

Fig. 56a–d. Incisions for resection of the cervical esophagus. **a** Incision along the anterior border of the sternocleidomastoid muscle (simple resection). **b** Unilateral collar incision. **c** Trapdoor incision (extended resection). **d** Full collar incision with U-shaped extensions (extended resection)

Steps in procedure:

(1) Exposure of the esophagus in the neck (see 2.1.1)
(2) Exploration to determine tumor extent
(3) Division of the esophagus below the cricopharyngeal muscle and above the thoracic inlet, or
(4) Extension of the skin incision for resection of the cervical viscera
(5) Division of the superficial cervical fascia
(6) Release of the sternocleidomastoid muscle from the clavicle
(7) Resection of the omohyoid muscle
(8) Dissection of the submental and submandibular lymph node groups in the antero-inferior direction
(9) Exposure of the digastric muscle (sparing the hypoglossal nerve)
(10) Exposure of the accessory nerve
(11) Snaring and circumferential dissection of the internal jugular vein, carotid vessels, and vagus nerve
(12) Ligation of the superior thyroid artery, ascending pharyngeal artery, and possibly the lingual and inferior thyroid arteries
(13) Release of the strap muscles from the clavicle
(14) Transection of the trachea at the level of the thoracic inlet and intubation of the tracheal stoma through the field
(15) Thyroidectomy, preserving one lobe if possible
(16) Supra- or infrahyoid division of the pharynx and larynx
(17) Separation of the pharynx and cervical esophagus from the prevertebral fascia
(18) Division of the esophagus at the level of the thoracic inlet, or extension of the resection to the thoracic esophagus.

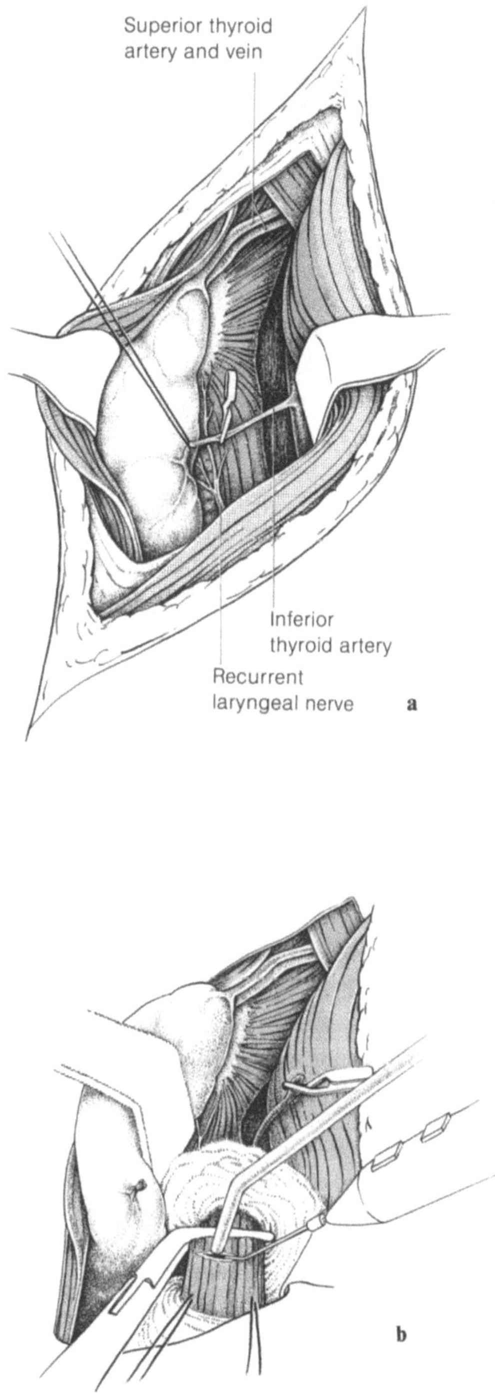

Fig. 57 a, b. Simple transverse resection of the cervical esophagus. Exploration of the tumor. **a** The inferior thyroid artery is ligated close to the thyroid gland, as it is a potential donor vessel for a free graft. **b** The esophagus is divided below the tumor with the electrocautery

6.4.2.1 *Exploration of the Tumor*

Operative technique: The esophagus is exposed (see 2.1.1). If a simple transverse resection is proposed, it should be considered that one of the two thyroid arteries is a potential donor vessel for a free graft (see 4.2.2). An adequate segment of this artery is exposed, ligated close to the thyroid, occluded proximally with a small clamp, and then divided (Fig. 57 a). With the aid of a binocular loupe, the recurrent laryngeal nerve is sought between the trachea and esophagus (watch for variations; see 2.1.1) and is traced to its site of entry into the larynx. The esophagus is palpated between the trachea and vertebral column to localize the neoplasm. Intraoperative esophagoscopy is helpful if doubt exists. The esophagus distal to the tumor is freed from its loose connective tissue attachments, and the anterior surface is carefully separated from the membranous wall of the trachea by patty dissection. When the esophagus has been freed circumferentially, it is snared with a rubber tape, avoiding injury to the contralateral recurrent nerve. The tape is pulled forward and upward to elevate the esophagus slightly away from the prevertebral fascia. A finger or dissecting patty is used to further separate the esophagus bluntly from the prevertebral fascia, carrying the dissection upward until the tumor-bearing segment of the esophagus, whose extent is determined by palpation, is cleared. Success in accomplishing this is considered to confirm resectability. If it is found that the tumor has penetrated the esophageal wall and invaded the prevertebral fascia, resectability becomes questionable. If the tumor extent is uncertain, the esophagus should be exposed from the opposite side using the same technique.

If tumor infiltration of surrounding structures is confirmed, the operation may be terminated without harm, since no essential structures have been sacrificed.

6.4.2.2 Simple Transverse Resection of the Esophagus

If the exploration reveals a small carcinoma and the patient is too ill to undergo extensive surgery, dissection of the esophagus from the prevertebral fascia is carried superiorly until the horizontal fibers of the cricopharyngeal muscle are recognized. The esophagus is pulled laterally with the rubber tape, and its anteromedial surface is bluntly separated from the trachea with the index finger or a dissecting patty, proceeding from below upward. Once the plane between the trachea and esophagus has been established, it should be possible to perform the transection as high as the cricoid, where the trachea is joined to the esophagus by the cricopharyngeal muscle. Difficulty in isolating the esophagus from the trachea may be due to tumor infiltration of the tracheal wall. In that case the plan for a simple transverse resection must be abandoned in favor of an extended resection. Blunt mobilization of the cervical esophagus is carried down past the thoracic inlet and into the posterior mediastinum to gain additional esophageal length for the resection. At this time the limits of the resection are defined. A gauze strip soaked in Clorpactin solution is packed around the esophagus in the thoracic inlet to prevent bacterial infection of the posterior mediastinum and tumor cell dissemination when the esophagus is opened. The esophagus is first engaged with two heavy traction sutures below the proposed site of transection to keep it from retracting into the chest. A right-angle clamp is placed on the esophagus above that site, and the esophageal wall facing the operator is opened transversely with the electrocautery or scalpel (Fig. 57 b). Residual secretions are aspirated from the esophagus, and the mucosa is cleaned with dissecting patties soaked in antiseptic solution before the rest of the wall circumference is divided. The cervical stump is occluded with a clamp, pulled laterally downward, and openly divided just below the cricopharyngeal muscle after first partially opening the wall and cleaning the lumen as described above. Both recurrent nerves are preserved with this technique.

6.4.2.3 Removal of the Cervical Lymph Nodes

If the tumor is resectable and an extended esophageal resection is proposed that includes removal of the cervical viscera, the skin incision must be extended accordingly (see 6.4.2, Fig. 56 c,d). The entire skin flap is dissected upward to the mandible (Fig. 58 a,b). The platysma is left on the skin flap; removing it does not improve tumor clearance but may jeopardize the viability of the flap [45].

The rest of the procedure depends on whether a "classic" (i.e. radical) or "functional" cervical lymph node dissection is planned. We do not favor the classic lymph node dissection with removal of the sternocleidomastoid, omohyoid, digastric and stylohyoid muscles, internal jugular vein, accessory nerve, cervical plexus, and submandibular gland for esophageal carcinoma, because it

Fig. 58 a, b. Functional lymph node dissection in the neck. **a** The skin, subcutaneous tissue, and platysma are dissected free. **b** The soft tissues have been reflected upward (and for clarity the superficial connective tissue and cervical fasciae removed) to demonstrate the surgical anatomy of the region ▷

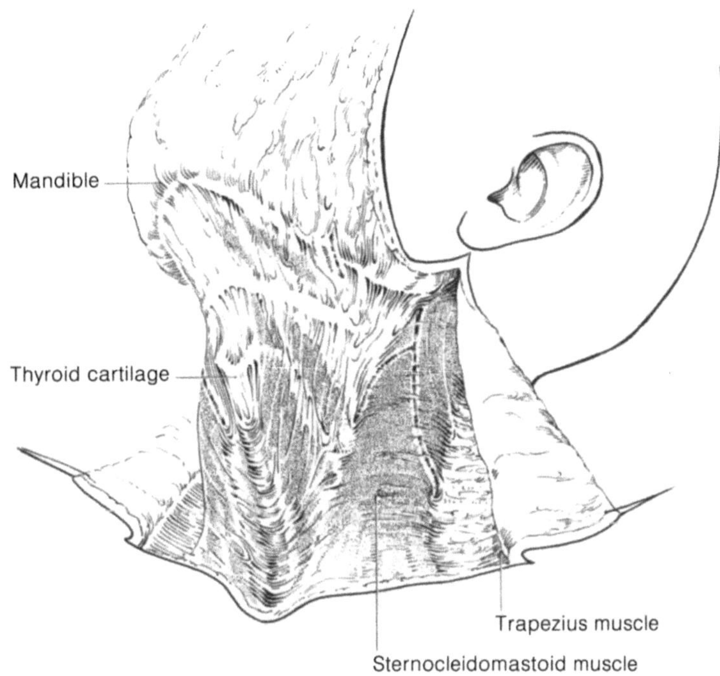

Mandible
Thyroid cartilage
Trapezius muscle
Sternocleidomastoid muscle

a

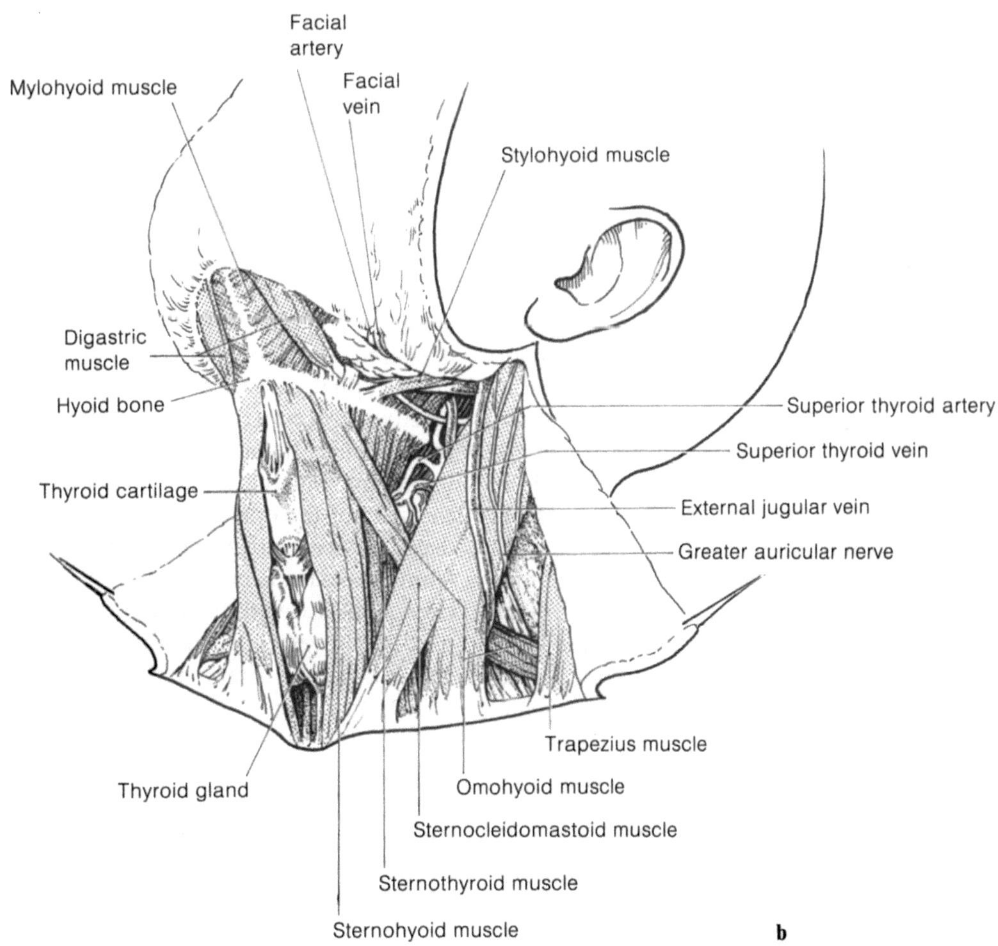

Facial artery
Facial vein
Mylohyoid muscle
Stylohyoid muscle
Digastric muscle
Hyoid bone
Superior thyroid artery
Superior thyroid vein
Thyroid cartilage
External jugular vein
Greater auricular nerve
Trapezius muscle
Thyroid gland
Omohyoid muscle
Sternocleidomastoid muscle
Sternothyroid muscle
Sternohyoid muscle

b

has not been proved that this mutiliating procedure improves the late result. The technique of the classic lymph node dissection is described fully in volume V/3 of this series [11].

Lam et al. [29] modified the lymph node dissection by removing only the sternocleidomastoid muscle and internal jugular vein on the side facing the tumor and then covering the exposed common carotid and internal carotid arteries with the levator scapulae or scalenus medius muscle following wide mobilization and division of the external carotid artery.

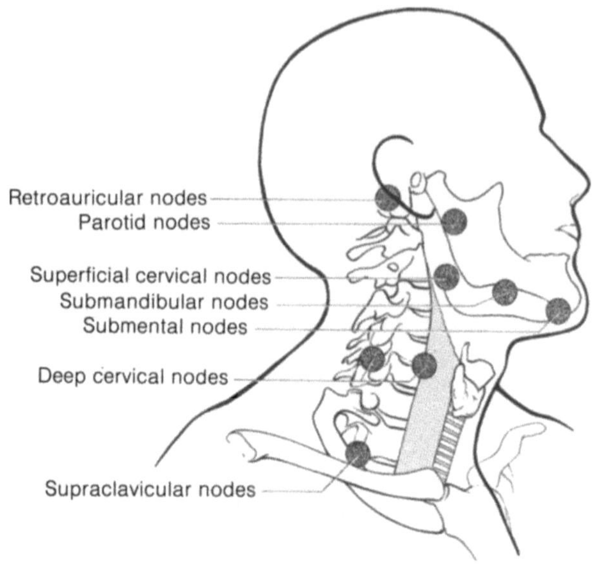

Fig. 59. Lymph node groups of the cervical region (schematic drawing)

We prefer the functional lymph node dissection (Fig. 59), in which the superficial cervical fascia is incised along the boundaries of the operative field. The veins crossing the field are divided. The superficial cervical fascia is incised along the anterior border of the sternocleidomastoid. From there the fascia, with the veins coursing upon it, is dissected back to the anterior border of the trapezius muscle, proceeding from above downward and sparing the great auricular nerve, until the fascia is attached only to the contents of the greater supraclavicular fossa. At this point the sternocleidomastoid muscle is mobilized and held aside with a blunt retractor for further dissections, or is divided 1 cm above its sternoclavicular origin and reflected superiorly. This technique is simpler, gives better exposure, and generally does not lead to functional loss.

The dissection is carried from above downward and from laterally to medially until finally the lymph node packet is left adherent to the strap muscles, the larynx, or the trachea. The submandibular fossa is opened a thumb's width below the mandible (Fig. 60 a). Maintaining this clearance avoids injury to the marginal branch of the facial nerve, which passes below the mandible in about 20% of cases. The facial artery arising from the external carotid is exposed and ligated with its accompanying veins. The vascular stumps may be retracted superiorly so that the inferior branch of the facial nerve can be positively identified and kept out of the field. The fat, connective tissue, and lymph nodes around the submandibular gland are bluntly dissected downward and medially from the gland without difficulty. As lymph nodes may be embedded in the glandular tissue, concurrent removal of the gland should be considered. As the dissection is carried farther anteriorly, the submental lymph node group with its accompanying connective tissue is dissected free and reflected downward. This group is continuous inferiorly with the lymph nodes around the digastric muscle. As the muscle is dissected free in the direction of the internal jugular vein (Fig. 60 b), attention is given to the hypoglossal nerve, which runs behind the intermediate tendon of the digastric. At this stage the proximal part of the neurovascular sheath lies exposed. The accessory nerve is sought posterolateral to the sheath; it courses deeply about a thumb's breadth below the mastoid process, where it is recognized by its posteroinferior course. The nerve is snared and dissected free. Now the connective and lymphatic tissue can be removed as far as the mastoid process (Fig. 60 c). After the greater supraclavicular fossa has been cleared of connective tissue and fat, the nodal packet dissected free at the start of the operation is pulled anteriorly. The deep cervical fascia, now exposed, is separated from the scalenus muscles, carefully preserving the cervical plexus with the phrenic nerve, the brachial plexus, the vessels of the thyrocervical trunk, and the subclavian artery and vein. The omohyoid muscle is resected. Now the lymph node packet

Fig. 60a–d. Functional lymph node dissection in the neck. **a** The submental and submandibular groups of nodes are dissected free. The sternocleidomastoid muscle is divided and reflected upward. **b** The lymphatic drainage tracts around the digastric muscle are removed, sparing the hypoglossal nerve. **c, d** see p. 304 ▷

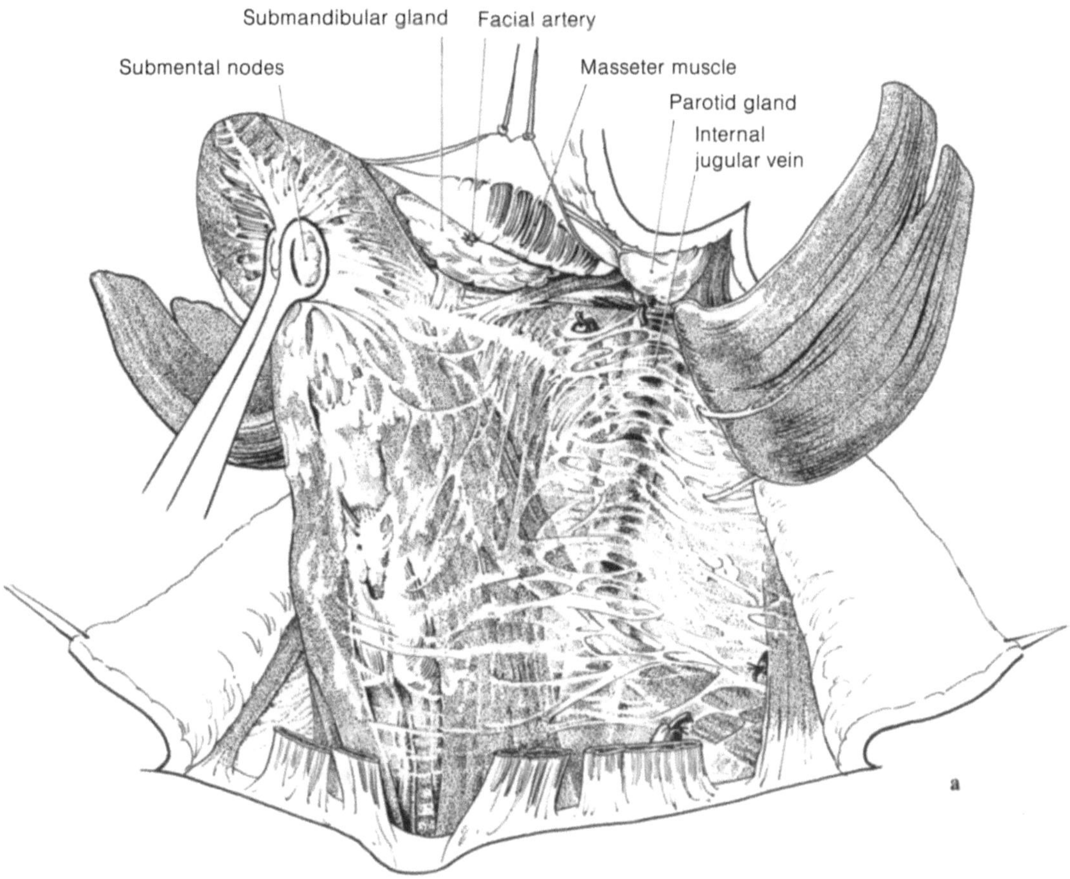
Submandibular gland
Facial artery
Submental nodes
Masseter muscle
Parotid gland
Internal jugular vein

a

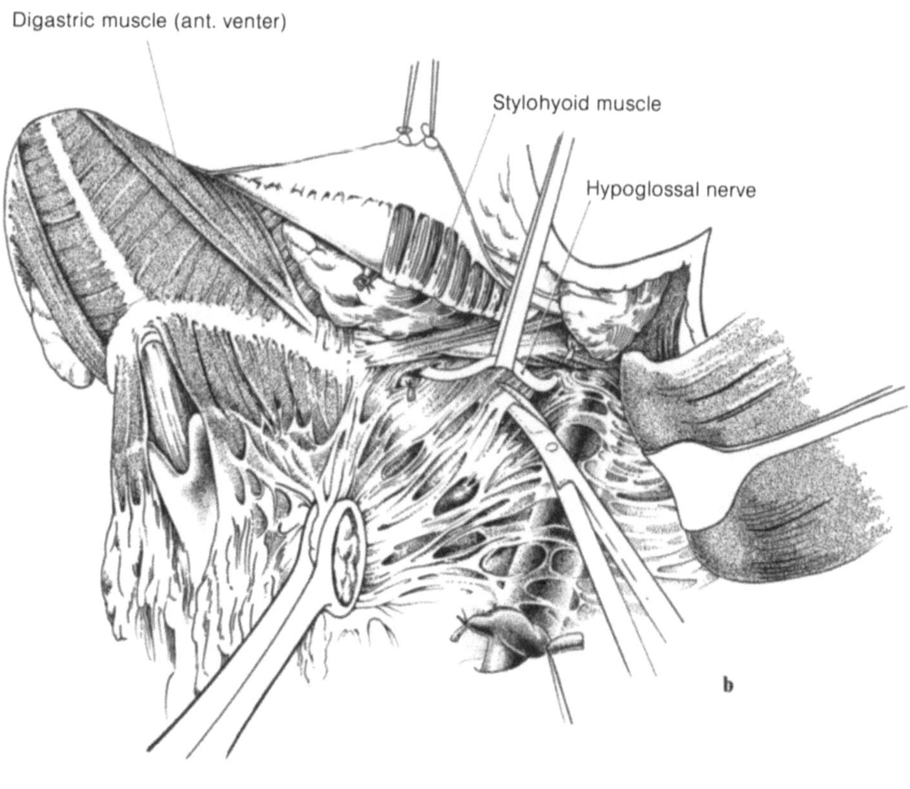
Digastric muscle (ant. venter)
Stylohyoid muscle
Hypoglossal nerve

b

Fig. 60. c The accessory nerve is exposed and protected. **d** Exposure of the neurovascular sheath

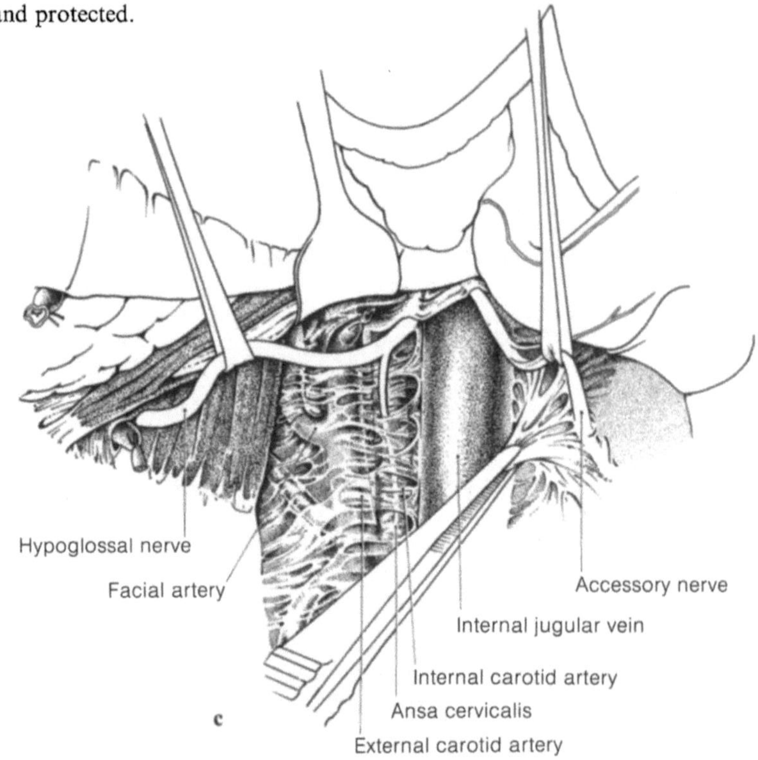

c

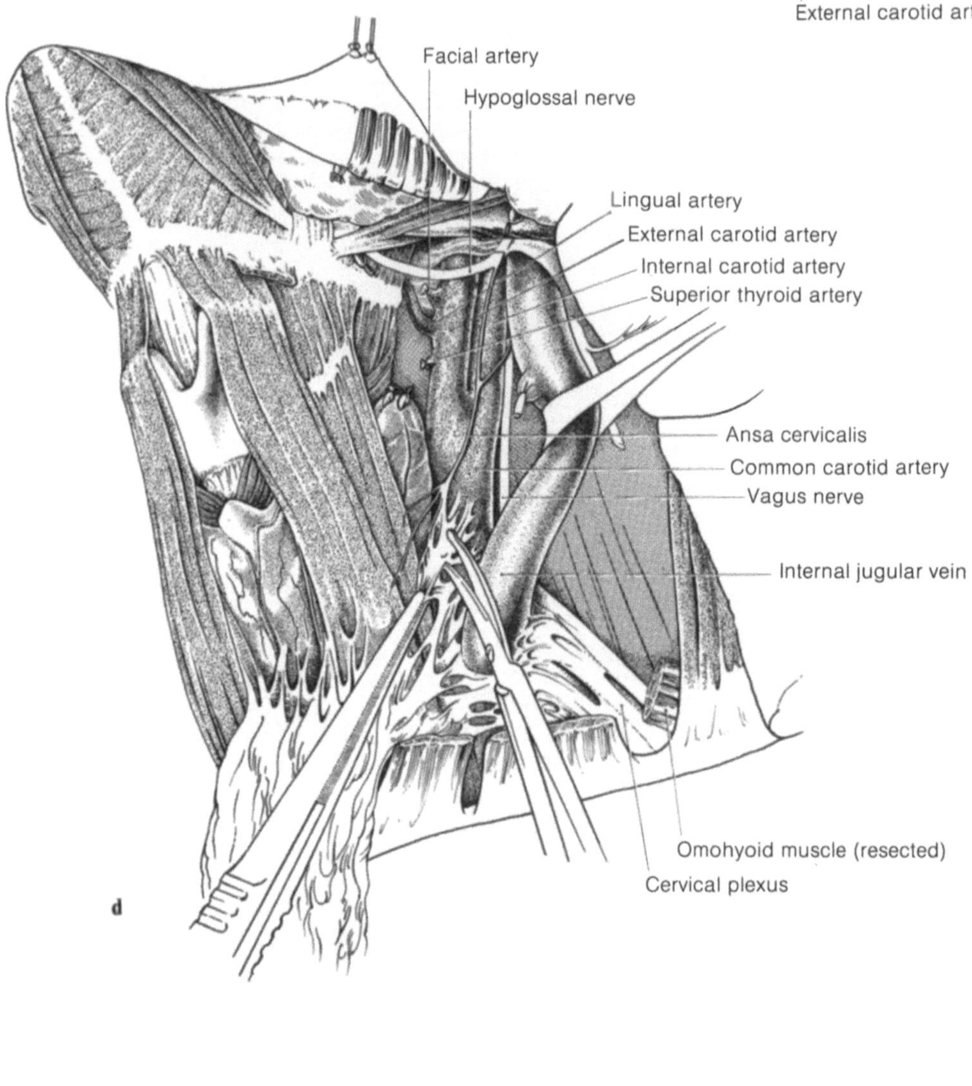

d

that has been pulled anteriorly is severed from its attachments to the carotid vessels, the internal jugular vein, and the vagus nerve (Fig. 60 d). These structures are carefully freed of lymph nodes and connective tissue about their whole circumference. The dissection is facilitated by snaring the structures individually and elevating them from their bed. If the internal jugular vein and vagus nerve are found to be infiltrated by lymph node metastases, they are resected if the involvement is unilateral. This produces recurrent nerve palsy on the affected side, but this is inconsequential if a laryngectomy is planned.

If involvement is bilateral, at least one side must be freed from tumor by sharp dissection. If a lymph node is so firmly fixed to one of the carotid vessels that it cannot be removed even on the subadventitial plane, the external carotid artery may be ligated proximal and distal to the site of involvement and resected without danger of late sequelae. With infiltration of the internal carotid artery or common carotid artery, the involved vascular segment is completely or partially resected under the protection of an intraluminal shunt, and the defect is repaired with a venous patch graft or interpositional vein graft. It should be added, however, that involvement of this extent generally signifies inoperability.

If the thyroid arteries were not previously divided during exploration of the tumor, and if the thyroid gland or one of its lobes is to be resected, the inferior thyroid artery, superior thyroid artery, and ascending pharyngeal artery are divided, proceeding from below upward. If a free graft is to be used for restoration of continuity, the artery that will be anastomosed to the graft is not ligated proximally, but is simply occluded with a small vascular clamp. Ligation of the lingual artery depends on the level of the resection in the pharynx. If the resection is to include the hyoid bone, the lingual artery must be ligated and divided. Following dissection of the neurovascular sheath, the entire lymph node packet will be adherent to the strap muscles and can be removed en bloc with the larynx, hypopharynx, and cervical esophagus.

The technique of dissection is essentially the same on both sides. On the left side, however, attention must be given to the thoracic duct when dissecting the lymph nodes in the supraclavicular area. The thoracic duct ascends from the thorax behind the subclavian artery, runs laterally upward behind the internal jugular vein, then arches downward and enters the junction of the internal jugular vein and subclavian vein from the posterior side (Fig. 61). It is located by tracing medially the vascular sheath behind the internal jugular

Fig. 61. The termination of the thoracic duct

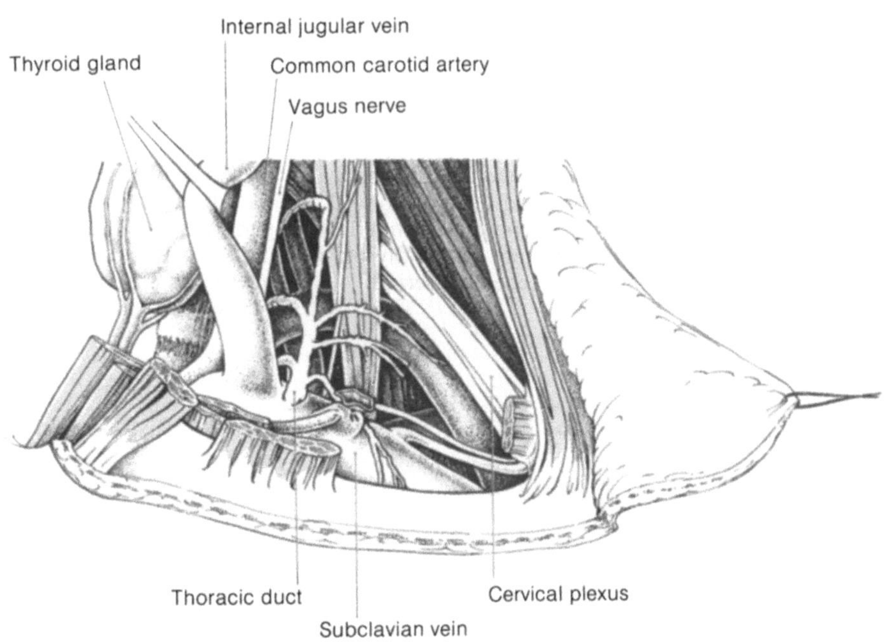

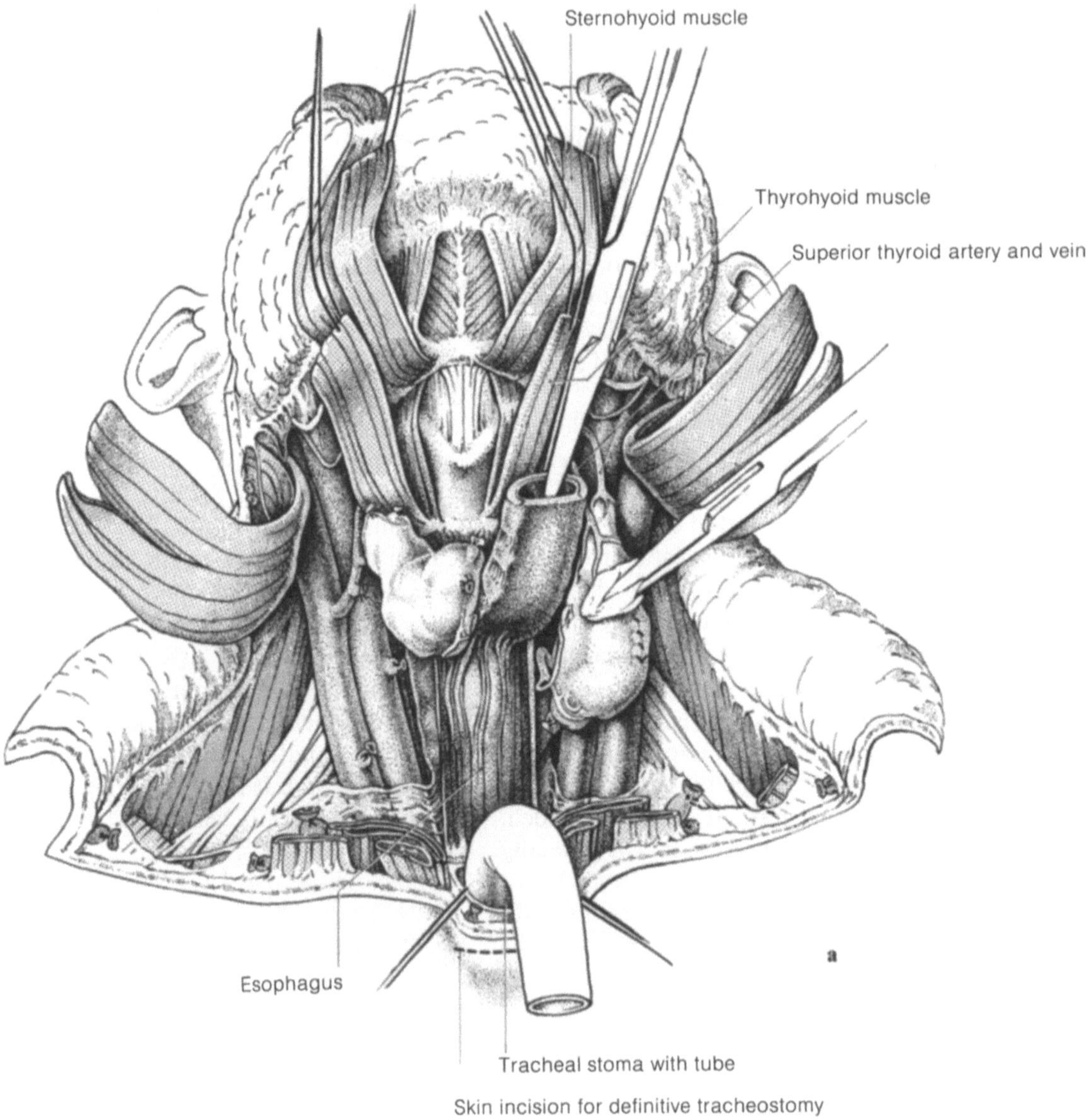

Fig. 62 a–d. Extended resection of the cervical esophagus. **a** Division of the trachea and construction of a tracheostomy. The strap muscles are divided inferiorly and reflected upward. The right lobe of the thyroid is included in the resection; the left lobe is preserved. **b** Incisions for infrahyoid and suprahyoid resection of the larynx. A functional lymph node dissection has been performed on the left side, and a classic lymph node dissection with resection of the sternocleidomastoid and internal jugular vein has been performed on the right side. **c,d** see p. 308

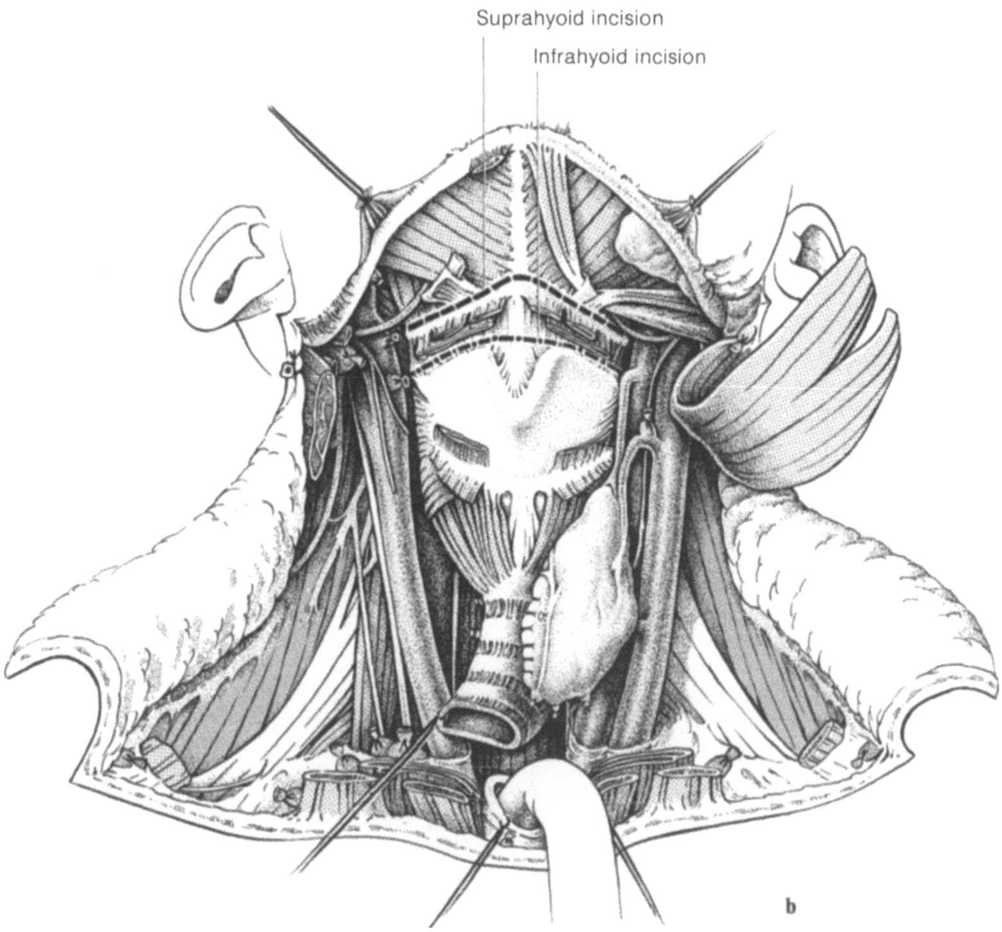

vein. If the duct is injured at operation, it must be ligated to prevent lymphatic fistula.

6.4.2.4 Division of the Trachea and Tracheostomy

The tracheostomy is begun by bluntly mobilizing the skin down past the manubrium. If tumor infiltration of the trachea closely approaches the thoracic inlet, the manubrium is partially resected to achieve an additional safety margin for tumor removal. A circular piece of skin matching the tracheal diameter is excised at the proposed level of transection of the trachea. The strap muscles are bluntly separated in the midline and dissected off the underlying trachea and thyroid. Their sternal attachments are severed with the electrocautery and reflected upward. The trachea is separated from the esophagus (if not previously done during the exploration) and encircled with a snare. After the trachea has been suctioned several times through the endotracheal tube, the tube is unseated, and the anterior wall of the trachea is incised at the level of the skin incision between two tracheal rings. The tube is pulled back past the incision, the remaining tracheal wall is divided with a scissors or scalpel, and the distal trachea is intubated through the operative field with a sterile Woodbridge tube (Fig. 62 a). The tube is seated and connected by sterile extension tubing to the anesthesia machine. The proximal lumen of the tracheal stump is covered with an antiseptic-soaked compress to avoid infection of the operative area. The distal stoma is sewn into the skin incision with a circumferential row of interrupted sutures.

6.4.2.5 Preservation of the Thyroid

Resection of the cervical viscera generally includes removal of the thyroid. In view of the fact that

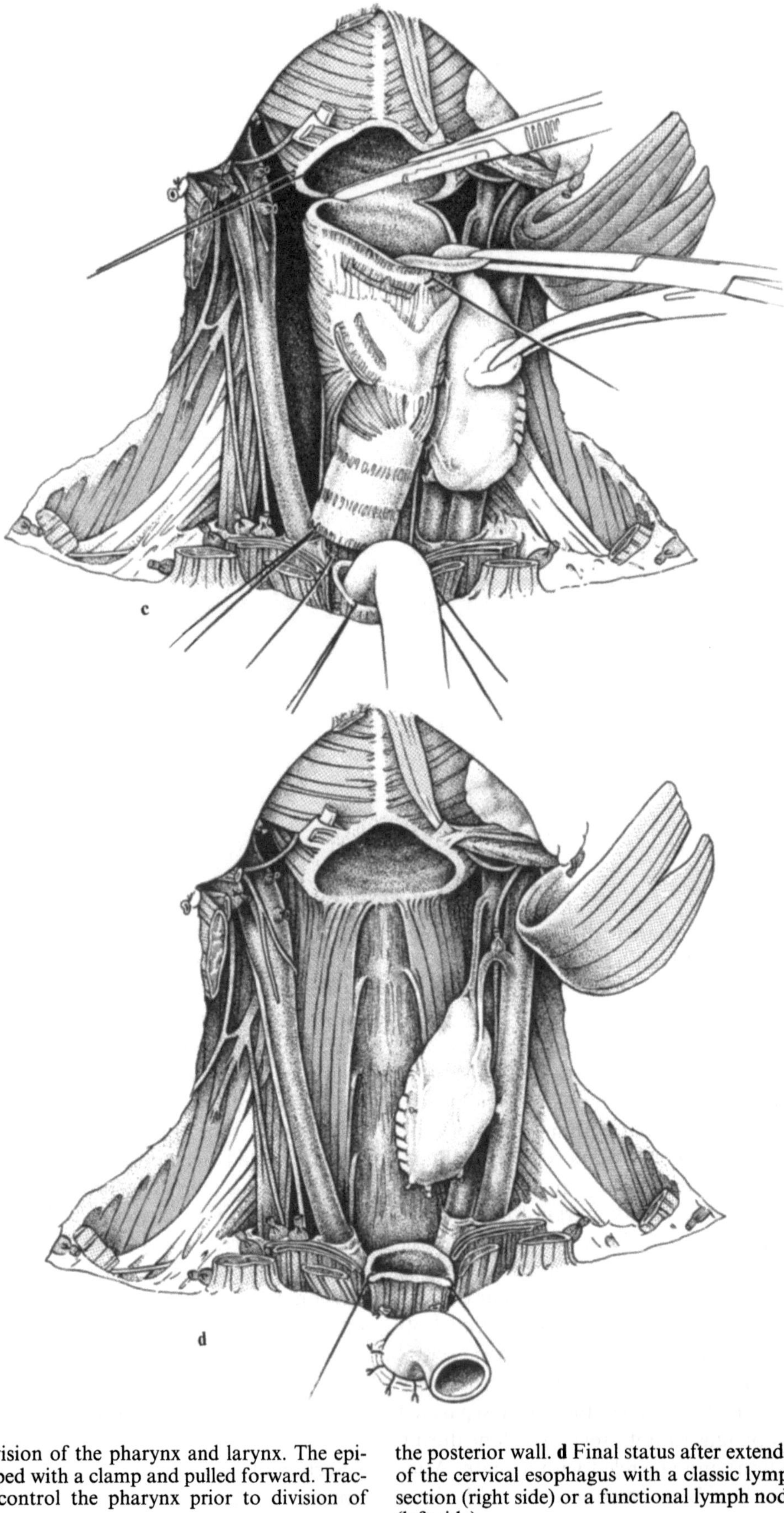

Fig. 62. c Division of the pharynx and larynx. The epiglottis is grasped with a clamp and pulled forward. Traction sutures control the pharynx prior to division of the posterior wall. **d** Final status after extended resection of the cervical esophagus with a classic lymph node dissection (right side) or a functional lymph node dissection (left side)

even this extensive resection is palliative in many cases, it would seem reasonable to preserve at least one thyroid lobe and the parathyroids on one side so that the patient will be spared the troublesome sequelae of thyroidectomy and parathyroidectomy [8]. It is advisable in this regard, though not essential, to preserve the blood supply to the thyroid via the superior or inferior thyroid artery as well as its venous drainage (especially on the side away from the tumor) during the exploratory and lymphatic dissection phase of the operation.

The detached strap muscles with their adherent lymph node packets are dissected upward from the thyroid body on the side that is to be preserved. The thyroid is divided through the isthmus, and the cut surface is closed with a ligature or running suture. Using a finger or dissecting patty, the lobe to be preserved is bluntly freed from its connective tissue attachments with the trachea from the medial side and reflected laterally so that it remains attached by one nutrient vessel (Fig. 62 b). The recurrent nerve may be ignored, since the larynx is to be removed.

6.4.2.6 Resection of the Larynx, Hypopharynx, and Cervical Esophagus (v. Hacker, Gluck, Soerensen)

The esophagus was already separated posteriorly from the prevertebral fascia as far as the hypopharynx during the exploratory phase of the procedure. This blunt dissection is continued superiorly to the level of the hyoid bone. Inferiorly, the esophagus is mobilized circumferentially beyond the thoracic inlet. The level of the laryngeal resection depends on the location of the tumor (Fig. 62 b). If it extends past the cricopharyngeal muscle, the hyoid bone should be included in the resection. For a *suprahyoid* resection the hyoid bone is engaged with a traction suture and pulled forward and downward. This maneuver places the mylohyoid, digastric, hypoglossus, and stylohyoid muscles on stretch, and these are severed from their attachments on the superior border of the hyoid bone. The epiglottis, now exposed, is grasped with a forceps and pulled forward and downward. Now the surgeon can inspect the interior of the pharynx and evaluate the cranial extent of tumor spread. Residual mucus within the larynx and pharynx is aspirated, and the mucosa is cleaned with dissecting patties soaked in antiseptic. The incision is extended into the lateral walls of the pharynx, formed by the inferior constrictor muscle, leaving only the posterior pharyngeal wall intact (Fig. 62 c). The posterior wall is divided in stepwise fashion back to the prevertebral fascia. The proximal stump is held with two or three traction sutures to prevent upward retraction of the mucosa. Once the last connective tissue attachments have been divided between the pharynx and the prevertebral fascia, the entire specimen can be pulled anteriorly, as it is only tethered distally by the cervical esophagus.

The *infrahyoid* resection begins by severing the sternohyoid and thyrohyoid muscles from the inferior margin of the hyoid bone. The muscles are bluntly dissected from the thyrohyoid membrane, which likewise is divided below the hyoid bone. The thyroid cartilage is pulled forward and downward with a small, sharp hook until the epiglottis is visualized. It is grasped with a clamp and also pulled anteroinferiorly. The lateral and posterior walls of the pharynx are divided as described above.

Two heavy traction sutures are placed in the esophagus close to the thoracic inlet. Then the superior mediastinum around the esophagus is packed with gauze soaked in antiseptic, and the esophagus is occluded just above the intended line of resection with a rubber-shod clamp. The esophageal wall facing the operator is opened transversely, and the lumen is suctioned and cleansed with patties soaked in Clorpactin. Then the distal transection is completed, and the specimen is removed en bloc (Fig. 62 d). The next step is restoration of alimentary continuity.

It should be added that it is simpler and perhaps better to remove the thoracic esophagus concurrently as far as the gastric inlet by blunt dissection (see 6.6.2) and then bring the stomach up for anastomosis to the pharynx. The stomach can be transposed into the former bed of the esophagus.

6.4.2.7 Extension of the Cervical Resection to the Upper Thoracic Esophagus or Entire Esophagus

For carcinomas that originate from the cervical esophagus and extend to the thoracic inlet, removal of the cervical esophagus must be combined with removal of at least the supraaortic segment, and preferably of the entire esophagus [3, 15, 39]. It is true that the cervical and upper thoracic esophagus can be removed by adding an upper median sternotomy or left parasternotomy to the cervical incision, resecting the esophagus, and restoring continuity with a free intestinal graft (see 7.6). But the difficulties and dangers associated with this approach, which relate particularly to the necessity of performing an intrathoracic anastomosis, make this procedure unattractive. It is safer in these cases to perform a total esophagectomy without thoracotomy (see 6.7) and restore continuity by advancing the stomach (see 7.3).

For esophageal carcinomas at the thoracic inlet and above the aortic arch, Ong [39] recommends the cervical-transsternal approach of Waddel [58], which is said to give the best exposure for an extensive resection. The skin is divided on the midline from the cervicotomy to the umbilicus. The peritoneum is not incised initially. The xyphoid process is removed, and the sternum is split with an oscillating saw. The left innominate vein is divided. The left common carotid artery is freed and retracted laterally. At this point there is free access to the superior mediastinum, and the tumor-bearing esophagus can be dissected free under vision. The abdomen is entered by incising the peritoneum, and the lower esophagus is bluntly mobilized, transected close the cardia, and extracted superiorly.

We are hesitant to utilize this procedure. If one wishes to expose the supraaortic portion of the esophagus through an anterior approach, this can be satisfactorily accomplished through a high, partial sternotomy to the level of the third or fourth interspace. Convalescence after this procedure is easier than with a full sternotomy. For carcinomas of the supraaortic esophagus whose main bulk is distal to the thoracic inlet, we perform the resection through a right thoracotomy, bluntly mobilize the esophagus at the hiatus, and transect the esophagus at the esophagogastric junction. After its exposure in the neck, the mobilized esophagus is extracted superiorly and divided just below the cricopharyngeal muscle.

6.5 Esophageal Resection through a Right Thoracic Approach

All or part of the abdominal and thoracic portions of the esophagus can be resected through a right thoracic approach. The resection can be performed at any level and is not constrained by the esophageal blood supply (see 6.1). The only major constraint is that the esophagus should not be mobilized for more than 3 cm past the line of resection, as this might compromise blood flow to the area of the future anastomosis.

For benign disease, we incise the pleura over the esophagus and reflect it back during the resection so that it can be reapposed later over the esophageal bed. For carcinoma, we remove the pleura overlying the esophagus together with the paraesophageal lymph nodes bordering the area of the resection. We feel that an extensive posterior mediastinectomy [3, 17, 32, 33] is appropriate only for T1-stage neoplasms [57].

Steps in procedure:

(1) Right thoracotomy and exposure of the esophagus (see 2.1.2)
(2) Incision of the mediastinal pleura at the anterior border of the azygos vein
(3) Division of the crossing of the azygos vein
(4) Snaring of the esophagus distal to the neoplasm
(5) Circumferential mobilization of the esophagus with its surrounding connective tissue and lymph nodes down to the cardia
(6) Division of the esophagus from the stomach and closure of the hiatus (if required)
(7) Further circumferential mobilization of the esophagus to the thoracic apex
(8) Completion of lymph node removal in the esophageal bed
(9) Division of the esophagus at the thoracic apex or exteriorization of the esophagus at the neck

Preoperative preparation: Antiseptic preparation of the pharynx, removal of teeth involved by caries or periodontal infection; prophylactic antibiotics (see Chap. C); intestinal lavage if reconstruction is planned in the same sitting.

Instruments: Basic set, extra thoracic set, EEA, GIA, TA.

Position and approach: Posterolateral thoracotomy in the 4th–6th interspace. A double thoracotomy may be performed through one skin incision if required (see Chap. B).

Operative technique: The chest is entered, and the lung is displaced anteriorly with a broad retractor. For benign disease the esophagus is exposed as described in 2.1.2, snared, and progressively exposed in the proximal and distal directions. At this time we try to preserve the azygos vein and the main vagus nerve trunks.

If carcinoma exists, it is necessary to determine its extent and its relationship to the trachea, the right hilar structures, the pericardium, the right atrium, and the aorta. To do this, it may be necessary first to expose the esophagus just in the area of the neoplasm. If the carcinoma is freely movable, the mediastinal pleura is incised just anterior to the azygos vein (Fig. 63 a). The pleural incision is continued inferiorly to the hiatus and superiorly to the crossing of the azygos vein. The pleura does not need to be incised farther cephalad if the resection is to be limited to the lower intrathoracic esophagus. If total esophagectomy is planned, the azygos vein is elevated from the esophagus and divided close to the vertebral column if proximity of tumor appears to justify removal of the vein (Fig. 63 b). On the other hand, if visible tumor extensions are several centimeters away from the azygos vein, it is sufficient to mobilize the vein so that the esophagus can be extracted from beneath it. The pleural incision is then continued to the pleural apex, keeping close to the vertebral column. Anteriorly, the mediastinal pleura is divided longitudinally below the tumor at its reflection between the esophagus and inferior pulmonary ligament. This incision may be extended proximally beyond the hilum to the pleural dome to define the anterior limit of the resection, but we prefer to snare the esophagus distal to the tumor and divide the pleura anteriorly when the resection is carried out. In any case the pleura is left attached to the esophagus. The dissection is carried distally to the hiatus (Fig. 63 c). All lymph nodes in the bed of the esophagus are removed. The esophagus is pulled cephalad to identify its attachments to the hiatus. The pleura, the underlying fatty tissue, the esophagophrenic membrane, and finally the peritoneal reflection are divided on the anterolateral side of the esophagus, opening the peritoneal cavity. During mobilization of the esophagus, attention is given to the branch of the left gastric artery that runs anteriorly upward and to the branch of the inferior phrenic artery that runs posteriorly. Both are ligated to ensure that their distal portion will not retract into the abdomen and cause unrecognized hemorrhage.

If the tumor has infiltrated a hiatal crus or the diaphragm, these structures must be included in the resection with a margin of 1–2 cm.

The esophagus having been freed from its hiatal attachments, the cardia can be delivered into the thorax (Fig. 63 d). The esophagus is occluded at the esophagocardial junction with the T-50 stapling instrument and transected proximal to the staple line with a scalpel along the edge of the instrument (Fig. 63 e). Both cut ends are wiped clean with antiseptic-soaked patties. The stapler is released, the stomach is allowed to retract into the abdomen, and the hiatus is closed with continuous or interrupted sutures. A condom is slid over the esophageal stump and secured with a heavy tie to avoid spillage of infectious material during the rest of the operation (Fig. 63 f).

If a transpleural esophageal reconstruction is planned during the same sitting (see 7.2.2.2.3), the hiatus is not closed. If the stomach is to serve as the esophageal substitute, we staple the esophagus with the TA instrument as described above, but we do not transect it until it has been completely mobilized. In that way the esophagus can be used to pull the stomach upward into the chest.

The esophageal stump is grasped with a forceps, pulled cephalad, and progressively freed from the posterior mediastinum as far as the pleural dome. Arteries entering the esophagus posteriorly are coagulated or ligated. The periesophageal connective tissue and the lymph nodes within it are taken with the esophagus. It is common to find adhesions in the area of the neoplasm; these may be due to inflammation or tumor infiltration. Structures that appear fixed to the tumor, such as the pericardium, should be included in the resection unless their removal would be incompatible with life or would necessitate a major extension of the resection (e.g., to portions of the lungs).

In cases of this kind, where the extent of disease has been underestimated during exploration, the tumor is bluntly or sharply dissected from adjacent structures. Subsequent esophageal replacement must be done by the subcutaneous or retrosternal route to avoid obstruction of the tract by local recurrence and to enable high-dosage radiation to be delivered to the tumor site if required.

When the tumor has been freed circumferentially, it is wrapped in a compress soaked in Clorpactin solution, and stay sutures are used to hold the compress in place.

During mobilization of the upper thoracic portion of the esophagus, attention must be given to the thoracic duct, which is closely related to the left wall of the esophagus at the level of the aortic arch. If the duct is injured, it must be ligated proximally and distally to avoid chylothorax. If the contralateral pleura has been entered or has been included in the resection, the defect should be repaired with sutures whenever possible. A drain is inserted at the end of the procedure only if there

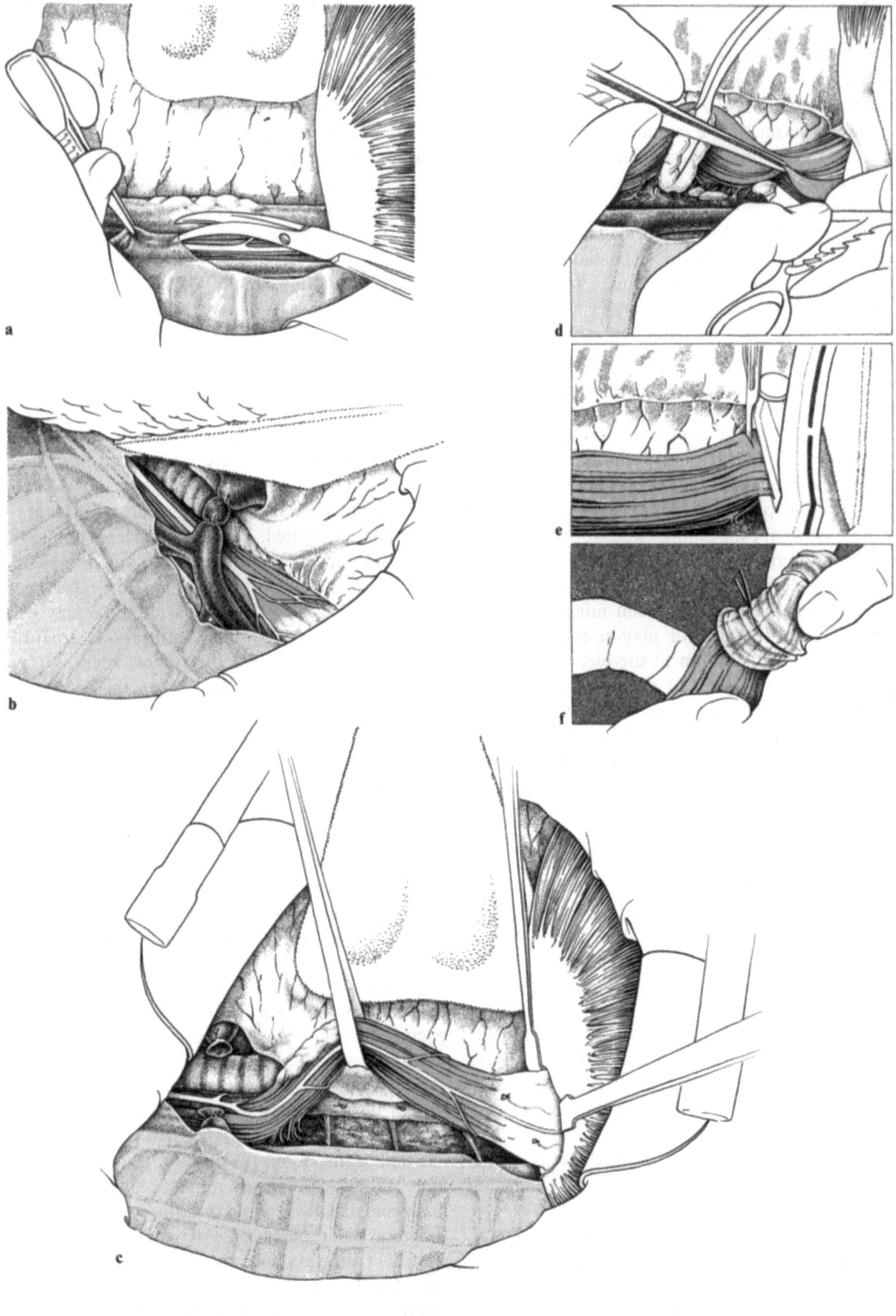
a
b
c
d
e
f

◁ **Fig. 63a–f.** Esophageal resection through a right thoracotomy. **a** Mediastinal pleura is incised along the azygos vein. **b** Azygos vein is ligated. **c** Esophagus is freed circumferentially. **d** Cardia is advanced into the chest through the enlarged esophageal hiatus. **e** The esophagus is stapled near the cardia and transected. **f** A condom is slipped over the end of the esophagus

is radiologic evidence of a contralateral pneumothorax.

When the dissection of the esophagus has reached the apex of the chest, the pleura is divided at its superior reflection, and the esophagus is bluntly mobilized beyond the thoracic inlet. The surgeon should stay close to the muscular wall of the esophagus at this time to avoid injury to the recurrent nerve and brachial vessels.

For construction of an intrathoracic anastomosis, the esophagus is pulled inferiorly, the wall facing the surgeon is opened with the electrocautery, and the lumen is cleaned with dissecting patties soaked in antiseptic. If a stapled anastomosis is desired, a pursestring suture and two guide sutures should be placed (see 1.3.3.2) and the EEA instrument introduced before the posterior wall is divided.

The esophagus is easily manipulated by its residual posterior wall, and the anvil of the EEA instrument glides over it easily into the lumen. The guide sutures are removed, and the pursestring suture is closed around the central rod of the EEA instrument before the posterior wall of the esophagus is divided.

If a cervical esophagostomy or cervical anastomosis is proposed, the esophagus is exposed through a right or left cervicotomy (see 2.1.1) and exteriorized (Fig. 64). With benign disease, the extent of the esophageal resection corresponds to the extent of the disease. For carcinoma below the aortic arch, the line of resection is level with the superior border of the clavicle; for carcinoma above the aortic arch, the line of resection is at the cricopharyngeal muscle.

If a two-stage procedure is planned, it is essential that an adequate remnant of esophagus be left to construct an end esophagostomy (see 2.2.2). With carcinoma above the aortic arch, it will be necessary to resect the cervical esophagus secondarily to the hypopharynx at the time of reconstruction.

For a tumor that requires concomitant resection of the cervical viscera, the procedure is continued as described in 6.4.3.2 and 6.4.2.6 after completion of the thoracic phase, although basic questions of resectability should be addressed.

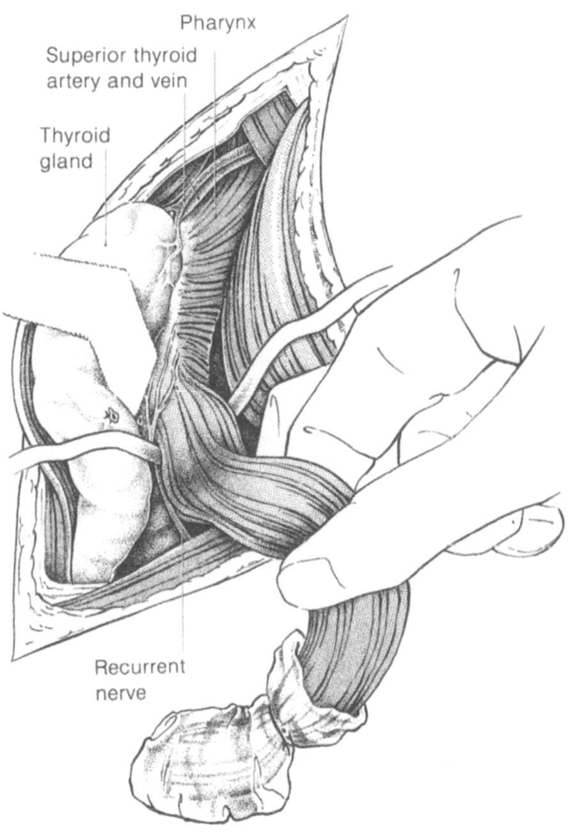

Fig. 64. The esophagus is exteriorized at the neck through a left cervicotomy along the anterior border of the sternocleidomastoid muscle

6.5.1 Posterior Mediastinectomy

Posterior mediastinectomy represents an attempt to apply the general rules of tumor surgery, i.e., en bloc resection of the affected organ and regional lymph nodes, to the esophagus [3, 17, 32]. While this approach may be justified for gastric and colorectal cancer, we feel that anatomic factors such as the lymphatic drainage of the esophagus and its proximity to vital structures contraindicate its use in the esophagus, especially when one considers that the late results of en bloc resection are no better than those of our "limited" resection. We also consider the risk of the procedure to be exorbitant in terms of injury to adjacent structures

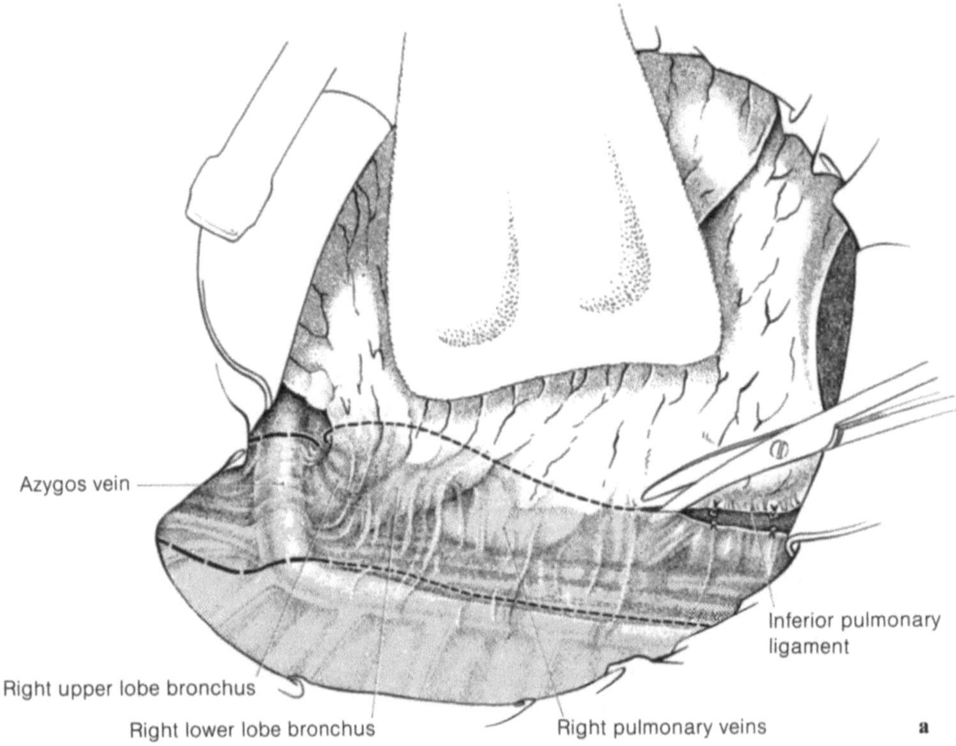

Azygos vein
Inferior pulmonary ligament
Right upper lobe bronchus
Right lower lobe bronchus
Right pulmonary veins

a

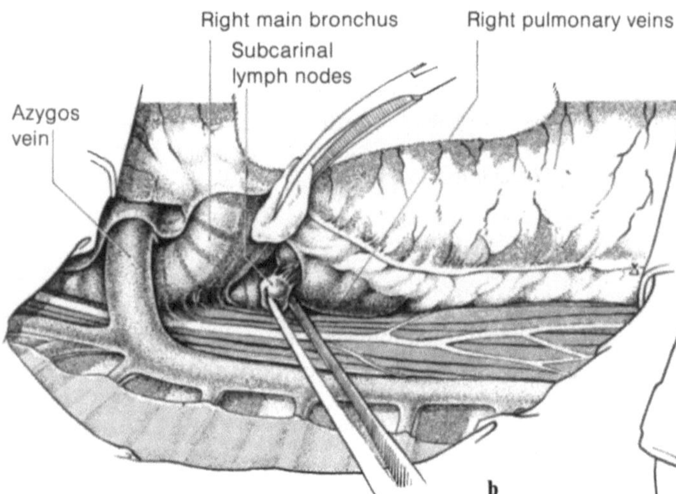

Right main bronchus
Right pulmonary veins
Subcarinal lymph nodes
Azygos vein

b

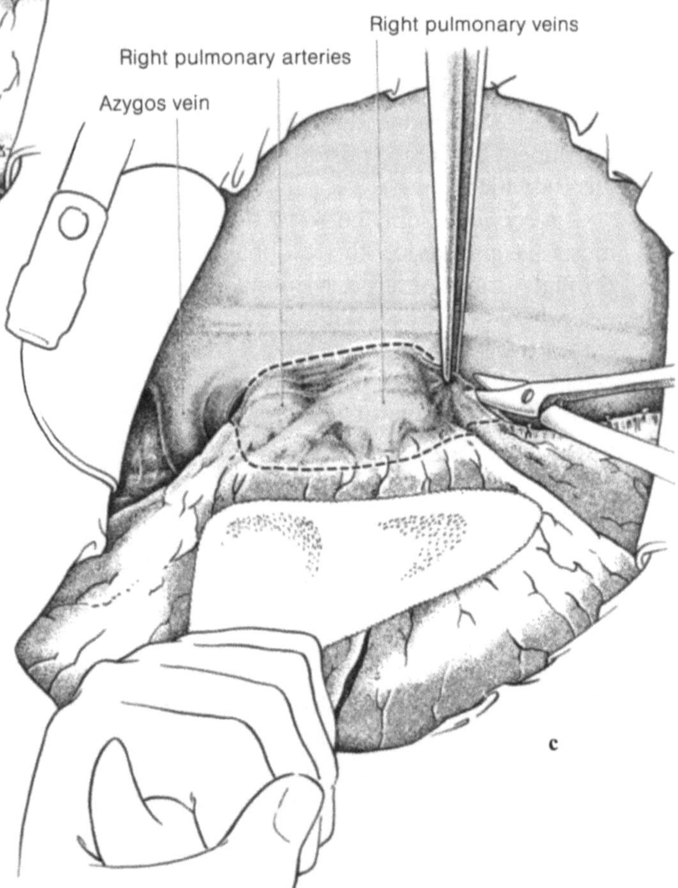

Right pulmonary veins
Right pulmonary arteries
Azygos vein

c

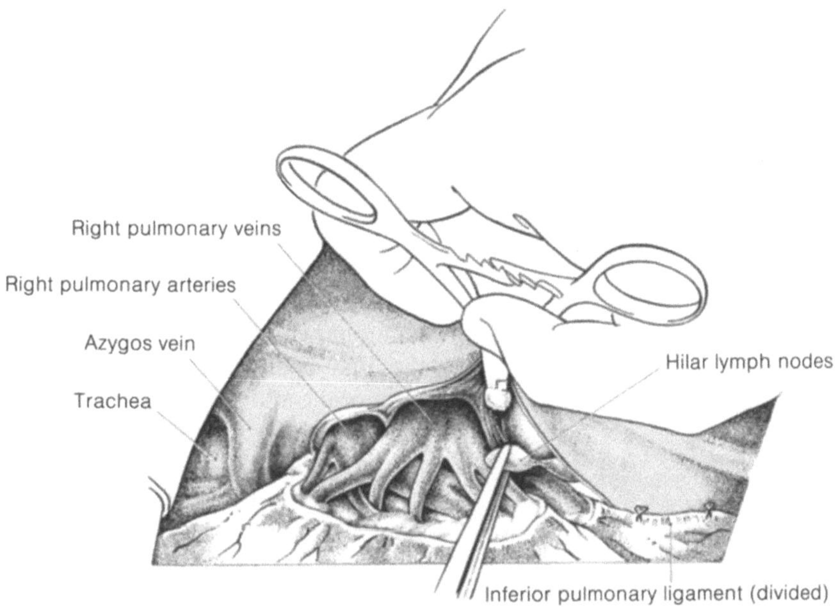

d

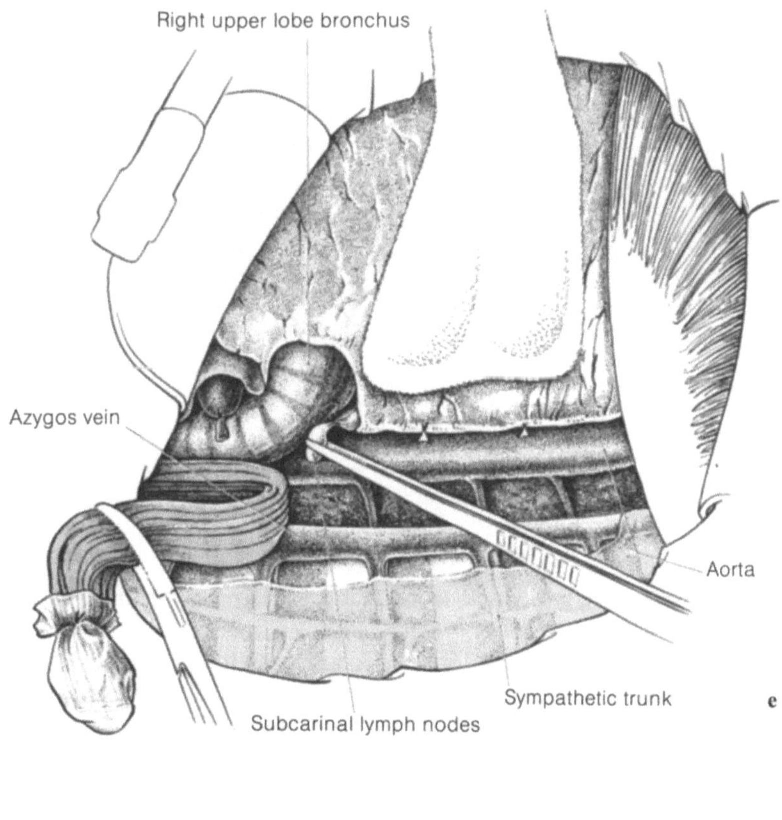

e

Fig. 65 a–e. Right posterior mediastinectomy. **a** Posterior extent of the mediastinectomy (broken lines). The lung is retracted anteriorly. The lower part of the inferior pulmonary ligament is divided. **b** Removal of the subcarinal nodes. **c** Anterior extent of the mediastinectomy (broken lines). The lung is retracted posteriorly. **d** The pulmonary hilum is dissected free from the anterior side. **e** Lymph nodes in the esophageal bed are removed as far as the contralateral pleura. The lung is retracted anteriorly and prolonged operating time, although we cannot cite statistical data to support this concern.

Preoperative preparation, instrumentation, position and approach: See 6.5.

Steps in procedure:

(1) Division of the inferior pulmonary ligament close to the lung
(2) Removal of the connective tissue and lymph nodes in the pulmonary hilum from the posterior and anterior sides
(3) Incision of the mediastinal pleura to the thoracic apex along the course of the azygos vein
(4) Resection of the azygos vein segment crossing the esophagus
(5) Incision of the mediastinal pleura along the pericardium
(6) Mobilization and snaring of the esophagus distant from the tumor
(7) Dissection of the esophagus inferiorly to the cardia
(8) Transection of the esophagus at the cardia
(9) Mobilization of the esophagus to the thoracic apex
(10) Removal of all lymph nodes and connective tissue as far as the contralateral pleura
(11) Blunt mobilization of the esophagus in the thoracic inlet
(12) Division of the esophagus at the thoracic apex or exteriorization of the esophagus at the neck

Operative technique: The lung is mobilized, and the inferior pulmonary ligament is divided close to the lung as far as the inferior pulmonary vein. The vessels coursing in the ligament are cauterized or ligated (Fig. 65 a). The lung is retracted anteriorly, and the pleura is incised over the pulmonary hilum to its superior border. The pleura is separated from the pulmonary veins and right main bronchus in the direction of the esophagus by blunt patty dissection. The hilar lymph nodes, the first of which is usually encountered below the inferior pulmonary vein, are removed along with the connective tissue surrounding them. Removal of the tracheobronchial nodes is continued along the main bronchus to the bifurcation (Fig. 65 b). When the hilar structures have been completely isolated from the posterior side, the lung is retracted posteriorly, and the pleura is incised from below upward, in continuity with the pulmonary ligament incision, to the superior border of the hilum (Fig. 65 c). The pleura is elevated medially from the pulmonary veins and adjacent arteries by patty dissection and incised along the pericardium or superior vena cava. Care is taken to spare the phrenic nerve, which courses anterior to the pulmonary arteries and veins. After removal of the hilar nodes from the anterior side, the structures of the hilum must be freed from all surrounding tissues (Fig. 65 d). Then the lung is again retracted anteriorly, and the pleura is incised along the anterior border of the azygos vein. As the incision is continued upward, the azygos vein is divided and ligated at the start of its arcuate portion. As the superior intercostal veins unite with the azygos above the site of division, they must be individually ligated and divided as the incision proceeds; the incision is placed about 1 cm lateral to the pleural reflection from the esophagus to the vertebral column. On reaching the thoracic apex, the esophagus and periesophageal connective tissue are bluntly separated from the prevertebral fascia with a dissecting patty.

Anteroinferiorly, the pleura is incised just above the hiatus at its pericardial reflection. If the tumor is attached to the pericardium, the latter must be included in the resection with an adequate margin. The defect is then repaired by direct suture or with a dural patch to prevent later cardiac herniation or tamponade. Defects less than 2 cm in size do not require repair. The esophagus is encircled and snared. The dissection is continued close to the pericardium as far as the inferior pulmonary veins. Then the mobilized segment of esophagus is pulled cephalad until the esophagogastric junction appears in the hiatus. The pleura around the hiatus is incised, and the structures fixing the cardia are divided between ligatures until the abdomen is reached. The esophagus is cleared circumferentially in the hiatus, whereupon it is transected at the esophagogastric junction as described in 6.5 and reflected superiorly. At this point a clear view is obtained of the structures adjoining the esophagus, such as the contralateral pleura and the aorta. The tissues left behind during the initial blind mobilization of the esophagus are removed as far as the left pleura, and the aortic adventitia is resected. The dissection is carried superiorly as the esophagus, the periesophageal tissue, and the paraesophageal lymph nodes are progressively separated from the prevertebral fascia, aorta, and left pleura (Fig. 65 e). The pleura dissected from the posterior aspect of the hilum is included in the resection and left attached to the esophagus. The nutrient vessels of the esophagus are coagulated or ligated. The stump of the azygos vein, severed posteriorly, is encountered over the pulmonary hilum. It is divided close to its insertion into the vena cava and is left attached to the specimen. During separation of the esophagus from the aortic arch, care is taken that the left recurrent laryngeal nerve is not injured as the periesophageal tissue is dissected from the aorta. The delicate connections between the esophagus and trachea are bluntly separated while the paratracheal lymph nodes are removed. When the pleural dome is reached, the pleura is divided over the esophagus, and the latter is bluntly mobilized into the thoracic inlet. The rest of the procedure depends on whether a cervical or intrathoracic anastomosis is to be performed (see 6.5).

6.5.2 Esophageal Resection with Proximal or Total Gastrectomy

For squamous cell carcinoma of the abdominal esophagus or adenocardinoma of the cardia, it is necessary to extend the resection distally to include part or all of the stomach. The extent of the esophageal resection depends on the nature and size of the tumor. For adenocardinoma, the line of esophageal resection is at the level of the inferior pulmonary veins. We perform this procedure through separate abdominal and left or right thoracic incisions and restore continuity by the interposition of jejunum or by a Roux-en-Y anastomosis. For squamous cell carcinoma of the abdominal esophagus, a margin of at least 6 cm should be maintained above the visible and palpable superior edge of the tumor. Akiyama [3] routinely uses an esophagotomy to determine the proximal tumor extent. One may elect to remove the entire thoracic esophagus in these cases to ensure a radical resection or to avoid an intrathoracic anastomosis. Continuity may be restored by uniting the gastric remnant to the esophagus or by interposing a segment of small bowel or colon, depending on the length of the defect.

6.5.2.1 Esophageal Resection with Proximal Gastrectomy through an Exclusive Right Thoracic Approach

Belsey and Hiebert [7] advocate this approach for squamous cell cancers of the abdominal to midthoracic portions of the esophagus, reporting that it permits the stomach to be elevated consistently to the azygos vein and frequently to the apex of the chest so that radical margins can be secured.

As there is no need to reposition the patient for laparotomy, operating time is shortened considerably. The lesser curvature of the stomach is included in the resection to remove the major tumor-bearing lymph nodes and to eliminate the part of the stomach that is most poorly vascularized after ligation of the left gastric artery.

Preoperative preparation and instruments: See 6.5.

Position and approach: Right lateral position, posterolateral thoracotomy through the fifth interspace (see Chap. B, 4.3.4).

Operative technique: The esophagus is mobilized from the upper limit of the resection (6 cm above the superior edge of the tumor) inferiorly to the hiatus, and its attachments to the diaphragm are divided (Fig. 66 a). The stomach is mobilized through the enlarged hiatus by sequentially dividing the short gastric arteries, the gastrophrenic ligament, the gastrosplenic ligament, and the greater and lesser omenta. If the trunk of the left gastric artery is visible on the lesser curvature, it is ligated and divided before its bifurcation into ascending and descending rami. Care is taken to preserve the gastroepiploic arcade on the greater curvature in order to spare the gastric blood supply. If the stomach can be mobilized to the proposed line of resection on the esophagus, then the lesser curvature, cardia, and possibly the fundus are resected. The gastric remnant is fashioned into a tube whose proximal end is anastomosed end-to-end to the esophagus (Fig. 66 b). Pyloroplasty is not possible, but this is of no functional consequence owing to the shortened, tubelike configuration of the gastric remnant.

6.5.2.2 Esophageal Resection with Proximal or Total Gastrectomy through a Thoracoabdominal Approach

It does not matter whether the thoracic or abdominal phase of the operation is done first, or whether the laparotomy and thoracotomy employ common or separate incisions. We prefer separate abdominal and thoracic incisions to avoid the alteration of respiratory mechanics that can result from incision of the diaphragm, and we generally begin with the abdominal phase (see Chap. B).

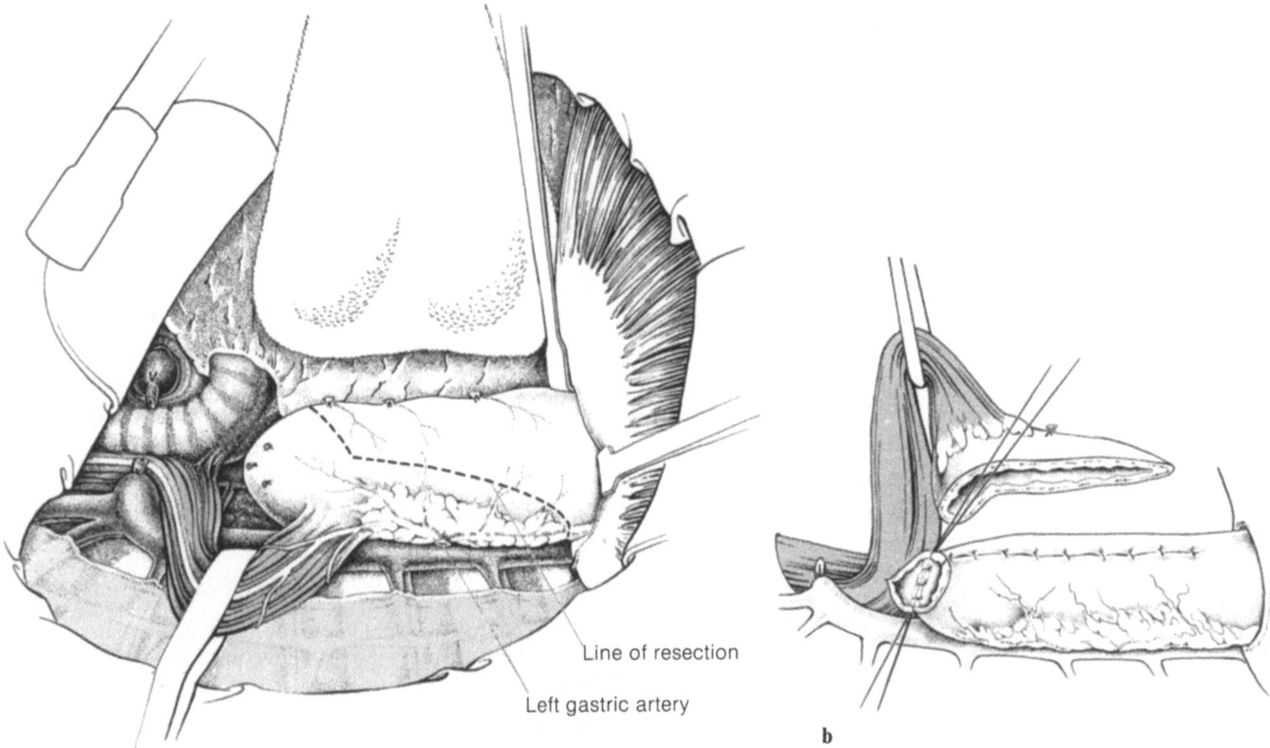

a b

Fig. 66a, b. Extension of thoracic esophagectomy to the proximal stomach through an exclusive thoracic approach. **a** The fundus and proximal body of the stomach are pulled into the thorax through the enlarged hiatus. **b** The esophagus is anastomosed to a tube constructed from the gastric remnant

6.5.2.2.1 Esophageal Resection with Proximal Gastrectomy

Preoperative preparation and instruments: See 6.5.

Position and approach: Upper midline laparatomy extended around the left side of the umbilicus; posterolateral thoracotomy through the sixth interspace (see Chap. B, 4.3.3).

Operative technique: The abdomen is entered and explored for organ metastases that would contraindicate resection. The line of the gastrectomy generally runs along the superior border of the pancreas, corresponding to the distribution of the left gastric artery and left gastroepiploic artery (Fig. 67 a). The esophagus is exposed and encircled with a snare. The vagus nerve trunks are severed to gain additional length so that the esophagus can be pulled inferiorly and anterolaterally. The lesser omentum is incised close to the liver, the left gastric artery is palpated, and its bifurcation into ascending and descending branches is identified. The site for ligating the artery depends on the proposed level of the resection through the lesser curvature and the importance placed upon removal of associated lymphatic pathways and other radical surgical considerations (see 6.5.2.3). Next the stomach is freed from its posterior adhesions with the retroperitoneum, and the gastrophrenic ligament and proximal part of the gastrosplenic ligament with its short gastric vessels are progressively divided as far as the hilum of the spleen. The proximal part of the stomach is now freely movable and can be divided along the superior border of the pancreas after occlusion of the distal gastric remnant with the TA stapler. The oral stump is wrapped in a glove and retracted superiorly. The esophagus is replaced with a sufficiently long segment of jejunum or colon (see 7.4, 7.5) whose aboral lumen is anastomosed in isoperistaltic fashion to the anterior wall of the stomach. After manual enlargement of the hiatus, the oral end of the esophageal substitute is fixed to the proximal gastric stump. A pyloroplasty is indicated due to sacrifice of the vagus nerve branches (Fig. 67 b). The operative area is drained, the abdomen closed, and the patient repositioned for thoracotomy. After the esophagus has been mobilized to the level proposed for the resection, the proximal gastric stump with attached esophageal substitute is pulled into the chest. The esophagus is transected, and continuity is restored by anastomosis to the substitute.

If a peptic stricture exists at the esophagogastric junction, extensive mobilization of the proximal stomach is not required. Additionally, the vagus nerve branches should be preserved. The esophagus is exposed and snared. Both vagus nerve trunks are dissected off the

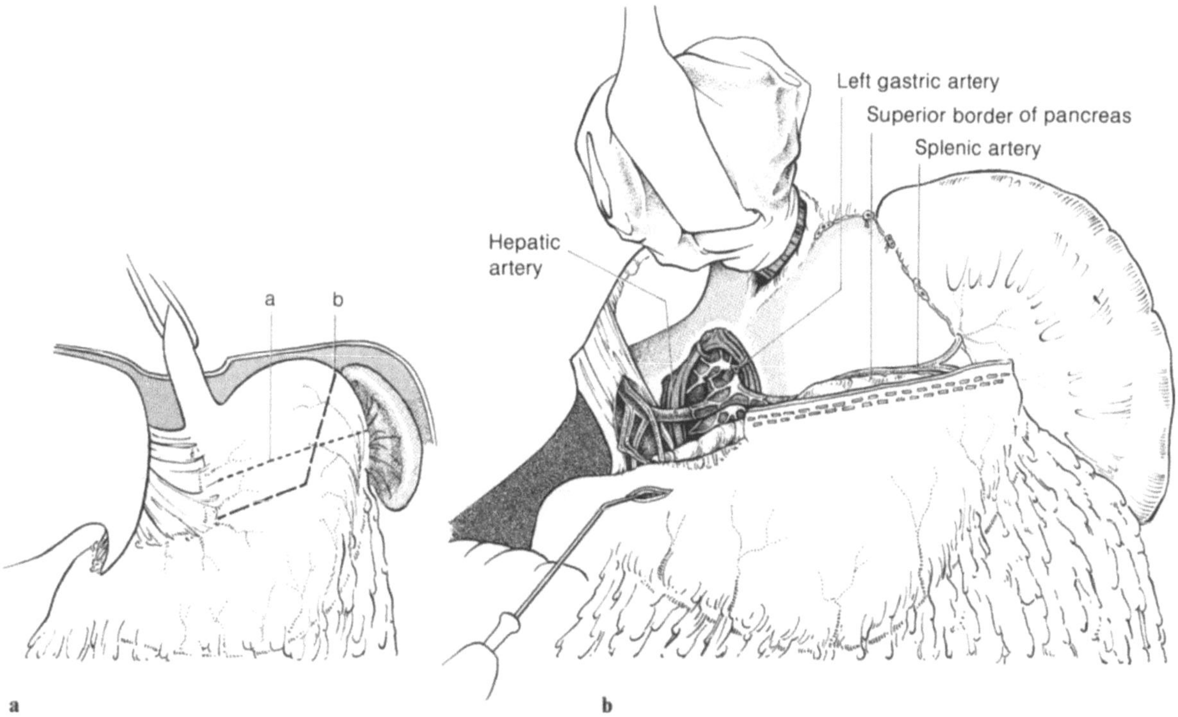

a b

Fig. 67 a, b. Extension of thoracic esophagectomy to the proximal stomach through a thoracoabdominal approach (schematic). **a** Extent of the gastric resection. *a* Resection line of Holle (1968), *b* resection line of Akiyama (1981). **b** Pyloroplasty is performed after the fundectomy and lymph node dissection

esophagus and likewise snared. The cardia is exposed and clamped a short distance below the stricture with a Satinski clamp, and the stomach is transected above it. Further resection of the esophagus corresponds to that for carcinoma. The resection may be limited to the immediate area of the stricture if there appears to be no advantage in removal of the entire thoracic esophagus with subsequent reconstruction by a cervical anastomosis.

The stomach can be used as the esophageal substitute following proximal gastrectomy by first mobilizing the entire stomach (see 7.3) and performing a pyloroplasty. The abdomen is closed, the chest is entered, and the esophagus is exposed to the proposed line of the resection (see 6.5). Then the proximal stomach is divided with adequate margins so as to leave a tubular remnant that can be anastomosed to the proximal stump of the esophagus. An antireflux procedure is indicated if the entire stomach has not been advanced into the chest, because the lower the position of the esophagogastric anastomosis within the chest, the greater the risk of subsequent reflux disease. We prefer to manage these cases by the isoperistaltic interposition of small bowel.

6.5.2.2.2 Esophageal Resection with Total Gastrectomy. We feel that total gastrectomy with removal of the spleen, greater omentum, and distal esophagus to the level of the inferior pulmonary veins is the operation of choice for adenocarcinoma of the cardia. We do not consider fundectomy [23, 24] to be adequate even if gross or frozen-section examination shows no involvement of the zone I and II groups of nodes along the right gastroepiploic and right gastric arteries [57]. The technique of fundectomy for carcinoma of the cardia is described fully in volume VII/1 [61].

Preoperative preparation and instruments: See 6.5.

Position and approach: Upper midline laparotomy extended around the left side of the umbilicus; right posterolateral thoracotomy in the 6th–7th interspace (see Chap. B, 4.3.3).

Operative technique: The abdomen is entered and explored for organ metastases. The triangular ligament of the liver is severed from its attachment to the retroperitoneum, and the left lobe of the liver is displaced medially with a broad retractor. The local extent of the carcinoma can now be as-

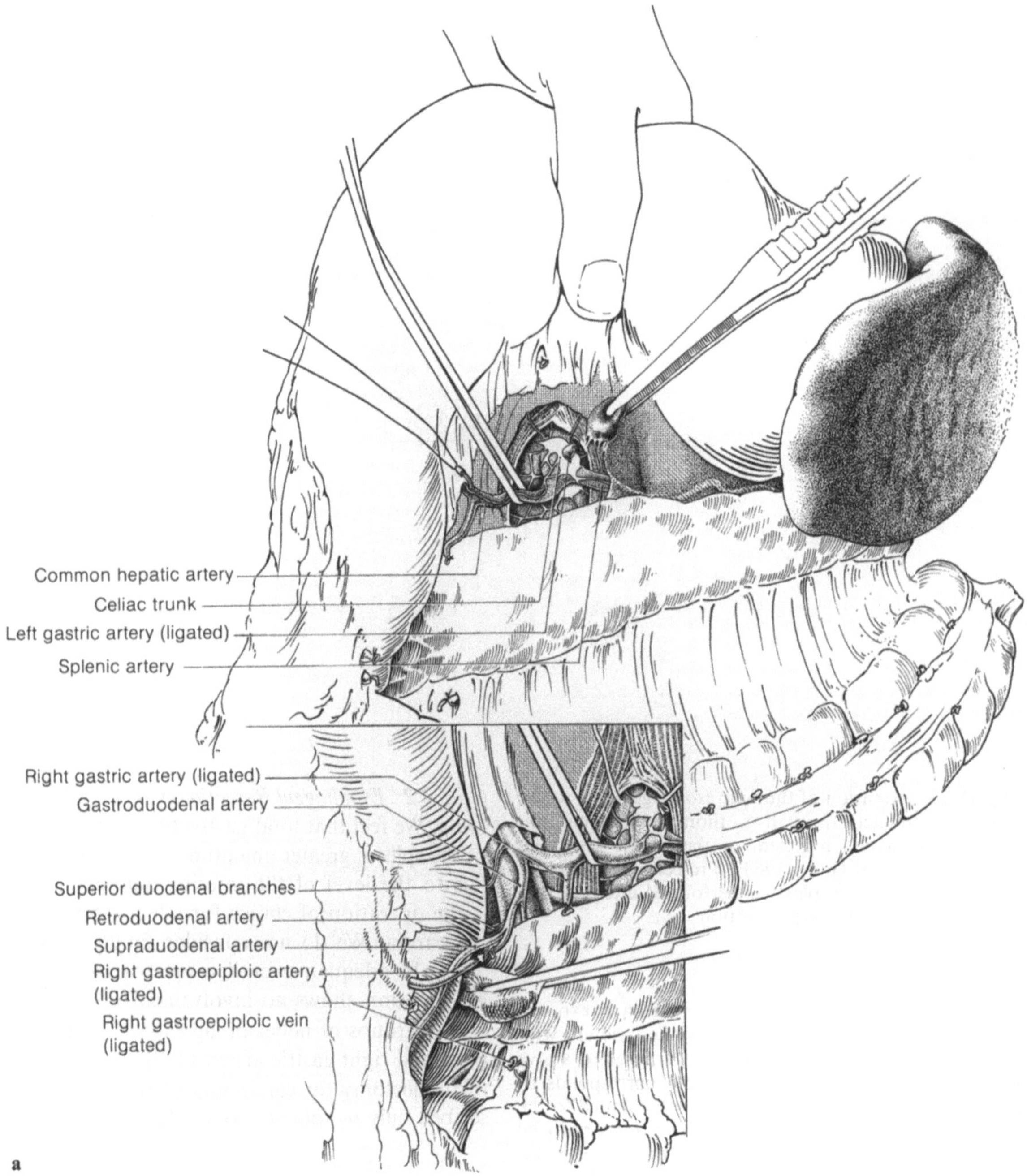

Fig. 68a–c. Resection of the thoracic esophagus with total gastrectomy. **a** Lymph node dissection. The greater omentum has been severed from the transverse colon, and the stomach reflected superiorly. All lymphatic tissues between the right renal artery, common hepatic artery, superior margin of the pancreas, and posterior abdominal wall are removed to the celiac trunk. **b** The esophagus is exposed circumferentially in the enlarged hiatus. The lesser omentum is divided. The stomach has been transected just distal to the pylorus. **c** Division of the splenic vessels from the posterior side

Steps in procedure:

(1) Detachment of the left hepatic lobe from the diaphragm
(2) Assessment of resectability
(3) Division of adhesions between the greater omentum and colon
(4) Mobilization of the posterior wall of the stomach
(5) Dissection of the pylorus from the posterior side
(6) Ligation of the right gastroepiploic artery and vein and right gastric artery
(7) Resection of the prepancreatic fascia and all lymphatic tissue between the right renal artery, common hepatic artery, superior pancreatic border, and posterior abdominal wall to the celiac trunk
(8) Ligation of the left gastric artery close to its origin
(9) Division of the lesser omentum distant from the stomach
(10) Postpyloric transection of the stomach with the GIA instrument
(11) Removal of lymph nodes in the hepatoduodenal ligament
(12) Snaring of the esophagus and blunt mobilization through the enlarged hiatus into the chest
(13) Freeing of the spleen from the retroperitoneum and ligation of the splenic vessels
(14) Transection of the esophagus at the cardia with the GIA instrument

certained. Wide infiltration of the diaphragm or involvement of the major vessels contraindicate resection. If only the left hepatic lobe is infiltrated by tumor, the involved portion is removed by a lobectomy or wedge resection.

If the extent of disease cannot be ascertained by inspection and palpation, the carcinoma must be exposed. This requires opening the omental bursa, which is necessary in any case as a prelude to the gastrectomy.

The greater omentum is pulled upward to demonstrate its attachments to the transverse colon; these attachments are severed with electrocautery from the duodenocolic ligament to the phrenocolic ligament. Larger, isolated blood vessels are divided between Pean clamps and ligated. The omental bursa is entered, and the posterior wall of the stomach is bluntly cleared of retrogastric adhesions in the direction of the cardia and fundus. The degree of involvement of the posterior gastric wall is determined, and the relation of the carcinoma to adjacent organs is evaluated. If the tumor is resectable, the dissection is carried past the left colic flexure to the splenocolic ligament, and the spleen is freed from its adhesions with the retroper-

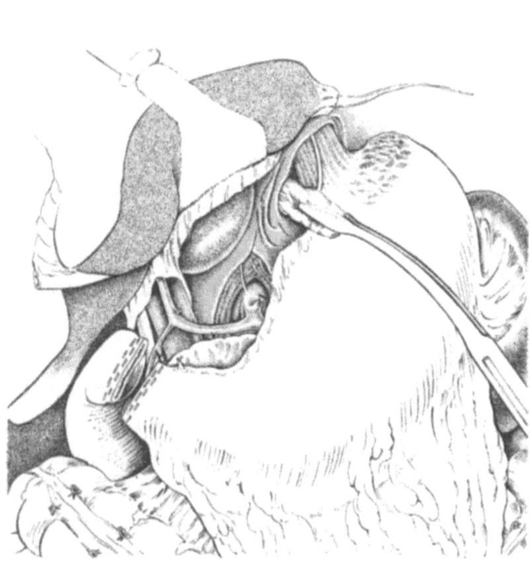
b

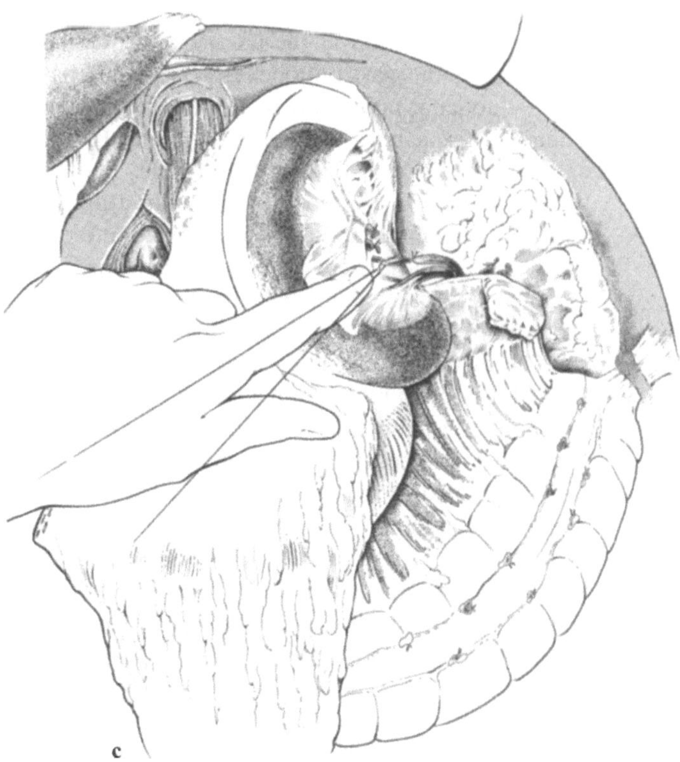
c

itoneum. The stomach is pulled downward with a grasping forceps, making the gastrophrenic ligament tense. This ligament is divided with the electrocautery or scissors until the esophagus is reached. Then the stomach and greater omentum are reflected superiorly, and the dissection is continued around the greater curvature toward the pylorus (Fig. 68 a). The right gastroepiploic artery is palpated and divided close to its origin from the gastroduodenal artery. The right gastroepiploic vein is identified and ligated just before its entry into the superior mesenteric vein. Now the prepancreatic fascia at the inferior border of the pancreas is freed and mobilized upward. At the superior border of the pancreas the common hepatic artery is snared, and the right gastric artery is identified at its origin and divided. All lymphatic tissue between the splenic artery, common hepatic artery, superior margin of the pancreas, and posterior abdominal wall is removed as far as the celiac trunk.

There the left gastric artery is identified and ligated at its origin. Splenic artery ligation also may be required, in which case it is recommended that the distal third of the pancreas be removed. We avoid pancreatic fistula in these cases by covering the cut surface of the pancreas with an isoperistaltic loop of jejunum mobilized by the Roux-en-Y technique.

The posterior wall of the pylorus and the duodenal bulb are dissected from the head of the pancreas in the direction of the lesser curvature. The branches of the gastroduodenal artery that pass to the duodenal bulb must be ligated at this time. Then the stomach is pulled inferiorly, and the lesser omentum is opened near the pylorus. The dissection is carried around the lesser curvature toward the duodenum until the latter is circumferentially cleared about 2 cm distal to the pylorus. The stomach is transected immediately distal to the pylorus with the GIA stapling instrument (Fig. 68 b). The distal cut end is cleaned with antiseptic-soaked dissecting patties and covered with a surgical sponge. A rubber glove is slipped over the gastric stump and secured with a ligature. The next step is removal of the lymph nodes in the hepatoduodenal ligament. The dissection proceeds toward the cardia and includes the lesser omentum and the lymph nodes therein. When the cardia is reached, the stomach is pulled inferiorly, and the peritoneum over the esophagus is divided proximal to the carcinoma. The esophagus is encircled and snared with a soft Penrose drain. The stomach is freed from remaining adhesions in the direction of the spleen until the hilum of the spleen can be encircled. If the splenic vessels have not already been ligated at their origin, the spleen is retracted anteromedially, and the splenic artery and vein are individually divided close to the tail of the pancreas, which should not be injured (Fig. 68 c). At this point the entire specimen is tethered only by the esophagus.

The esophagus is bluntly mobilized in the hiatus, which is manually enlarged. The esophagus is then grasped just above the tumor with a right-angle forceps and divided distal to the forceps with the GIA instrument.

When the esophageal substitute has been mobilized and continuity restored within the abdomen (see Sect. 7), the oral end of the substitute is fixed to the esophageal stump with stay sutures, and the abdomen is drained and closed.

The patient is repositioned for thoracotomy. The esophagus is mobilized as far as the inferior pulmonary veins or azygos vein, depending on the level of the resection (see 6.5). The substitute is pulled into the chest through the enlarged hiatus, carefully sparing the vascular arcades, the esophagus is transected, and continuity is restored by an end-to-end or end-to-side anastomosis. The esophageal substitute is fixed to the hiatus and to the cut surface of the mediastinal pleura with several interrupted sutures. A chest tube is placed at the intrathoracic anastomosis, and the thoracotomy is closed.

6.6 Esophageal Resection through a Left Thoracic Approach (Garlock, Ohsawa, Sweet)

Esophageal resection through a left thoracic approach follows the same basic principles as the right-sided procedure (see 6.5). The esophagus can be resected at any level. Resections for benign and malignant disease are largely the same, except that carcinoma additionally requires removal of the overlying pleura and accessible lymph nodes. We do not routinely perform an extensive posterior mediastinectomy like that recommended by the French school [32, 33].

Extension of the resection to include the cervical esophagus or a proximal or total gastrectomy follows the same indications and technique as the right-sided procedure. A separate laparotomy and left thoracotomy are commonly used to resect adenocarcinoma of the cardia and squamous cell carcinoma of the abdominal esophagus that do not show significant upward extension past the hiatus on endoscopic or radiologic examination. For adenocarcinoma we resect the esophagus as far as the inferior pulmonary vein, perform total gastrectomy, and additionally remove the greater omentum and spleen. For squamous cell carcinoma we resect the esophagus below the aortic arch and perform a proximal gastrectomy, or we perform a subtotal esophagectomy and place the anastomosis in the neck. We favor resection of the abdominal and entire thoracic esophagus from the left side with an intrathoracic or cervical anastomosis for squamous cell cancers that extend farther into the thoracic portion of the esophagus than preoperative studies indicated. We prefer the left approach when it appears that significant pleural thickening on the right side would hinder a right approach and lead to postoperative complications.

6.6.1 Technique of Abdominothoracic Esophageal Resection from the Left Side

Preoperative preparation and instruments: See 6.5.

Position and approach: Left posterolateral thoracotomy in the 4th–6th interspace (see Chap. B, 4.3.4); a left double thoracotomy through one skin incision is also possible (see Chap. B, 4.3.5).

Steps in procedure:

(1) Incision of the mediastinal pleura from the anterior edge of the aorta to the hiatus
(2) Snaring of the esophagus
(3) Circumferential exposure of the esophagus to the cardia
(4) Transection of the esophagus at the cardia
(5) Mobilization of the esophagus below the aortic arch
(6) Mobilization of the esophagus to the apex of the chest
(7) Blunt dissection of the esophagus beyond the thoracic inlet (if required)
(8) Removal of lymph nodes in the esophageal bed
(9) Transection of the esophagus at the thoracic apex or exteriorization of the esophagus at the neck

Operative technique: For benign disease the esophagus is exposed below the aortic arch as described in 2.1.2, snared, and progressively mobilized in the direction of the hiatus. For carcinoma it is necessary first to determine the extent of the tumor and its relation to the trachea, the right hilar structures, the pericardium, and the aorta. Initially this may require exposing just the portion of the esophagus that is involved by tumor. If the carcinoma is freely movable, the mediastinal pleura is incised at the anterior border of the aorta and at its junction with the pericardium (Fig. 69 a). This pleura is left attached to the esophagus after the latter has been dissected from the aorta, vertebral column, and right pleura, and it is removed with the specimen.

The pleural incision extends inferiorly to the hiatus and superiorly to the aortic arch. It terminates there or at the level of the inferior pulmonary veins if resection of only the distal (cardia carcinoma) or the distal and middle thoracic segments of the esophagus is proposed. The dissection is carried distally to the hiatus. As blood vessels entering the esophagus become tense, they are coagulated or ligated and divided. The lymph nodes in the bed of the esophagus are included in the resection. When the hiatus is reached, the esophagus is pulled superiorly to demonstrate its attachments with the diaphragm. The pleura, the underlying fatty tissue, the esophagophrenic membrane, and finally the peritoneal reflection are divided until the abdominal cavity is opened. As the esophagus is circumferentially freed, attention is given to the anterior, ascending branch of the left gastric artery and to the posterior branch of the inferior phrenic artery. Both must be ligated to ensure that their distal ends will not retract into the abdomen and cause undetected bleeding.

If the tumor has infiltrated a hiatal crus or the diaphragm, these structures must be included in the resection with a margin of 1–2 cm.

When the esophagus has been freed from its hiatal attachments, the cardia is delivered into the chest. The esophagus is occluded at the esophagocardial junction with the TA stapler and transected along the upper edge of the instrument with a scalpel. Both cut ends are cleaned with patties soaked in antiseptic. The stapler is released, the stomach is returned to the abdomen, and the hiatus is closed with continuous or interrupted sutures. A condom is slid over the esophageal stump and secured with a heavy ligature to avoid spillage of infectious material into the field.

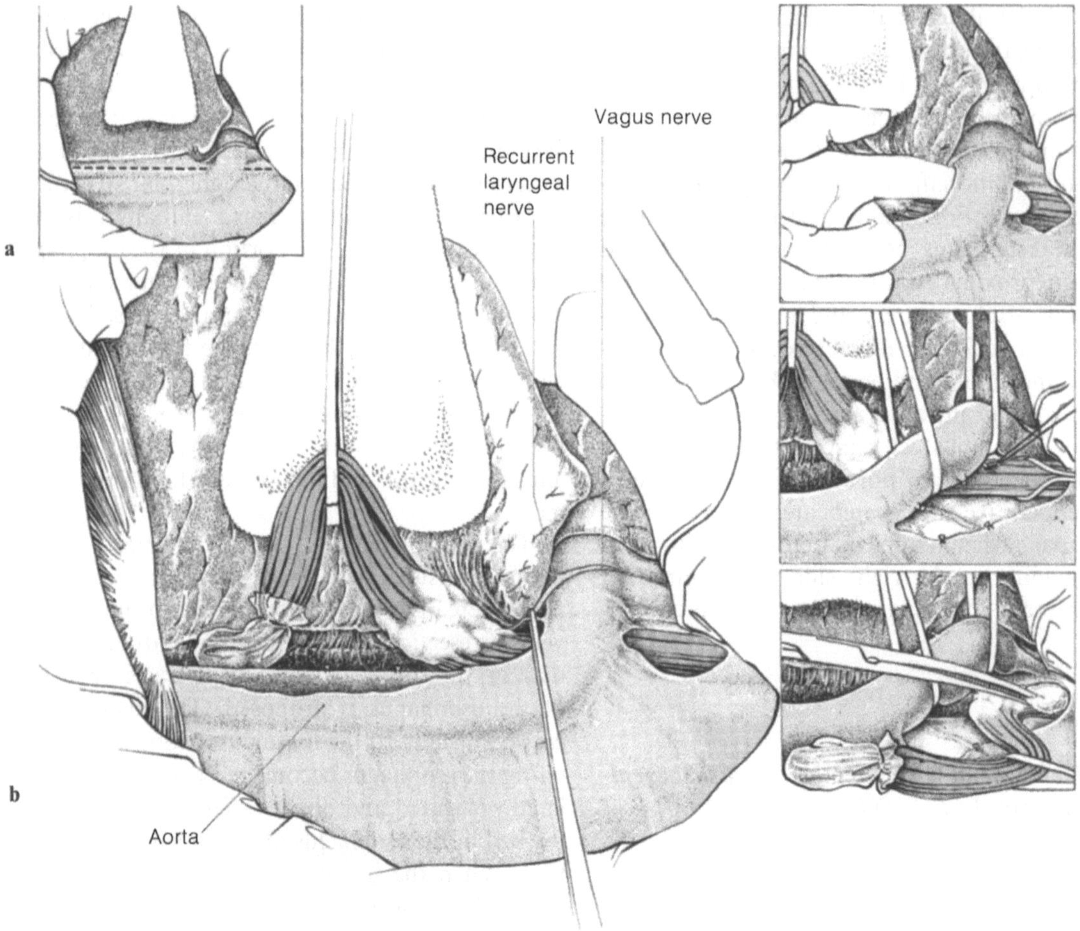

Fig. 69a–e. Esophageal resection through the left thoracic approach. **a** Mediastinal pleura is incised between the aorta and esophagus (broken line). **b** The tumor-bearing esophagus is freed circumferentially to the aortic arch. **c** A finger is passed beneath the aortic arch to mobilize the esophagus. **d** The aortic arch is snared, and vessels passing from the arch to the esophagus are ligated. **e** The esophagus, mobilized superiorly to the thoracic apex, is extracted from beneath the aortic arch

If a transpleural esophageal reconstruction is planned for the same sitting (see 7.2.2.2.3), the hiatus is not closed. For reconstruction by stomach, we staple the esophagus with the TA instrument as described above but do not transect it until it has been completely mobilized. In that way the esophagus can be used to pull the stomach into the chest.

The esophageal stump is elevated, pulled superiorly, and progressively freed from the posterior mediastinum as far as the aortic arch (Fig. 69 b).

Mobilization of the esophagus below the aortic arch is identical for benign and malignant disease. First the pleura above the aortic arch is divided and separated from the esophagus by patty dissection. The esophagus is pulled distally to make its fibrous and vascular attachments with the aorta tense so that they can be cauterized or ligated and divided. Now the aorta can be elevated with a hook and the dissection carried farther cephalad. Elevation of the aorta may require mobilization of the aortic arch and interruption of the highest intercostal artery, with care taken to preserve the spinal artery. The recurrent nerve should be exposed at this stage so that it can be more easily protected. When the posterior surface of the aorta has been largely cleared, it is encircled with the finger (Fig. 69 c) and mobilized past the border of the esophagus. The aorta is snared with tapes and gently pulled inferiorly; this is done carefully to avoid compromising the left ventricular outflow tract. The remaining connections between the aorta and esophagus are divided under vision (Fig. 69 d). Now the esophagus is bluntly freed from the posterior mediastinum beyond the aortic arch, encircled proximal to the aortic arch; and snared with a soft Penrose drain.

With lateral traction on the drain, the attachments between the esophagus and trachea are made tense and are divided. Now the esophagus can be extracted from beneath the aortic arch by pulling it from above and pushing it from below. In the area of the pleural dome, the pleura is divided at its superior reflection, and the esophagus is bluntly mobilized beyond the thoracic inlet (Fig. 69 e). The surgeon should stay close to the muscular wall of the esophagus to avoid injury to the recurrent nerve and brachial vessels.

Adhesions due to inflammation or tumor infiltration are commonly found in the area of the neoplasm. Structures that appear fixed to the tumor, such as the pericardium, should be included in the resection unless their removal would be incompatible with life or would necessitate a major extension of the resection (e.g., to portions of the lungs). In cases where the extent of disease has been underestimated in the initial phase of the operation, the tumor is dissectly bluntly or sharply from adjacent structures. Subsequent esophageal replacement must be done by the subcutaneous or retrosternal route to avoid obstruction of the tract by local recurrence and to leave open the option of high-dosage postoperative irradiation.

When the tumor has been freed circumferentially, it is wrapped in a compress soaked in Clorpactin solution, and stay sutures are used to hold the compress in place.

During mobilization of the upper thoracic part of the esophagus, attention must be given to the thoracic duct, which is closely related to the left wall of the esophagus at the level of the aortic arch. If the duct is injured, it must be ligated proximally and distally to avoid chylothorax. If the contralateral pleura has been entered or has been included in the resection, the defect is repaired with sutures whenever possible. A drain is inserted at the end of the procedure only if there is radiologic evidence of a contralateral pneumothorax.

The level of the esophageal resection depends both on the location of the tumor and on the type of anastomosis that is planned. For an intrathoracic anastomosis, the esophagus is pulled inferiorly, the wall facing the surgeon is opened with the electrocautery, and the lumen is cleaned with dissecting patties soaked in antiseptic. If a stapled anastomosis is desired, it is recommended that a pursestring suture and two guide sutures be placed (see 1.3.3.2) and the EEA instrument introduced before the posterior wall is divided. The esophagus is easily manipulated by its residual posterior wall, and the anvil of the EEA instrument glides over it easily into the lumen. The guide sutures are removed, and the pursestring suture is closed around the central rod of the EEA instrument before the posterior wall of the esophagus is divided.

If a cervical esophagostomy or cervical anastomosis is proposed, the esophagus is exposed through a right or left cervicotomy (see 2.1.1) and exteriorized. With benign disease, the extent of the esophageal resection corresponds to the extent of the disease. For carcinoma distal to the aortic arch, the line of resection is level with the superior border of the clavicle. For carcinoma above the aortic arch, the line of resection is at the cricopharyngeal muscle. If a two-stage procedure is planned, it is essential that an adequate remnant of esophagus be left for construction of an end esophagostomy (see 2.2.2). With carcinoma above the aortic arch, it will be necessary to resect the cervical esophagus secondarily to the hypopharynx at the time of reconstruction.

For a tumor that requires concomitant resection of the cervical viscera, the procedure is continued as described in 6.4.3.2 and 6.4.2.6 after completion of the thoracic phase, although basic questions of resectability still must be addressed.

6.6.2 Esophageal Resection with Proximal or Total Gastrectomy

Extension of the esophageal resection to include the cardia for benign disease or to include a proximal or total gastrectomy for malignant disease can be accomplished through an exclusive left thoracic approach with or without phrenotomy; through a combined abdominothoracic approach with division of the cartilaginous costal arch, phrenotomy, and upper oblique laparotomy; or through separate abdominal and thoracic incisions. We prefer to employ a separate laparotomy and thoracotomy (see Chap. B, 4.3.6).

The technique of the extended resection through a left thoracic approach is identical to that for the right-sided approach (see 6.5.2).

Steps in procedure:

(1) Division of the inferior pulmonary ligament close to the lung
(2) Removal of lymphatic and connective tissue from the anterior and posterior sides of the hilum
(3) Dissection of the mediastinal pleura and adventitia from the anterior border of the aorta to the esophageal hiatus
(4) Snaring of the esophagus
(5) Mobilization of the esophagus distally to the cardia
(6) Transection of the esophagus close to the cardia with the GIA instrument
(7) Mobilization of the esophagus below the aortic arch
(8) Incision of the mediastinal pleura on both sides of the supraaortic esophagus to the thoracic apex
(9) Mobilization of the esophagus to the thoracic apex
(10) Blunt dissection of the esophagus past the thoracic inlet (if required)
(11) Resection of the connective and lymphatic tissue in the esophageal bed as far as the contralateral pleura
(12) Transection of the esophagus at the thoracic apex or exteriorization of the esophagus at the neck

Fig. 70a–c. Left posterior mediastinectomy. **a** Extent of the mediastinectomy (broken lines). The lung is retracted anteriorly. The inferior pulmonary ligament is divided close to the lung parenchyma. **b** All connective and lymphatic tissues are removed from the pulmonary hilum. **c** The hilum is dissected free from the anterior side ▷

6.6.3 Posterior Mediastinectomy

Besides resection of the esophagus, posterior mediastinectomy involves removal of the overlying pleura, the aortic adventitia, the mediastinal connective tissue as far as the contralateral pleura, and the hilar and tracheal lymph nodes.

Preoperative preparation, instruments, position and approach: See 6.5 and 6.6.1.

Operative technique: The inferior pulmonary ligament is divided close to the lung as far as the inferior pulmonary vein. The lung is retracted anteriorly, and the pleura over the pulmonary hilum is incised in continuity with the pulmonary ligament incision as far as the superior border of the hilum (Fig. 70 a).

The pleura is dissected from the inferior pulmonary vein, the bronchus, and the pulmonary artery in the direction of the esophagus by blunt patty dissection. The tracheobronchial lymph nodes are removed along with the connective tissue surrounding the pulmonary artery, pulmonary vein, and bronchus. The lymphadenectomy is continued medially to the bifurcation, removing as many of the subcarinal nodes as possible (Fig. 70 b). The lung is retracted posteriorly, and the pleura is incised from below upward, in continuity with the pulmonary ligament incision, to the superior border of the hilum. The pleura is dissected free as far as the pericardium, sparing the phrenic nerve, and is removed. The resection must include any connective and lymphatic tissue that remains among the hilar structures (Fig. 70 c). Then the lung is again retracted anteriorly, and the pleura and underlying adventitia are dissected inferiorly from the anterior edge of the aorta to the hiatus and superiorly beyond the aortic arch to the apex of the chest, sparing the recurrent nerve.

The anterior limit of the pleural resection is defined by its pericardial reflection. The esophagus is snared, freed from its hiatal attachments as previously described, and pulled cephalad. In contrast to the standard procedure (see 6.6.1), the resection includes the periesophageal tissue as far as the pleura of the opposite side. The thoracic duct is removed only if lymph nodes are found in its course. When the inferior border of the aortic arch is reached, the esophagus is mobilized below it. The adventitia of the aorta is included in the resection. When the divided esophagus has been pulled from beneath the aorta, the dissection is continued to the thoracic apex, and the esophagus is bluntly mobilized into the thoracic inlet.

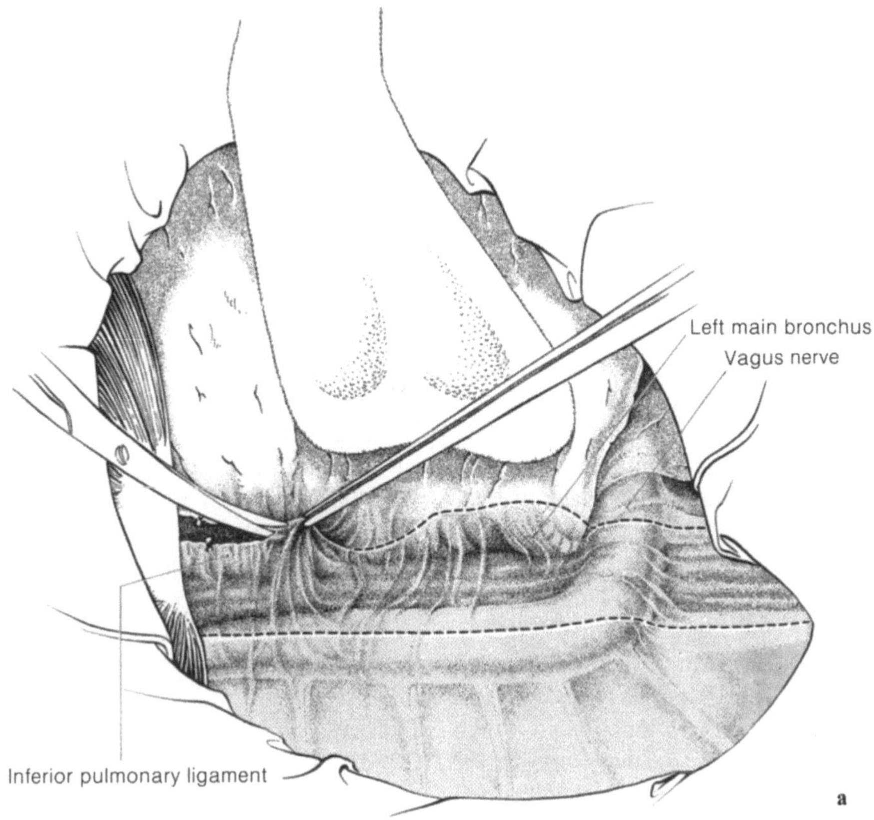
Left main bronchus
Vagus nerve
Inferior pulmonary ligament

a

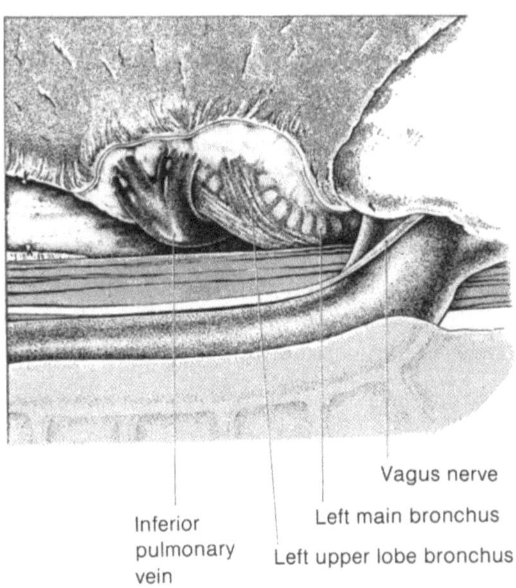
Vagus nerve
Left main bronchus
Inferior pulmonary vein
Left upper lobe bronchus

b

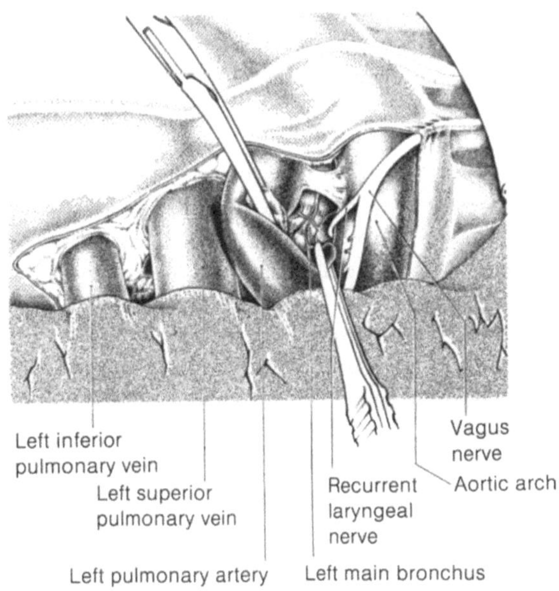
Left inferior pulmonary vein
Left superior pulmonary vein
Left pulmonary artery
Recurrent laryngeal nerve
Left main bronchus
Vagus nerve
Aortic arch

c

6.7 Esophagectomy without Thoracotomy [1, 12, 56]

Blunt dissection [12, 56] or "eversion stripping" [1, 2] of the esophagus is made possible by the fact that long portions of the esophagus in the posterior mediastinum are enclosed by loose connective tissue. The blood vessels of the thoracic esophagus (see 1.1.3) do not pose a serious obstacle to the procedure. If the threadlike arteries or veins are torn during the dissection, they will become occluded by thrombosis within a few minutes, possibly aided by compression with gauze rolls. The blood loss is less than about 500 ml [27].

The major advantage of this procedure over transthoracic resection is the elimination of thoracotomy, which reduces risks and shortens operating time by about 1 h [53]. The exclusive cervicoabdominal approach can be tolerated even by high-risk patients with impaired pulmonary function.

Resection without thoracotomy [2] is indicated for carcinomas of the hypopharynx, cervical esophagus, or esophagogastric junction in which the tumor and its lymphatic drainage can be resected under vision, CT shows no mediastinal lymph node involvement, and total esophagectomy is desired due to possible intramural tumor spread or to facilitate reconstruction. It may also be used in patients with scleroderma or a long, nondilatable esophageal stricture without significant periesophagitis, or after a failed reconstruction of the cervical esophagus where the transfer of stomach or bowel is planned for restoration of continuity.

Esophagectomy without thoracotomy is not appropriate for the treatment of esophageal varices [27], because endoscopic sclerotherapy is far less invasive and offers comparable efficacy. The value of the procedure in carcinoma of the thoracic esophagus is open to question, since it cannot remove tumor that has spread beyond the boundaries of the esophagus, nor can it provide removal of regional nodes [2]. However, we feel that the relatively poor late results of transthoracic resection for esophageal carcinoma [14] make this argument less convincing, and we would emphasize the advantage of "shelling out" the carcinoma without fear of injury to adjacent organs. If comparative prospective studies were to show that the postoperative mortality of esophagectomy without thoracotomy were significantly below that of transthoracic resection, which is still in the range of 10%–30% according to reports in the European and American literature [5, 9, 20, 34, 43, 51], this would offer a strong argument in its favor. So far, the results of uncontrolled studies [19, 41, 53] indicate a lower rate of complications after esophagectomy without thoracotomy, but no reduction of hospital mortality. This raises the general question of the advisability of surgical resection, whose superiority over radiotherapy for esophageal carcinoma has not been proven in comparative studies [13, 14]. Another option for advanced malignant strictures is endoscopic intubation (see Sect. 5), which is associated with a low rate of postoperative complications.

A convenient instrument for eversion stripping of the esophagus is the Babcock vein stripper. Blunt dissection of the esophagus is usually performed manually. As early as 1913, Denk [12] described an esophageal dissector, since modified [26], that is supposed to simplify blunt removal of the esophagus and especially the digital separation of fibrous tissue strands in the subcarinal area, which are thought to result from prior lymphangitis. Another advantage of mobilizing the esophagus with the dissector is that it avoids the reduction of cardiac output that can occur in manual dissection when the hand, inserted into the posterior mediastinum, presses the heart against the sternum.

Preoperative preparation: Antiseptic preparation of the oropharynx, prophylactic antibiotics (see Chap. C), extraction of teeth involved by caries or periodontal infection.

Instruments: Basic set, Babcock stripper or esophageal dissector, GIA or TA-55 stapling instrument.

Position and approach: Upper midline laparotomy extended around the left side of the umbilicus; right or left cervicotomy along the anterior border of the sternocleidomastoid muscle (Fig. 71 a).

Fig. 71 a–d. Esophagectomy without thoracotomy. ▷ **a** Cervical (*a*) and abdominal (*b*) incisions. **b** Stripping of the esophagus with a Babcock acorn-tipped probe. The esophagus has been partially mobilized manually through the cervical and abdominal incisions. The esophagus is transected in the neck, and its upper end is tied around the probe. **c** Eversion stripping of the esophagus. The tape (*a* attached to the stripper can be used to pull a gauze roll into the wound bed for compression. **d** Blunt manual dissection of the entire thoracic esophagus

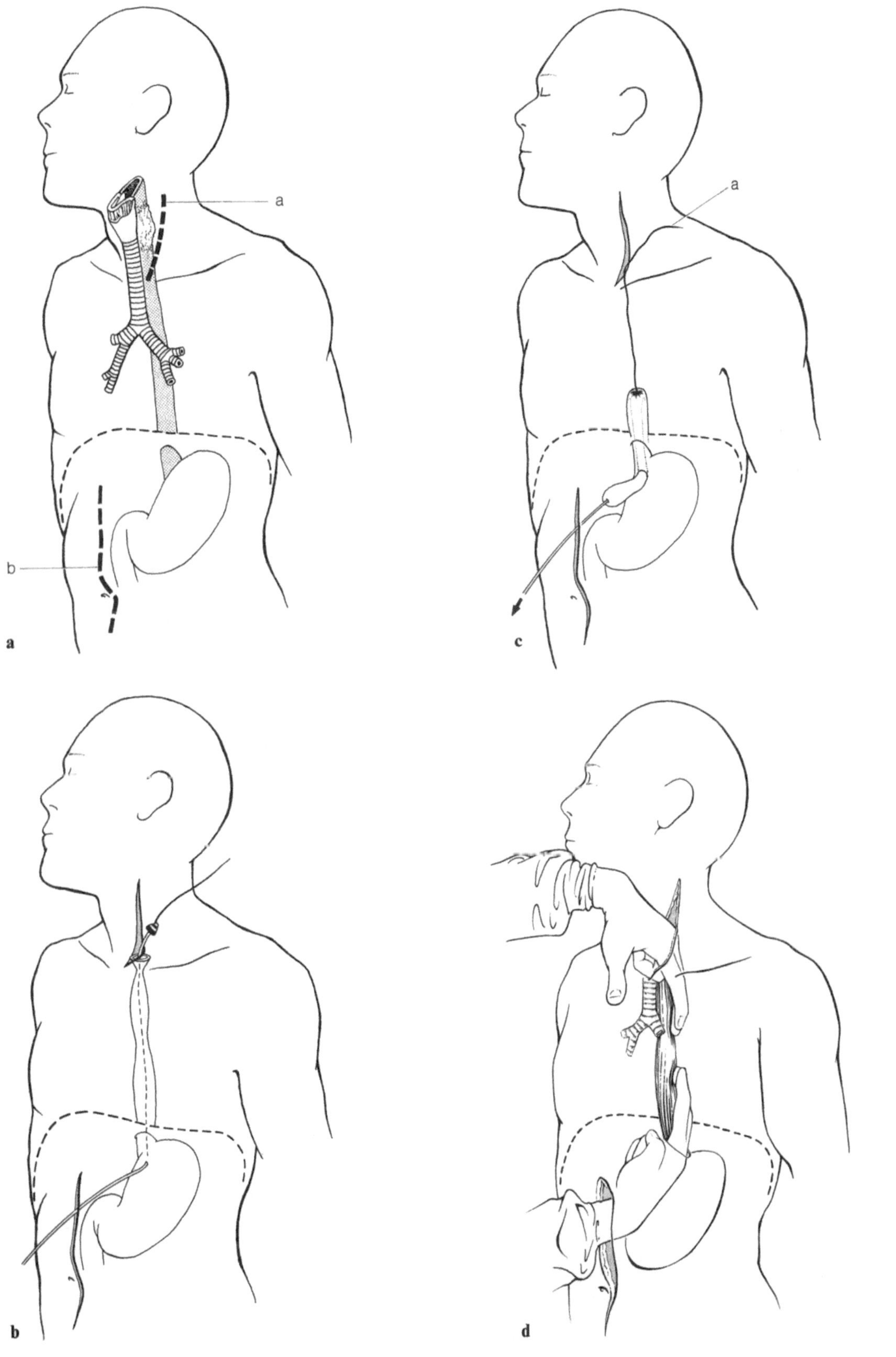
a
b
a
a
c
b
d

Steps in procedure:

(1) Laparatomy and separation of the left hepatic lobe from the diaphragm
(2) Snaring of the abdominal esophagus
(3) Manual, circumferential mobilization of the esophagus through the hiatus
(4) Exposure and snaring of the cervical esophagus
(5) Manual, circumferential mobilization of the esophagus in the thoracic inlet
(6) Cervical esophagotomy
(7) Insertion of the Babcock probe into the esophagus
(8) Incision of the cardia, extraction of the tip of the Babcock probe
(9) Fixation of the cervical esophagus around the Babcock probe with a heavy tie
(10) Transection of the cervical esophagus
(11) Gradual extraction of the Babcock probe through the gastrotomy, everting and exteriorizing the esophagus
(12) Resection of the esophagus with the GIA instrument

Operative technique: The abdomen is entered, the triangular ligament of the liver is divided, and the hepatic left lobe is retracted medially with a broad retractor. The peritoneum over the esophagus is incised, and the esophagus is exposed and encircled with a snare. Both vagus nerve trunks are identified and severed. They are bluntly mobilized about a hand's breadth into the hiatus. For eversion stripping, this concludes the abdominal phase of the operation.

For blunt dissection of the esophagus, the hiatal crura are exposed with a dissecting patty, and the hiatus is manually enlarged. We usually find it necessary to divide the right or left crus between ligatures before a hand can be passed into the posterior mediastinum. The enlarged hiatus is held open with two retractors so that the posterior mediastinum can be visualized. Both vagus nerve trunks are identified and generally are divided.

It may be desirable to avoid the side-effects of truncal vagotomy, especially in benign disease. This can be done by snaring the two main vagus nerve trunks, severing their branches to the esophagus, and performing a selective proximal vagotomy. The esophagus is removed by stripping as described below. In this technique the cardia and lesser curvature must be resected to the level of the "crow's foot," because the blood flow in this area is marginal, and there is a danger of gastric wall necrosis. It should also be determined whether the mobilized stomach has sufficient length to reach the neck.

The ascending branches of the left gastric artery and inferior phrenic artery are ligated or clipped and divided. The rest of the dissection is performed blindly. One hand pulls the esophagus downward and keeps it under tension, while the index finger of the other hand, staying close to the muscular wall, frees the esophagus from its connective tissue attachments while avulsing its vascular supply. Usually the esophagus can be mobilized transhiatally to the level of the bifurcation. Close attention should be given to the blood pressure and pulse rate at this time due to the potential for cardiac compression by the hand in the posterior mediastinum. We advise continuous intravascular monitoring of the blood pressure via the radial artery.

After the abdominal phase is completed, the esophagus is exposed through a cervicotomy and snared (see 2.1.1). For eversion stripping, it is sufficient to mobilize the esophagus to the thoracic inlet. Then the cervical esophagus is opened, and the Babcock probe is inserted until its tip can be palpated in the cardia. It is brought out at that point through a small gastrotomy. The cervical esophagus is tied around the probe with a heavy ligature, and a tape is tied to the cap of the stripper (Fig. 71 b). Proximal to the ligature, the esophagus is occluded with a soft intestinal clamp and transected with the electrocautery. Both cut ends are wiped with antiseptic solution.

The abdominal viscera are carefully covered with towels soaked in antiseptic so that they will not come in contact with the everted mucosa of the esophagus, which must be considered contaminated. Now the stripper is pulled downward with a steady but gentle force, delivering the invaginated esophagus through the gastrotomy. Hemostasis can be aided by attaching gauze rolls to the tape and dragging them into the bed of the esophagus (Fig. 71 c).

For esophagectomy by blunt dissection (Fig. 71 d), mobilization of the esophagus is continued with the index finger down past the thoracic inlet and into the posterior mediastinum. If the thoracic inlet is so narrow that the esophagus cannot be mobilized to an adequate depth, access can be improved by splitting the manubrium or resecting the clavicle at its sternal attachment. However, in these cases we prefer to combine blunt dissection with eversion stripping as a means of completing the mobilization. A particularly vulnerable area during blunt dissection is the membranous trachea, and separation of the esophagus from the trachea must be done with extreme care to avoid tearing the membranous wall. The terminal portion in the area of the bifurcation should be dissected simultaneously or alternately through the abdominal and cervical fields until both dissections meet. Finally the esophagus is occluded with a ligature and transected at its abdominal or cervical end. The stump is cleaned with antiseptic solution, a tape is attached to it (or two gauze rolls for hemostasis), and the esophagus is extracted through the cervical or abdominal incision. About 10 min are allowed to pass to make certain there is no heavy bleeding from the esophageal bed, during which time the esophageal substitute can be prepared for transfer. If the substitute is to be routed through the esophageal bed, its proximal end is attached to the tape or to one of the gauze rolls, which is pulled upward through the cervicotomy. The use of a plastic sleeve can greatly facilitate passage of the transplant (see 7.2.2.3). Following the anastomosis, drains are inserted into the cervical and abdominal fields. The chest should be X-rayed while the patient is still in the operating room so that pneumothorax due to pleural entry can be promptly recognized and treated with a chest tube.

References

1. Ach (1931) Beiträge zur Ösophaguschirurgie. München (zit n DENK)
2. Akiyama H (1981) Esophagectomy without thoracotomy. Surg An 13:109
3. Akiyama H (1980) Surgery for carcinoma of the esophagus. Curr Probl Surg 17:1
4. Akiyama H, Kogure T, Hag I (1972) The esophageal axis and its relationship to the resectability of carcinoma of the esophagus. Ann Surg 176:30
5. Appelquist P (1972) Carcinoma of the esophagus and gastric cardia. Chir Scand Suppl 430
6. Bakamjian V (1968) Total reconstruction of the pharynx with a medially based deltopectoral skin flap. NY State J Med 68:2771
7. Belsey R, Hiebert CA (1974) An exclusive right thoracic approach for cancer of the middle third of the esophagus. Ann Thorac Surg 18:1
8. Buchanan G, Wesr TE, Woodhead JS, Lowry I (1975) Hypoparathyroidism following pharyngolaryngectomy. Clin Oncol 1:89
9. Cederquist C, Nielson J, Berthelsen A (1978) Cancer of the esophagus. Acta Cir Scand 144:227
10. Daffner R, Halber MD, Postlethwaith RW, Korobkin M, Thompson WM (1979) CT of the esophagus. Am J Roentgenol 133:1051
11. Deneke HJ (1980) Die oto-rhino-laryngologischen Operationen im Mund und Halsbereich. Springer, Berlin Heidelberg New York
12. Denk W (1913) Zur Radikaloperation des Ösophaguskarzinoms. Zentralbl Chir 40:1065
13. Earlam R, Cunha-Melo JR (1980) Oesophageal squamous cell carcinoma: II. A critical review of radiotherapy. Br J Surg 67:457
14. Earlam R, Cunha-Melo JR (1980) Oesophageal cell carcinoma: I. A critical review of surgery. Br J Surg 67:381
15. Ellis jr FH (1980) Esophagogastrectomy for carcinoma. Technical considerations based on anatomic location of lesion. Surg Clin North Am 60:265
16. Ellis TH, Maggs PR (1981) Surgery for carcinoma of the lower esophagus and cardia. World J Surg 5:527
17. Fekete F, Lortat-Jacob J (1981) Ösophagektomie von links. In: Allgöwer M, Harder F, Hollander LF, Peiper HJ, Siewert JR (Hrsg) Chirurgische Gastroenterologie 1. Springer, Berlin Heidelberg New York
18. Garlock JH (1938) The surgical treatment of carcinoma of the thoracic esophagus. Surg Gynecol Obstet 66:534
19. Garvin PJ, Kaminski DL (1980) Extrathoracic esophagectomy in the treatment of esophageal cancer. Am J Surg 140:772
20. Giuli R, Gignoux (1980) Treatment of carcinoma of the esophagus. Ann Surg 192:44
21. Gluck TH, Soerensen J (1922) In: Katz L, Blumenfeld F (Hrsg) Handbuch der speziellen Chirurgie des Ohres und der oberen Luftwege. Bd IV, Kabitzsch, Leipzig
22. Hegemann G (1959) Resektion und Rekonstruktion der Speiseröhre. Chirurg 30:501
23. Holle F (1968) Spezielle Magenchirurgie. Springer, Berlin Heidelberg New York
24. Holle F, Hart W, Parchwitz HV (1963) Die Fundektomie des Magens, neuere Erfahrungen und Modifikationen. Chir Praxis 7:351
25. Hopkins SM, Van den Berg HJ (1968) Segmental resection for carcinoma of the esophagus. Arch Surg 96:936
26. Kunath U (1980) Ein Instrument zur stumpfen Dissektion der Speiseröhre. Chirurg 51:738
27. Kunath U (1981) Ergebnisse und Erfahrungen mit der Ösophagektomie durch stumpfe Dissektion. Chirurg 52:706
28. Lam KH, Wong J, Lim STK, Ong GB (1980) Surgical treatment of carcinoma of the hypopharynx and cervical esophagus. Ann Acad Med 9:317
29. Lam KH, Wong J, Lim STK, Ong DS (1981) Pharyngogastric anastomoses following pharyngolaryngoesophagectomy: Analysis of 157 cases. World J Surg 5:509
30. Le Quesne LP, Ranger D (1966) Pharyngolaryngectomy with immediate pharyngogastric anastomosis. Br J Surg 53:105
31. Lewis J (1946) The surgical treatment of carcinoma of the esophagus with special reference to a new operation for growth of the middle third. Br J Surg 34:18

32. Lortat-Jacob J, Maillard JN (1961) Les oesophagectomies. Encycl Medico-Chirurgeale 18 we Seguir Paris-6
33. Lortat-Jacob JL, Maillard JN, Richard CA, Fekete F, Launois B (1970) Surgical treatment of cancer of the esophagus. Brit J Clin Pract 24:13
34. McKeown KC (1981) Resection of midesophageal carcinoma with esophagogastric anastomosis. World J Surg 5:517–525
35. Nakayama K (1966) Persönliche Erfahrungen in der Ösophaguschirurgie. Langenbecks Arch Chir 316:300
36. Nakayama K, Yamamoto K, Tamiya T (1964) Experience with free autografts of the bowel with a new venous anastomosis apparatus. Surgery 55:796
37. Ohsawa T (1933) Surgery of the oesophagus. Arch Jpn Chir 10
38. Ong GB, Lam KH, Lau WF, Wong J (1981) Radical exstirpation of carcinoma of the Ösophagus. In: Häring R (Hrsg) Chirurgie des Ösophaguskarzinoms. Edition Medizin Weinheim Deerfield Basel
39. Ong GB, Lam KH, Lam PH, Wong J (1978) Resection for carcinoma of the superior mediastinal segment of the esophagus. World J Surg 2:497
40. Ong GB, Lee TC (1960) Pharyngogastric anastomosis after esophagopharyngectomy for carcinoma of the hypopharynx and cervical esophagus. Br J Surg 48:193
41. Orringer MB, Sloan H (1978) Esophagectomy without thoracotomy. J Thorac Cardiovasc Surg 76:643
42. Pichlmaier H (1981) Operationsindikation zur Ösophagusresektion. In: Häring R (Hrsg) Chirurgie des Ösophaguskarzinoms. Edition Medizin Weinheim Deerfield Basel
43. Pichlmaier H, Müller JM, Neumann G (1984) Ösophagus und Kardiakarzinom. Deutsches Ärzteblatt 81:33
44. Pichlmaier H, Müller JM, Wintzer G (1978) Ösophagusersatz. Chirurg 49:65
45. Schwemmle K (1980) Die allgemeinchirurgischen Operationen am Halse. Springer, Berlin, Heidelberg New York
46. Seidenberg B, Rosenak SS, Hurwitt ES, Som ML (1959) Immediate reconstruction of the cervical esophagus by a revascularized isolated jejunal segment. Ann Surg 149:162
47. Sheppard HW (1977) Surgery for the post-cricoid carcinoma. Report on 23 cases in which replacement by stomach was attempted. J Otolaryngol 6:271
48. Siewert R, Peiper HG (1976) Taktik und Technik in der operativen Behandlung des Cardia-Carcinoms. Chir Praxis 21:597
49. Silver CE (1981) Surgical treatment of hypopharyngeal and cervical esophageal carcinoma. World J Surg 5:499
50. Silver CE (1976) Gastric pull-up operation for replacement of the cervical position of the esophagus. Surg Gynecol Obstet 142:243
51. Skinner D (1984) Resection for cancer of the esophagus. 1st International Congress of OESO, Paris 17.–19.5.1984
52. Sörensen J (1930) Die Mund- und Halsoperationen. Urban & Schwarzenberg, Berlin Wien
53. Steiger Z, Wilson RF (1981) Comparison of the results of esophagectomy with and without a thoracotomy. Surg Gynecol Obstet 153:653–656
54. Sweet RH (1945) Transthoracic resection of the esophagus and stomach for carcinoma. Ann Surg 121:272
55. Tanner NC (1949) The present position of carcinoma of the esophagus. Postgrad Med J 23:109
56. Turner GG (1936) Carcinoma of the Ösophagus. The question of its treatment by surgery. Lancet I:130
57. UICC (1919) TNM Klassifikation der malignen Tumoren. 3. Aufl. Springer, Berlin Heidelberg New York
58. Waddell WR, Scannel JG (1952) Anterior approach to carcinoma of the superior mediastinal and cervical segments of the esophagus. J Thorac Surg 9:663
59. Withers EH, Franklin JD, Madden JJ, Lynch JB (1979) Pectoralis maior myocutaneous island flap for reconstruction of the head and neck. Head Neck Surg 1:293
60. Wookey H (1942) The surgical treatment of carcinoma of the pharynx and upper esophagus. Surg Gynecol Obstet 75:499
61. Zenker R, Bary S v, Feifel G et al. (1975) Die Eingriffe am Magen und Zwölffingerdarm. In: Zenker R, Berchtold R, Hamelmann H (Hrsg) Die Eingriffe in der Bauchhöhle. Springer, Berlin Heidelberg New York (Allgemeine und spezielle chirurgische Operationslehre, 3. neubearb. Aufl. Bd. VII/1, S 93

7 Reconstruction of the Esophagus

CONTENTS

7.1 Selection of an Organ for Esophageal Reconstruction

The ideal method of esophageal replacement would relieve dysphagia completely and permanently with no adverse side-effects, would be suitable for replacing all or part of the esophagus in any age group with an acceptable postoperative morbidity and mortality, would allow for a one-stage resection and reconstruction, and would be practicable by surgeons with average skills or by surgeons in training. At at present time no method of esophageal replacement satisfies all these criteria. Consequently the surgeon must know a variety of reconstructive techniques along with their advantages and disadvantages so that he can select the optimum approach for a given situation and can change to a different procedure if anatomic constraints make it necessary to abandon the original plan.

7.1.1 Nonvisceral Reconstruction of the Esophagus

The oldest known method of esophageal reconstruction is the antethoracic skin tube, which was first used by Bircher [12] in 1894 to bridge the gap between an esophagostomy and gastrostomy. Today the dermatoplasty is used only by otorhinolaryngologic surgeons for replacement of the cervical esophagus [5, 95, 96]. The various techniques are described in volume V/1 of this series [15]. In our view the prolonged operating time, the high rate of local complications such as fistula formation and stricturing, and repeated reports of carcinoma formation are strong arguments against the use of this method. However, Japanese authors have recently described favorable results with segmental esophageal replacement using a pedicled myocutaneous flap (e.g., pectoralis muscle) that is fashioned into a tube and placed subcutaneously or covered over with Thiersch grafts. So far, attempts to reconstruct the esophagus with fascia lata, dura, or aorta [33, 56] or with prosthetic materials [11, 70, 81, 93] have been unsuccessful. Positive results have been achieved with extracorporeal bypass tubes (see 2.4) for interim use in two-stage reconstructions and in cases where the severity or level of the stricture prevents the use of an endoesophageal tube.

7.1.2 Visceral Reconstruction of the Esophagus

7.1.2.1 Stomach

Generally the stomach will retain an adequate blood supply if the right gastric and right gastroepiploic vessels are preserved [39]. Suitably mobilized, the stomach will extend as high as the larynx when brought up by the subcutaneous, retrosternal, or transpleural route. Additional length can be gained by performing Kocher's maneuver to mobilize the duodenum. Since only one anastomosis is required, the operation can be performed simply, quickly, and safely.

Because the pulled-up stomach assumes the shape of an elongated tube, there is little danger that the transplant will become kinked or twisted as there is when jejunum or colon is used. A previous gastric resection, but not gastrostomy, makes the stomach unfit for use as an esophageal substitute. With adenocarcinoma of the esophagogastric junction, we feel that a total gastrectomy is indicated; with squamous cell carcinoma of this region, at least a fundectomy is advised. In the latter case a high intrathoracic esophagogastrostomy can always be performed. The gastric remnant can frequently be anastomosed to the cervical esophagus, but it rarely has sufficient length for anastomosis to the pharynx.

The reflux of gastric contents into the esophagus or pharynx can lead to esophagitis, regurgitation, and aspiration. If the entire stomach is transposed into the chest, the incidence of reflux is less than 5% even after several years' follow-up [22, 62]. But if most of the gastric pouch is retained within the abdomen, it will be exposed intermittently to high positive pressures. Since the intrathoracic portion of the stomach is in an area of negative and low positive pressures, an orally directed pressure gradient develops which promotes upward flow of gastric juices. A drainage procedure [52] or antireflux repair [13, 41] can provide sufficient palliation in these cases to minimize the importance of the adverse pressure gradient, at least in cancer patients whose life expectancy is limited to a few years. With benign disease, on the other hand, the danger of reflux esophagitis raises a more serious objection to using the stomach as an esophageal substitute [85]. We rarely recommend this type of reconstruction in children and adolescents.

Distention of the intrathoracic stomach after eating can lead to diminished respiratory capacity in the first months after surgery [44], but this does not appear to have major clinical significance. The intrathoracic stomach increasingly assumes a tubular shape with passage of time and ceases to interfere with respiration [59]. The construction of a "reversed gastric tube" from the greater curvature [8, 19, 25] offers the advantage of keeping at least part of the gastric reservoir within the abdomen. The portion of the antrum, pylorus, or duodenum that is united to the esophagus does not produce acid. This, plus the lack of antiperistalsis in the tube, should eliminate the danger of peptic reflux esophagitis [20, 26]. The small diameter of the tube does not compromise pulmonary function, even when placed transpleurally. And because the tube grows with the patient, the procedure is suitable even for children and adolescents. The use of stapling instruments (TA, GIA) has greatly shortened the formerly long operating time of this procedure and has decreased the risk of leakage from the long suture line, although this risk is still higher than when the whole stomach is transposed. A prior gastric resection precludes use of the reversed gastric tube procedure, and a previous gastroenterostomy limits its application. While the procedure is widely utilized at present, our knowledge of its late results is based entirely on individual case reports, so we cannot assess its suitability for benign disorders. A major disadvantage of the procedure, especially in children, is the virtual necessity of performing a splenectomy, for even the reimplantation of splenic tissue, vaccines, and prophylactic antibiotics are not entirely effective in preventing eventual postsplenectomy sepsis [36].

7.1.2.2 Jejunum

The vascular anatomy of the proximal small intestine greatly limits its routine use for total esophageal replacement. In only about half of cases do vessels of adequate size arise from the superior mesenteric artery and form large, uninterrupted marginal arcades sufficient to enable the jejunum to be advanced into the neck [4, 22, 23, 98]. In principle the transplant, which takes a tortuous course along its mesenteric attachment, can be lengthened and straightened by means of radial incisions [15], by resecting excess intestine from the loop [59], or by uniting the proximal part of the transplant to the internal mammary vessels [4] or to the inferior or superior thyroid artery, but even these measures cannot always ensure a favorable disposition of the vessels. Moreover, reconstruction with jejunum requires that two additional intestinal anastomoses be performed. This increases the risk of leakage and prolongs the operating time. The jejunal vessels are delicate, and venous return from the transplant is easily compromised by pressure. Thus, use of the jejunum as a total esophageal substitute should be considered only if other options are unavailable.

Good results have been obtained with free or pedicled jejunal grafts for segmental esophageal replacement. The lumen of the graft clostly matches that of the esophagus, and the segment retains its peristaltic activity after transplantation [53, 64]. Thus the graft can restore an effective sphincteric mechanism and prevent reflux when transplanted into the lower third of the esophagus in the isoperistaltic position [50]. When anastomosed to a stomach with insufficient drainage and intact vagal innervation, the jejunal segment is vulnerable to peptic ulceration due to the low acid resistance of the jejunal mucosa. Generally this problem can be avoided by performing a vagotomy (usually done anyway during the esophageal resection) and by adding a pyloroplasty to improve gastric emptying.

In cases requiring replacement of the entire stomach along with the distal esophagus, we feel that the procedures of choice are the interposition of isoperistaltic jejunum [24, 46] and the Roux-en-Y procedure [73], both employing at least a 40-cm limb of bowel.

7.1.2.3 Colon

In principle, a gap of any length between the pharynx and stomach can be bridged with an interposed segment of ascending colon [42, 71], transverse colon [37, 92], or descending colon [61]. Adequate blood flow is provided by large arterial and venous trunks and by marginal vascular arcades that run close to the bowel wall. The right colon shows the most pronounced variations in its vascular pattern. The superior mesenteric artery gives off three branches to the right side of the colon in only about 25% of cases. In 4% these branches are absent, and in another 5% there are discontinuities in the marginal arcades on the right side [6, 99]. The left colon, based on the left colic artery or one of the sigmoid arteries, has a more dependable blood supply, can span a considerable distance, and has a caliber similar to that of the esophagus [86]. On the other hand, the left flexure is not bridged by arcadian vessels in 7% of cases [76]; this must be considered if the surgeon wishes to use part of the transverse colon to increase the length of the transplant. The vascular supply must always be assessed intraoperatively by transillumination, and in doubtful cases the vessels that are to be ligated should be clamped off to be sure there is adequate blood flow to the proposed transplant. We do not consider it necessary to evaluate the vascular pattern preoperatively by selective angiography of the superior or inferior mesenteric artery.

The peristaltic activity of the isolated colon is directional but not propulsive. Thus the segment should be placed so that it forms a straight but tension-free conduit. A transplant that is too long is predisposed to kinking, torsion, and pregastric statis, which may necessitate surgical revision. Therefore we always perform the esophagocolic anastomosis first, check the length of the interposed segment, and resect any excessive bowel before anastomosing the distal end of the transplant to the stomach. Manometric and radiologic proof of peristalsis in the isolated colon segment [34, 53] as well as the clinical experience of frequent eructation and fetid breath odor in patients with an antiperistaltic transplant [10, 22] have clearly demonstrated the superiority of the isoperistaltic colon interposition over the antiperistaltic. Reflux-related complaints, especially peptic ulceration in the interposed colon, are uncommon regardless of whether the segment is placed in the iso- or antiperistaltic position. The pathogenesis of these complaints remains unclear, although major importance is ascribed to delayed gastric emptying secondary to truncal vagotomy during the esophageal resection. A drainage procedure seems appropriate, therefore. The tubular shape of the colon segment does not compromise pulmonary function in adults, even with transthoracic placement. However, marked dilatation of the transpleurally routed colon with recurring episodes of respiratory embarrassment have been reported in children even months after the operation [68], especially if a short length of esophagus was left intact distally [94] to preserve the sphincteric mechanism of the cardia. A disadvantage of colon compared with other portions of the alimentary tract is its physiologic colonization by bacteria, which can become disseminated and incite a local infection even after meticulous preoperative cleansing of the bowel. Whereas esophagogastrostomy requires only one anastomosis, colon interposition requires three. Other disadvantages are the potential for diverticular, polypoid, or inflammatory changes in the colon of older patients, rendering it unfit as an esophageal substitute, and the fact that disease is more likely to develop in interposed colon than in stomach or small bowel.

7.1.3 Recommendations on the Selection of an Esophageal Substitute

We believe that isoperistaltic stomach is best for replacing esophagus that has been resected for squamous cell carcinoma at any level, followed by colon and jejunum. In cases where the stomach has been resected for adenocarcinoma of the esophagogastric junction, reconstruction with interposed jejunum [24, 46] or a Roux-en-Y loop [73] is the procedure of choice. Segmental esophageal replacement for benign disease can be similarly accomplished by transplanting a free or pedicled graft of jejunum or colon. We prefer to use jejunum because its lumen matches that of the esophagus, and because it is free of microorganisms. We believe that the left colon is best suited for total esophageal reconstruction in benign disease, followed by the other parts of the colon, the jejunum, and finally the stomach.

7.2 Placement of the Esophageal Substitute

7.2.1 Intraabdominal Placement of the Esophageal Substitute

An isolated bowel segment for interposition esophagoplasty is always placed in the retrocolic position. The segment with its vascular pedicle may be brought up in front of or behind the stomach for delivery into the thorax. Regardless of how the bowel is placed in the chest, we always bring it up behind the stomach, as this shortens the distance traversed by the vascular pedicle and lessens the danger of strangulation from gastric distention. The incision of the lesser omentum required for the subcutaneous or retrosternal route is of no consequence.

7.2.2 Thoracic Placement of the Esophageal Substitute

7.2.2.1 Selection of Procedure

The subcutaneous route for esophageal reconstruction (Fig. 72 a) poses the fewest risks to the patient. Because the transplant is placed beneath the skin, disruption of the suture line or necrosis of the transplant is easily recognized. If the viability of the transplant is in doubt, it can be checked by making a small skin incision. Even if the transplant becomes necrotic, there is no danger of the infection spreading to the mediastinum. The transplant bypasses the narrow part of the thoracic inlet and can be removed with a minimum of intervention. The procedure for creating the subcutaneous tunnel is technically straightforward, and there is no danger of pleural entry as there is with the substernal route. The disadvantages of the subcutaneous route are its length and the poor cosmetic result, which is particularly objectionable in young patients. The superficial position of the transplant makes it vulnerable to compression and minor trauma. Also, kinking of the tube at the sternal margins (especially the inferior) can impede the progression of food, which is already more sluggish than when other routes are used.

The retrosternal route (Fig. 72 b) is more direct than the subcutaneous, and there are no angulation problems at the sternal margins. The cosmetic and functional result is excellent. However, infectious complications are a more serious concern due to the potential for spread to the mediastinum and pleural space. Even so, the retrosternal route is still considered to be the best route for total esophageal reconstruction [74]. The danger of compression of the transplant in the thoracic inlet can be

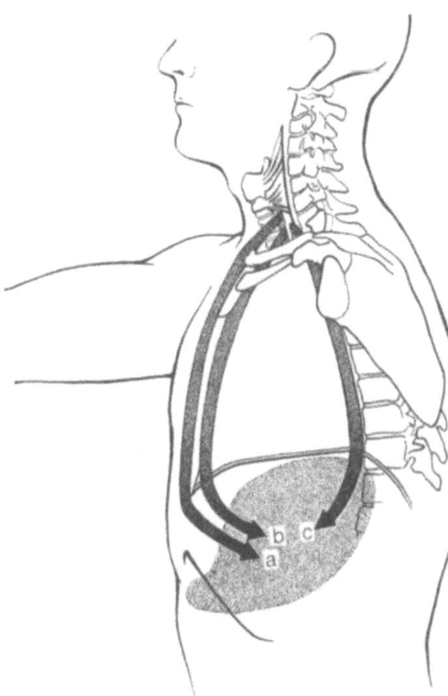

Fig. 72. Thoracic routes of esophageal reconstruction. *a* Subcutaneous route, *b* retrosternal route, *c* intrathoracic route

minimized by notching or dividing the short strap muscles of the neck or, if necessary, by partial resection of the manubrium. Other dangers are inadvertent pleural entry with pneumothorax during creation of the retrosternal tunnel, and indrawing and kinking of the transplant by negative pressure in the chest cavity [54]. A chest X-ray should always be obtained after the operation is concluded.

The intrathoracic route (Fig. 72 c) through the esophageal bed is anatomically and physiologically favorable and is the only option available when an intrathoracic anastomosis is proposed. In the left thoracic approach the esophageal substitute may be routed in front of or behind the aortic arch, depending on the level of the anastomosis. Unless the esophagus is bluntly dissected, it is necessary to enter the pleural cavity. In the event of anastomotic leak or necrosis, infection can spread freely in the thorax and produce an overwhelming sepsis.

7.2.2.2 Creation of the Tunnel

Ordinarily the tunnel for the esophageal substitute is created after preparation of the transplant and exposure of the cervical esophagus or cervicostomy. Creating the tunnel before isolating the transplant is advantageous in that it permits any bleeding in the tunnel to be controlled by compression. But if the substitute is found to be shorter or more bulky than expected, it may be necessary to select a different route, and for that reason we recommend that the tunnel be created after the transplant has been mobilized.

7.2.2.2.1 Subcutaneous Route. If the abdominal part of the operation has been performed through an upper midline laparotomy, the incision is extended past the xiphoid process to the inferior edge of the body of the sternum. At this time the peritoneum is incised only to the inferior border of the xiphoid process, as it will be needed to cover the bone edges after resection of the xiphoid. If the jejunal or colon segment has been mobilized through a paramedian incision in the midabdomen, an additional incision about 5–7 cm long must be made over the xiphoid process, which is then severed from its muscular and connective-tissue attachments with the electrocautery to the angle of the costal arch. The epigastric vessels anastomose in that area with the internal mammary vessels; bleeding from one of these vessels is not uncommon and will require suture ligation. Next

Fig. 73. Creation of a subcutaneous tunnel for the esophageal substitute. The xiphoid process is resected and the cut edge covered with peritoneum

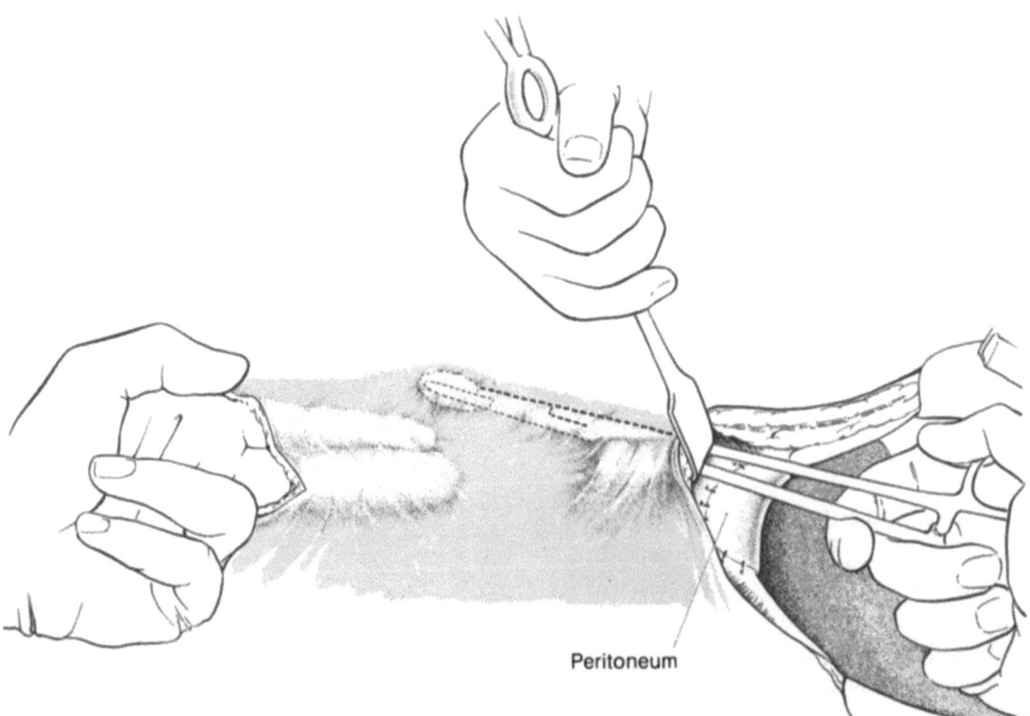

the peritoneum is separated from the posterior surface of the xiphoid process, and the xiphoid is resected with a bone shears or ronguer, leaving a concave cut edge. To protect the esophageal substitute from injury, the peritoneal tissue previously dissected free is reflected over the cut edge of the xiphoid and tacked to the periosteum with a few sutures. The subcutaneous tunnel is now created by blunt dissection from above and below, keeping the fingers in contact with the sternal periosteum (Fig. 73). With a short thorax, the dissection may be continued until the fingertips touch. With a longer thorax, a sponge stick is passed upward until it reaches the finger inserted from above. The skin and subcutaneous tissue are elevated over a width of 8–10 cm to ensure that the tunnel will not compress the transplant. If the dissection is started directly on the sternal periosteum and continued to the costal cartilage, there should be no significant bleeding as the subcutaneous tissue is mobilized.

7.2.2.2.2 Retrosternal Route. The retrosternal route through the anterior mediastinum is bounded anteriorly by the sternum, laterally by the right and left mediastinal pleura, posteriorly by the anterior surface of the pericardium, and superiorly by the great vessels or by the fat and connective tissue covering them.

We begin the dissection inferiorly by separating the peritoneum from the anterior diaphragm to expose the foramen of Morgagni. The xiphoid process is freed from its lateral attachments, and the peritoneum and anterior attachments of the diaphragm are separated from its posterior surface by finger dissection. At this point a thin fascia is encountered which encloses the lower end of the anterior mediastinal space; it is divided. The epigastric vessels coursing in this area are retracted laterally. Now a finger is passed cephalad, keeping on the posterior surface of the sternum and carefully pushing the right and left mediastinal pleura aside. When an adequate space has been developed, a second finger is introduced, and the tunnel is enlarged. The dissection should proceed carefully, with care taken not to injure the pleura. Small pleural leaks are of minor importance, and pleural entry rarely will require subsequent tube drainage. It is essential that the patient be X-rayed while still in the operating room, prior to extubation, so that a pneumothorax can be promptly recognized. If a larger leak develops, portions of the esophageal substitute may be drawn into the chest through the opened pleura, with a potential for kinking and necrosis of the transplant [31, 54]. Large pleural injuries should be repaired under vision through a sternotomy [31]. When the tunnel cannot be developed further through the abdominal field, the dissection is continued from the cervical side. A finger is passed through the cervicotomy into the anterior superior mediastinum. The finger keeps against the posterior surface of the manubrium and then the body of the sternum and does not deviate from the midline. The mediastinal pleura and large veins are carefully displaced laterally and posteriorlly as the finger is advanced. The dissection is continued inferiorly until the finger enters the space previously developed from below (Fig. 74). The sternum is then elevated anteriorly with a pair of Roux retractors placed on its superi-

Fig. 74. Creation of a retrosternal tunnel for the esophageal substitute. Most of the interior of the tunnel can be visualized with fiberoptic illumination

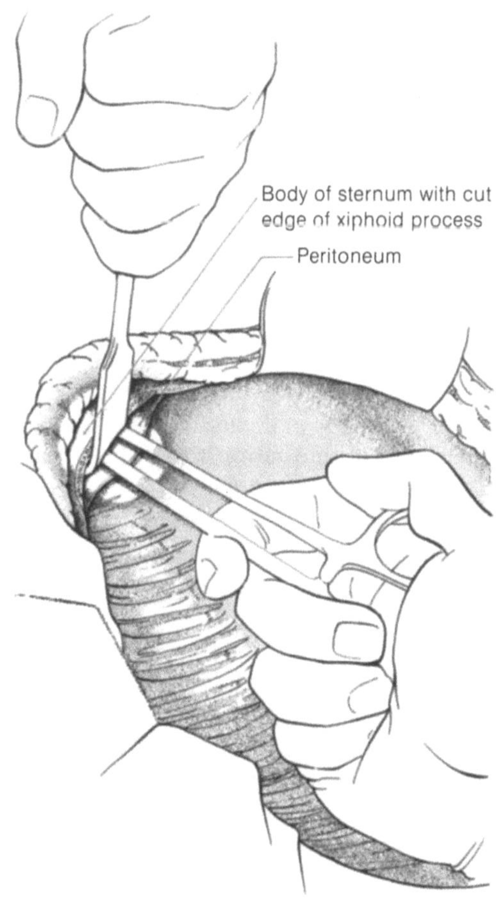

or and inferior edges, and the dissection is continued laterally with the finger or with a long sponge stick until sufficient space has been cleared to accommodate the transplant. At least part of the dissection can be performed under vision by the use of fiberoptic lighting. If the thoracic inlet is too narrow for creation of the retrosternal tunnel, a portion of the manubrium sterni may be resected.

7.2.2.2.3 Transpleural Route. The space for transpleural placement of the esophageal substitute is created by the excisional phase of the operation. When the resection is performed through a right thoracic approach, the esophageal substitute is placed in the posterior mediastinum between the spinal column and lung. For an anastomosis that is to be performed in the neck or thoracic apex following a left-sided approach, the esophageal substitute may be brought up anterior or posterior to the aortic arch. We prefer to place it in front of the aortic arch, as this makes it easier to perform an anastomosis in the apex of the chest.

7.2.2.3 Pull-Through of the Substitute

A similar pull-through technique is used for subcutaneous, retrosternal, and extrapleural routes that have been developed by blunt dissection. We assist the maneuver by using a plastic sleeve that is about 50 cm long, 15 cm wide, and open at both ends. The esophageal substitute is mobilized and is passed behind the stomach through the lesser omentum when a segment of intestine is used. A heavy traction suture is placed through its proximal end. To facilitate pull-through and removal of the plastic sleeve, we moisten the inside and outside of the sleeve and carefully slip it over the esophageal substitute (Fig. 75 a). The traction thread is brought out through the proximal opening of the sleeve, which is then sealed with a heavy tape about 5 cm above the transplant. Residual sleeve is turned back, and the tape is tied over it again. With a long clamp passed through the tunnel from above, the holding tape is grasped and pulled into the cervical field. The position of the transplant within the sleeve is carefully checked to be sure it is not twisted. Then the transplant is carefully slipped into the tunnel with one hand while the other hand exerts gentle upward traction on the tape. The plastic sleeve should glide through the tunnel with very little resistance. If the resistance seems excessive, the sleeve should be withdrawn and the tunnel widened. When the proximal end of the sleeve presents in the cervical incision, it is pulled forward until the upper edge of the transplant appears (Fig. 75 b). Then the top of the sleeve is cut off. Before removing the sleeve, the operator makes certain that the transplant is correctly positioned. While still inside the sleeve, the organ can be rotated, straightened, or withdrawn without risk of injury to its vascular pedicle. When the stomach is used without mobilization of the duodenum, the greater curvature will face laterally as it does in situ. If a Kocher maneuver has been performed, the stomach should be rotated slightly so that its greater curvature faces anterolaterally. When intestine is used, the segment should be reasonably straight as it traverses the tunnel, and there should be no redundant bowel in the pregastric position. When necessary adjustments have been made, the plastic sleeve is removed through the cervicotomy, and the anastomosis is prepared.

In transpleural reconstructions, the esophageal substitute does not need to be protected with a plastic sleeve as it is drawn into position. The esophagus is severed from the stomach as required, the opening in the stomach is oversewn, and the cut end of the esophagus is sealed with a condom to prevent soilage. The transplant is then fixed to the distal stump of the esophagus with a stay suture so that it can be pulled into the thorax when the abdominal phase of the operation is completed. When stomach is to be used for the reconstruction, it is sufficient to place a staple line at the proposed site of the resection with the TA instrument during the abdominal phase. Then, when the esophagus has been adequately mobilized through a thoracic approach and prepared for resection, it can be used to pull the stomach into the thorax.

Fig. 75a, b. Passing the esophageal substitute through the subcutaneous tunnel. **a** The tubed stomach is encased in a plastic sleeve to avoid injury to its vascular arcades during the transplantation. **b** When the upper border of the stomach presents in the cervical field, the sleeve is removed ▷

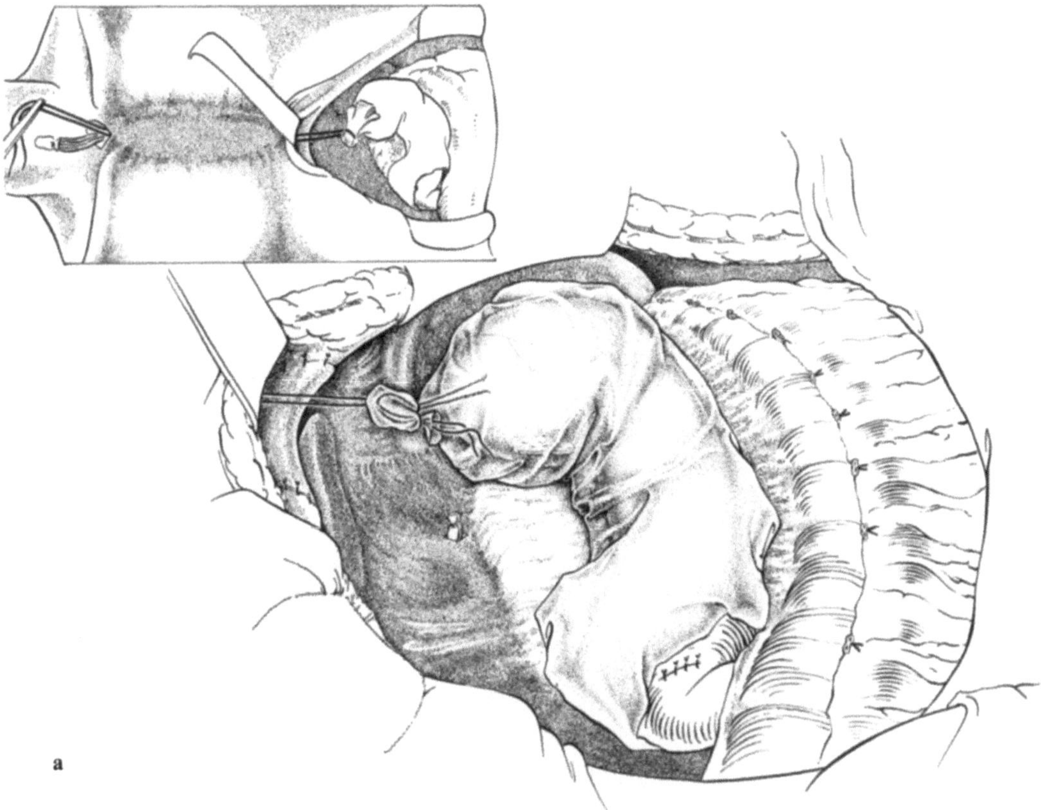

a

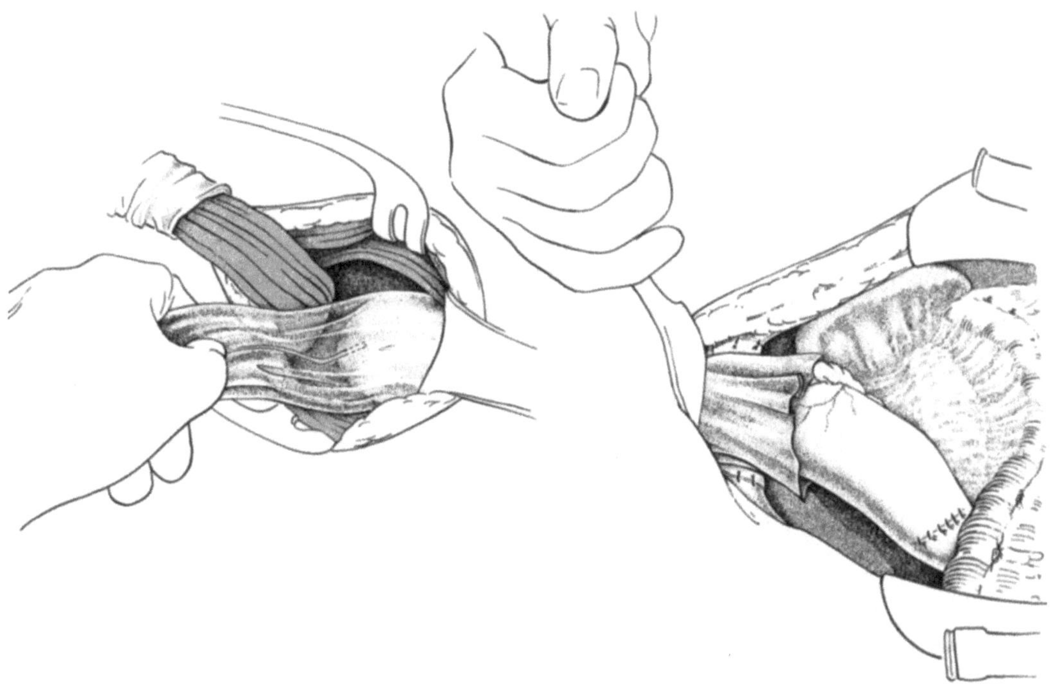

b

Fig. 76. a Isoperistaltic total gastric esophagoplasty of Kirschner. The left gastric artery, inferior phrenic artery, left gastroepiploic artery, and short gastric arteries must be divided (×) for mobilization of the stomach. **b** The esophagus is transected, a pyloroplasty is performed, and the stomach, supplied by the right gastroepiploic artery and right gastric artery, is pulled up for the anastomosis

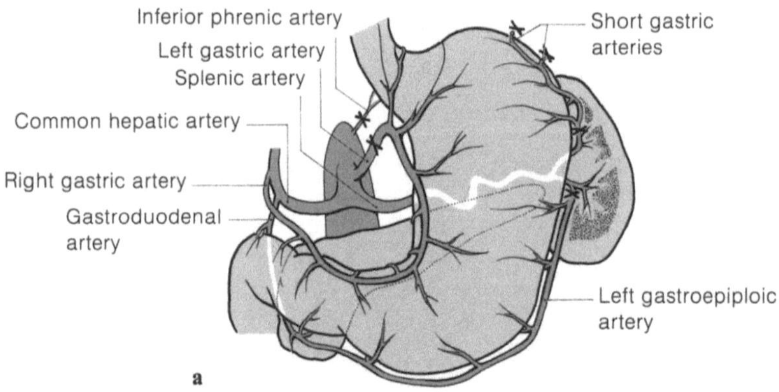

a

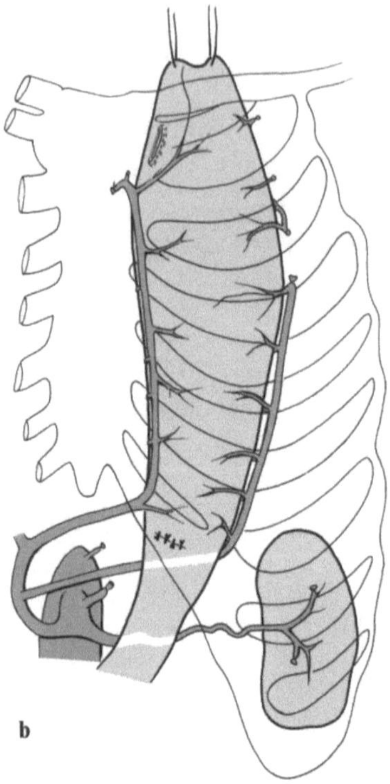

b

7.3 Use of the Stomach as an Esophageal Substitute

Of the many ways in which the stomach can be used to replace all or part of the esophagus, three standard methods have found wide clinical application in the last 10–15 years, as they satisfy most of the criteria stated in 7.1. They are: 1) the isoperistaltic total gastric esophagoplasty of Kirschner [39] (Fig. 76 a,b); 2) its modification (Fig. 77) by total fundectomy as performed by Holle et al. [30] or by resecting portions of the lesser curvature and fundus and fashioning the rest of the stomach into an isoperistaltic tube, as practiced by Akiyama et al. [2] and Kakegawa et al. [35]; and 3) the reversed greater curvature gastric tube, originated by Beck and Carrel [8] and successfully modified for clinical use by Heimlich and Winfield [25] and Gavriliu [19] (Fig. 78 a,b).

The reversed gastric tube procedure of Fink [17], the reversed anterior wall gastric tube of Hirsch [28], the isoperistaltic subtotal gastric esophagoplasty with gastrojejunostomy of Deucher and Widmer [15], the isoperistaltic greater curvature gastric tube of Yamagishi et al. [97], and the isoperistaltic greater curvature tube of Rutkowski [75], recently revived by Postlethwait [66] for the palliation of nonresectable esophageal carcinoma, are either of purely historical interest or have not gained wide clinical application because of their functional deficiencies or technical complexity.

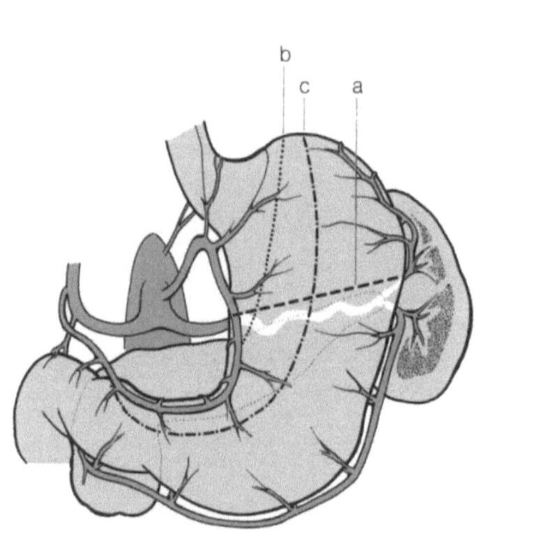

Fig. 77. Modification of the isoperistaltic gastric esophagoplasty by fundectomy (*a*) and by the creation of a limited (*b*) or extended (*c*) gastric tube

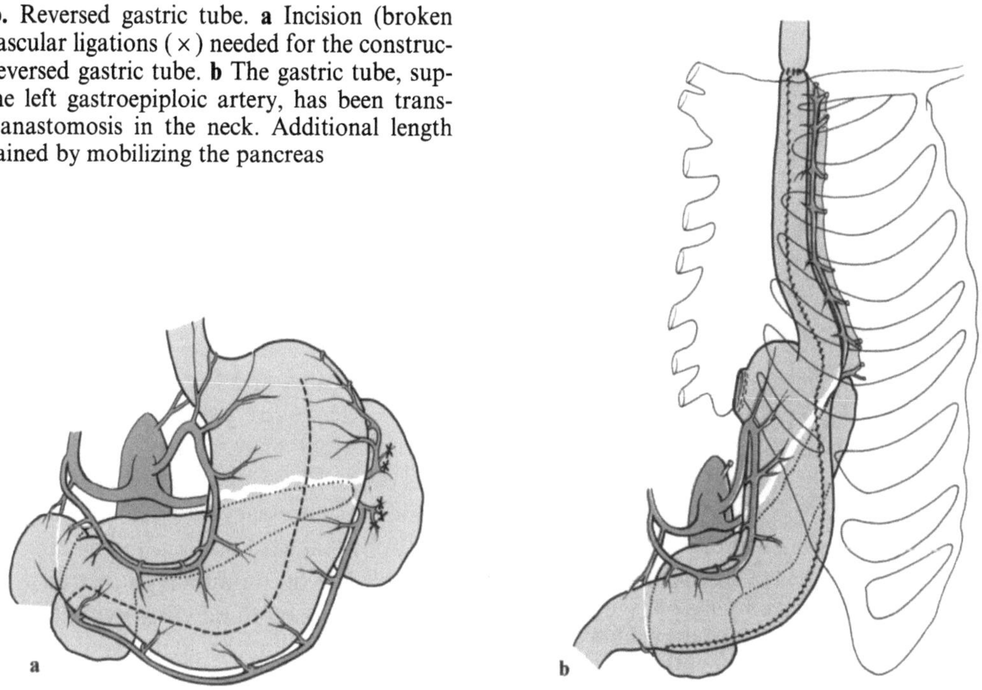

Fig. 78 a, b. Reversed gastric tube. **a** Incision (broken line) and vascular ligations (×) needed for the construction of a reversed gastric tube. **b** The gastric tube, supplied by the left gastroepiploic artery, has been transposed for anastomosis in the neck. Additional length has been gained by mobilizing the pancreas

7.3.1 Blood Supply of the Mobilized Stomach

The arterial supply of the lesser curvature of the stomach is derived from the arcades of the right gastric artery, arising from the common hepatic, and the left gastric artery, arising from the celiac trunk (Fig. 76 a). Branches of these vessels are further distributed to parts of the gastric fundus and distal esophagus. The greater curvature of the stomach is supplied by the right gastroepiploic artery arising from the gastroduodenal and by the left gastroepiploic artery arising from the splenic. Short gastric arteries from the splenic supply the fundic region on the greater curvature side. The major arteries interanastomose with one another through an extensive intramural vascular network. As early as 1920, Kirschner [39] showed experimentally that one of the four major arteries is sufficient to supply the entire stomach. Now that the Kirschner operation has been reintroduced by Ong [60] and is gaining popularity, there is renewed interest in determining which of the main arteries can be ligated without seriously compromising blood flow to the stomach and especially to the fundic region, which is most commonly used for anastomosis. Studies on this question utilizing the injection of various dyes and contrast media into the individual arteries of cadaveric stomachs [2, 7, 78, 90] differ in some of their findings, and they fail to take into account the situation that is created by transposition of the stomach for esophageal replacement. There is general agreement, however, that preserving the left gastric artery, right gastric artery, and right gastroepiploic artery is almost always sufficient to maintain adequate blood flow to the stomach. Stelzner and Kunath [87] caution that division of the short gastric arteries in elderly patients can in itself seriously compromise blood flow to the fundus. It is possible to improve fundic perfusion (Fig. 79) by ligating the trunk of the splenic artery and its perihilar branches in the splenic parenchyma, thereby redirecting flow from the right and left gastroepiploic arteries into the short gastric vessels, but this procedure is technically complex, rarely necessary, and makes it necessary to resect the spleen and in some cases the tail of the pancreas.

When the left gastric artery is ligated and divided near its origin from the celiac trunk proximal to its main bifurcation, the flow from the right gastric and right gastroepiploic arteries generally will be sufficient to supply the entire stomach. However, Stelzner and Kunath [87] found that this reduces perfusion by 10% compared with the case where

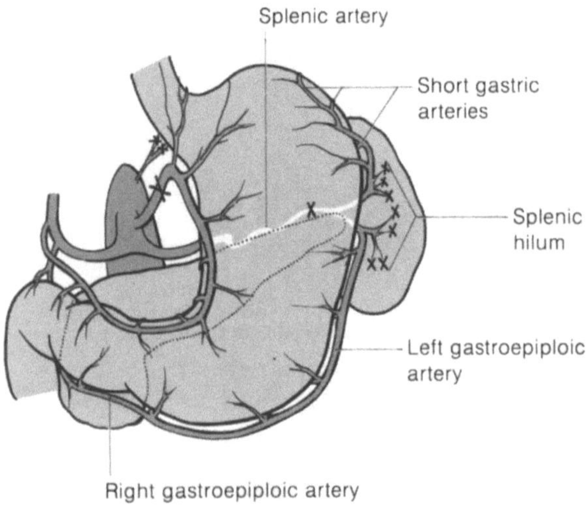

Fig. 79. Method of improving the blood supply to the gastric fundus for a whole-stomach esophagoplasty. The splenic artery is divided proximal to its main bifurcation and distally at its hilar branches (×) thereby redirecting flow from the left and right gastroepiploic arteries to the short gastric vessels

three main arteries are preserved, posing a threat to the viability of the fundic region. This led them to recommend that the fundus be resected routinely along with the lower end of the esophagus. This conflicts with the anatomic studies of Akiyama et al. [2], Barlow et al. [7], and Thomas et al. [90], who always found adequate fundic perfusion except when the vascular system showed significant arteriosclerotic disease. We do not believe that a general recommendation for fundectomy is justified.

When the right gastroepiploic artery alone is preserved, Stelzner and Kunath [87] state that only the antrum and body of the stomach have a satisfactory blood supply. On the other hand, Thomas et al. [90] found that the vascular supply to the fundus was intact in three-fourths of cases, although circulation along the lesser curvature was diminished. In microangiographic studies, the authors found that this was due to a smaller number of intramural anastomoses in the area of the lesser curvature. The authors concluded that there was no anatomic basis for preserving the gastric arcade on the left side.

The clinical relevance of these anatomic studies is limited, as vascular filling is not a very good indicator of local oxygen consumption or energy metabolism. The stomach can tolerate more than a 60% reduction in its blood flow before hypoxic damage to its cellular metabolism becomes apparent. Until we have studies on regional oxygen supply and energy metabolism before and after mobilization or transplantation of the stomach and how they correlate with complications in the underperfused area, we must continue to rely on clinical experience. The experience of numerous authors [1, 2, 16, 38, 59, 60] as well as our own indicates that the entire stomach maintains a satisfactory blood supply when the trunk of the left gastric artery is ligated and the right gastric and gastroepiploic arteries are preserved. Consequently, fundectomy alone or combined with resection of portions of the lesser curvature is indicated only when considered necessary to ensure a radical removal of esophageal carcinoma [2]. The effect the tubed stomach has on pulmonary function when placed transpleurally in these cases remains unclear. We feel, however, that this factor is of no consequence when decompression by nasogastric tube is maintained for a sufficient length of time. In some cases the lesser curvature will be found to be quite short and cannot be adequately straightened because of its vascular arcade. Here we recommend dividing the right gastric artery a handswidth above the pylorus and then resecting the lesser curvature, cardia, and adjacent fundus from that point.

When reconstruction is performed with a reversed gastric tube [19, 25], the remaining stomach derives its blood supply from the right and left gastric arteries and short gastric vessels. The tube itself is supplied by the arcade of the left and right gastroepiploic arteries. To ensure an adequate blood supply, flow is redirected from the splenic artery to the left gastroepiploic by removing the spleen close to its hilum. This procedure necessarily entails sacrifice of the spleen.

7.3.2 Mobilization of the Whole Stomach through an Abdominal Approach (Kirschner's Isoperistaltic Total Gastric Esophagoplasty [39]*)*

Preoperative preparation: Perioperative antibiotics, intestinal lavage (see Chap. C).

Instruments: Basic set, extra sets II and V, set VII as required, GIA, TA, EEA.

Position and approach: Midline laparotomy extended around the left side of the umbilicus.

Steps in procedure:

(1) Inspection of the gastric and gastro-epiploic arcades
(2) Stepwise division of the gastrocolic ligament 1–2 cm below the gastroepiploic arcade
(3) Separation of retrogastric adhesions
(4) Division of the gastrosplenic ligament
(5) Ligation of the short gastric arteries
(6) Detachment of the left lobe of the liver from the diaphragm
(7) Division of the gastrophrenic ligament and snaring of the esophagus
(8) Ligation of the left gastric artery near its origin
(9) Stepwise division of the lesser omentum 1–2 cm above the gastric arcade
(10) Transection of the esophagus with the GIA instrument
(11) Dissection of the pylorus from the posterior side, preserving the right gastric artery and vein and the right gastroepiploic artery and vein
(12) Exteriorization of the mobilized stomach to confirm sufficient length for the anastomosis
(13) If necessary, Kocher's maneuver to gain length
(14) If necessary, fundectomy or tubularization of the stomach to gain length or extend the resection

Operative technique: The abdomen is entered through a midline incision, the greater omentum is pulled downward, and the vascular supply of the stomach is inspected and palpated. Special attention is given to the gastroepiploic arcade. If the right gastroepiploic artery extends only slightly past the midpoint of the greater curvature and there is no well-defined left portion of the arcade, or a gap of several centimeters exists between the arcade and the lowest short gastric artery, the blood flow to the fundic region will be precarious after gastric mobilization unless the left gastric artery can be preserved. As it is not always possible to gain sufficient length for a high intrathoracic or cervical anastomosis without ligating the trunk of the left gastric artery, one should consider using a different organ for esophageal replacement when these circumstances exist.

Mobilization of the stomach may be started from above and proceed downward or vice versa. We prefer to start at the lower end of the greater curvature, near the pylorus, and progress upward. The gastrocolic ligament is made tense by gentle traction on the transverse colon and is divided about 1–2 cm inferior to the gastroepiploic arcade (Fig. 80 a), opening the omental bursa. Adhesions between the ligament and transverse mesocolon are cleared by blunt dissection. Starting from the opening in the bursa and keeping the same distance from the gastroepiploic arcade, the gastrocolic ligament is progressively divided and ligated between clamps. This should be done in small steps so that the greater curvature does not become plicated and prevent adequate straightening of the stomach. When the level of the spleen is reached, the greater curvature is raised and connective-tissue adhesions between the stomach and retroperitoneum are divided. The index finger of one hand is then carefully passed laterally between the posterior gastric wall and the tail of the pancreas, displacing the tail and the splenic vessels on its superior border posteriorly. As the finger crosses the greater curvature, it is raised to pick up the gastrosplenic ligament, which is divided in steps. Injury to the splenic hilum or capsule is not unusual at this stage as a result of distal traction on the stomach. In these cases we always try to preserve the spleen and to control bleeding with fibrin glue and collagen fleece, or if necessary with coapting parenchymal sutures. The greater curvature having been freed past the hilum, the short gastric arteries are divided in the gastrosplenic ligament. These vessels may exhibit bifurcation-like interanastomoses. We feel that these connections should be preserved even if they limit the distensibility of the fundus. We do not recommend dividing the splenic vessels in the hilum and at the upper edge of the tail of the pancreas to direct more flow from the gastroepiploic arcade to the short gastric arteries (see 7.3.1). Exposure of the cardia and hiatus is now increased by dividing the triangular ligament of the liver and displacing the left lobe of the liver mediad with a curved retractor (Fig. 80 b). The stomach is pulled downward to make the gastrophrenic ligament tense. The ligament is avascular and can be divided with a scissors (Fig. 80 c). When the dissection has reached the lateral wall of the esophagus, the peritoneum over the esophagus is divided transversely, and the esophagus is encircled with the finger and snared with a rubber tape. The stomach is reflected upward, and its posterior surface is freed from remaining avascular adhesions with the pancreas

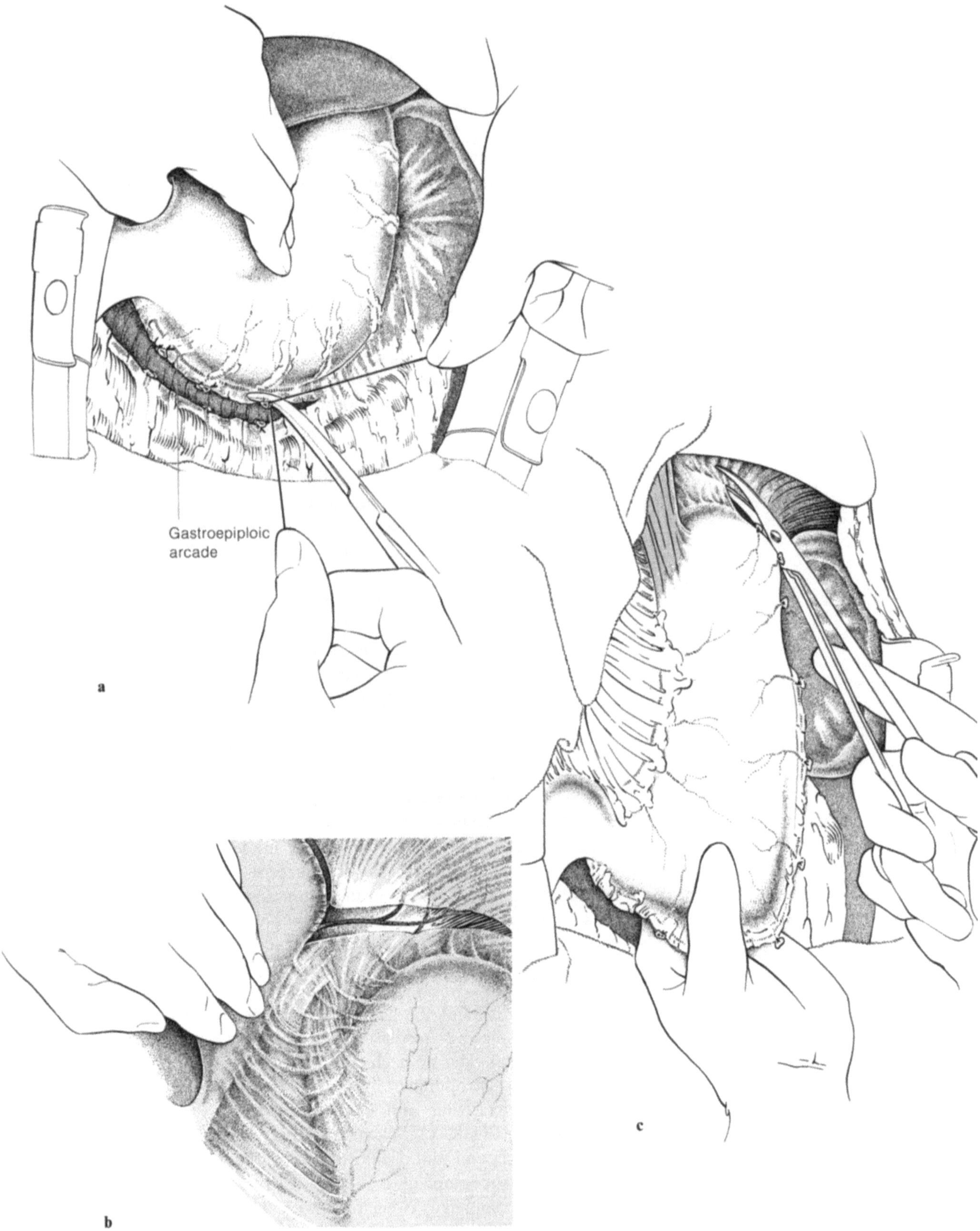
Gastroepiploic arcade
a
b
c

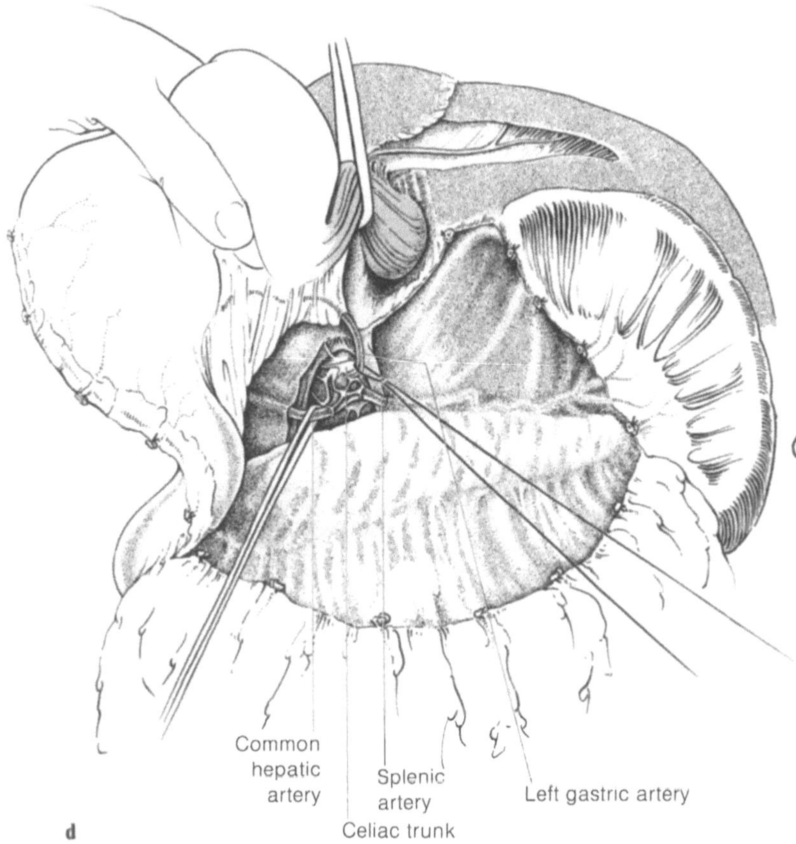

d

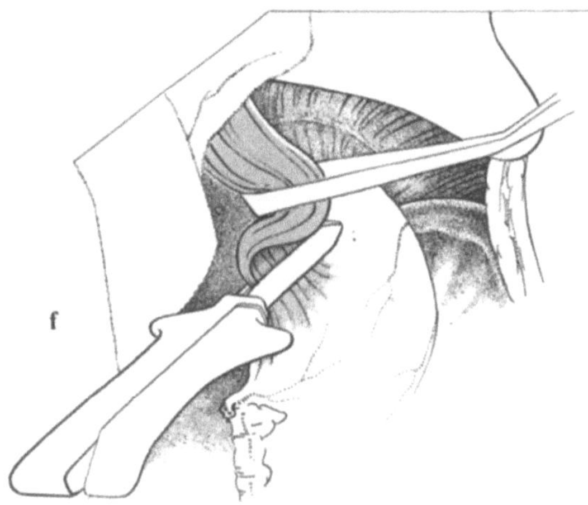

f

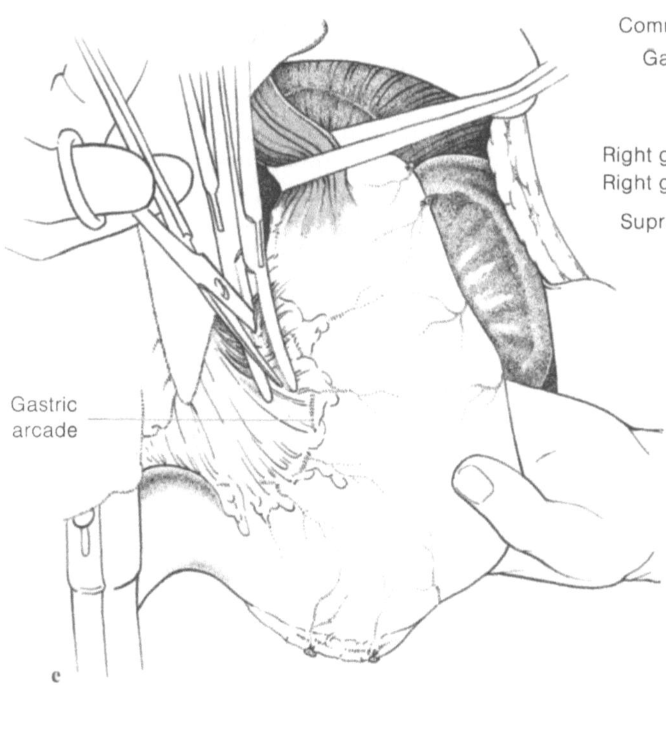

e

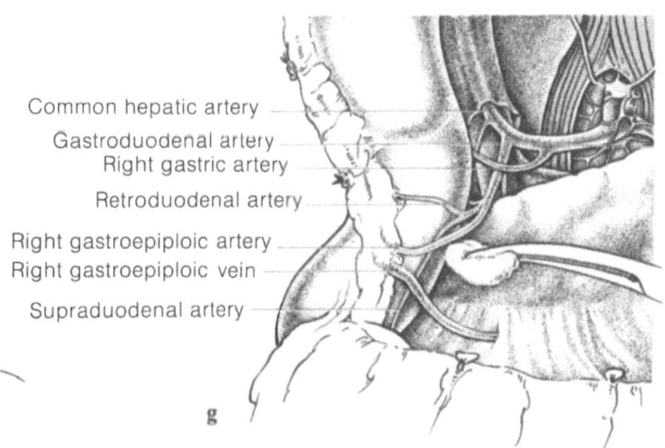

g

Fig. 80a–g. Isoperistaltic total gastric esophagoplasty. **a** The gastrocolic ligament is divided below the gastroepiploic arcade. **b** The triangular ligament of the liver is divided, and the left hepatic lobe is retracted medially to give access to the cardia. **c** The gastrophrenic ligament is divided. **d** The left gastric artery is divided close to its origin. **e** The lesser omentum is divided above the gastric arcade. **f** The esophagus is transected with the GIA instrument. **g** The pylorus is dissected free from the posterior side. (For clarity, overlying connective tissue has been removed to show the vascular supply of this region)

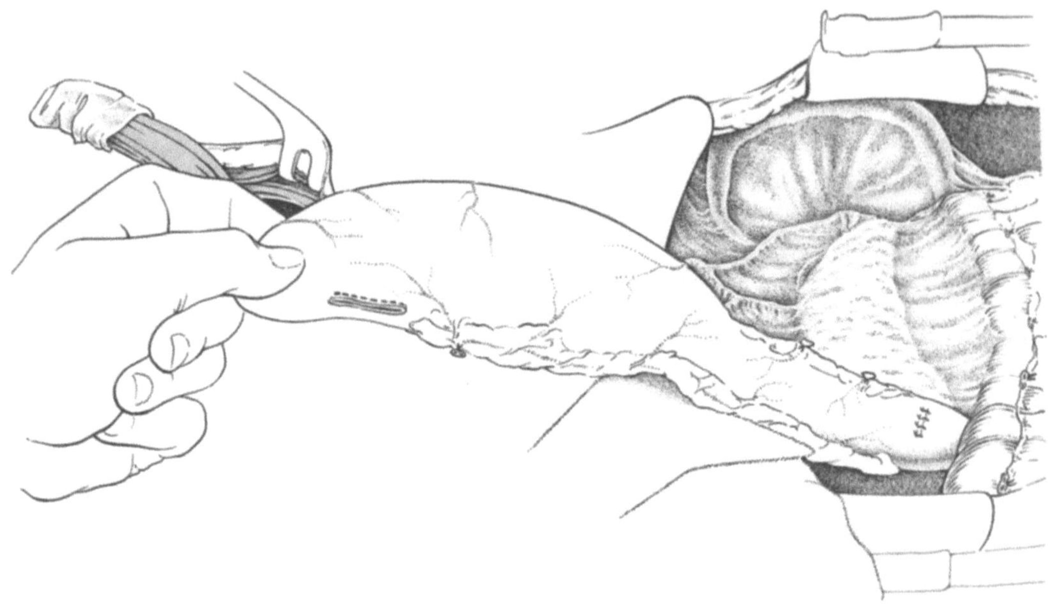

Fig. 81. The mobilized stomach is exteriorized and brought up to the cervicotomy to confirm sufficient length for the anastomosis

and retroperitoneum. The left gastric artery is identified. It is located at the superior border of the pancreas, level with the proximal third of the greater curvature. To make certain the ligature is placed on the trunk of the left gastric artery, proximal to its main division, the course of the vessel is palpated until its bifurcation is identified close to the stomach, and the vessel is divided proximal to that site. The artery can be ligated directly at its origin from the celiac axis by snaring it and dissecting it free until the axis is reached (Fig. 80 d). The stomach is now turned downward, and the esophagus is pulled laterally with the rubber tape so that the lesser omentum is made tense. It is divided 1–2 cm from the gastric arcade (Fig. 80 e). On reaching the antrum, the surgeon palpates the right gastric artery, which ascends posterolaterally, to protect it from inadvertent harm. The dissection terminates at the level of the pylorus. The esophagus is then transected at its distal end with the GIA instrument (Fig. 80 f). The stump of the esophagus is covered with a condom to prevent soilage of the field. The opening in the stomach is covered with a surgical sponge soaked in antiseptic. Then the stomach is reflected medially upward so that the antrum is slightly tense, and the pylorus is cleared posteriorly by patty dissection (Fig. 80 g). The right gastroepiploic artery and vein are encountered just below and lateral to the pylorus, where they diverge. The artery is visible behind the proximal duodenum at its site of origin from the gastroduodenal. The vein runs downward and medially to the cleft between the neck and uncinate process of the pancreas, where it drains into either the middle colic or superior mesenteric vein. It is important to note that this vein provides the main venous drainage of the mobilized stomach, and if it is damaged during the dissection or transposition, the viability of the stomach may be jeopardized.

The stomach having been mobilized, it is picked up between the thumb and index finger at its highest point (the "pinching up" maneuver) and is exteriorized over the anterior surface of the chest (Fig. 81) to confirm sufficient length. If the stomach is too short to reach the desired level of the anastomosis, its mobility can be increased by performing the Kocher maneuver on the duodenum.

The abdominal part of the operation generally concludes by performing a drainage procedure.

7.3.3 *Modifications of the Kirschner Operation*

We regard isoperistaltic gastric esophagoplasty with fundectomy or the creation of a gastric tube as modifications of the Kirschner operation, since the technique of gastric mobilization is identical and is simply followed by the removal of part of the stomach.

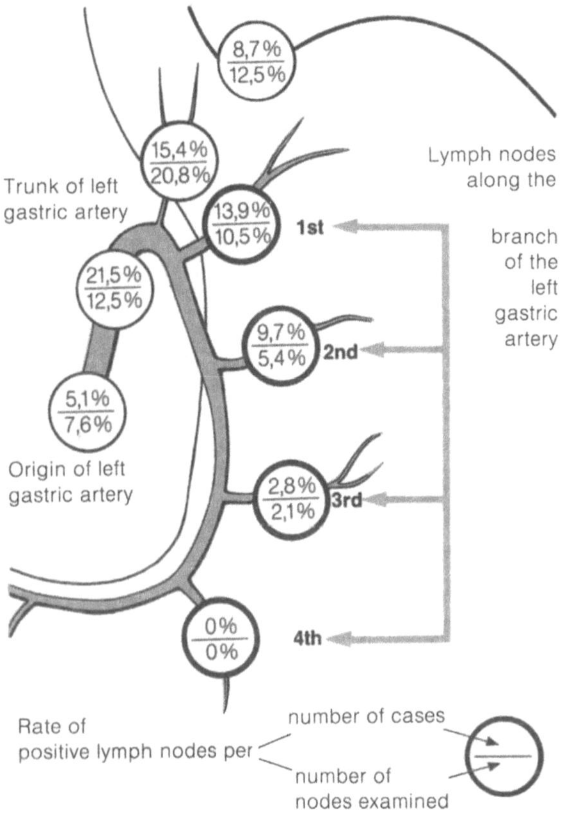

Fig. 82. Rates of positive lymph nodes in the distribution of the left gastric artery in 128 patients with squamous cell carcinoma of the thoracic or abdominal esophagus (modified from Akiyama et al. [1])

7.3.3.1 Fundectomy

Fundectomy was described by Holle et al. [30] for the treatment of ulcers close to the gastric cardia. We do not consider it to be an adequate procedure for adenocarcinoma of the cardia, which we manage by total gastrectomy. Fundectomy is appropriate, however, as part of the resection for squamous cell carcinoma of the distal esophagus. A vascular indication for fundectomy is recognized but is infrequent. The two methods differ in the extent of the resection. For carcinoma the line of the resection extends from the level of the splenic hilum on the greater curvature to the junction of the right and left gastric arteries on the lesser curvature, just below its midpoint. This ensures the removal of any positive lymph nodes along the course of the left gastric artery. Fundectomy for vascular problems begins at the greater curvature, also near the splenic hilum, and ends just below the cardia on the lesser curvature. The goal of this resection is removal of the fundic region supplied by the short gastric arteries on the greater curvature side. The stomach may be divided between Nakayama clamps, between the staple lines of the TA instrument, or with the GIA instrument.

7.3.3.2 Creation of an Isoperistaltic Gastric Tube

A gastric tube may be fashioned for the purpose of extending the resection to lymph nodes along the left gastric artery, decreasing the volume of the stomach, or increasing the length of the residual stomach while safely preserving its blood supply. Akiyama et al. [2] showed that intraabdominal lymph node involvement from locally resectable carcinoma of the thoracic esophagus rarely extends beyond the third branch of the left gastric artery (Fig. 82). This led the authors to advise prophylactic removal of this area for all esophageal carcinomas located distal to the thoracic inlet. It has been our experience that the reduction of gastric volume, which is relevant only in transpleural reconstructions, is of minor importance. When the transposed stomach is placed in a straightened position with no excess and decompression is maintained for an adequate period after surgery, we have seen no clinically significant compromise of pulmonary function. However, we do consider tubularization of the stomach to be of significant benefit in terms of lengthening the transplant and eliminating areas around the cardia that may be underperfused after the stomach is mobilized.

7.3.3.2.1 Fashioning a Gastric Tube to Extend the Resection [2]. With the stomach mobilized (see 7.3.2), the left gastric artery is sought at the lesser curvature. Its third branch is identified, and the artery is ligated distal to it. The line of resection is determined by picking up the highest point of the fundus between the thumb and index finger (Fig. 83 a). The line extends from the tip of the thumb to the site of ligation of the left gastric artery and includes the cardia, the fundus adjacent to the cardia, and approximately half of the lesser curvature. Removal of this area is most easily accomplished with a stapling instrument.

7.3.3.2.2 Fashioning a Gastric Tube to Gain Length [35]. With the stomach mobilized (see 7.3.2), the

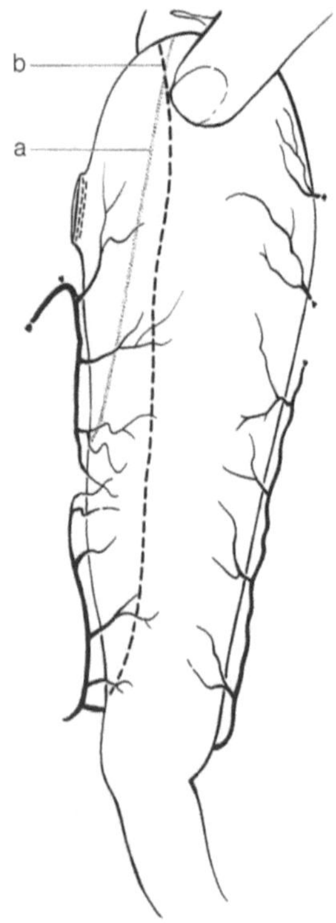

Fig. 83. Modification of the isoperistaltic gastric esophagoplasty. *a* Tubularization of the stomach to extend the resection. The line of resection (dotted) extends from the highest point on the fundus to the third branch of the left gastric artery. *b* Tubularization to gain length. The line of resection (dashed) extends from the highest point on the fundus to the prepyloric antrum

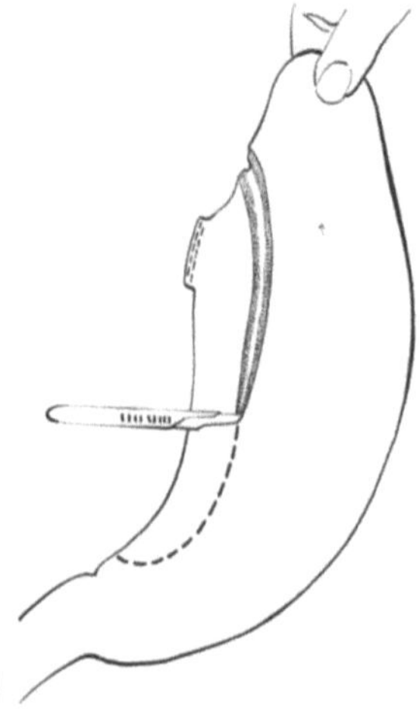

84

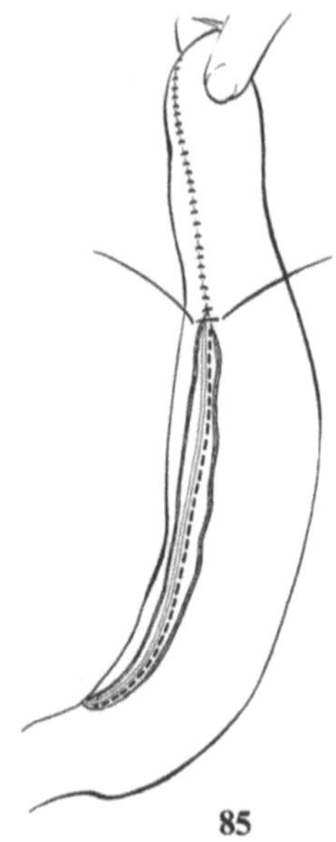

85

Fig. 84. Lengthening the isoperistaltic gastric tube by separate incision of the seromuscularis and mucosa. The seromuscular coat is divided, sparing the mucosa

Fig. 85. Lengthening the isoperistaltic gastric tube by separate incision of the seromuscularis and mucosa. The tubed stomach is stretched out, and the mucosa is divided with a stapler. The seromuscularis is reapproximated with sutures

right gastric artery is identified just above the pylorus and is divided. The line of resection extends parallel to the greater curvature from that point. This leaves a tubular gastric remnant (Fig. 83 b) whose width approximates that of the prepyloric antrum. The resection may be performed with the GIA or TA instrument. Sugimachi et al. [88] note that an additional 4–5 cm of length can be gained by dividing the layers of the gastric wall individually. The first incision is made just through the seromuscular layer of the anterior and posterior walls of the stomach along the proposed line of resection (Fig. 84). Then the stomach is stretched out, and in that position the submucosa and mucosa are divided with a stapling instrument. Finally the muscular layer is closed over the staple line with interrupted inverting sutures (Fig. 85).

7.3.4 Mobilization of the Stomach through a Thoracic Approach

7.3.4.1 Left Thoracic Approach

Oshawa [57] treated carcinoma of the distal esophagus and cardia by resecting the lower third of the esophagus and gastric fundus entirely through a left thoracic approach and using the gastric remnant to restore continuity.

Preoperative preparation: Perioperative antibiotics, intestinal lavage (see Chap. C).

Instruments: Basic set; extra sets II, V, and VII as required; TA, GIA.

Position and approach: Left thoracotomy in the 7th or 8th interspace.

Operative technique: Resectability is confirmed, and the esophagus is mobilized as far as the inferior pulmonary

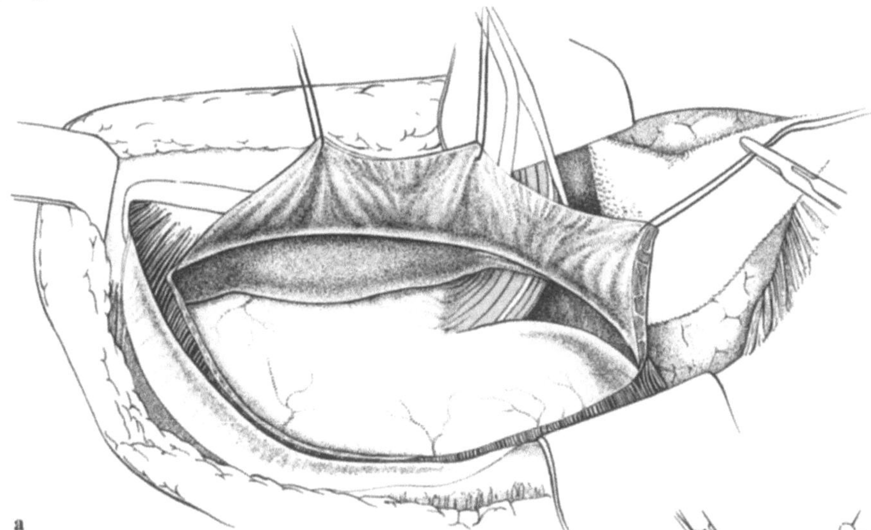

a

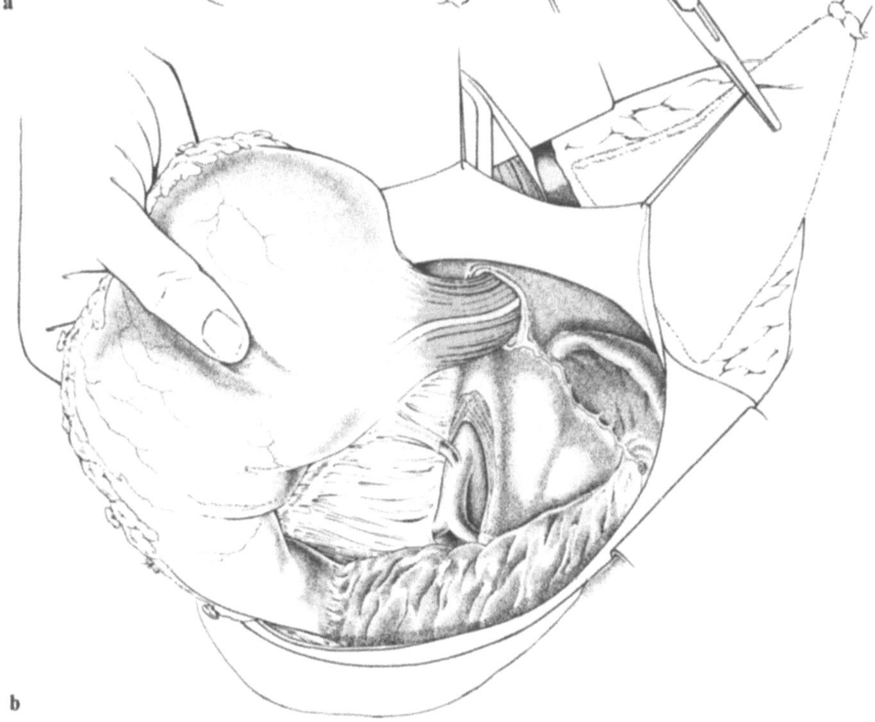

b

vein or aortic arch, depending on the extent of disease (see 2.1.2). Then the diaphragm is divided, and the stomach is mobilized. Oshawa [57] performed the phrenotomy through the tendinous center, but this denervates a portion of the diaphragm resulting in postsurgical respiratory impairment. Ellis [16] spares the nerves by making a curved phrenotomy 1 cm from the costal arch (Fig. 86 a).

Fig. 86 a, b. Mobilization of the stomach through a thoracic approach. **a** Entering the abdomen through a paracostal phrenotomy gives sufficient exposure for mobilization of the stomach. **b** The gastrocolic ligament is divided to expose the left gastric artery

The authors state that both approaches give adequate exposure of the upper abdomen for mobilization of the stomach. It is difficult, however, to perform a Kocher maneuver or carry out a drainage procedure on the pylorus. The technique for mobilizing the stomach is similar to that in the abdominal approach, except that the dissection proceeds downward from above. The esophagogastric junction is freed from its attachments with the hiatus, and the gastrophrenic ligament is divided. Then the posterior surface of the stomach is freed from its attachments with the peritoneum. The gastrosplenic ligament and the short gastric arteries contained therein are divided 1–2 cm from the stomach while carefully preserving the spleen and its vascular pedicle. The left gastroepiploic artery is ligated and divided as close as possible to its origin from the splenic artery. The dissection is continued distally outside the gastroepiploic arcade to the level of the pylorus. If lymph nodes are found at the splenic hilum, the spleen should be removed. Occasionally the tail of the pancreas will also have to be resected to ensure radical margins. The greater curvature is elevated, and remaining adhesions between the stomach and retroperitoneum are divided. The left gastric artery is identified by palpation at the superior border of the pancreas, level with the upper third of the gastric lesser curvature, and is divided well proximal to its main bifurcation (Fig. 86 b). Any lymph nodes found at the celiac trunk or along the common hepatic or left gastric artery are removed. The lesser omentum is divided as far as the pylorus, preserving the gastric arcade. When the whole stomach has been mobilized, its proximal portion is transected with a stapling instrument, the line of the resection depending on the location of the tumor (see 7.3.3.1 and 7.3.3.2.1).

When a central phrenotomy is used, the gastric remnant can be advanced into the thorax right away. If a crescent-shaped phrenotomy has been made, it is first necessary to stretch the esophageal hiatus or divide one crus of the hiatus before the stomach can be delivered into the chest. If the length of the gastric remnant is insufficient to permit a tension-free anastomosis at the desired level, Kocher's maneuver must be performed. As noted earlier, this can be difficult through the thoracic approach, and it might be better to reposition the patient and perform a laparotomy so that the Kocher maneuver and pyloroplasty can be accomplished more easily. With the stomach adequately mobilized, the esophagus is transected at the designated level, and the esophagogastrostomy is performed. The phrenotomy is closed with sutures, and the pulled-up stomach is fixed to the hiatus with several interrupted sutures. A chest tube is inserted, and the thoracotomy is closed.

7.3.4.2 Right Thoracic Approach

Resection of the esophagus and proximal stomach and reconstruction with the residual stomach in one operation through an exclusive right thoracic approach is recommended by Belsey and Hiebert [9] and is described in 6.5.2.1.

7.3.5 Reversed Gastric Tube

Preoperative preparation: Prophylactic antibiotics, intestinal lavage as required (see Chap. C).

Instruments: Basic set; extra sets II, V, and VII if required; TA, GIA; Ch 32–36 stomach tube.

Position and approach: Upper midline laparotomy extended around the left side of the umbilicus.

Steps in procedure:

(1) Inspection of the gastroepiploic arcade
(2) Mobilization of the spleen from the posterior side, ligation of the hilar vessels close to the parenchyma
(3) Mobilization of the pancreas as far as the aorta from the posterior side
(4) Division of the gastrophrenic ligament
(5) Measurement of the necessary length of the reversed gastric tube
(6) Division of the gastrocolic ligament 1–2 cm below the gastroepiploic arcade, or detachment of the greater omentum from the colon
(7) Separation of retrogastric adhesions
(8) Ligation of the right gastroepiploic artery at the proposed oral end of the gastric tube
(9) Incision of the stomach to a depth of 3–4 cm at right angles to the greater curvature
(10) Insertion of a stomach tube (Ch 32–36) along the greater curvature
(11) Division of the greater curvature along the tube with the GIA instrument
(12) Closure of the gastric defect; oversewing of staple lines on the stomach or newly constructed gastric tube (optional)
(13) Use of the greater omentum (optional) to cover the staple line on the gastric tube
(14) Injection of methylene blue to test the integrity of the gastric tube

Operative technique: The vascular pattern along the greater curvature is examined. The reversed gastric tube procedure should be considered only if there is a continuous arcade from the left gastroepiploic artery through the right gastroepiploic artery to the pylorus (Fig. 87 a). If the arcade is found to be intact, the spleen is displaced medially

Fig. 87 a–e. Reversed gastric tube. **a** The tube is formed by an incision parallel to the greater curvature. **b** The gastrocolic ligament is severed below the gastroepiploic arcade, and the splenic vessels are ligated close to the parenchyma from the posterior side. **c** The pancreas is mobilized laterally to the aorta. **d** The greater-curvature tube is cut from the rest of the stomach with the GIA instrument. A large-caliber stomach tube is positioned along the greater curvature and held in place with clamps to serve as a stent for construction of the reversed gastric tube. **e** The staple line on the reversed gastric tube is covered with greater omentum ▷

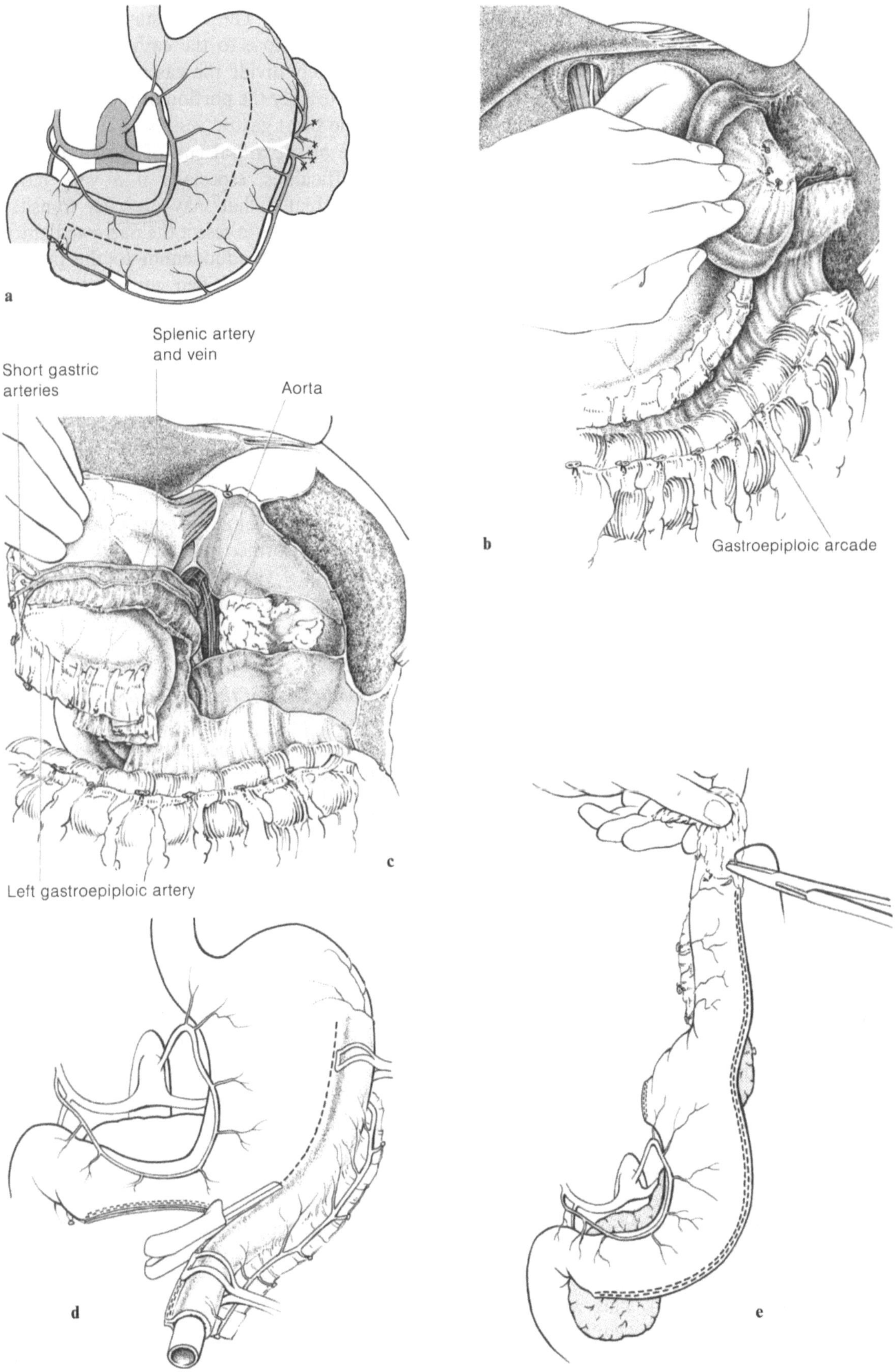
a
b
Gastroepiploic arcade
Splenic artery
and vein
Short gastric
arteries
Aorta
c
Left gastroepiploic artery
d
e

from its bed and freed from its adhesions with the diaphragm and retroperitoneum.

The vessels in the splenic hilum are divided as close to the parenchyma as possible, proceeding from below upward, and the spleen is removed (Fig. 87 b). The stomach is pulled laterally, and the peritoneum is incised over the tail of the pancreas. The pancreas is freed from its posterior connective-tissue attachments by blunt finger dissection, carried as far as the aorta (Fig. 87 c). The attachments between the pancreas and kidney are usually dense and must be sharply divided. Two or three small arterial branches are usually found at the inferior border of the pancreas; these must be ligated when the pancreas is mobilized. Then the stomach is pulled downward, and the gastrophrenic ligament is divided. The necessary length of the reversed gastric tube can be measured with a string placed at the site on the greater curvature that will form the base of the tube. The incision for the oral end of the tube is usually placed about 5 cm proximal to the pylorus, although the pylorus and proximal duodenum may be included in the antiperistaltic tube and continuity restored by gastroduodenostomy; this provides an additional 6–10 cm of tube length.

Now the decision is made whether to wrap the gastric tube in a sleeve of omentum, as suggested by Gavriliu [20], or follow the example of Heimlich [26] and avoid this step. Gavriliu [20] detaches the greater omentum from the colon and fashions an omental flap that is about 10 cm wide and 5 cm longer than the gastric tube. He uses the flap to cover both the gastric tube and the anastomosis. Heimlich [26] leaves the greater omentum on the transverse colon and divides the gastrocolic ligament about 1–2 cm below the gastroepiploic arcade. With the greater curvature mobilized, the stomach is elevated, and the avascular attachments between its posterior wall and the retroperitoneum are divided. The right gastroepiploic artery is divided at the level of the proposed line of resection, usually several centimeters proximal to the pylorus. At the same location an incision is made 3–4 cm into the lumen of the stomach between two Nakayama clamps. The proximal clamp is removed, and the gastric contents are aspirated. A 32 to 36 Ch size tube is inserted into the opened lumen and advanced along the greater curvature to the esophagus (Fig. 87 d). This will serve as a stent to ensure a lumen of adequate caliber as the gastric tube is formed. Soft clamps are used to hold the catheter in place and make the gastric wall slightly tense. The GIA stapling instrument is now applied close to the catheter and is used to progressively divide the gastric wall to the desired level, usually the portion of the stomach supplied by the short gastric vessels.

Closure of the antral end of the stomach can present difficulties, especially if a very narrow channel is created that may obstruct transit. In these cases it is best to resect the narrowed antrum and anastomose the duodenum to the proximal gastric remnant [20]. When construction of the gastric tube is completed, Gavriliu [20] places an omental flap over the staple line and sutures it to the wall of the tube (Fig. 87 e). Before the gastric tube is brought up for anastomosis to the cervical or thoracic esophagus, watertightness is confirmed by injecting methylene blue solution into it under pressure. To conclude the abdominal part of the operation, a temporary gastrostomy is performed for postoperative decompression. Pyloroplasty is not performed routinely [20, 26] and is indicated only if vagotomy was done as part of the esophageal resection.

7.3.6 Mobilization of the Duodenum

For esophageal reconstruction with isoperistaltic stomach, additional length can be gained by performing the Kocher maneuver to mobilize the duodenum. This maneuver is not indicated routinely, for even without it the stomach generally can be apposed without tension to the cervical esophagus or pharynx. This eliminates the danger of impaired biliary flow that can result from the Kocher maneuver.

Operative technique: The duodenum is retroperitoneal from about the middle of its first portion almost to the duodenojejunal flexure. Its blood vessels enter from the medial side, arising from the right gastric, gastroduodenal, and pancreaticoduodenal arteries. The veins parallel the arteries and terminate in the superior mesenteric vein and portal vein. The peritoneum at the lateral edge of the duodenum can be divided from the first segment around the superior flexure to the third segment without endangering the duodenal blood supply (Fig. 88 a,b). The duodenum can then be bluntly mobilized medially together with the common bile duct and the underlying head of the pancreas. The posterior surface of the pancreas is freed from the renal capsule and inferior vena cava as far as the

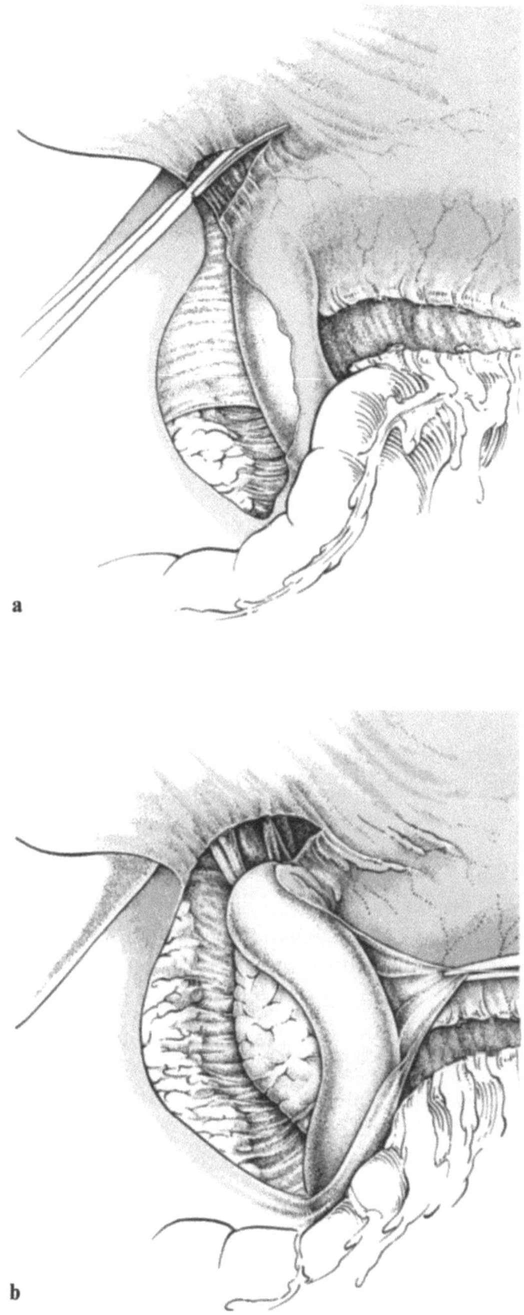

Fig. 88a, b. Kocher's maneuver für mobilizing the duodenum. The peritoneal coat is divided along the lateral border of the duodenum

aorta. The mobilization is continued to the point where the duodenum is crossed by the superior mesenteric vein. When the maneuver is completed, transposition of the stomach should bring the pyloric region to within a few centimeters of the esophageal hiatus.

7.3.7 *Drainage Procedures after Truncal Vagotomy*

Truncal vagotomy is a part of most esophageal resections. The result of this is gastric atony and hypertonicity of the pyloric sphincter, at least in the initial weeks after surgery. This has prompted recommendations that truncal vagotomy be followed by a drainage procedure in the form of a pyloroplasty [52] or pylorotomy [67]. However, other authors [10, 18, 85, 89] caution against a drainage procedure, noting that it provokes gastroduodenal reflux and that longitudinal incision of the pylorus destroys the intramural vascular network and can compromise blood flow to the lesser curvature. These authors also state that the effects of vagotomy in the pulled-up stomach are not comparable to the effects in situ. They argue that transposing the stomach rotates the plane of the pylorus in such a way that a food bolus encounters the pyloric opening at right angles, and the food is unable to escape into an atonic reservoir like that provided by the fundus and body of the unmobilized stomach. As an alternative to pyloroplasty, they recommend stretching the postvagotomy "spastic pylorus" with a finger invaginated through the gastric or duodenal wall or with a transgastric dilator. We personally use pyloroplasty quite often in cases where the whole stomach is transposed. The alternative procedure of pyloromyotomy is more technically demanding in adults with a normally developed pyloric muscle and is associated with a higher failure rate due to overlooked muscle fibers. Not infrequently, the procedure must be converted to a pyloroplasty due to injury of the mucosa.

7.3.7.1 *Pyloroplasty*

Operative technique: In the original technique of Heineke-Mikulicz [52] a longitudinal incision is made through the full thickness of the pylorus, extending about 3 cm proximally into the antrum and a similar distance distally into the duodenum.

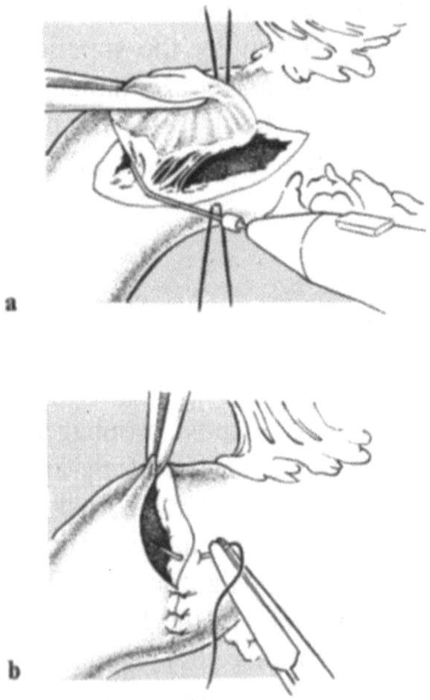

Fig. 89a, b. Heineke-Mikulicz pyloroplasty [52]. **a** Elliptical excision of the pyloric muscle. **b** Transverse closure of the pylorotomy with inverting sutures

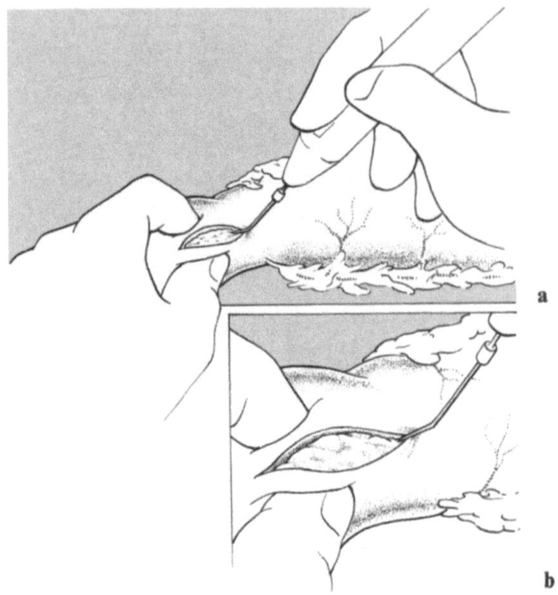

Fig. 90a, b. Pyloromyotomy. The seromuscular coat is incised with the electrocautery

Bleeding from the mucosa and muscle is controlled by coagulation, and arterial bleeders are suture ligated. The incision is closed transversely. Since the original technique can lead to the formation of side pockets where chyme becomes collected, Allgöwer and Burri [3] eliminated redundant tissue by using an elliptical incision. We follow their suggestion by excising an oval-shaped piece of pyloric muscle, but we do not extend the excision into the stomach and duodenum if the pylorus is intact and unstenosed (Fig. 89 a). Bleeding from the muscle and mucosa is carefully controlled, and the defect is closed transversely with interrupted sutures (Fig. 89 b). We place the central suture first to avoid pyloric distortion. Two or three additional sutures are then placed on each side to complete the closure.

7.3.7.2 Pyloromyotomy

Operative technique: The pylorus is grasped between the thumb and index finger to form a bulge of anterior-wall muscle. The serosa and outermost muscular layer are carefully divided with the electrocautery. A dissecting patty is used to push the muscular edges apart, and residual muscle bundles are picked up with a small clamp and divided with the cautery (Fig. 90). The submucosa will bulge forward slightly when reached. Following the plane between the submucosa and muscularis with the small clamp, the surgeon picks up the remaining muscle bundles and divides them. Myotomy in the normal adult pylorus is substantially more difficult than in the spastic pylorus of the newborn. If the mucosa is inadvertently opened, it is better to convert to a pyloroplasty than attempt to repair the mucosa.

7.3.8 Bringing Up the Stomach for Anastomosis

Options and techniques for the subcutaneous, retrosternal, and transpleural placement of an esophageal substitute were described in 7.2. When using the stomach for reconstruction, we prefer the retrosternal route. However, the transpleural route is indicated if an intrathoracic anastomosis is planned. When the anastomosis is to be placed in the apex of the chest following an esophageal resection through a left-sided approach, the transplant should be positioned in front of the aortic arch.

7.3.9 Esophagogastrostomy

The anastomosis between the stomach and esophagus can be performed manually and, at most levels, mechanically using the EEA stapling instrument. We consider a mechanical anastomosis to be superior when performed at a technically favorable site (see 1.3.1).

7.3.9.1 Site of the Anastomosis in the Stomach

In the reversed gastric tube procedure and also when the whole isoperistaltic stomach is used, the esophagogastric anastomosis is constructed at the highest point using an end-to-end technique. When the gastric fundus has been resected, an end-to-end anastomosis may be performed at the highest point of the resection plane, or the esophagus may be anastomosed in end-to-side fashion to the anterior stomach wall.

7.3.9.2 Esophagogastrostomy with the EEA Instrument

The technique of mechanical esophagogastrostomy is described fully in 1.3.3.2, so here we shall review only the essentials. We use the straight or curved EEA instrument with a 25-mm cartridge, depending on the site of the anastomosis. A pursestring suture is placed in the esophagus on the proposed line of resection using the ASP 50 instrument or a manual all-coats technique. A second pursestring suture about 1.5 cm in diameter is placed in the stomach at the proposed anastomotic site, and an opening is made at its center. The stapling instrument is passed either transorally into the esophagus or transabdominally or transthoracically into the stomach through a gastrotomy and is opened. The structures to be united are fixed between the anvil and cartridge by tightening the pursestring sutures around the central rod of the stapler, and the instrument is fired. After removal of the stapler, the anastomosis is tested for watertightness, and the gastrotomy through which the EEA instrument was introduced is closed with the TA stapler.

7.3.9.3 Manual Esophagogastrostomy

The techniques for manual esophageal anastomosis are described in 1.3.2. We prefer the two-layer technique with a continuous mucosa-to-mucosa suture and construct the anastomosis in end-to-end fashion at the highest point of the mobilized stomach (see 1.3.2.3).

7.3.9.3.1 End-to-Side Esophagogastrostomy. The end-to-side anastomosis is generally placed on the anterior stomach wall [13, 41, 84]. The posterior esophagogastrostomy [58] is more technically difficult and appears to offer no functional advantages. The stomach must be adequately mobilized for an end-to-side anastomosis, which is placed 2–5 cm below its highest point.

Operative technique: The stomach is grasped at its highest point with two Babcock clamps spaced about 10 cm apart and is stretched out. The esophagus, still closed, is placed over the anterior wall of the stomach to determine the level of the anastomosis in the gastric wall. The anastomosis should be positioned 2–5 cm from the highest point on the stomach. The lateral sides of the esophagus are fixed to the highest point with a pair of interrupted sutures to suspend the stomach from the esophagus, and the Babcock clamps are removed. The esophagus is reflected upward, and two or three additional fixation sutures are placed between the two corner threads. Then the actual anastomosis is performed. The technique is the same as for an end-to-end anastomosis (see 1.3.2.3). A single- or double-layer technique, either inverting or end-on, may be employed.

7.3.10 Methods of Reinforcing the Esophagogastrostomy and Preventing Reflux

Esophagogastrostomies are more prone to leakage than other types of gastrointestinal anastomosis. An intrathoracic leakage is often fatal. This fact, plus the high incidence of gastroesophageal reflux that occurs when only part of the stomach is transposed into the chest, has prompted surgeons either to remove tension from the anastomosis by fixing the transplant to adjacent tissue or to cover and protect the anastomotic suture line with surrounding material (see 1.6) or with the stomach itself. When the stomach is used for this purpose, an antireflux mechanism is also created. While we appreciate the benefits of transplant fixation, we question the value of techniques that "cover up" the anastomosis. We feel that the best protection for an anastomosis is a well-perfused, tension-free transplant that is anastomosed in watertight fashion using flawless technique. There is no conclusive evidence that covering or reinforcing an anastomosis significantly lowers the incidence of disruption. We personally do not reinforce either a cervical or intrathoracic esophagogastrostomy with surrounding material or with the stomach itself. However, we do approve of simple, fast reinforcement techniques as long as their purpose is not to salvage a poorly constructed anastomosis or a poorly perfused transplant. We feel that it is better in these cases either to discard the transplant and obtain another, or else defer the anastomosis, construct separate gastrostomy and esophagostomy, and restore alimentary continuity in a later operation. If only a small part of the prepyloric region is left in the abdomen after the stomach has been transposed, late esophageal reflux disease will develop in fewer than 5% of cases. Reflux, then, does not pose a major clinical problem following the resection of esophageal carcinoma and reconstruction by stomach. When the resection has been performed for benign disease, on the other hand, such as a peptic stricture at the esophagogastric junction, a large part of the stomach remains in the abdomen following esophagogastrostomy. Reflux esophagitis is inevitable unless an antireflux procedure is added. Generally, however, we prefer to use an interposed segment of jejunum or colon in these cases rather than stomach.

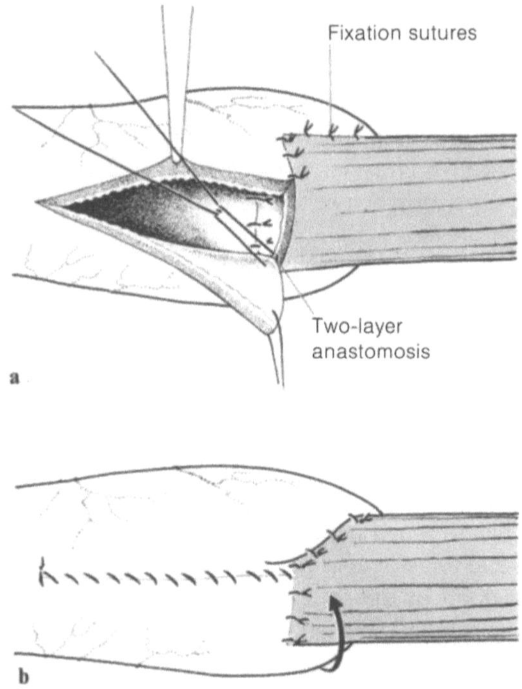

Fig. 91 a, b. "Continent" esophagogastrostomy. **a** A two-layer anastomosis is performed between the esophagus and the body of the stomach. Fixation sutures appose the greater curvature to the posterior wall of the anastomosis. **b** The anterior wall of the anastomosis is covered by imbricating the body of the stomach over the esophageal suture line

7.3.10.1 Fixation of the Transplant

Tension can be removed from the anastomosis by fixing the gastric wall to surrounding structures with a few interrupted sutures. In a transpleural reconstruction, the stomach can be anchored to the divided layers of the mediastinal pleura or to the prevertebral fascia. Fixation to the deep cervical muscles or prevertebral fascia is possible when the stomach is placed subcutaneously or retrosternally, although we consider fixation to be unnecessary in those cases.

7.3.10.2 Using Portions of the Stomach to Reinforce an End-to-End Anastomosis and Prevent Reflux

7.3.10.2.1 Inkwell Anastomosis. An "inkwell" or telescopic anastomosis (see 1.6.5) is constructed by invaginating the esophagogastrostomy suture line. The seromuscular layer of the stomach is grasped about 3 cm below the anastomosis (depending on the amount of material available) and is stitched to the muscular coat of the esophagus an equal distance above the anastomosis using simple interrupted sutures. A circular row of 6–8 of these sutures is sufficient to invaginate the anastomosis and the esophagus above it into the stomach. Coverage with the stomach wall protects the anastomosis, and the intragastric part of the esophagus creates a barrier against reflux.

7.3.10.2.2 Continent Anastomosis. The "continent" anastomosis was described by Lortat-Jacob and Fekete [47] for uniting the esophagus to the fundectomized stomach. The anastomosis is performed using an open technique. After resection of the fundus, traction sutures are placed in the lesser curvature of the gastric remnant and at the center of its anterior and posterior walls. When the sutures are pulled apart, the opening in the stomach assumes a triangular shape. The esophagus is now apposed to the greater curvature side of the triangle so that a flush fit is obtained. The posterior side of the esophagus is fixed to the greater curvature with three interrupted sutures placed about 2 cm from the cut edge. Then the posterior part of the anastomosis is constructed in two layers, the innermost layer formed by mucosa-to-mucosa sutures. When the posterior part of the anastomosis has been completed, the sutures are continued around the anterior side in circular fashion (Fig. 91 a). The mucosa is closed first with simple interrupted sutures. The final suture meets with the longitudinal opening in the stomach and is placed in the fashion of a three-point stitch. The second layer of the anastomosis unites the muscular coat of the esophagus to the seromuscular coat of the stomach and is performed with inverting sutures. The longitudinal opening that remains in the stomach is likewise closed in two layers. As in the inkwell anastomosis, the wall of the stomach is

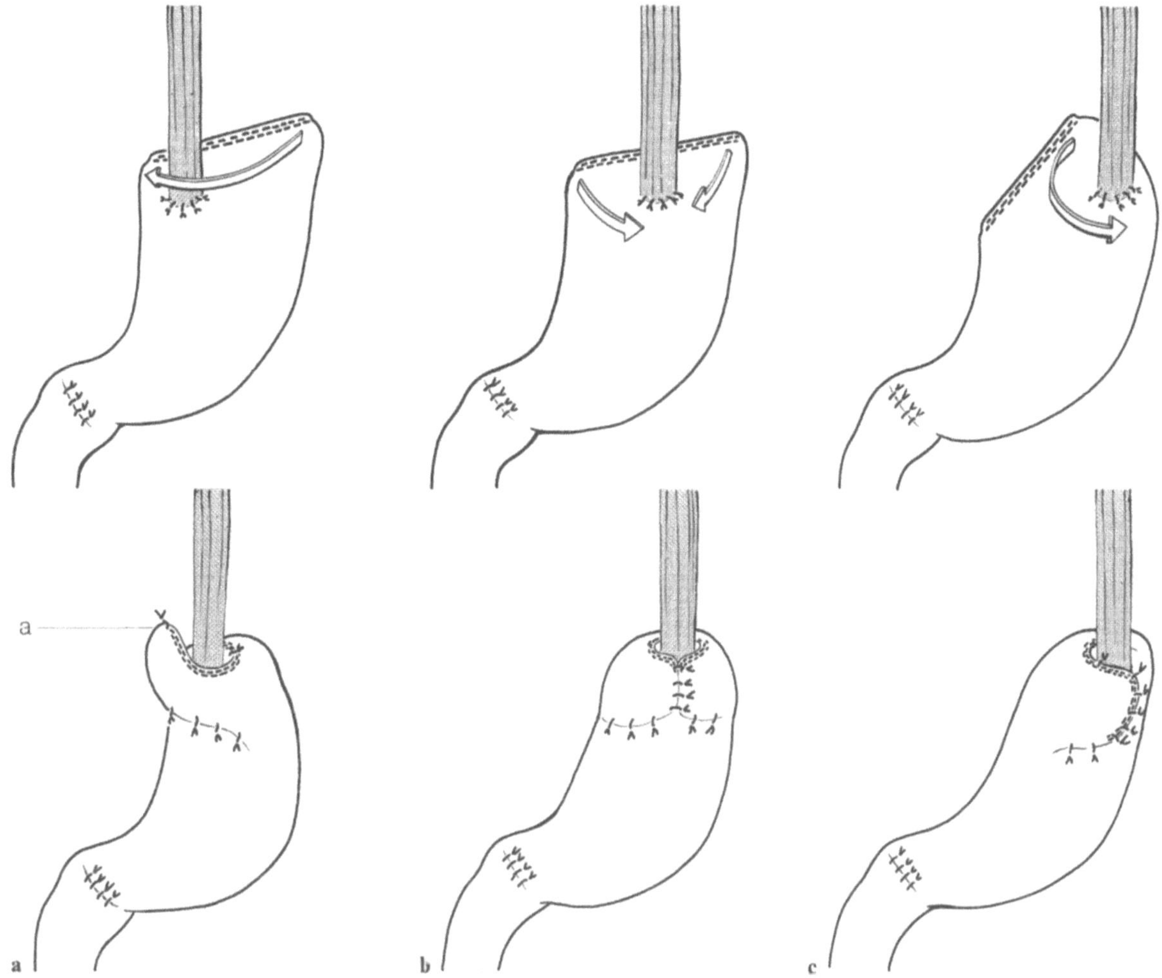

grasped 2–3 cm from the anastomosis and advanced over the lower end of the esophagus, which becomes invaginated into the gastric lumen (Fig. 91 b). The stomach wall is fixed to the esophagus with a circumferential row of interrupted sutures.

Fig. 92a–c. Methods of reinforcing an end-to-side esophagogastrostomy and preventing reflux. **a** An anastomosis placed near the lesser curvature is covered with the greater curvature portion of the gastric stump. The projecting corner of the pouch *a* is fixed to the mediastinal border. **b** A centrally placed anastomosis is covered with portions of the greater and lesser curvatures. **c** An anastomosis placed toward the greater curvature side is covered with portions of the greater and lesser curvatures

7.3.10.3 Using Portions of the Stomach to Reinforce an End-to-Side Anastomosis and Prevent Reflux

The techniques for constructing an end-to-side esophagogastrostomy and preventing reflux are basically the same as for an end-to-end anastomosis. The suture line is covered with portions of the stomach, and a 3- to 5-cm long intragastric segment of esophagus is created to function as an antireflux valve. In all the techniques for end-to-side esophagogastrostomy, the part of the stomach that overlaps the anastomosis is fixed not to the esophagus itself but to other parts of the stomach. This provides a more secure suture line and eliminates the danger of esophageal fistula in the event a suture tears out. If the anastomosis has been placed near the lesser curvature [41], the remaining greater curvature lateral to the anastomosis is turned over the esophagus toward the lesser curvature so that the corner of the pouch is above the oral border of the fundus (Fig. 92 a). In that position the corner is stitched to the cut edge of the mediastinum. The wrap is additionally secured anteriorly with interrupted seromuscular stitches.

If the anastomosis has been placed at a more central position in the anterior stomach wall [13], the wrap is made with portions of the greater and lesser curvatures, which are united in front of the esophagus with simple interrupted sutures (Fig. 92 b). The lower edge of the wrap is fixed to the anterior stomach wall with additional interrupted sutures so that the anastomosis will not slip out of the cuff.

Finally, if the anastomosis has been placed on the greater curvature side, its anterior portion is covered by the projecting remnant of the lesser curvature (Fig. 92 c). The wrap brings the proximal end of the gastric cut edge to the left side of the anastomosis. The gastric pouch formed by this maneuver is fixed to the greater curvature and anterior wall of the stomach with interrupted sutures.

7.3.10.4 Other Methods of Protecting the Anastomosis and Preventing Reflux

The methods described above are technically simple, yet they are effective in protecting the suture line and preventing reflux. We feel that there is no need to resort to more complicated procedures such as Franke's anterior gastric wall flap, the pad procedure of Gohrbrandt, Watkin's esophageal wall flap, etc.

7.4 Use of the Small Intestine as an Esophageal Substitute

The jejunum is used almost exclusively for reconstructions of the esophagus with small intestine. We know of only one reported case where an interposed segment of ileum was used [29]. At one time it was thought that the ileocolon would be excellent for interposition between the stomach and esophagus owing to the natural valvular mechanism at the ilcocolic junction [23]. However, since it has been shown that a 12- to 15-cm segment of jejunum interposed isoperistaltically can prevent reflux of gastric contents into the esophagus by virtue of its propulsive peristaltic activity [50], the direct and indirect sequelae of an ileocecal resection, such as bacterial proliferation in the distal small intestine and impaired reabsorption of bile acids and vitamin B_{12}, do not justify interposition of the ileocolon. Because small intestine retains its peristaltic activity when transplanted, interposed, or transposed, there is no question that isoperistaltic placement of the jejunum [73] is superior to antiperistaltic [69]. The only exception to this rule is the interposition of a short antiperistaltic segment in the gastric reconstruction procedure of Schrader et al. [79], where it is desirable for the antiperistaltic transplant to delay transit.

There are basically three ways in which the small intestine can be used as an esophageal and/or gastric substitute.

Transplantation: A segment of jejunum can be resected with its vascular pedicle and freely transplanted into the thorax or neck, where its vessels are anastomosed to local donor vessels [82].

Interposition: A jejunal segment can be mobilized on a vascular pedicle and interposed between the cut ends of the esophagus, between the esophagus and stomach [73], or between the esophagus and duodenum following gastrectomy [46]. The isolated jejunal loop, originally used by Roux [73] with a side-to-side esophagojejunostomy, end-to-side jejunogastrostomy, and side-to-side jejunojejunostomy to bypass the unresected esophagus (Fig. 93 a), has become the standard operation for esophageal replacement with small intestine when the stomach is preserved, although modern techniques employ end-to-end esophagojejunal and jejunojejunal anastomoses (Fig. 93 b). The procedures described by Longmire et al. [46], Gütgemann et al. [24], Schrader et al. [79], Maki [49], and Schreiber et al. [80] are derived from Seo's gastric reconstruction procedure [83], which preserves duodenal transit and uses an isolated jejunal loop with an end-to-side esophagojejunostomy and end-to-end jejunoduodenostomy.

Transposition: The jejunum, transected distal to the ligament of Treitz, can be mobilized sufficiently to be brought up to the thoracic or cervical esophagus without further disrupting its continuity. The cut end of the proximal jejunal segment is anastomosed to the side of the mobilized segment. Herzen [27] united the pulled-up jejunum to the gastric reservoir through a side-to-side jejunogastrostomy (Fig. 93 c), but Yudin [98] considered this unnecessary and omitted the gastroenterostomy (Fig. 93 d). For functional reasons both methods are seldom used today, and then only as palliative operations for the bypass of malignant strictures, especially those involving the lower third of the esophagus. Schlatter [78] advocated an end-to-side esophagojejunostomy following gastrectomy and duodenal closure. This method formed the basis for the reconstructive procedures that are currently used with gastrectomy and defunctionalization of the duodenum [21, 32, 84].

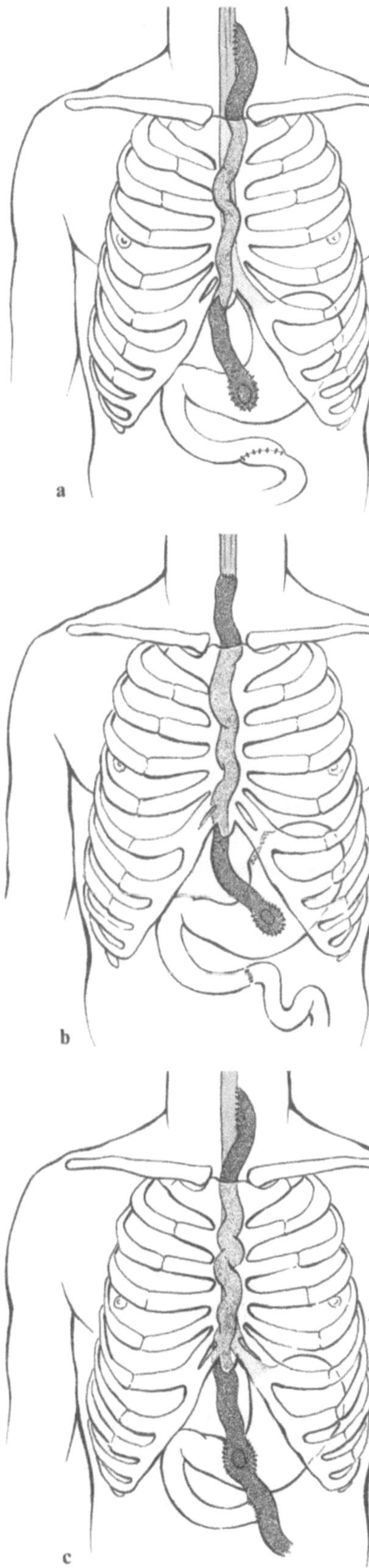

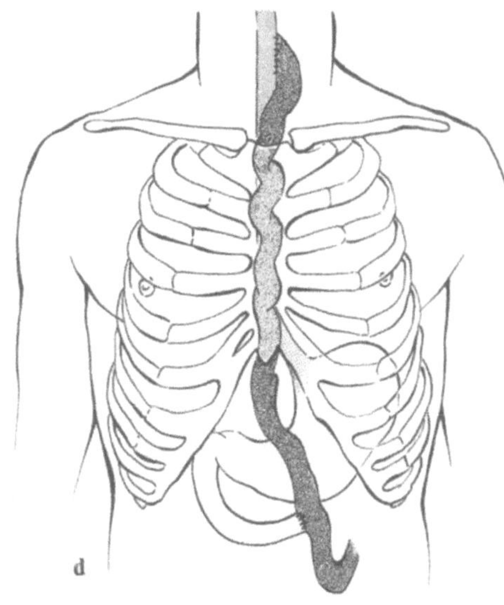

Fig. 93a–d. Methods of reconstructing the esophagus with small intestine. **a** Roux's original method of esophagojejunogastrostomy for bypass of the unresected esophagus [73]. **b** Roux's isoperistaltic jejunal interposition following esophageal resection [73] (currently the standard method for replacing the whole esophagus with small intestine). **c** Herzen's bypass operation with a side-to-side jejunogastrostomy [28]. **d** Yudin's isoperistaltic transposition of the jejunum [98]

7.4.1 Blood Supply of the Mobilized Jejunum

The proximal small intestine derives its blood supply from the superior mesenteric artery and is drained by the jejunal branches of the superior mesenteric vein. The distribution pattern of the first four or five jejunal arteries beyond the ligament of Treitz is the main determinant of whether the jejunum can be used to replace a lengthy portion of the esophagus, i.e., can be elevated to a site above the inferior pulmonary veins. Generally speaking, a sufficiently long segment of jejunum can be mobilized for intrathoracic anastomosis to the esophagus following the resection of a cardia carcinoma, for segmental replacement of peptic strictures of the lower esophagus, and for free transplantation. If the primary jejunal arteries arising from the superior mesenteric are of reasonably large caliber and form well-defined marginal arcades that are peripherally situated (Fig. 94 a), it is virtually certain that a sufficiently long vascular pedicle can be developed to elevate the jejunum as far as the neck. On the other hand, if many

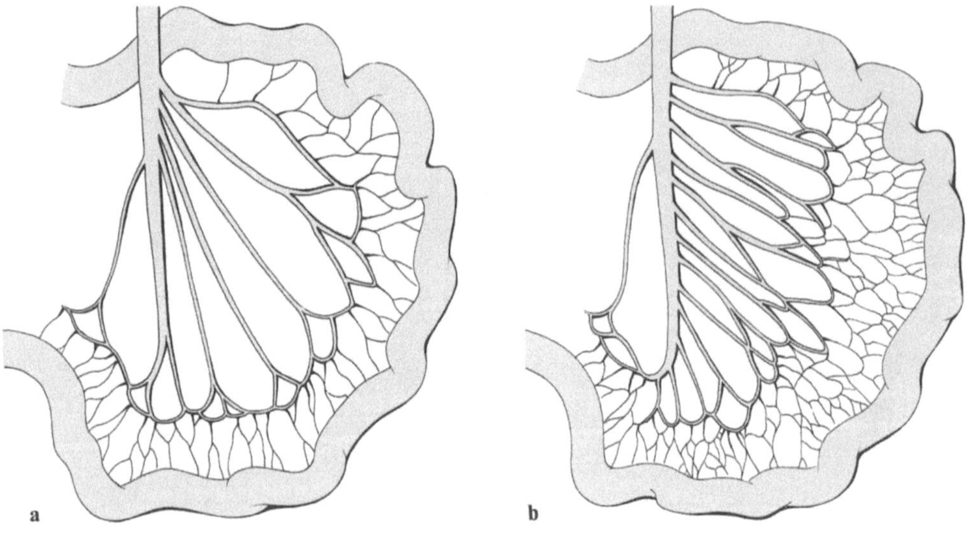

Fig. 94a, b. Vascular supply of the jejunum. **a** Favorable vascular pattern for jejunal reconstruction of the esophagus: A few main branches of large size arise from the superior mesenteric artery and form marginal arcades close to the bowel. **b** Unfavorable vascular pattern for jejunal reconstruction of the esophagus: Numerous small-caliber branches arise from the superior mesenteric and form arcades close to the parent vessel

separate branches of small size arise from the superior mesenteric artery; if the anastomoses between the jejunal arteries are numerous, poorly developed, and proximally situated (Fig. 94 b); or if there is a defect in the continuity the marginal arcade, the jejunum is considered unfit for replacing a long segment of esophagus. The mesentery of the first jejunal loop is usually short and should not be mobilized. Only the second and third loops should be considered. Their suitability is determined by inspecting the primary arteries and the arcades. If the mesentery is thickened, it can be difficult to evaluate the marginal arcades, and in these cases it is necessary to expose the jejunal arteries that are to be ligated and temporarily occlude them with rubber-shod clamps. We maintain the occlusion for 5 min and then check for the telltale signs of vascular insufficiency: discoloration, hyperperistalsis, and lack of arterial pulsations. In borderline cases the jejunum should not be mobilized.

The venous drainage of the jejunal segment is no less important than its arterial supply and is particularly sensitive to external compression because of the low intravenous pressure. The small veins run parallel to the arterial arcades. The collecting veins may course separate from the arcades in the mesentery. Special care must be taken to preserve these vessels during the mobilization and transplantation phases of the procedure.

Anatomic constraints determine the usefulness of the jejunum as an esophageal substitute. There are ways of correcting anatomic deficiencies to some extent, such as radial incision of the mesentery, the resection of redundant bowel, and local vascular anastomoses. But these techniques should be reserved for cases where a problem of length or blood flow is noted after the loop has been mobilized; they should not be used to correct a primarily unfavorable disposition of the vessels.

7.4.2 Mobilization of an Isolated Jejunal Loop for Segmental or Total Reconstruction of the Esophagus (and Stomach)

Preoperative preparation: Perioperative antibiotics, intestinal lavage as required (see Chap. C).

Instruments: Basic set; extra sets II and V; TA, GIA, EEA.

Position and approach: Midline laparotomy extended around the umbilicus.

Steps in procedure:

(1) Inspection of the vascular supply of the proximal jejunum by transillumination
(2) Identification of the vessels supplying the jejunal loop to be isolated
(3) If desired, temporary occlusion of the arteries to be ligated with Bulldog clamps
(4) Incision of the peritoneal layers of the mesentery at the proximal line of resection
(5) Selective division of the vessels in the mesentery
(6) Transection of the jejunum with the GIA instrument at the proximal line of resection
(7) Division of the proximal arcade
(8) Division of the mesentery to the proposed mesenteric pedicle
(9) Identification of the distal line of resection
(10) Division of the peritoneal layers and mesenteric vessels toward the vascular pedicle of the segment to be isolated
(11) Transection of the jejunum with the GIA instrument at the distal line of resection
(12) Reanastomosis of the small bowel anterior to the vascular pedicle of the isolated segment
(13) Closure of the mesenteric incision

Operative technique. After the abdomen is entered, the greater omentum and transverse colon are reflected superiorly, wrapped in moist gauze pads, and held aside. The loops of small intestine are retracted downward to the right so that the ligament of Treitz can be identified. The first loop of jejunum is picked up, stretched out between the thumb and index finger of both hands, and the vascular supply of the proximal loops is inspected by transillumination (Fig. 95 a). The proximal line of transection should be at least 10–15 cm below the ligament of Treitz. The length of the jejunal segment to be isolated is determined by the distance that must be spanned. Generally a segment about 15 cm long is sufficient to perform a segmental replacement of the esophagus without gastrectomy [50]. Shorter segments have been shown to allow some regurgitation. We prefer a somewhat longer length for interpositions. If it is necessary to reconstruct the stomach as well as the lower esophagus, a 15- to 20-cm length of small intestine proximal to the vascular pedicle is usually sufficient to enable an anastomosis to be performed up to the level of the pulmonary veins. Because the segment distal to the vascular pedicle is not isolated, and its mesentery may be left intact, it can provide the total length of slightly more than 40 cm needed to create an adequate substitute gastric reservoir and antireflux valve.

Generally two or three loops of jejunum are needed to replace the whole esophagus. These are supplied by the 4th or 5th jejunal artery following division of the 2nd, 3rd, and if necessary the 4th arteries. This is not a rigid guideline, however, and selection of the jejunal segment will depend on the anatomic situation. After it has been determined which jejunal vessels will serve as the pedicle and which must be divided, and after any trial occlusion has been done to confirm the viability of the segment, both peritoneal layers of the mesentery are incised with the scalpel between two vasa recta at the proposed proximal line of the resection (Fig. 95 b), and the vessels coursing in the mesentery to their insertion in the small bowel are selectively divided between small clamps (Fig. 95 c). The jejunum itself is transected with the GIA stapling instrument (Fig. 95 d). Both ends of the segment are wrapped with gauze pads soaked in antiseptic to avoid spillage of septic material during the rest of the dissection. Then the cranial arcade is divided between clamps. Keeping 1–2 cm proximal to the arcade, the mesentery is incised to the base of the proposed mesenteric pedicle as the primary vessels supplying the arcades are individually ligated and divided. The dissection should not be carried too close to the arcades so that a narrow, protective rim of mesentery is preserved. The primary vessels should be divided sufficiently proximal to their bifurcations into arcades so as not to impair the passage of blood, but they should not be ligated so far from the bifurcations that a long, blind stump is created that may promote clot formation. The dissection terminates 1–2 cm from the origin of the primary vessel supplying the segment. The surgeon now defines the distal limit of the resection–generally 10 cm aboral to the vascular pedicle. Care is taken not to make the segment too long if the stomach has been preserved; otherwise there may be redundant bowel above the distal anastomosis. The situation is different if the stomach has been resected and it is necessary to reconstruct it as well. In these cases we provide about an additional 35-cm length of interposed bowel, which requires no special mesenteric dissection since the preexisting length of the

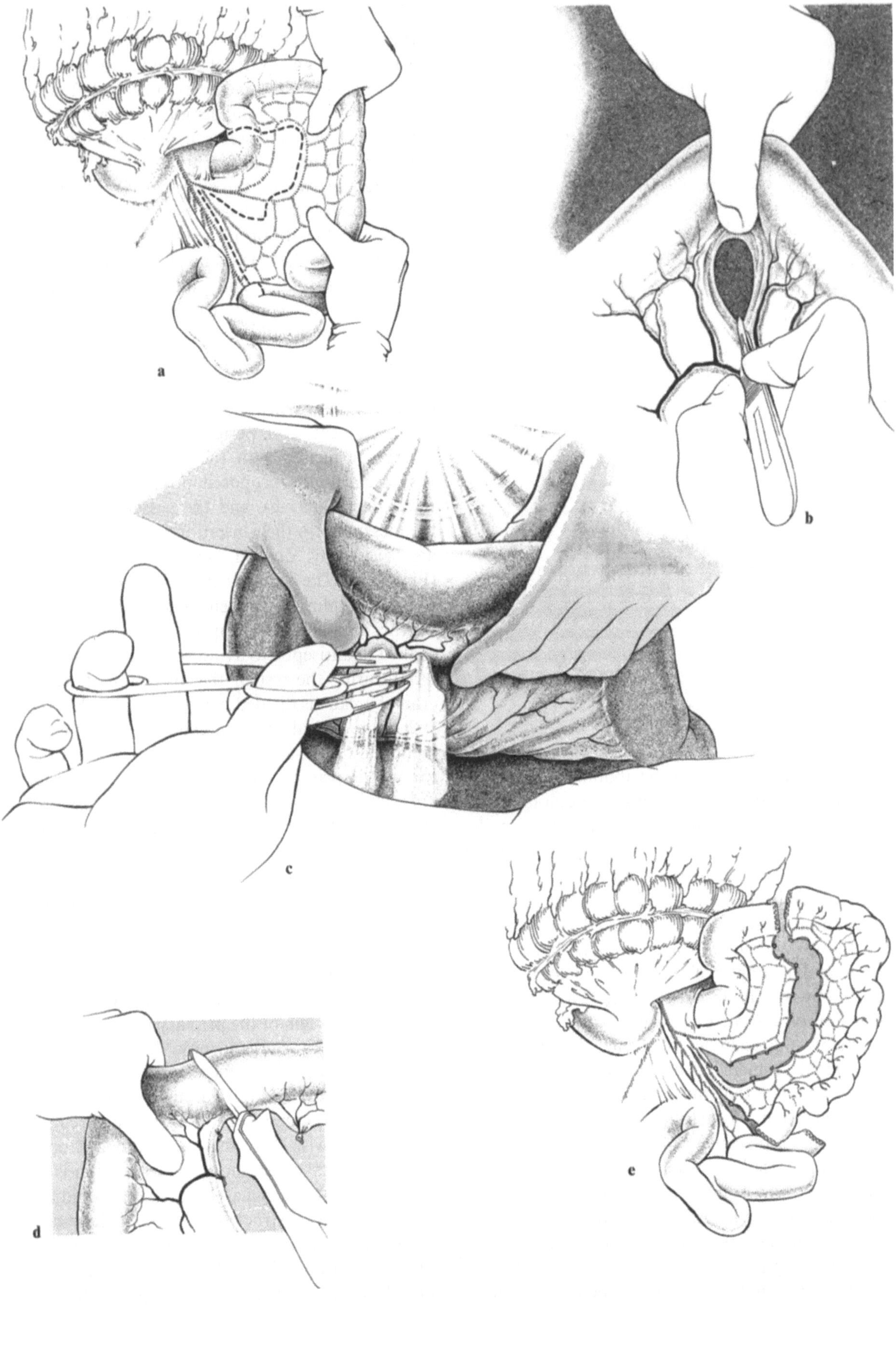
a
b
c
d
e

◁ **Fig. 95a–e.** Mobilization of an isolated loop of jejunum for replacement of the whole esophagus. **a** The proximal coils of jejunum are transilluminated to evaluate their vascular pattern. The limits of the segment to be isolated (broken line) are defined. **b** The peritoneal layers of the mesentery are divided between two vasa recta. **c** The jejunum is dissected free at the proposed site of transection. The vessels on the line of resection are selectively ligated and divided. **d** The jejunum is transected with the GIA instrument. **e** Isolated jejunal segment ready for transplantation

mesentery is sufficient. The segment is mobilized by dividing both peritoneal layers with the scalpel, as before, and individually ligating the mesenteric vessels. The bowel is transected with the GIA instrument. The mesentery is incised in a straight line down to the root of the vascular pedicle to ensure if possible that there is no overlap between the blood supplies of proximal and distal segments. This completes the mobilization of the jejunal segment (Fig. 95 e). The degree of coiling of the segment on its mesentery should be assessed to determine if there is a need to straighten the segment to avoid stasis.

7.4.3 Mobilization of a Y Loop for Partial or Total Reconstruction of the Esophagus (and Stomach)

Preoperative preparation, instruments, position and approach: See 4.3.

Operative technique: The initial steps of mobilizing a Y loop for partial or total reconstruction of the esophagus are identical to those for mobilizing an isolated loop (Fig. 96 a). The major difference is that the bowel is not divided distally, and the proximal cut end is anastomosed to the side of the mobilized jejunal segment (Fig. 96 b).

7.4.4 Technical Complications and their Remedies

The following complications may be associated with replacement of the whole esophagus by jejunum:

(1) Plication of the interposed segment by a too-short mesentery
(2) Excessive coiling of the jejunum on its mesentery that may obstruct transit following placement in the chest
(3) Insufficient blood supply.

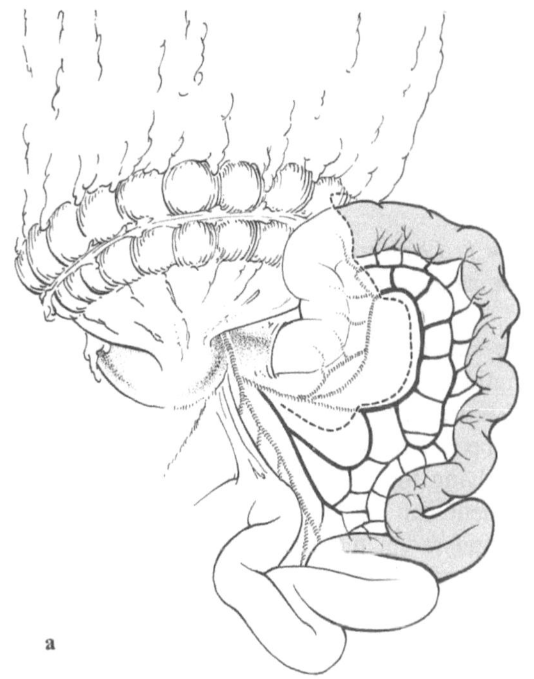

a

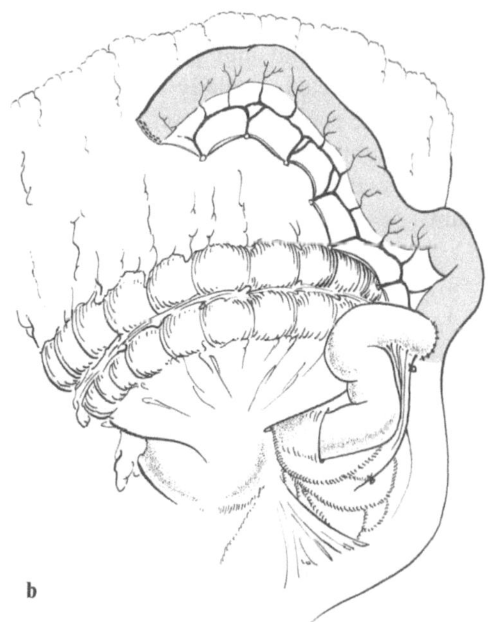

b

Fig. 96a, b. Mobilization of a Y loop of jejunum for esophageal replacement. **a** The vascular pattern of the proximal jejunum is inspected by transillumination, and the line of transection in the bowel and mesentery (broken line) is determined. **b** The Y loop is ready for transposition. Small bowel continuity has been restored by an end-to-side jejunojejunostomy. The mesenteric incision has been closed with interrupted sutures

In many cases an isolated loop of jejunum can be salvaged by radial incision of the mesentery [15], mobilization of the cecum [63], the resection of redundant intestine [59], and by anastomosing the jejunal arteries to regional blood vessels [4].

7.4.4.1 Lengthening the Mesentery with a Radial Incision

The radial incision is the simplest method of lengthening and straightening a loop of jejunum. However, it is possible only when the mesentery has been divided too far from the marginal arcade supplying the segment. In these cases the jejunal segment can be lengthened and straightened by making radial incisions in the mesentery toward the vascular arcades (Fig. 97 a,b).

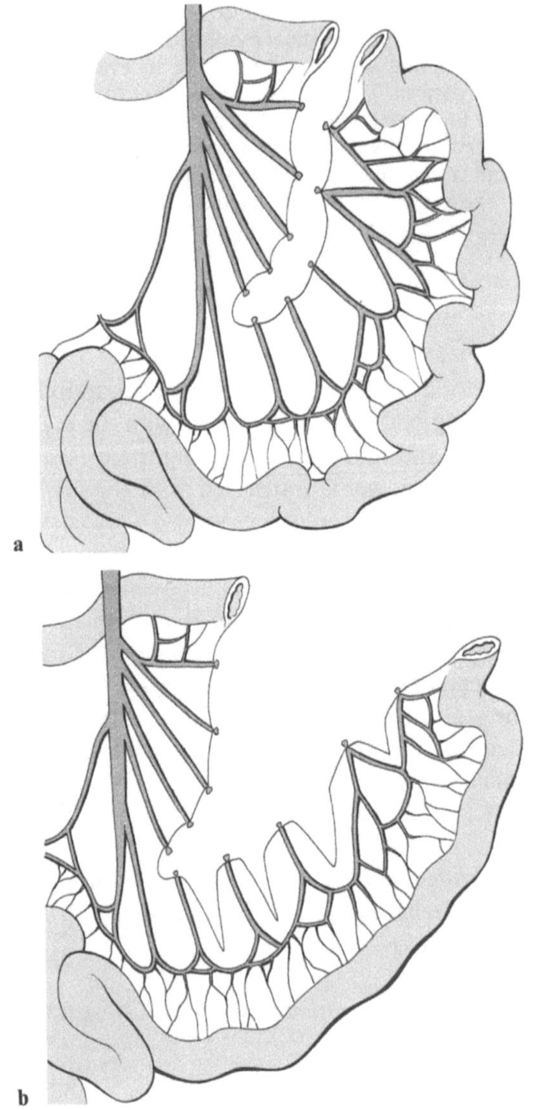

Fig. 97a, b. Radial incision of the mesentery to lengthen the jejunal segment

7.4.4.2 Mobilization of the Cecum

Petrov [63] pointed out that 10–20 cm of additional length can be gained if the cecum is also mobilized and the parietal and posterior peritoneum below it is dissected medially toward the spine. In this way the root of the mesentery is freed and can be brought upward with the entire mass of bowel loops, including the mobilized segment of jejunum.

7.4.4.3 Resection of Redundant Jejunum

The limiting factor in terms of the length of an interposed jejunal segment is its mesentery. As the mesentery is straightened out, the attached loops of jejunum will tend to remain coiled, creating a potential obstruction to transit. The loop of small intestine can be straightened by dividing the vasa recta of a redundant segment close to the bowel wall and then resecting the redundant intestine with the GIA instrument (Fig. 98). The continuity of the transplant is restored by an end-to-end anastomosis. While this technique is effective in straightening the interposed segment, the need for an extra anastomosis increases the operative risk.

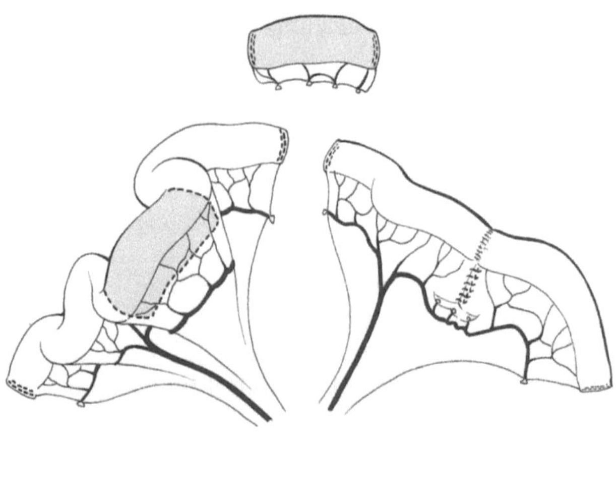

Fig. 98. Resection of redundant jejunum to straighten the transplant

7.4.4.4 Anastomosis of Jejunal Arteries to Intrathoracic Vessels

An artery at the oral end of the transplant that has questionable blood flow can be anastomosed to a local blood vessel using microsurgical technique. The internal mammary artery or epigastric artery make suitable donor vessels for a subcutaneous reconstruction. A transplant placed transpleurally or retrosternally may be anastomosed to the inferior thyroid artery, the thyrocervical trunk, the external carotid artery or its first division, or to the superior thyroid artery. In all cases venous return is through the vascular pedicle of the jejunal segment; a venous anastomosis is not performed. If venous return is impaired, we would advise against taking further measures to salvage the transplant, and we would prefer to use an alternative procedure. If the arterial connection becomes occluded 2–3 weeks after the interposition, capillary ingrowth by that time should be sufficient to nourish the jejunal segment [45, 65].

The proximal jejunal artery is anastomosed to an artery in the neck using the same technique as for the free transplantation of a jejunal patch (see 4.3.2). For anastomosing the jejunal artery to the internal mammary artery in a subcutaneous reconstruction, the skin incision must be extended over the sternum to the neck. The subcutaneous tissue is reflected past the costochondral junction of the ribs, and the cartilaginous attachments of the second and third ribs are resected within their perichondrium. The internal mammary artery coursing posteriorly on the pleura is separated from the pleural surface, ligated inferiorly, occluded proximally, and mobilized with a small vascular clamp for a length of 2–3 cm in preparation for the anastomosis. The anastomosis may be performed with the aid of a binocular loupe or operating microscope, depending on the size of the vessels (see 4.3.2).

7.4.5 *Restoration of Bowel Continuity*

After mobilization of the jejunal segment as an isolated or Y loop, continuity of the small intestine is restored by reanastomosing the proximal and distal cut ends or by anastomosing the proximal cut end to the side of the jejunum below the vascular pedicle. Both anastomoses can be performed with the EEA stapling instrument. In the Y-loop procedure for replacement of the distal esophagus and stomach, the instrument can be used for both the jejunojejunostomy and esophagojejunostomy simply by making an incision in the antimesenteric portion of the small bowel. However, we continue to prefer manual anastomoses of the small intestine because of their high efficacy and low cost.

7.4.5.1 End-to-End Anastomosis

The cut ends of the jejunum, which are either stapled shut or occluded with rubber-shod clamps, are approximated such that their mesentery is in front of the vascular pedicle of the isolated loop (Fig. 99 a). The mesenteric border is cut away from the bowel for about 1–3 cm at each end. Then the bowel ends are apposed and held together with a pair of laterally placed guide sutures, which are immediately tied. The posterior surface of the bowel is presented by passing one of the guide sutures behind the bowel and pulling the threads to rotate the area of the anastomosis into view. We perform the posterior part of the anastomosis first, starting with a central suture and placing inverting sutures laterally from it toward the guide threads (Fig. 99 b). When this row has been completed, the guide suture is passed back in the opposite direction to bring the anterior surface of the bowel into view. The GIA staple lines at the bowel ends are excised with a scissors or electrocautery, and mucosal bleeding points are coagulated. The lumina, held open by the guide threads, are cleaned with dissecting patties soaked in antiseptic. Then the posterior part of the anastomosis is completed with a continuous mucosa-to-mucosa suture line (Fig. 99 c). When we reach a corner thread, we interrupt the continuous suture with an additional holding suture so that stricturing will not occur when the suture is tightened. We then continue the mucosal-to-mucosa suture around the anterior side (Fig. 99 d). The seromuscular layers are approximated over the mucosa with simple interrupted threads (Fig. 99 e). We check the patency of the anastomosis with the thumb and index finger and then close the mesenteric incision with interrupted sutures to the root of the mesentery.

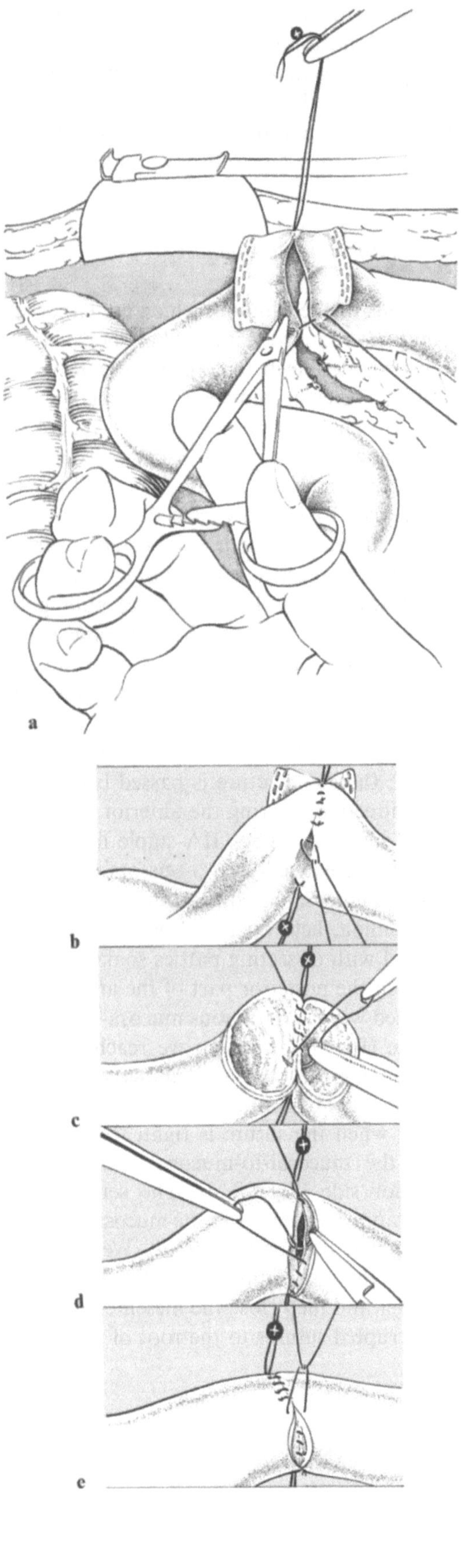

Fig. 99 a–e. Restoring small bowel continuity by an end-to-end jejunojejunostomy. **a** The bowel segments are approximated and tacked together. **b** The posterior sides are united with interrupted seromuscular stitches. **c** A continuous mucosa-to-mucosa suture completes the posterior part of the anastomosis. **d** The anterior mucosal suture is applied. **e** Interrupted seromuscular sutures complete the anterior wall of the anastomosis

7.4.5.2 End-to-Side Anastomosis

The proximal cut end of the first jejunal loop is anastomosed to the side of the middle jejunum about 10–20 cm below the superior edge of the vascular pedicle. The anastomosis is not constructed in T-shape fashion but at an acute angle in the direction of the flow. The technique is like that for an end-to-end anastomosis.

7.4.6 Intraabdominal Transfer of the Mobilized Segment

In cases that require replacement of the stomach as well as the esophagus, the previous resection will have included the greater omentum, so it is necessary only to bring the jejunal segment up behind the transverse colon through an incision in the transverse mesocolon. Care must be taken at this time to avoid injury to the midcolic vessels. Their course is determined by transillumination, and the mesocolon is incised lateral to them. The incision is enlarged somewhat with the fingers, and the loop of jejunum is drawn through the opening. If the stomach has not been resected, it is still necessary first to identify the midcolic artery, incise the transverse mesocolon lateral to it, and bluntly enlarge the opening. Then, in thin patients, it is usually sufficient to divide the lesser omentum proximal to the gastric arcade, separate any adhesions between the posterior gastric wall and retroperitoneum, and form a tunnel behind the stomach and colon by blunt dissection for passage of the jejunal loop. If the mesocolon and greater omentum are thickened, it is better either to detach the greater omentum from the transverse colon or to make about a 10-cm incision in the gastrocolic ligament and develop the retrocolic and retrogastric tunnels separately. As the jejunum is pulled upward, great care should be taken to avoid twisting of its vascular pedicle. We do not narrow the incision in the transverse mesocolon with sutures, nor do we fix the vascular pedicle to it for fear of obstructing the venous drainage of the segment.

If a Y loop has been constructed, it is now brought up as a bypass or substitute for anastomosis to the esophagus. When an isolated segment is used and the stomach is retained, jejunogastrostomy is performed after transection of the esophagus and vagotomy, and a pyloroplasty is added. If the stomach has been resected, the aboral end of the jejunal loop is anastomosed to the duodenum in end-to-end fashion.

7.4.7 Jejunogastric Anastomosis

When an esophageal stricture is to be bypassed with an isolated loop of jejunum, vagotomy is recommended to protect the jejunal mucosa. The peritoneum is incised over the esophagus, which is then encircled with the finger and snared with a soft rubber tape or drain. Both vagus nerve trunks are identified and divided. If the esophagus is to be resected, it is snared and transected below the esophagogastric junction. The surgeon must be sure that no squamous epithelium is left distal to the site of transection. Because this tissue is susceptible to the effects of acid, residual areas of squamous epithelium form sites of predilection for ulcers and perforations.

After bluntly mobilizing the esophagus into the thorax, we divide it immediately distal to the esophagogastric junction with the GIA instrument. We cover the distal stump of the esophagus with a condom and secure it with a heavy ligature. We then allow it to retract into the thorax. If the isolated loop is to be placed intrathoracically, it can be tied to the ligating thread for subsequent elevation into the chest. We place the anastomosis in the anterior wall of the body of the stomach. If a stapled anastomosis is desired, the stomach is opened 7–10 cm distal to the proposed site between 2 guide sutures, and the EEA instrument is introduced. The rest of the procedure follows the technique described in 1.3.3.2. If the lower esophagus can be reconstructed by an intraabdominal esophagojejunostomy after gastrectomy, the esophagojejunal anastomosis is performed first. The EEA instrument may be introduced through the oral or aboral lumen of the isolated segment or through a separate antimesenteric incision. In the first case the anastomosis is performed in end-to-side fashion. In the two latter cases either an end-to-end or end-to-side anastomosis may be used. If the jejunal segment has already been opened for construction of the esophagojejunostomy, it is better to utilize that opening as access for the jejunogastric anastomosis than to make a separate gastrotomy for insertion of the EEA instrument.

Our usual policy is to perform the jejunogastric anastomosis manually. The distal end of the loop is grasped by its occluding staple line and pulled to the proposed anastomotic site on the anterior wall of the stomach. We first place a guide suture on one lateral side, tie it, and leave its ends uncut. Starting from that suture, we begin the posterior part of the anastomosis with an interrupted row of inverting seromuscular stitches. The last suture serves as a second holding thread. The stomach is opened about 3 mm from the suture line and its contents evacuated. Mucosal bleeding points are controlled by coagulation or von Haberer suture ligatures. Then the staple line at the aboral end of the isolated segment is excised with the electrocautery, residual mucus is suctioned from the jejunal orifice, and both the jejunal lumen and the gastric lumen about the anastomotic site are cleaned with dissecting patties soaked in antiseptic solution. The continuous mucosa-to-mucosa suture is started posteriorly at the level of one corner thread, is interrupted by a stay suture at the second corner thread, and is then continued on the anterior side. Finally the seromuscular layers are united with an interrupted suture line started centrally.

After completion of the jejunogastrostomy, we perform a drainage procedure on the stomach to prevent stasis-related damage to the jejunal mucosa by gastric fluids. Our favorite drainage procedure is the Heineke-Mikulicz pyloroplasty (see 7.3.7.1).

7.4.8 Jejunoduodenal Anastomosis

The anastomosis between the distal end of the isolated jejunal loop and the duodenal stump, like the jejunogastrostomy, can be performed with the EEA instrument inserted through an incision on the antimesenteric side of the isolated loop (see 1.3.3.2). For this and other gastrointestinal anastomoses, we prefer a two-layer manual anastomosis that includes a continuous mucosa-to-mucosa suture.

7.4.9 Bringing Up the Mobilized Loop of Jejunum for Anastomosis to the Esophagus

Preparation of the jejunum for transfer completes the abdominal phase of the operation. The techniques for subcutaneous, retrosternal, and transpleural placement of the transplant are described in 7.2. Because a loop of jejunum is generally used for the segmental replacement or bypass of the distal esophagus or for interposition within the thoracic esophagus, the transpleural route is generally used.

7.4.10 Esophagojejunostomy

The esophagus may be anastomosed to the jejunal segment using an end-to-side or end-to-end technique. Neither technique is essentially superior to the other. As in all esophageal anastomoses, we recommend use of the EEA instrument where technically feasible.

7.4.10.1 Esophagojejunostomy with the EEA Instrument

For an end-to-side anastomosis, the EEA instrument can be introduced through the oral or aboral lumen of the interposed segment or through an incision in its antimesenteric side. Only the latter two cases allow an end-to-end anastomosis to be performed. The technique is described in 1.3.3.2. After the stapling is completed, the incision in the jejunum or its oral lumen, as the case may be, is closed with inverting sutures or with the TA stapler.

7.4.10.2 Manual Esophagojejunostomy

The suturing techniques are identical for an end-to-end and end-to-side anastomosis. We favor a two-layer technique like that used for any anastomosis involving the esophagus (see 1.3.2.3). For an end-to-side anastomosis, the length of the incision for opening the jejunum depends on the width of the esophagus. In the end-to-end anastomosis, the luminal size of the jejunum is predetermined. If its lumen is substantially larger than that of the esophagus and cannot be adequately reduced by using an oblique, plicating suture technique in the transplanted segment, congruity can be established by making a 1- to 1.5-cm incision in the anterior esophageal wall.

7.4.11 Methods of Reinforcing the Esophagojejunostomy

We feel that the same principles apply to the reinforcement of an esophagojejunal anastomosis as to the esophagogastric or esophagocolic anastomosis (see 7.3.10). The technical complexity of some methods must be weighed against the lack of proven efficacy in reducing the incidence of anastomotic leak.

7.4.11.1 Fixation of the Transplant

In a transpleural reconstruction, the anastomosis can be protected from tension by fixing the jejunal wall or an avascular area of the mesenteric pedicle to the divided layers of the mediastinal pleura or to the prevertebral fascia with a few interrupted sutures. This type of protection is unnecessary for a transplant that is placed subcutaneously or retrosternally.

7.4.11.2 Covering the Anastomosis with Adjacent Tissue

Methods of covering the anastomosis with pleura or greater omentum are described in 1.6. We consider these techniques to be unnecessary.

7.4.11.3 Reinforcing the Anastomosis with the Wall of the Esophageal Substitute

7.4.11.3.1 Inkwell Anastomosis. In this technique the suture line of the esophagojejunostomy is protected by invagination. The seromuscular layer of the mobilized loop of jejunum is grasped about 3–5 cm from the anastomosis (depending on the amount of material available) and stitched to the esophageal muscularis with interrupted sutures. A circumferential row of 6–8 of these sutures invaginates the anastomosis and the esophagus above it into the jejunal loop (see 1.6.5).

7.4.11.3.2 Reinforcing the End-to-Side Anastomosis. Various techniques are known for reinforcing the end-to-side esophagojejunostomy [80, 84], but their usefulness is limited for intrathoracic anastomoses, and they are of no value for cervical anastomoses. For an end-to-side esophagojejunostomy placed in the mid- to upper esophagus, usually there is only enough residual jejunum to form a wrap over the anterior or posterior side of the anastomosis and secure it with a few interrupted sutures.

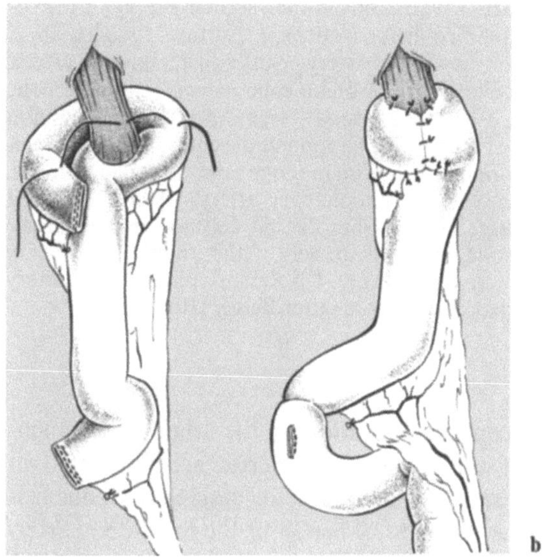

△

Fig. 100. a Reinforcement of an end-to-side esophagojejunostomy by jejunoplication. The excess jejunum is passed behind the esophagus and sutured to the esophagus and to itself with interrupted sutures. **b** The completed jejunal wrap

7.4.11.3.3 Jejunoplication. The antimesenteric side of the jejunal loop is anastomosed to the esophagus [80] about 15 cm from the oral end of the loop. The projecting segment is then wrapped around the anastomosis in circular fashion (Fig. 100 a,b). In any given case it must be determined how the segment can be best positioned to avoid tension on the mesentery. Generally the segment can be wrapped counterclockwise around the anastomosis. The plication is fixed to the esophagus and to the jejunum with simple interrupted sutures. The wrap should not be made too tight, and mesenteric strangulation must be avoided. A partial wrap may be performed if the projecting bowel segment is too short for a 360° wrap.

Another type of jejunoplication was described by Siewert et al. [84] for constructing a gastric substitute and reinforcing the anastomosis with a loop of jejunum pulled up in continuity with the rest of the bowel. The same technique can be applied, with slight modifications, to an isolated or Y loop of jejunum. The loop is grasped about 20 cm from its proximal end, and that point is pulled up to the level of the proposed anastomosis. A

Fig. 101 a–d. Jejunoplication in the construction of a substitute gastric reservoir. **a** The posterior part of the jejunojejunostomy is constructed by a two-layer suture technique. **b** The anterior wall of the gastric substitute is closed in one layer, leaving a stoma for the esophageal anastomosis. **c** The esophagus is anastomosed to the anterior wall of the gastric substitute in end-to-side fashion. **d** The anastomosis is covered by jejunoplication

▽

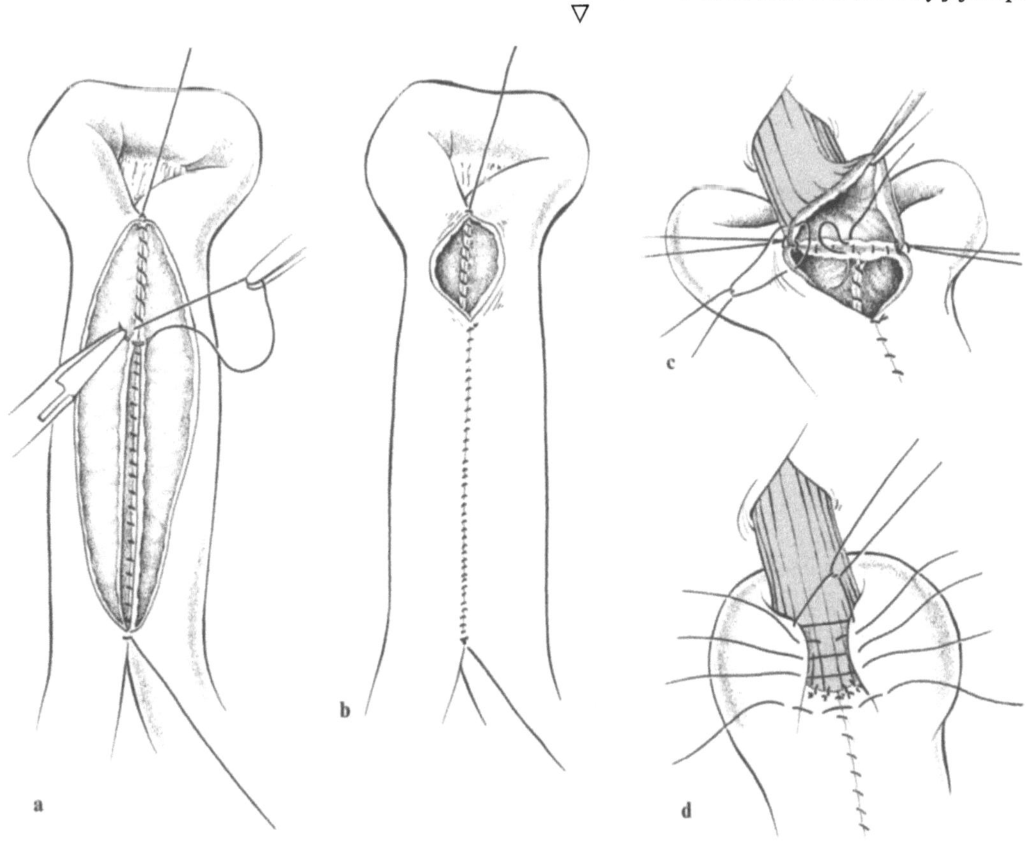

segment about three fingers wide is defined at the top of the loop, and a stay suture is placed just below that site to tack the two limbs of the loop together. A second stay suture is placed from the proximal end of the descending limb to an opposing point on the ascending limb so that two parallel segments of the pulled-up loop, each about 10 cm in length, are juxtaposed. Starting from one of the stay sutures, the adjacent walls of the jejunum are united by a continuous suture line extending to the other stay suture. Then the jejunum is incised 2 mm to the right and left of the suture line, converting the two separate lumina into one large tube. The posterior part of the anastomosis is completed with a continuous mucosa-to-mucosa suture (Fig. 101 a). The newly formed anterior wall is also closed in two layers (Fig. 101 b). An opening about 3–4 cm long is left at the upper end of the enteroenterostomy for anastomosis to the cut end of the esophagus using a one- or two-layer technique (Fig. 101 c). Siewert recommends that vertical mattress sutures be used for the posterior part of the anastomosis. The upper part of the jejunal loop is positioned behind the esophagus for the esophagojejunostomy, although it does not need to be fixed there. After completion of the esophagujejunostomy, the right and left sides of the upper loop are approximated in front of the anastomosis and united with 4 or 5 serosa-to-serosa sutures (Fig. 101 d). A "four-point" suture is used that engages both edges of the jejunum as well as the anterior wall of the pulled-up jejunal loop on the right and left sides of the vertical suture line.

7.5 Use of the Colon as an Esophageal Substitute

7.5.1 Blood Supply of the Mobilized Colon Segment

The anatomy of the colon and its blood supply are favorable for the creation of a free transplant or an isolated segment for partial or total esophageal replacement. The anatomic subdivision of the large intestine into an ascending, transverse, and descending colon does not correlate precisely with the surgical isolation of a segment for total esophageal replacement, because only the transverse colon would be long enough for that purpose. Thus, when the ascending or descending colon is used for interpositon, it is always necessary to mobilize one flexure and a portion of the transverse colon. However, the critical factor in the isolation of a colon segment is not the length of the bowel, but the vascular pedicle and the mesenteric attachment. The arterial supply of the colon from the ileocecal valve to the Canon-Böhm point near the left flexure is derived from branches of the superior mesenteric artery, which in most cases communicates directly with the inferior mesenteric artery supplying the descending colon and sigmoid. The most common variations in the origin and branching of the main colic arteries are illustrated in Fig. 102 a–f. A critical factor besides anatomic features is the state of health of the mesenteric arteries. Arteriosclerotic narrowing in older patients more commonly affects the inferior mesenteric artery than the superior mesenteric. The branches of the main colic arteries terminate directly or after further ramification in a marginal arcade that runs close to the bowel from the cecum to the sigmoid. If a main artery branches before joining the marginal arcade, it must be ligated proximal to the bifurcation when the segment is mobilized. This forms a secondary marginal arcade that contributes to the blood flow through the segment. Due to conflicting data from different authors, the literature provides only an approximate guide as to the areas of the colon in which the marginal arcade is well developed and continuous, and the areas where it is apt to be discontinuous. Thus, for example, prevalence figures from 1% [99] to 32% [51] are reported for the absence of a connection between the superior and inferior mesenteric arteries. The overall impression is that the marginal arcade of the left half of the colon is more consistent than on the right, with the greatest variability on the left side occurring in the junctional area between the left and middle colic arteries, and on the right side between the right colic and ileocolic arteries. We emphasize that the primary vessel and the marginal arcade should always be evaluated jointly. Adequate pulsation of the marginal artery at the proposed site of anastomosis of the colon segment to the esophagus says nothing about the viability of the segment unless the vascular connections that are to be divided have been tested by temporary occlusion. Vigorous pulsation at the proximal end of the intended transplant and the absence of cyanosis signify adequate circulation. Potential risk factors in terms of the venous drain-

Fig. 102 a–f. Variations in the vascular supply of the colon (modified from Netter). *1* Aorta, *2* duodenum, *3* superior mesenteric artery, *4* inferior mesenteric artery, *5* ileocolic artery, *6* right colic artery, *7* middle colic artery, *8* left colic artery, *9* sigmoid artery. **a** Common origin of the right colic and middle colic arteries. **b** Common origin of the right colic and ileocolic arteries. **c** Absence of the middle colic artery, which is replaced by a large branch from the left colic. **d** Absence of the right colic artery. **e** Branch of the middle colic artery to the left colic flexure. **f** Accessory middle colic artery to the left colic flexure (after Belsey [10]) ▷

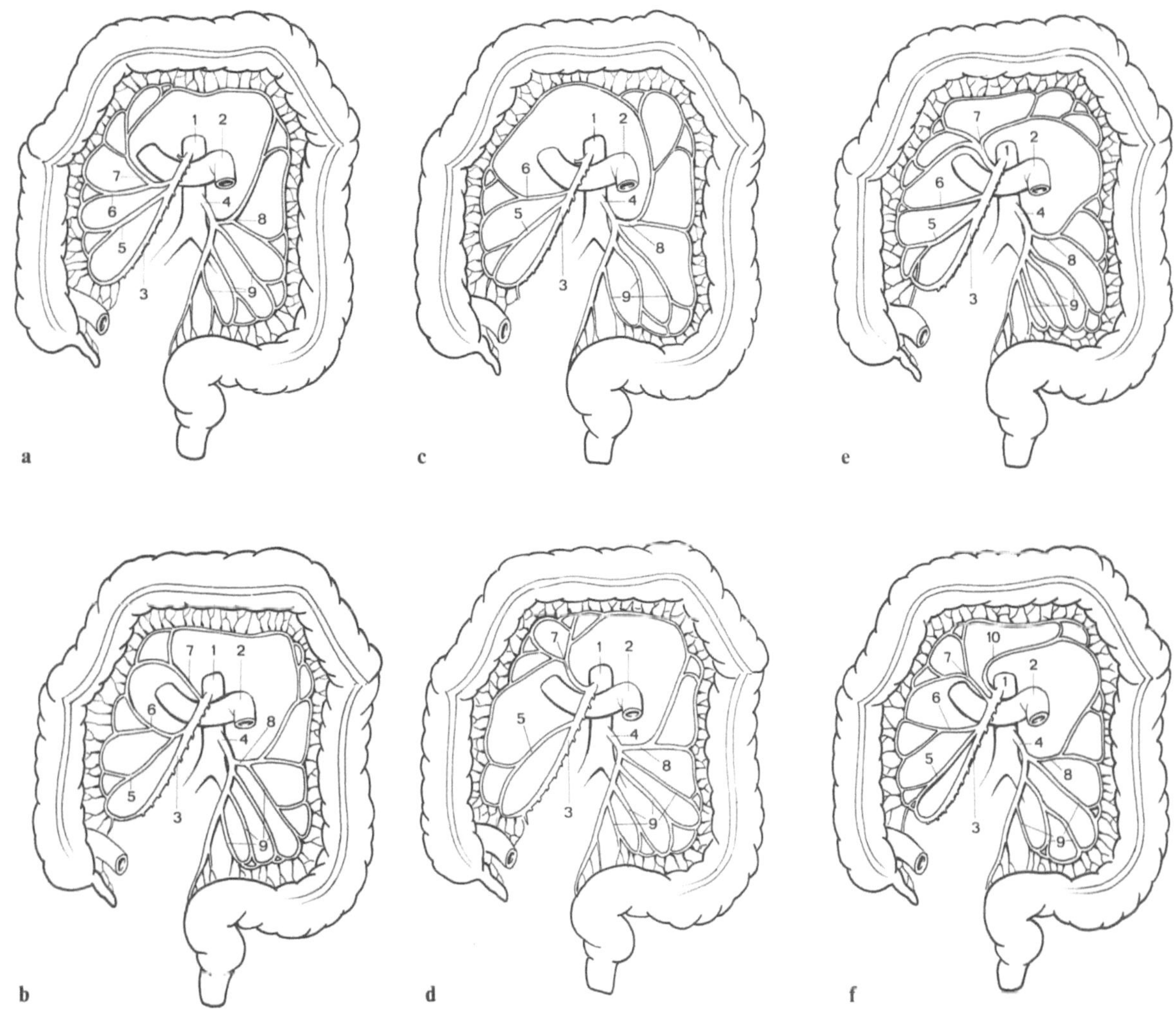

age of a colon transplant are, in decreasing frequency, the dichotomic arrangement of the veins of the right colon, the absence of a venous arcade along the ascending colon, a deficient caliber of the left colic vein, and an incomplete arcade in the transverse mesocolon [40].

7.5.2 Mobilization of an Isoperistaltic or Antiperistaltic Colon Transplant

Preoperative preparation: Prophylactic antibiotics, preoperative intestinal lavage (see Chap. C).

Instruments: Basic set, extra thoracic set, GIA, TA, EEA.

Position and approach: Midline laparotomy.

7.5.2.1 Mobilization of a Left Colon Isoperistaltic Transplant Based on the Left Colic Artery or Sigmoid Artery

The left colon transplant comprises the descending colon, left flexure, and as much of the transverse colon as the length of the interposition requires. The left colon is the most versatile colon segment for partial or total esophageal replacement and, in our estimation, the first choice for colon esophagoplasty (Fig. 103 a,b). Occasionally this part of the colon may be unfit for use in older patients, as it is more likely to contain diverticula or polyps than other segments, and the inferior mesenteric artery is more likely to be narrowed by arteriosclerosis.

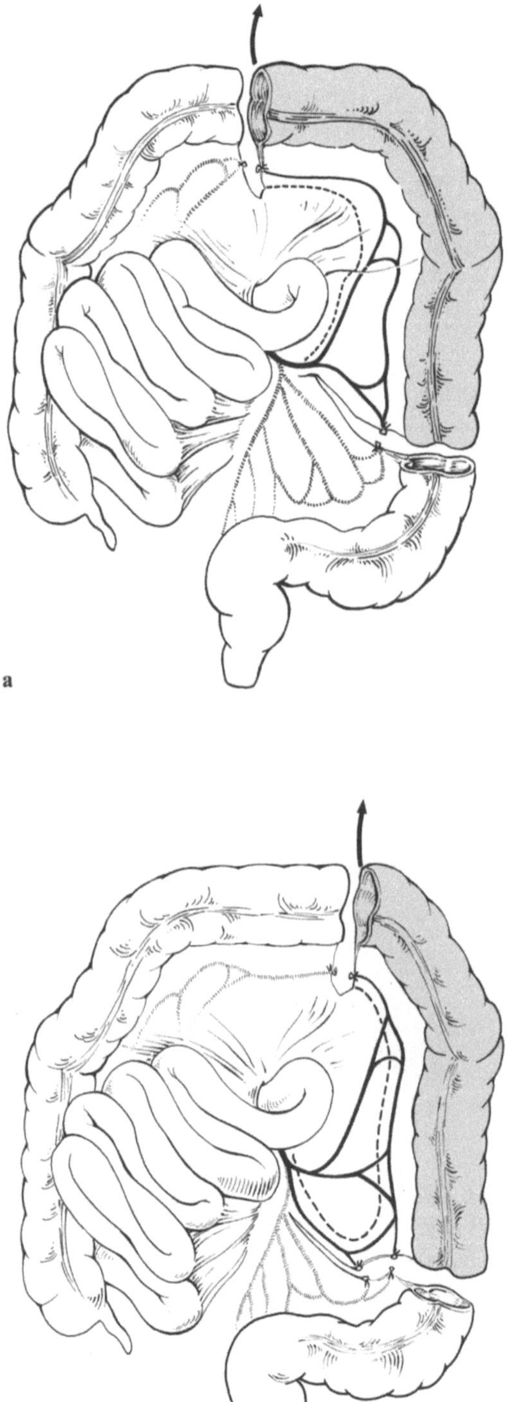

a

b

Fig. 103. a Mobilization of a left colon isoperistaltic transplant based on the left colic artery (schematic). **b** Mobilization of a left colon isoperistaltic transplant based on the sigmoid artery (schematic)

Steps in procedure:

(1) Inspection of the inferior mesenteric artery, descending colon, and transverse colon and their vascular arcades
(2) Detachment of the greater omentum from the transverse colon
(3) Division of the fascia fusion layer of Toldt
(4) Division of the splenocolic ligament
(5) Blunt mobilization of the descending colon and its vascular supply as far as the abdominal midline
(6) Identification of the main artery supplying the segment to be isolated (inferior mesenteric, sigmoid) using transillumination
(7) Determination of the proximal and distal sites of colon transection
(8) Incision of the peritoneal layers of the mesocolon along the proposed line of resection
(9) Selective ligation of the vessels in the mesentery on the line of the resection
(10) Clearing of the proposed proximal and distal sites of colon transection
(11) Transection of the colon at both sites with the GIA instrument
(12) Restoration of colon continuity by end-to-end anastomosis in front of the vascular pedicle of the isolated segment

Operative technique: The greater omentum is reflected superiorly, and the small intestine is covered with a moist gauze pad and displaced downward to the right. Then the left colon from the sigmoid to the midtransverse colon is examined for abnormalities, and the pulsations of the inferior mesenteric artery are palpated in the mesosigmoid about 2–3 fingerwidths above the aortic bifurcation. If the segment appears suitable, the attachments between the transverse colon and greater omentum are made tense and are divided while preserving the marginal arcades of the transverse colon and the middle colic artery. The descending colon is pulled medially to expose the white fusion line of Toldt, and the peritoneum along this line is divided with a scissors (Fig. 104 a). Rarely this layer may contain small vessels that require coagulation. When the left flexure is reached, it is mobilized from the lateral side. The splenocolic ligament is made tense by gentle downward traction on the descending and transverse colon, avoiding injury to the spleen. This ligament is divided between clamps, as it main contain vessels of large caliber. Starting from the peritoneal incision, the descending colon is freed from its loose posterior adhesions with a sponge stick while carefully preserving the underlying ureter, the left kidney, and the adrenal gland. The descending colon and its vessels can be mobilized without difficulty as far as the abdominal midline (Fig. 104 b), recapitulating the situation in utero. At this point the left colon is attached only to the medial layer of the peritoneum, which carries its vascular pedicle. The mobilized colon segment is now held up, and its mesentery is transilluminated to evaluate its vascular pattern. If the marginal arcade is discontinuous and is not satisfactorily bridged in that area by the branches of a main artery, the segment should not be used. If the arcade is continuous over the length of the segment, the mesentery on both sides of the vessels that are to be divided is incised with a scalpel so that the vessels can be temporarily occluded with soft vascular clamps. The occlusion should be maintained for about 10 min to confirm the adequacy of the blood supply. It should be noted, however, that temporary clamping is not a completely reliable indicator of transplant viability. Bringing up the colon segment for interposition profoundly alters the circulatory conditions in the transplant, and only a very copious blood supply with unimpaired drainage can ensure complication-free healing. The length of the segment to be isolated depends on the distance that must be spanned. This can be estimated or measured with a string, taking into accout the route that will be used for the reconstruction. The transplant may derive its arterial supply from the ascending or descending branch of the left colic artery or from the first sigmoid artery, depending on the caliber of the vessels. From that point the string is laid along the mesenteric attachment of the colon, and the proximal line of resection is determined. If this site appears satisfactory in terms of vascular supply, it is marked with a rubber-shod clamp. If only about a 15-cm segment is needed for replacement of the lower esophagus,

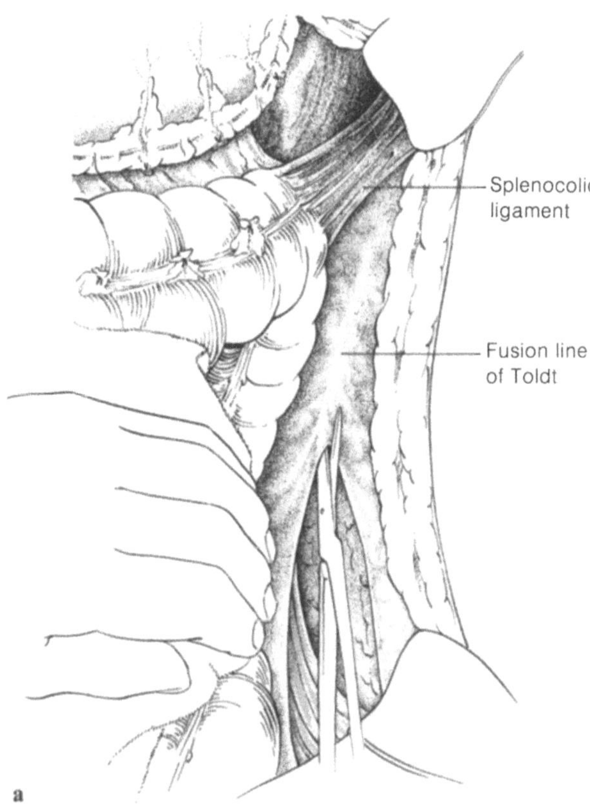

a

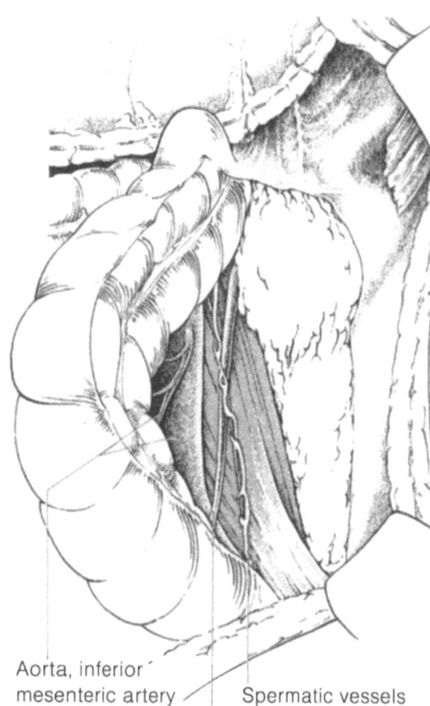

b

Fig. 104. a Mobilization of the left colon. The lateral attachment of the colon along the line of Toldt is divided, and the splenocolic ligament is severed. **b** The left colon is bluntly mobilized to the abdominal midline the descending colon is divided just distal to or between the ascending and descending branches of the left colic artery. Then the transverse colon is divided near the left flexure, leaving the right branch of the middle colic artery intact. When a long transplant is needed, Stelzner [86] recommends dividing the descending colon between the ascending and descending branches of the left colic artery. The colon also may be transected below the descending branch or distal to the first sigmoid artery [10]. Then, depending on the required length of the transplant, the transverse colon may be divided close to the right flexure or oral to it. In this case the middle colic artery is divided proximal to its point of division.

After the limits of the resection have been established, the mesocolon is transilluminated, and its serosal coat is incised with a scalpel. Distally the incision is carried over the marginal arcade to the base of the pedicle, i.e., to the origin of the artery that will supply the transplant. Proximally the incision is carried over the marginal arcade of the middle colic artery and then parallel to it. It is continued toward the vascular pedicle, preserving branchings of the middle colic artery close to the primary marginal arcade so they they can function as a "secondary" arcade. When the incisions have been completed, the colon is skeletonized at its proposed sites of transection, clearing about a 3-cm area at each site. The marginal arcades and the vessels in the marked area are cleared of fatty tissue by patty dissection so that the arteries and veins can be divided. Now the fatty tissue, which contains only a few small vessels, is divided with a scissors or electrocautery along the line previously drawn with the scalpel. This technique requires only a few selective ligations, the operating time is short, and little tissue remains that is prone to necrosis. Division of the mesentery with progressive ligation of the cut edges is less favorable, as it leads to plication and occasionally stasis in the venous limb. We do not transect the bowel proximally and distally until the mesentery has been divided down to the vascular pedicle. By dividing the colon after the pedicle has been mobilized, contamination is reduced. Gauze pads soaked in antiseptic are placed over the oral and aboral ends of the mobilized segment, and colon continuity is restored.

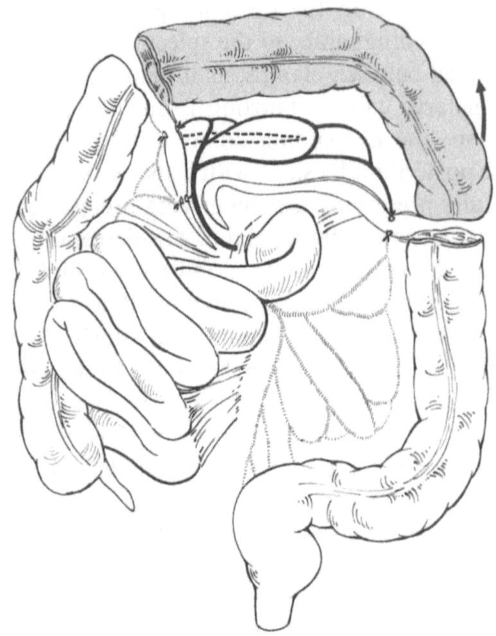

Fig. 105. Mobilization of a left colon antiperistaltic transplant based on the middle colic artery (schematic)

7.5.2.2 Mobilization of a Left Colon Antiperistaltic Transplant Based on the Middle Colic Artery

This transplant comprises the middle and left portion of the transverse colon, the left flexure, the descending colon, and also the proximal sigmoid colon if additional length is required (Fig. 105). The disadvantages of placing a colon segment in the antiperistaltic position were previously noted (see 7.1.2.3). The antiperistaltic left colon transplant is indicated only if the middle colic artery is very well developed, the left colic artery shows significant arteriosclerotic occlusion, and the marginal arcade of the ascending colon is discontinuous. The transverse and descending colon are mobilized as described in 7.5.2.1, except that the middle colic artery must be isolated to supply the transplant.

7.5.2.3 Mobilization of a Right Colon Isoperistaltic Transplant Based on the Middle Colic Artery

This segment includes the terminal ileum, cecum (with appendix removed), ascending colon, right

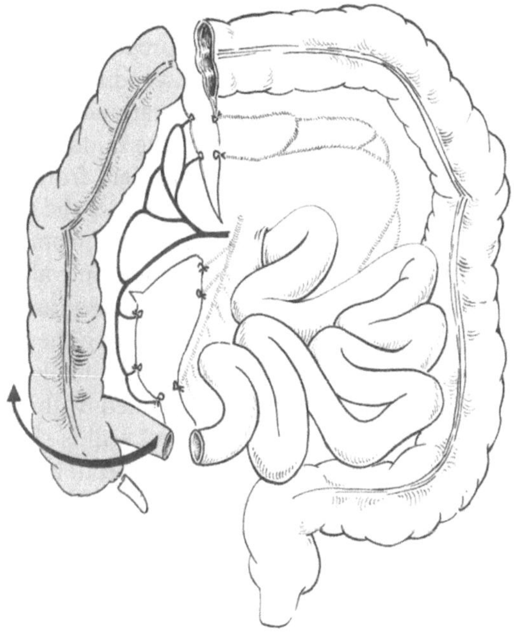

Fig. 106. Mobilization of a right colon isoperistaltic transplant based on the middle colic artery (schematic)

flexure, and proximal part of the transverse colon (Fig. 106). It can provide an isoperistaltic transplant as long as the left colon transplant described above. It is used when the descending colon is abnormal or diseased. An advantage of this transplant is that the caliber of the terminal ileum closely matches that of the esophagus. On the negative side, the marginal arcade may be poorly developed in the area between the ileocolic and right colic arteries. In addition, the cecum is bulky and may be unsightly when placed subcutaneously. There is disagreement as to whether the ileocecal valve should be regarded as an effective antireflux mechanism [23] or as a potential obstacle to the passage of food [63]. In the series of Scanlon and Stealy [77], no swallowing difficulties were reported in association with isoperistaltic interposition of the ileocolon. The ileocecal valve has been shown to retain its competence as a reflux barrier even when considerable external pressure is applied to the upper abdominal contents [23].

Operative technique: After general inspection of the colon, the middle colic artery is palpated. If it is found to be well developed, the greater omentum is detached from the transverse colon. The ascending colon is pulled medially to expose its attachment at the white line of Toldt, and the peritoneum is divided along that line with a scissors. The right flexure is mobilized from the lateral side. The hepatocolic ligament is made tense by gentle downward traction on the ascending and transverse colon and is divided between clamps, as it may contain large-caliber vessels. Starting from the peritoneal incision, the ascending colon is freed from its loose posterior attachments. Care is taken to preserve the second and third portions of the duodenum superiorly and the ureter inferiorly. The ascending colon and its vessels are mobilized to the vascular root at about the level of the abdominal midline. At this point the right colon is attached only to the medial layer of the peritoneum, which carries its vascular pedicle. The mobilized bowel segment is now held up, and its mesentery is transilluminated to evaluate its vascular pattern. Scanlon and Stealy [77] advise that particular attention be given to the calibers of the right colic and ileocolic arteries. They state that if both vessels are large, it is unlikely that the middle colic artery will be able to sustain the right colon. The most common pattern is for the middle, right, and ileocolic arteries to arise separately from the superior mesenteric. It is also common for the right and middle colic arteries or the middle colic and ileocolic arteries to display a common origin. If the terminal ileum is to be included in the transplant, the ileocolic artery must be divided near its origin. The mesentery on both sides of the vessel is incised close to the origin of the ileocolic artery and proximal to the bifurcation of the middle colic artery, and both arteries are occluded for about 10 min with a soft vascular clamp. While the effects of the occlusion are being observed, the appendix can be removed and its stump buried. The terminal ileum is transected 5–10 cm proximal to the ileocecal valve. The transverse colon is transected a handswidth distal to the junction of the middle colic artery with its marginal arcade. Using transillumination, the line of division of the mesocolon is marked with a scalpel. Starting from the small bowel, the line crosses the branch of the ileocolic artery that is distributed to the ileum. The incision continues along this vessel and over the main trunk of the ileocolic artery, then follows its branch to the colon (Fig. 107). The descending branch of the right colic artery is reached along the marginal arcade. If the right colic artery is found to have a common origin with the middle colic artery, it usually will not be necessary to ligate the middle colic. If the right colic and middle

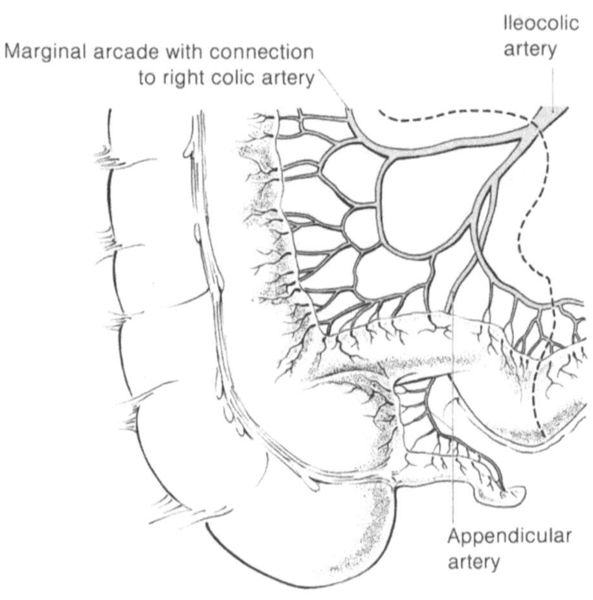

Fig. 107. Vascular supply of the ileocecal region with the proposed line of resection (dashed) for mobilization of the right colon

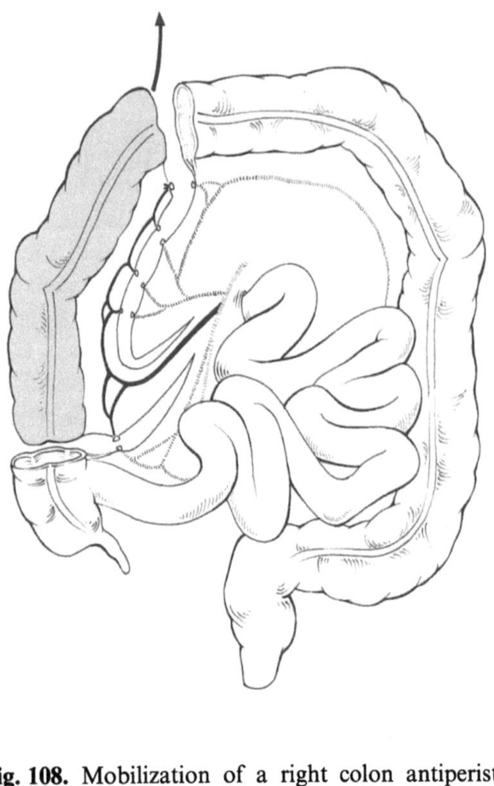

Fig. 108. Mobilization of a right colon antiperistaltic transplant based on the right colic artery

colic arteries have separate origins, the incision follows the branch to the first bifurcation, crosses it, and is continued along the ascending branch of the right colic artery to the marginal arcade and thence to the first branch of the middle colic artery, following the artery to its origin from the superior mesenteric. At the aboral end of the proposed transplant, the mesentery is incised from the bowel wall over the marginal arcade and along the left branch of the middle colic artery as far as its origin. The arteries and veins along the line of the incision are identified and individually divided. Then the mesocolon is divided with the scissors or electrocautery, the bowel wall is skeletonized at the proposed sites of transection, and the transections are performed with the GIA instrument. As the ileocecal region is a site of predilection for circulatory problems in the transplant, it is best to exclude the ileocolon if a satisfactory reconstruction can be accomplished without it.

7.5.2.4 Mobilization of a Right Colon Antiperistaltic Transplant Based on the Right Colic Artery

The segment to be mobilized consists of the ascending colon, right flexure, and portions of the transverse colon (Fig. 108). The disadvantages of an antiperistaltic transplant were noted previously. The technique for mobilizing the right colon and right flexure is the same as described in 7.5.2.3, except that the segment is based on the right colic vessels.

7.5.2.5 Mobilization of a Transverse Colon Isoperistaltic Transplant Based on the Middle Colic Artery

A transverse colon segment based on the middle colic artery (Fig. 109) is easily mobilized and is excellent for replacing the lower esophagus or occasionally even the whole esophagus when interposed in the isoperistaltic position. The segment should be at least 15 cm long in order to prevent gastroesophageal reflux. Including both flexures in the transplant creates a situation identical to that described for mobilization of the left or right colon.

Operative technique: The greater omentum is detached from the transverse colon. The latter is held up and its mesentery transilluminated to evaluate the course of the middle colic artery and its marginal arcades. The necessary length of the transplant is determined. For an isoperistaltic reconstruction, the colon is divided proximally as far as necessary from the trunk of the middle colic artery. If the right flexure is to be included in the transplant, first the ascending colon is mobilized and the hepatocolic ligament is divided from the lateral side. The entire ascending colon should be mobilized, regardless of how much of it is to be included in the transplant, as this will be necessary in any case to reestablish the continuity of the large bowel. Distally the colon is divided several centimeters from the trunk of the middle colic artery. Under transillumination, the line of division is marked with a scalpel in the serosa of the transverse mesocolon. At each end of the proposed segment the incision runs from the bowel over the marginal arcade and turns toward the middle colic artery, following its branches and then its main trunk to its origin from the superior mesenteric. The vessels along the incision line are separately ligated and divided. The bowel wall is skeletonized at the designated sites, and the mesocolon is divided along the preplaced incision line with the scissors or electrocautery. Then the bowel segment is resected with the GIA instrument.

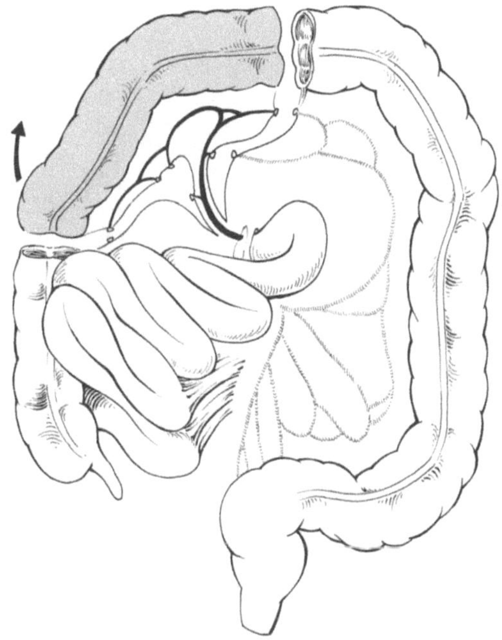

Fig. 109. Mobilization of a transverse colon isoperistaltic transplant based on the middle colic artery

7.5.3 Restoration of Bowel Continuity

After mobilization of the colon segment, bowel continuity is reestablished by an end-to-end anastomosis between the ileum and transverse colon or between the remaining parts of the colon. The anastomosis is performed in front of the vascular pedicle of the isolated segment. Whereas the ileum is mobile enough to be anastomosed without further measures, a tension-free reanastomosis of the two colon halves will require mobilization of one flexure or of an entire division of the colon, depending on the length and position of the isolated segment. The right or left colic flexure is mobilized from the lateral aspect. The ligaments that unite the colon to the liver or to the spleen are divided between clamps and ligated. After division of the lateral attachment along the line of Toldt, both parts of the colon are bluntly freed from their retroperitoneal attachments until their stapled ends can be approximated without tension. The anastomosis is performed like a small bowel anastomosis, using a two-layer technique with a continuous mucosa-to-mucosa suture (see 7.4.6.1). If significant luminal discrepancy exists, it can be corrected by incorporating transverse sutures in the larger member and longitudinal sutures in the smaller member or by making a 1- to 2-cm longitudinal incision in the antimesenteric side of the smaller member. When the anastomosis has been completed, its patency is checked by invaginating the anterior bowel wall through the suture line between the thumb and forefinger. The rest of the mesenteric incision is closed with simple interrupted sutures, making certain that the vascular supply is not damaged or caught in the suture line.

7.5.4 Intraabdominal Transfer of the Mobilized Colon Segment

The advantages and disadvantages of the pre- and retrogastric routes of transplantation were discussed in a previous section (see 7.2.1). We generally bring the colon segment up posterior to the stomach (Fig. 110). The omental bursa is already opened at this point due to the earlier detachment of the greater omentum from the transverse colon. The greater curvature of the stomach is held up, and its posterior wall is bluntly freed from adhe-

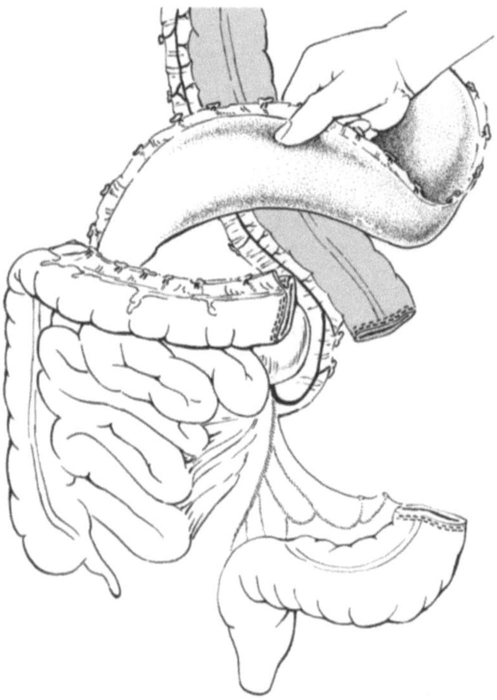

Fig. 110. Intraabdominal transfer of the mobilized colon segment. The left colon is brought up posterior to the transverse colon and stomach for the anastomosis

Fig. 111. Cologastric anastomosis. The posterior suture line is placed, the stomach is opened, and the stapled end of the colon segment is excised

sions with the retroperitoneum. We prefer to anastomose the colon to the anterior wall of the stomach, and for this it is necessary to divide the lesser omentum above the gastric arcade. This is not necessary if the colon is to be anastomosed to the posterior gastric wall and placed transpleurally. If the esophageal resection is planned for the same operation, it is recommended that the necessary abdominal phase be completed before the colon segment is transposed. The fewer manipulations are needed after the intraabdominal transfer of the segment, the lower the risk of injury to the segment.

7.5.5 Anastomosing the Colon to the Stomach

The cologastric anastomosis is performed before the transplant is elevated into position. We anastomose the colon to the center of the anterior wall of the body of the stomach. This procedure is technically simple and minimizes angulation of the intraabdominal part of the transplant. Before the anastomosis is started, the general course of the vascular pedicle is examined to make certain it is straight and untwisted. The anastomosis is either performed with the EEA stapling instrument (see 1.3.3.3) introduced through a gastrotomy or an antimesenteric incision in the colon, or it is performed manually in two layers, as we prefer

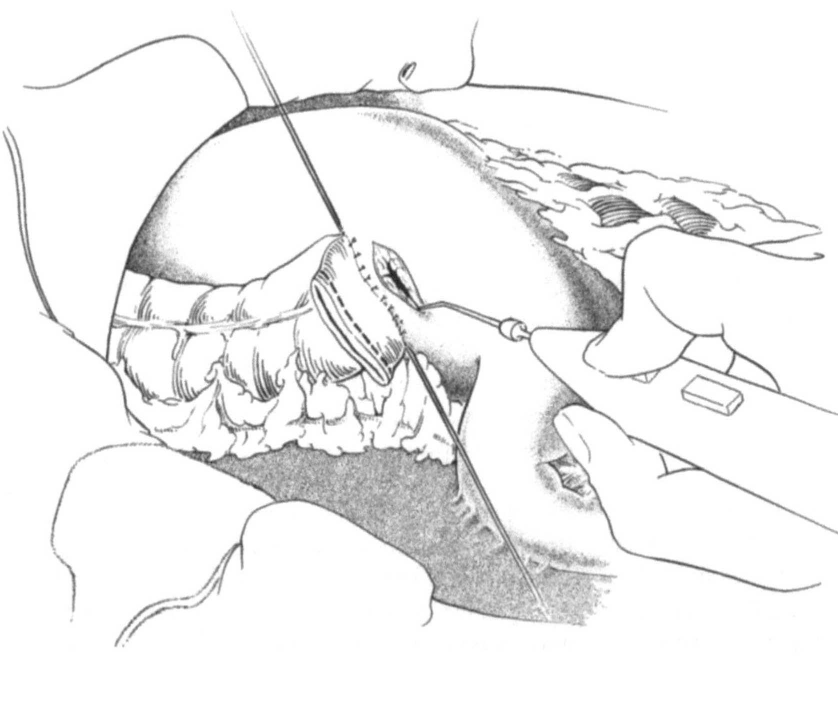

(Fig. 111). The gastrotomy or enterotomy made for insertion of the EEA instrument is closed with the TA stapler or with interrupted inverting sutures.

7.5.6 Bringing Up the Colon Segment for Anastomosis to the Esophagus

The technique for the subcutaneous, retrosternal, or transpleural placement of an esophageal substitute is described in 7.2. The transpleural route is indicated for segmental replacement of the lower esophagus. For a long colon interposition with a cervical anastomosis, we prefer the retrosternal route. Regardless of the route selected, the mesenteric attachment should be on the right side for an isoperistaltic reconstruction and on the left side for an antiperistaltic reconstruction.

7.5.7 Anastomosing the Colon to the Esophagus

After the colon segment has been pulled into position for the anastomosis, its proximal end should be closely inspected for signs of venous congestion or deficient arterial perfusion. If there is doubt as to the viability of the upper end of the transplant, it should be brought out as a stoma, either into the cervical incision next to the distal end of the esophagus or at a separate site. Alternatively, the posterior part of the anastomosis may be constructed and the anterior part sutured into the skin incision to create a stoma. The definitive esophagocolic anastomosis is then performed in a second operation 2–3 weeks later. If a single-stage operation is feasible, redundant bowel should be resected from the mobilized segment for an end-to-end anastomosis so that the substitute will be straight and free of tension. For an end-to-side anastomosis, several centimeters of redundant bowel is acceptable. Neither type of anastomosis is essentially superior to the other. Both can be performed mechanically (see 1.3.3.3) or manually (see 1.3.3.2). We prefer the manual technique in the neck and perform a two-layer anastomosis consisting of an outer row of interrupted inverting sutures and an inner, continuous suture row that incorporates only the mucosa and submucosa. When the anastomosis is completed, a soft Penrose drain is placed in the wound area, and the skin is closed without placing separate approximating sutures in the muscle or fascia.

7.5.8 Methods of Reinforcing the Esophagocolic Anastomosis

The same principles apply to reinforcement of the esophagocolic anastomosis as to other types of reconstruction. A well-perfused transplant united to the esophagus without tension by a flawless suture technique is the best safeguard against anastomotic disruption. Anastomoses at some levels can be covered over with pleura or portions of the greater omentum (see 1.4), although we do not recognize any indications for this. When the colon is transplanted by the transpleural route, the anastomosis can be protected from tension by fixing an avascular part of the mesentery to the mediastinal pleura or prevertebral fascia with a few interrupted sutures. This type of fixation is unnecessary when the subcutaneous or retrosternal route is used.

7.5.8.1 *Reinforcing an End-to-End Anastomosis*

The suture line of an end-to-end esophagocolic anastomosis can be covered by invagination (see 1.6.5). The colon segment is mobilized with about a 3-cm excess of bowel at its upper end, and the anastomosis is performed. Then the seromuscular coat of the colon segment is grasped a certain distance from the suture line, depending on the amount of excess bowel available, is advanced onto the muscular coat of the esophagus, and is fixed an equal distance above the suture line with a circumferential row of 6–8 sutures.

7.5.8.2 *Reinforcing an End-to-Side Anastomosis*

In theory at least, the same principles apply to reinforcing an end-to-side esophagocolic anastomosis as to an esophagojejunal anastomosis (see 7.4.11). However, limitations of space and of available redundant bowel generally allow only a limited plication that covers only the anterior side of the anastomosis. The redundant colon is placed over the suture line and fixed to the esophagus or adjacent structures with a few interrupted sutures. In a broad sense, the temporary ileostomy that has been described in connection with interposition of an ileocolic segment [48] represents another approach to anastomotic protection. Given sufficient material, the technique is applicable to other types of colon transplant (Fig. 112). After an end-to-side anastomosis has been performed

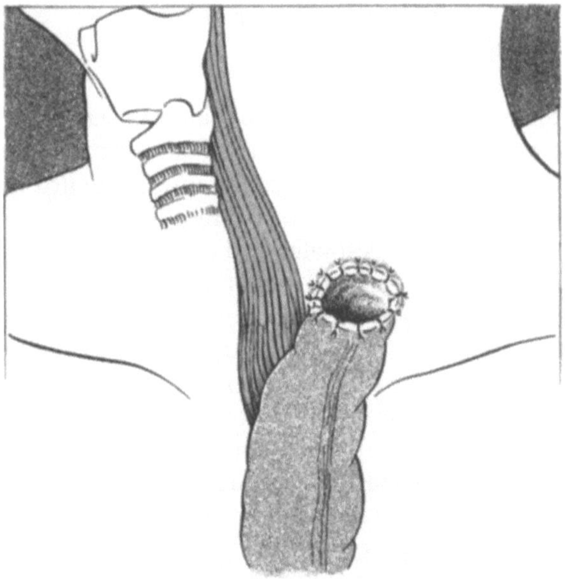

Fig. 112. A temporary colostomy is constructed following an end-to-side esophagocolic anastomosis

between the esophagus and colon segment, the upper end of the segment is brought out at the neck as a stoma. A stomach tube is passed through the stoma into the transplant to provide decompression and to make certain that the transplant is viable. If the stoma does not close spontaneously within a few weeks, it is excised and closed with sutures.

References

1. Akiyama H, Hiyama M, Hashimoto C (1976) Resection and reconstruction for carcinoma of the thoracic ösophagus. Br J Surg 63
2. Akiyama H, Miyazono H, Tsurumaru M, Hashimoto C, Kawamura T (1978) Use of the stomach as an esophageal substitute. Ann Surg 188:606
3. Allgöwer M, Burri C (1968) Zur Technik der Pyloroplastik. Chirurg 11:39
4. Androsov PI (1956) Blood supply of mobilized intestine used for an artificial esophagus. Arch Surg 73:917
5. Bakymjian VY (1968) Total reconstruction of pharynx with medially based deltopectoral skin flap. NY State J Med 68:2771
6. Baranofsky IE, Edelman S, Kreel J, Baens H (1960) Surgical techniques. The use of the left colon for esophageal replacement. J Mount Sinai Hosp NY 27:88
7. Barlow TE, Bentley FH, Waldner DN (1981) Arteries, veins and arteriovenous anastomoses in the human stomach. Surg Gynecol Obstet 93:657
8. Beck C, Carrel A (1905) Demonstration of specimens illustrating a method of formation of a prethoracic esophagus. Ill Med J 7:463
9. Belsey R, Hiebert CA (1974) An exclusive right thoracic approach for cancer of the middle third of the esophagus. Ann Thorac Surg 18:1
10. Belsey RHR (1981) Esophageal reconstruction. In: Keen G (ed) Operative Surgery and Management. Wright PSG Bristol London Boston
11. Berman EF (1952) The plastic esophagus. J Internat Coll Surg 18:695
12. Bircher E (1907) Ein Beitrag zur plastischen Bildung eines neuen Ösophagus. Zentralbl Chirurgie 34:1479
13. Chassin JL (1978) Esophagogastrectomy: Data favouring end-to-side anastomosis. Ann Surg 188:22
14. Daeneke HJ (1980) Die oto-rhino-laryngologischen Operationen im Mund- und Halsbereich. Springer, Berlin Heidelberg New York
15. Deucher F, Widmer A (1967) Speiseröhre. In: Brunner A, Zenker R (red. von) Die Eingriffe an der Brust und in der Brusthöhle. Springer, Berlin Heidelberg New York (Allgemeine und spezielle chirurgische Operationslehre, 2 neubearb Aufl, Bd VI/1, S 714)
16. Ellis FH JR (1980) Esophagogastrectomy for carcinoma. Technical considerations based on anatomic location of lesion. Surg Clin North Am 60:265
17. Fink F (1913) Über plastischen Ersatz der Speiseröhre. Zbl Chir 40:545
18. Fisher RD, Brawley RK, Kieffer RF (1972) Esophagogastrectomy in the treatment of carcinoma of the distal two-third of the esophagus. Ann Thorac Surg 14:6
19. Gavriliu D (1955) Direct visceral esophagoplastic. Chirurgica (Buc) 104
20. Gavriliu D (1975) Aspects of esophageal surgery. Curr Probl Surg 12:1
21. Graham RR (1940) Technique for total gastrectomy. Surgery 8:257
22. Grimes OF (1967) Surgical reconstruction of the diseased esophagus, Part I. Surgery 61:325
23. Grimes OF (1967) Surgical reconstruction of the diseased esophagus. Part II. Surgery 61:487
24. Gütgemann A, Schreiber HW, Bernhard A (1963) Erfahrungen mit der totalen Gastrektomie. Langenbecks Arch Klin Chir 303:73
25. Heimlich HJ, Winfield JM (1955) The use of a gastric tube to replace or bypass the esophagus. Surgery 37:549
26. Heimlich HJ (1975) Reversed gastric tube esophagoplasty for failure of colon, jejunum and prostetic interpositions. Ann Surg 182:154
27. Herzen P (1908) Eine Modifikation der Roux'schen Ösophagojejunostomie. Zb Chir 35:219
28. Hirsch M (1911) Plastischer Ersatz des Ösophagus aus dem Magen. Zbl Chir 38:1561
29. Hirsch DM, Neville WE (1968) Total esophageal replacement with a segment of ileum. J Thorac Cardiovasc Surg 55:211

30. Holle F, Hart W, Parchwitz HV (1963) Die Fundektomie des Magens. Neuere Erfahrungen und Modifikationen. Chir Praxis 7:351
31. Hong PW, Seel DJ, Dietrick RB (1967) The use of colon in the repair of benigne stricture of the esophagus. Pacific Med Surg 74:148
32. Hunt CJ (1952) Construction of food pouch from segment of jejunum as substitute from stomach in total gastrectomy. Arch Surg 64:601
33. Javid H (1952) Bridging of esophageal defects with fresh and preserved aortic grafts. Surg Forum 3:82
34. Jones EL, Booth DJ, Cameron JL (1971) Functional evaluation of esophageal reconstructions. Ann Thorac Surg 12:331
35. Kakegawa T, Tsuzuki T, Sasaki T (1973) Primary pharyngogastrostomy for carcinoma of the esophagus situated in the cervico thoracic segment. Surgery 73:226
36. Keller HW, Müller JM, Schmitz M, Brenner U (1984) Lebensbedrohliche Komplikationen nach Splenektomie. Leber Magen Darm 14:18
37. Kelling G (1911) Ösophagusplastik mit Hilfe des Quercolons. Zbl Chir 38:1209
38. Mc Keown KC (1981) Resection of midesophageal carcinoma with esophagogastric anastomosis. World J Surg 5:517
39. Kirschner MB (1920) Ein neues Verfahren der Ösophagusplastik. Langenbecks Arch Klin Chir 114:606
40. Kralik J, Turek K (1967) Die Wichtigkeit des venösen Abflusses aus dem zur Ösophagoplastik verwendeten Kolontransplantat. Zbl Chir 44:2772
41. Kügeler S (1978) Ein Beitrag zur Antirefluxplastik bei intrathorakaler termino-lateraler Ösophago-Gastrostomie. Der Chirurg 47:408
42. Lafargue P, Dufour R, Cabanie H, Chavannaz I (1951) Ileocolo-oesophagoplastice. Mem Acad Chir 77:420
43. Lam KH, Lim STK, Wong J, Lam SK, Ong GB (1979) Gastric histology and function in patients with intrathoracic stomach replacement after esophagectomy. Surgery 85:283
44. Linder F, Hecker WC (1962) Ösophagusersatz durch Colon. Der Chirurg 33:18
45. Longmire WP, Ravitch MM (1946) A new method for constructing an artificial esophagus. Ann Surg 123:819
46. Longmire WP, Beal JM (1952) Construction of an substitute gastric reservoir following total gastrectomy. Ann Surg 135:637
47. Lortat-Jacob JL, Fekete F (1961) Un procédé pour éviter le reflux après résection oesophage-gastrique. Surgery 50:600
48. Maingot R (1974) Abdominal operations. Appleton-Century-Grafts 6. Vol Englewood NY
49. Maki T (1969) Ergebnisse der totalen Gastrektomie beim Magenkarzinom. Langenbecks Arch Chir 325:450
50. Merendino KA, Dillard DH (1955) The concept of sphincter substitution by an interposed jejunal segment for anatomic and physiologic abnormalities at the esophago gastric junction. Ann Surg 142:486
51. Michels E (1982) Evaluation and research in physical therapy. Phys Therapy 62:6, 828
52. Mikulicz J (1888) Zur operativen Behandlung des stenosierenden Magengeschwürs. Arch Klin Chir 37:39
53. Miller H, Lam KH, Ong GB (1975) Observations of pressure waves in stomach, jejunal and colonic loops used to replace the esophagus. Surgery 78:543
54. Mullen DC, Postlethweith RW, Dillon ML (1970) Complications of substernal colon interposition. Am Surg 36:80
55. Nakayama K, Yazava C, Sakakibara N (1971) A report on three cases with carcinoma developing after antethoracic reconstructive surgery of the esophagus. Surgery 69:800
56. Neuhoff H, Ziegler JM (1922) Experimental reconstruction of the esophagus by granulation tubes. Surg Gynecol Obstet 34:767
57. Ohsawa T (1933) The surgery of the esophagus. Arch Jap Chir 10:605
58. Okada N, Kuriyama T, Umemoto H (1974) Esophageal surgery: A procedure for posterior invagination esophago-gastrostomy in one stage without positional change. Ann Surg 179:27
59. Ong GB (1971) Resection and reconstruction of the esophagus. Curr Probl Surg 8:1
60. Ong GB (1973) The Kirschner operation – A forgotten procedure. Brit J Surg 60:221
61. Orsoni P, Toupet A (1950) Utilization du colon descendant et de la partie gauche du colon transverse l'oesophagoplastice pour prethoracique. Presse méd 804
62. Paulino F (1969) Esophagectomy with high intrathoracic esophagogastric anastomosis for benign stenosis of the esophagus. In: Cooper P (ed) The craft of surgery, vol I. Little Brown Boston, p 453
63. Petrov BA (1959) Retrosternal artificial esophagus from jejunum and colon. Surgery 45:890
64. Pichlmaier H (1973) The pathophysiology of the esophagus and its replacement. In: Sörensen HP (ed) The function of the esophagus. Odense University Press
65. Popow WI, Filin WI (1961) Free translation of the intestine for the reconstruction of the esophagus. Zbl Chir 86:1745
66. Postlethwait RW (1979) Technique for isoperistaltic gastric tube for esophageal bypass. Ann Surg 189:673
67. Ramstedt C (1912) Zur Operation der angeborenen Pylorusstenose. Mschr Kinderheilk 11:409
68. Rehbein F (1976) Kinderchirurgische Operationen. Hippokrates, Stuttgart
69. Rienhoff WT (1946) Intrathoracic esophagojejunostomy to lesions of the upper third of the esophagus. South Med J 39:928
70. Rob CG, Bateman GH (1949) Reconstruction of the trachea and cervical esophagus. Br J Surg 37: 202
71. Roith O (1924) Die einzeitige antethorakale Ösophagoplastik aus dem Dickdarm. Deutsch 2. Chir 183:419
72. Rooney BP (1969) The blood supply of the colon in esophageal replacement. Br J Surg Sci 2:301
73. Roux C (1907) L'oesophago-jejuno-gastrostomose, nouvelle opération pour rétrécissement infranchissable de l'oesophage. Sem méd (Paris) 27:37

74. Rudler JC, Monod Broca PH (1951)Un cas d'oesophagoplastic palliative retrosternale avec l'iléocolon droit. Mem Acad Chir 77:747
75. Rutkowski M (1923) Oesophagoplastica totalis. Pol Przegl Chir
76. Sauerbruch F (1905) Anastomose zwischen Magen und Speiseröhre und die Resektion des Brustabschnitts der Speiseröhre. Zbl Chir 32:81
77. Scanlon EF, Stealy CJ (1970) The use of the ascending and right half of the transverse colon in esophagoplasty. Surg Gynecol Obstet 107:101
78. Schlatter C (1897) Über Ernährung und Verdauung nach vollständiger Entfernung des Magens beim Menschen. Brun's Breit Klin Chir 19:757
79. Schrader CP, Koslowski L, Fline U, Konold P (1971) Vergleichende tierexperimentelle Untersuchungen über die Bildung eines Nahrungsreservoirs, seines Ernährungstyps und seiner Auswirkung auf die Fettresorption. Langenbecks Arch Klin Chir 329:242
80. Schreiber HW, Eichfuss HP, Fahrtmann E, Eckat P (1975) Ösophagojejunostomie. Langenbecks Arch Chir 338:159
81. Schuring AE, Rag JW (1966) Experimental use of dacron as an esophageal prothesis. Am Otol Rhinol Laryngol 75:202
82. Seidenberg B, Rosenak SG, Hurwit EG, Jam ML (1959) Immediate reconstruction of the cervical esophagus by a revascularized isolated jejunal segment. Ann Surg 149:162
83. Seo T (1942) Technik der totalen Gastrektomie mit Ersatzmagen. Nippon Rinsko Geka Ikai Lasski (Jap) 6:4
84. Siewert JR, Peiper HJ, Jennewein HM, Waldeck F (1973) Die Oesophago-Jejunoplicatio. Chirurg 44:115
85. Skinner DB (1980) Esophageal reconstruction. Am J Surg 139:810
86. Stelzner F (1970) Der Ersatz der Speiseröhre durch das linke Colon. In: Breitner B (Hrsg) Chirurgische Operationslehre II Ergänzung 1970, Urban & Schwarzenberg, München Berlin Wien
87. Stelzner F, Kunath U (1977) Ergebnisse bei ösophago-intestinalen Anastomosen und Untersuchungen der Durchblutung des dafür mobilisierten Magens. Chirurg 48:651
88. Sugimachi K, Yaita A, Keo H, Natsuda Y, Inokuchi K (1983) A safer and more reliable operative technique for esophageal reconstruction using a gastric tube. Am J Surg 140:471
89. Sweet R (1950) Thoracic surgery. Saunders, Philadelphia London
90. Thomas DM, Langford RM, Russell RCG, Le Quesne LP (1979) The anatomical basis for gastric mobilization in total ösophagectomy. Br J Surg 66:230
91. Tomoda M (1962) Technik der totalen Gastrektomie mit Ersatzmagen. Chirurg 23:264
92. Vulliet H (1911) De l'oesophagoplastic et des divers modifications. Sem méd (Paris) 31:529
93. Watanabe K, Mark JBD (1971) Segmental replacement of the thoracic esophagus with a silastic prothesis. Am J Surg 121:238
94. Waterston DJ (1964) Colonic replacement of esophagus (intrathoracic). Surg Clin N Amer 44:1441
95. Withers EH, Franklin JD, Madden JJ, Lynch JB (1979) Pectoralis maior myocutaneous island flap for reconstruction of the head and neck. Head Neck Surg 1:293
96. Wookey H (1942) The surgical treatment of carcinoma of the pharynx and upper esophagus. Surg Gynecol Obstet 75:499
97. Yamagishi M, Ikeda N, Yonemoto T (1970) An isoperistaltic gastric tube. Arch Surg 100:689
98. Yudin S (1944) The surgical construction of 80 cases of artificial esophagus. Surg Gynecol Obstet 78:561
99. Zängl A (1964) Experimentelle und klinische Untersuchungen zur Gefäßversorgung der linken Colonhälfte. Wien Klin Wschr 47:76

8 Enucleation or Local Excision of Benign Tumors and Cysts of the Esophagus

CONTENTS

8.1 Frequency, Classification, Indication for Surgery

Benign tumors and cysts of the esophagus are causative in only 0.1% of patients who are treated for dysphagia [6]. Their prevalence even in large autopsy series is reported to be less than 0.5% [7]. Most solid tumors of the esophagus are of mesenchymal origin, and most cystic lesions are of epithelial origin. The most common benign esophageal tumor is the leiomyoma, accounting for 60%–85% of all benign neoplasms and up to 95% of all intramural benign neoplasms of the esophagus [3, 8]. Leiomyomas are followed in frequency by congenital or acquired cysts, lipomas and fibromas, and tumors of neurogenic or vascular origin. Adenomas, papillomas, lymphangiomas, myxofibromas, granular cell tumors, and amyloid tumors are rare.

A distinction is made therapeutically between pedunculated or sessile tumors of the esophageal mucosa and tumors that have an extramucosal, intramural localization. The latter types are extremely unlikely to undergo malignant change [4], so the indication for surgery is based on the tendency of the tumor to enlarge and on positive confirmation of its identity. Biopsy is contraindicated for hemangioma due to the potential for severe hemorrhage, and it is not advised for intramural tumors since the associated mucosal injury would complicate or prevent submucosal enucleation of the tumor.

8.2 Intramural Tumors

Given their smooth-muscle origin, leimyomas are most commonly encountered in the lower and middle thirds of the esophagus. Cysts also occur most frequently in the lower third [2, 3].

Both types of lesion are diagnosed radiographically. The role of esophagoscopy is to examine the mucosa so that the most appropriate surgical treatment–enucleation or resection–can be established preoperatively. If the mucosa has been injured by biopsy, it is recommended that the defect be allowed to heal before a surgical procedure is carried out. Mucosa that is ulcerated over the tumor (common with leiomyomas of the esophagogastric junction) will not heal spontaneously, and so esophageal resection becomes the primary treatment of choice.

8.2.1 Enucleation of a Tumor or Cyst from the Esophageal Wall

Preoperative preparation: See Chap. C.

Instruments: Basic set, extra thoracic set as required; stomach tube (Ch 32); gastroscope.

Position and approach: Tumors of the cervical esophagus are approached through an incision along the anterior border of the sternocleidomastoid muscle (see 2.1.1). For intrathoracic tumors, the level and side of the thoracotomy depends on the location and extent of the neoplasm. We prefer to approach tumors of the lower third of the esophagus through a left posterolateral thoracotomy in the sixth or seventh interspace. For tumors of the middle or upper thoracic esophagus, we perform a right posterolateral thoracotomy in the fourth or fifth interspace (see Chap. B).

Operative technique: The location of the tumor is established, and the involved portion of the esophagus is exposed and encircled with a snare (see 2.1.1 or 2.1.2). Small, soft tumors can be made

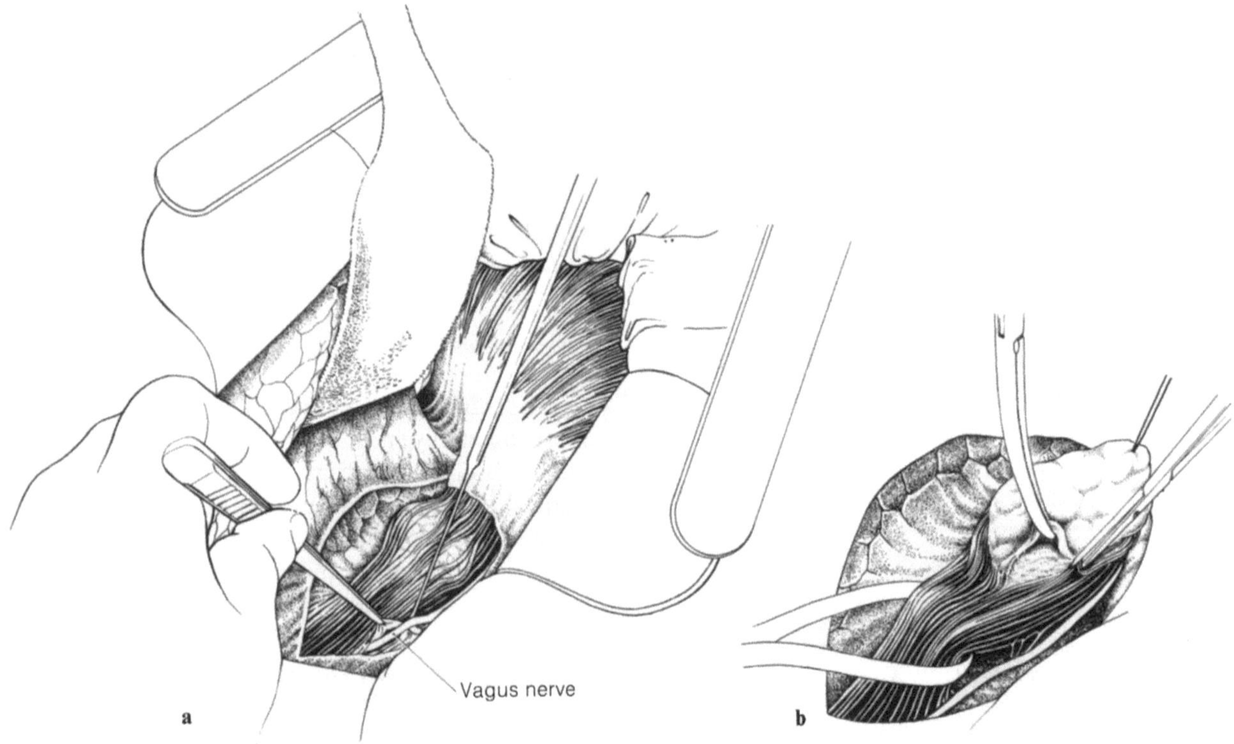

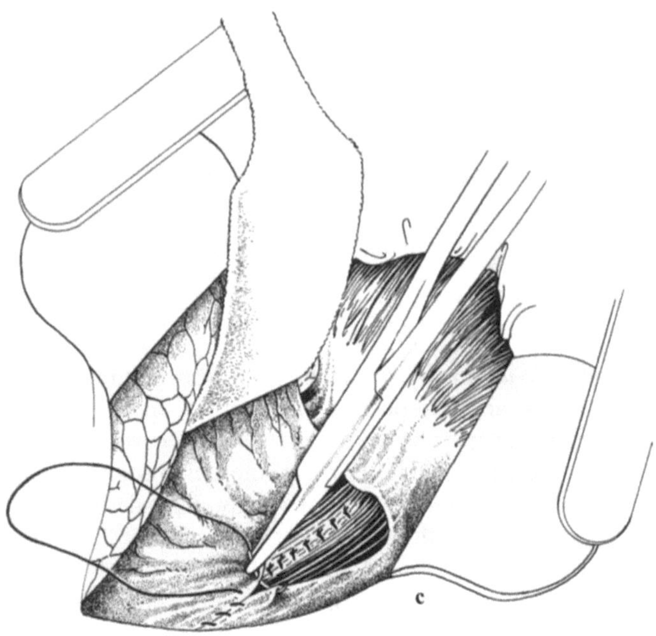

Fig. 113a–c. Enucleation of a benign intramural tumor of the esophagus. a The tumor is exposed. The vagus nerve is carefully dissected from the neoplasm. b The tumor is shelled out from the esophageal wall. c The mediastinal pleura is closed by continuous suture. If possible, the defect left by the enucleation is closed by reapproximation of the muscle and pleura

palpable by advancing the stomach tube into the esophagus. Gastroscopy may be performed if desired. Usually the tumor is covered by a thin muscular layer. This is bluntly split apart in the direction of its fibers, avoiding vagus nerve injury, until the tumor is visualized (Fig. 113 a). Most tumors are encapsulated, are not firmly adherent to the mucosa, and can be bluntly enucleated from the surrounding muscle with little difficulty. Dissecting the tumor from the mucosa requires special care and good exposure. Fibrous attachments between the tumor and mucosa are made tense by elevating the tumor and are divided close to the lesion with a scissors (Fig. 113 b). If a biopsy has been performed, inflammatory adhesions will exist between the mucosa and tumor. In these cases mucosal injury may be unavoidable during the enucleation, and the defect is closed at once by continuous suture. After removal of the tumor the muscularis is reapproximated over the surgical defect with several interrupted sutures, and the pleura is closed over it with a continuous suture (Fig. 113 c).

In all but a few cases, surgical removal of an esophageal cyst is conducted in the same fashion as for an intramural tumor. Very rarely a common wall may exist between the cyst and the esophagus [1], making it necessary to aspirate the cyst contents and sharply remove the portion of the cyst that is not fused to the esophagus. The raw surface left by the excision is covered over by muscularis or parietal pleura.

The removal of large leiomyomas may be followed by a disturbance of esophageal motility with pronounced dysphagic complaints. This led Lortat-Jacob [5] to suggest that an extramucosal esophagomyotomy be performed after the enucleation of these lesions.

8.2.2 Segmental Resection of the Esophagus for the Removal of a Benign Tumor

Rarely, ulceration of the mucosa can make it impossible to remove a leimyoma at the esophagogastric junction by enucleation, and primary segmental resection of the esophagus may be indicated (see I 6). The defect is reconstructed in the same sitting by the free interposition of a pedicled segment of jejunum (see 7.4).

8.3 Removal of Pedunculated or Sessile Tumors of the Mucosa

These tumors present an irregular, polypoid, or ulcerative shape on radiographs and can simulate a carcinoma. Endoscopic biopsy is mandatory and, in fact, represents the definitive treatment for small papillomas. Myxomas, lipomas, and their mixed forms occur almost exclusively in the cervical esophagus. Lesions displaying a pedicle with a narrow base can be removed endoscopically with a diathermy loop. Pedunculated masses with a broad base and sessile tumors are removed operatively after their location has been established.

Preoperative preparation, instruments, position and approach: See 8.2.1.

Operative technique: The esophagus is exposed in the area of tumor involvement and may be snared if required (see 2.1.1 or 2.1.2). Intraoperative esophagoscopy can be helpful in identifying the site of the lesion. The esophagus is opened with a vertical incision on the side opposite the tumor. We infiltrate the base of the tumor with saline solution (0.9%) to elevate it from the muscularis. An incision is made around the tumor, including a healthy tissue margin of several millimeters, then the lesion is carefully undermined and progressively removed. The resultant defect is closed transversely or longitudinally by continuous suture. The esophagus is splinted under vision with the stomach tube, and the esophagotomy is closed in two layers (see 1.3.2.2). In an intrathoracic procedure, the pleura is closed over the esophagus with a running suture. A soft Penrose drain is placed at the esophagotomy site in the neck, a chest tube is placed in the thorax, and the wound is closed in layers.

References

1. Andersen HA, Pluth JR (1974) Benign tumors, cysts and duplications of the esophagus. In: Payne WS, Olsen AM (eds) The esophagus. Lea and Febiger, Philadelphia, pp 225–237
2. Boyd DP, Hill LD (1957) Benign tumors and cysts of the esophagus. Am J Surg 93:252
3. Dillow BM, Neis DD, Sellers RD (1970) Leiomyoma of the esophagus. Am J Surg 120:615
4. Gray SW, Shandaleikis JE, Shepard D (1961) Smooth muscle tumors of the esophagus. Int Abstr Surg 113:205
5. Lortat-Jacob J (1950) Myomatoses localisées, myomatoses diffuses de l'oesophage. Arch Mal App Digest 39:519
6. Moersch HJ, Herrington SW (1967) Benign tumors of the esophagus. Ann Otol 53:800
7. Plachta A (1962) Benign tumors of the esophagus. Am J Gastroenterol 38:639
8. Seremetis MG, de Guzman VL, Lyons WS, Peabody JW (1973) Leiomyoma of the esophagus. Ann Thorac Surg 16:308

9 Esophagomyotomy

CONTENTS

9.1 Indications for Myotomy

Except in incompetence of the lower esophageal sphincter, myotomy continues to be the mainstay in the surgical treatment of esophageal motility disorders. Because myotomy does not restore normal motor function to the esophagus, but rather weakens it irreversibly, an accurate analysis of esophageal function is an essential prelude to the selection of patients for operative treatment.

9.2 Myotomy of the Upper Esophageal Sphincter

The upper esophageal sphincter is formed by the cricopharyngeal muscle, i.e., by the horizontal fibers of the constrictor pharyngis inferior. Abnormal function of this sphincter usually relates to a failure of temporal coordination [9, 10]. Although possessing the capability for normal relaxation, the upper esophageal sphincter closes before contraction of the pharynx is completed. The abnormal pressures associated with this premature closure promote diverticulum formation in the posterior pharyngeal wall, which has sparse muscular coverage, in the area of Killian's triangle just distal to the cricopharyngeal muscle. A situation analogous to achalasia of the lower esophageal sphincter, i.e., failure of relaxation of the cricopharyngeal muscle, has been demonstrated manometrically in only a few cases [2, 23]. While it is widely accepted that cricopharyngeal myotomy is effective as a treatment for localized as well as generalized esophageal motor dysfunction and can relieve cervical dysphagia in most patients, clinical results cast doubt on the value of myotomy in the treatment of central nervous system disorders [6, 16].

9.2.1 Technique of Cricopharyngeal Myotomy

Preoperative preparation: No special preparations are required.

Instruments: Basic set; Sengstaken tube (optional).

Position and approach: Unilateral Kocher collar incision on the left side or incision along the anterior border of the left sternocleidomastoid muscle (see 2.1.1).

Steps in procedure:

(1) The cervical esophagus is exposed (see 2.1.1)
(2) The cricopharyngeal muscle is identified
(3) The plane between the muscle and submucosa is defined with an Overholt clamp
(4) The cricopharyngeal muscle is divided between the jaws of the Overholt clamp with the electrocautery
(5) The myotomy site is inspected for mucosal defects and undivided muscle fibers (may be facilitated by passing a Sengstaken tube)
(6) The cervicotomy is closed

Operative technique: The cervical esophagus is exposed as described in 2.1.1. The cricopharyngeal muscle is identified after removal of the overlying connective tissue. If a diverticulum is present, it should not pose a major obstacle since all or most of the muscle bundles course below the neck of the diverticulum. Otherwise the cricopharyngeal muscle can be identified by the horizontal course of its slightly fusiform muscle bundles, which distinguish it from the flat, ascending fibers of the rest of the constrictor pharyngis inferior. Another distinguishing feature of the cricopharyngeal muscle is its palpable or visible origin at the cricoid cartilage.

The muscle is incised either on the posterior midline or anterolateral to it. The midline incision avoids injury to the recurrent nerve, which courses laterally. The electrocautery knife is swept carefully over the musculature with a minimum of pressure. The muscle is divided bundle by bundle, the bundles retracting laterally as they are severed so that the next deeper layer can be visualized. When the grayish white luster of the submucosa appears, an Overholt clamp is insinuated behind the muscle bundles and is used to spread them apart so they can be divided between the open jaws of the clamp (Fig. 114). The mucosa and submucosa will bulge into the defect as the myotomy proceeds.

The total length of the myotomy is 4–5 cm. It extends inferiorly to the esophageal musculature. Superiorly it may be carried about 1 cm into the oblique ascending fibers of the constrictor pharyngis inferior muscle to make sure the cervical high pressure zone is weakened [10], since we do consider this to be essential. The success of the myotomy depends mainly on its completeness. The search for undivided muscle bundles is greatly aided by passing a Sengstaken balloon tube and inflating it in the area of the myotomy. Remaining muscle fibers will stand out clearly in their horizontal course against the inflated bag and can be divided. If the lumen of the esophagus has been entered during the myotomy, the leak is immediately repaired by continuous suture. That is the only cases where we feel it necessary to place a small Penrose drain in the operative area before closing. The completeness of the myotomy is of crucial importance when the mucosa has been injured. If a high pressure zone remains due to the presence of uncut muscle fibers, there is a danger that the pressure will blow out the suture line. There should be little bleeding from the submucosa and divided muscle in an uncomplicated myotomy. Bleeding points on the muscle are coagulated, and any bleeding from the submucosa is controlled by compression.

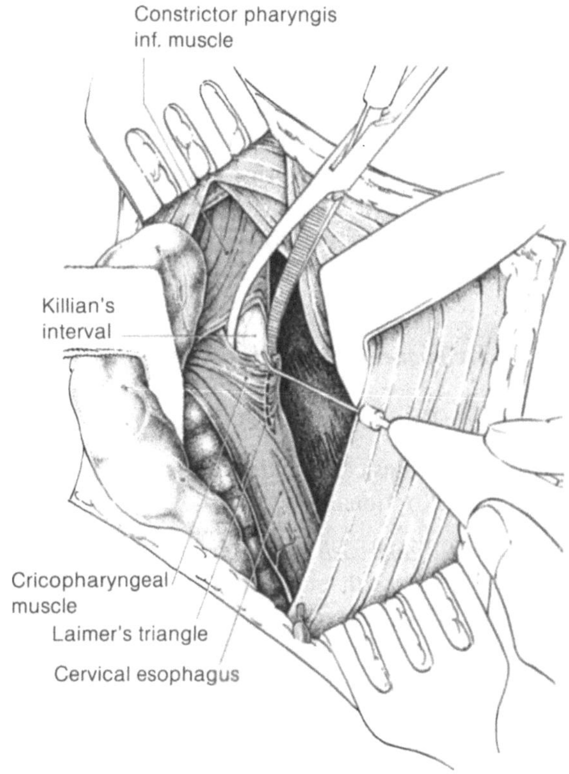

Fig. 114. Myotomy of the upper esophageal sphincter. The cricopharyngeal muscle is divided with the electrocautery

9.3 Extended Esophagomyotomy

9.3.1 Indications

Myotomy of the tubular esophagus should be reserved for the rare cases of idiopathic diffuse esophageal spasm, confirmed by manometry and radiography, that are unresponsive to medical therapy and are causing severe disability due to dysphagia, retrosternal pain, or cardiac irritation [9, 18, 19].

Esophageal manometry serves not only to confirm the diagnosis by the demonstration of prolonged, high-amplitude, nonperistaltic contractile waves with normal pressure in the lower esophageal sphincter but also to establish the length of the functional disturbance and thus of the myotomy. Typically the disorder involves the body of the esophagus between the lower sphincter and the aortic arch. The condition is frequently associated with a hiatal hernia, an effect rather than a cause of the diffuse spasm, and with an epiphrenic diverticulum. The diverticulum is always treated at the time the myotomy is performed. An antireflux procedure for treatment of hiatal hernia is indicated only if there is positive evidence of gastroesophageal reflux.

9.3.2 Technique of Extended Esophagomyotomy

Preoperative preparation: See Chap. C.

Instruments: Basic set, extra thoracic set; Sengstaken tube (optional).

Position and approach: Left posterolateral thoracotomy in the sixth or seventh interspace. If the area of diffuse spasm extends above the aortic arch, and there is no evidence of gastroesophageal reflux, it can be advantageous to use a right posterolateral incision in the fifth or sixth interspace (see Chap. B).

Operative technique: The esophagus is exposed in the proposed area of the myotomy and encircled with a soft Penrose drain (see 2.1.2). The esophagus is pulled superiorly by gentle traction on the drain until the esophagogastric junction presents in the hiatus. This maneuver is done only to evaluate the abdominal portion of the esophagus, since the lower esophageal sphincter will be spared. Care is taken not to injure the hiatal structures. The myotomy begins 3–5 cm proximal to the esophagogastric junction. The Sengstaken tube is passed through the esophagus and cardia and is inflated to distend the esophageal wall. The muscle bundles are spread apart with an Overholt clamp until the gray-white luster of the submucosa appears. The closed Overholt clamp is inserted between the mucosa and muscularis, opened, and the muscle fibers are progressively divided between the jaws of the clamp with an electrocautery knife. The incision is continued proximally and distally according to the proposed extent of the myotomy, following the plane between the muscle and submucosa (Fig. 115 a). After the myotomy is completed, the Sengstaken tube is inflated further to help locate any muscle fibers that have been missed. These are identified and divided (Fig. 115 b). The muscle wall can then be bluntly dissected laterally so that approximately half the circumference of the sub-

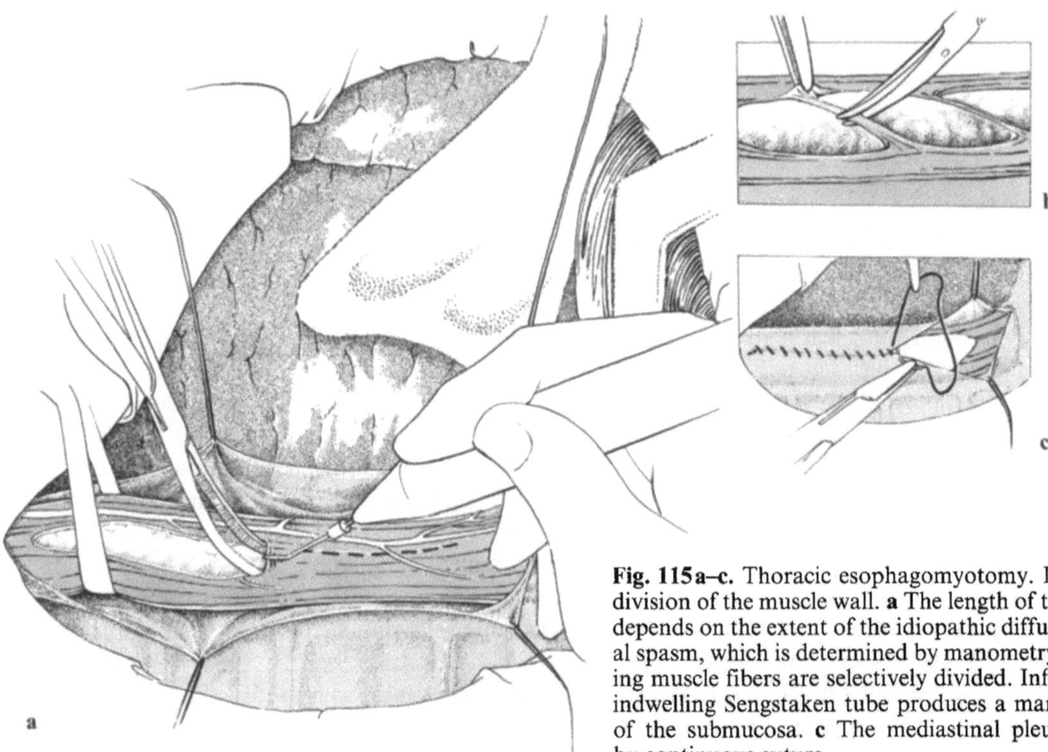

Fig. 115a–c. Thoracic esophagomyotomy. Longitudinal division of the muscle wall. **a** The length of the myotomy depends on the extent of the idiopathic diffuse esophageal spasm, which is determined by manometry. **b** Remaining muscle fibers are selectively divided. Inflation of the indwelling Sengstaken tube produces a marked bulging of the submucosa. **c** The mediastinal pleura is closed by continuous suture

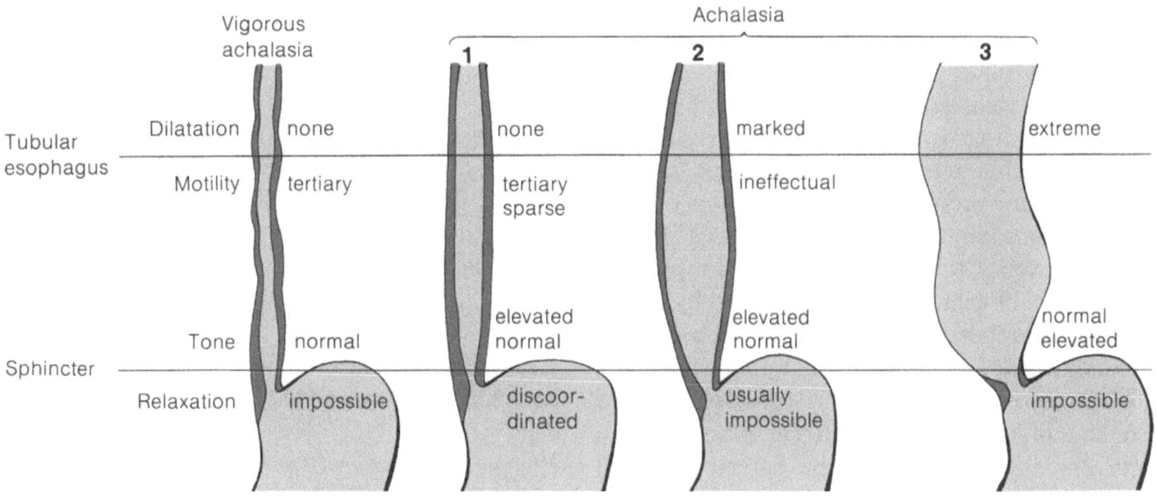

Fig. 116. The different forms of achalasia and their associated anatomic and functional pathology. (Modified from Herfahrth et al. [14])

mucosa is freed, permitting it to bulge widely through the muscular incision. This is done to aid the transit of ingested material and prevent eventual reapproximation of the divided muscular layers. Bleeding points on the muscle are selectively cauterized. Any defect in the mucosa should be repaired at once by continuous suture.

If gastroesophageal reflux existed preoperatively, an antireflux procedure is performed through the same approach or transabdominally (see 11.5 and 11.6). In each case the hiatal ring is palpated with the Sengstaken tube still in place. If there is room for more than one fingertip next to the dilated esophagus, the crural margins should be approximated behind the esophagus with two or three sutures. Then the mediastinal pleura is closed with a continuous suture (Fig. 115 c), a chest tube is inserted, the lung is inflated, and the thoracotomy is closed in layers.

9.4 Myotomy of the Lower Esophageal Sphincter

9.4.1 Indications

Myotomy of the lower esophageal sphincter and adjacent esophagus is employed in the classic form of achalasia, characterized by absence of propulsive peristalsis in the esophageal body and failure of the lower sphincter to relax in response to swallowing. It is also used to treat the hypermotile variant ("vigorous achalasia") and hypertonicity of the lower sphincter (Fig. 116).

9.4.2 Myotomy versus Dilatation

There continues to be controversy as to whether myotomy or dilatation should be the primary treatment of choice for patients with achalasia. It is generally accepted that myotomy is preferred in children, in patients who are psychotic or uncooperative, and in the rare cases where malignant disease of the esophagogastric junction cannot be excluded despite intensive diagnostic study. When we look at the many publications on both forms of treatment in an attempt to determine which should be applied first, the following facts emerge [1, 2, 3, 9, 17, 18, 19, 22]: Both treatments are associated with a low rate of complications and hospital mortality. Dilatation, even when performed repeatedly, is more easily tolerated than myotomy and therefore is appropriate in the presence of risk factors that would contraindicate major surgery. Also, dilatation is less costly and time-consuming than myotomy. The majority of authors report better late results with myotomy and fewer recurrences. Previous dilatation does not preclude myotomy, although the esophageal wall damage that invariably accompanies dilatation can complicate the surgical procedure and may even necessitate plastic enlargement of the esophagogastric junction, with an associated increase in operative risk. In patients with Stage 3 achalasia, neither treatment method can ensure the drainage of ingested material from the greatly enlarged "sigmoid" esophagus. The problem of gastroesophageal reflux is equivalent in both methods. The high reflux rates reported by some authors after myotomy presumably relate to errors of technique. Physicians at the Mayo Clinic [17], who have experience with the largest and longest-followed series of achalasia patients treated by operative and nonoperative methods, report a shift in emphasis away from forceful dilatation, which was initially used in more than 80% of cases, toward esophagomyotomy. Their current practice is to elect dilatation only when the patient's general condition does not permit a major operation. In the only prospective study to date comparing pneumatic dilatation with esophagomyotomy, Csendes et al. [8] noted significantly better long-term objective and subjective results after myotomy in 38 patients. How the above facts are weighted will determine whether myotomy or dilatation appears to be the more favorable primary therapy for achalasia. Myotomy is the only option to be considered for the "vigorous" form of the disease. However, the incision must include the part of the esophageal body that is affected by the functional disorder. We personally favor pneumatic dilatation under endoscopic control (see Sect. 10) as a primary treatment and reserve myotomy for patients who do not benefit from nonoperative dilatation or whose achalasia recurs.

9.4.3 Special Preoperative Preparations

The dilated esophagus must be carefully evacuated and cleaned prior to operation. If endoscopy has disclosed significant mucosal inflammation, the procedure should be postponed to avoid injury to the inflamed and fragile mucosa. Parenteral alimentation and antibiotics are maintained for a period of several days while the esophagus is irrigated and decompressed through a nasogastric tube.

9.4.4 Transabdominal or Transthoracic Approach for Myotomy of the Lower Esophageal Sphincter

Today the great majority of surgeons favor the transabdominal approach over the transthoracic, as it provides better exposure of the operative area, permits the entire abdomen to be inspected, and permits the myotomy to be extended several centimeters onto the stomach. There is no question that laparotomy is better tolerated by most patients than thoracotomy. Belsey [2], Ellis [9], and Payne and Olsen [19] use the transthoracic approach exclusively, emphasizing the advantages of good exposure, direct access to the esophagus, which requires little mobilization, and the ability to preserve hiatal structures.

9.4.5 Transabdominal Myotomy of the Lower Esophageal Sphincter [11, 13]

Preoperative preparation: See Chap. C and 9.4.3.

Instruments: Basic set; Sengstaken tube (optional).

Position and approach: Upper midline laparotomy.

Steps in procedure:

(1) Division of the peritoneal reflection over the abdominal esophagus
(2) Lateral retraction of the vagus nerve with a tape
(3) Snaring of the esophagus
(4) Development of the plane between the muscularis and submucosa of the abdominal esophagus with an Overholt clamp
(5) Longitudinal electrocautery incision of the muscle bundles of the lower esophageal sphincter between the blades of the Overholt clamp
(6) Inflation of the indwelling Sengstaken tube to check for uncut fibers
(7) If necessary, approximation of the hiatal margins
(8) Semifundoplication to cover the myotomy incision
(9) Closure of the abdomen

Operative technique: The abdomen is inspected, and if exposure of the cardia requires it, the left lobe of the liver is retracted anteromedially and the triangular ligament is detached from the diaphragm. The left lobe of the liver is displaced medially with a broad retractor. The stomach is grasped by its greater curvature and pulled downward. A stomach tube previously placed along the greater curvature will facilitate this maneuver. The peritoneal reflection covering the esophagogastric junction is transversely incised. The anterior vagus

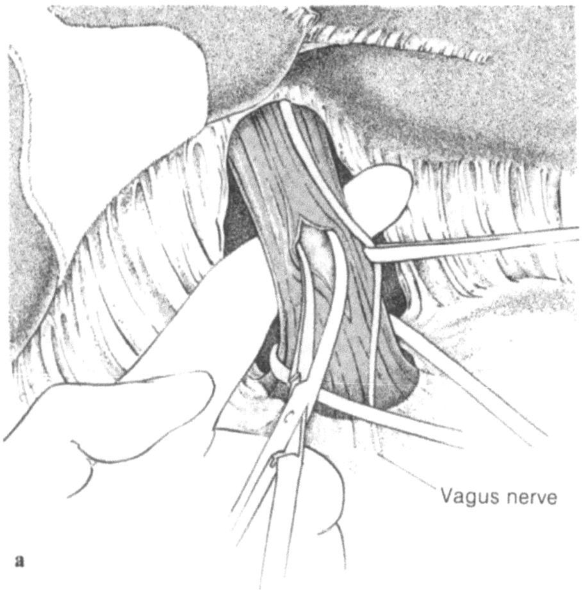

a

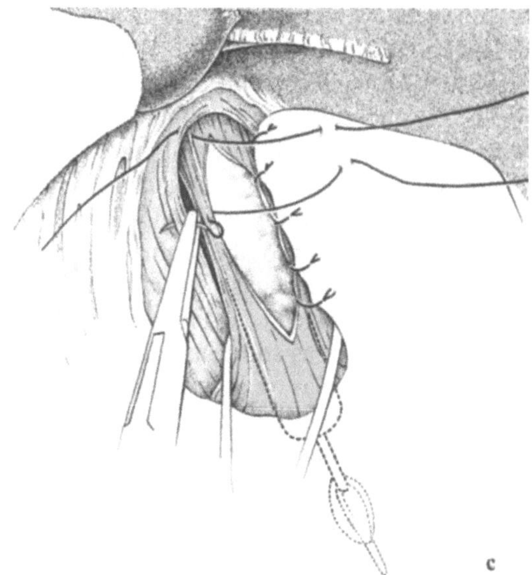

c

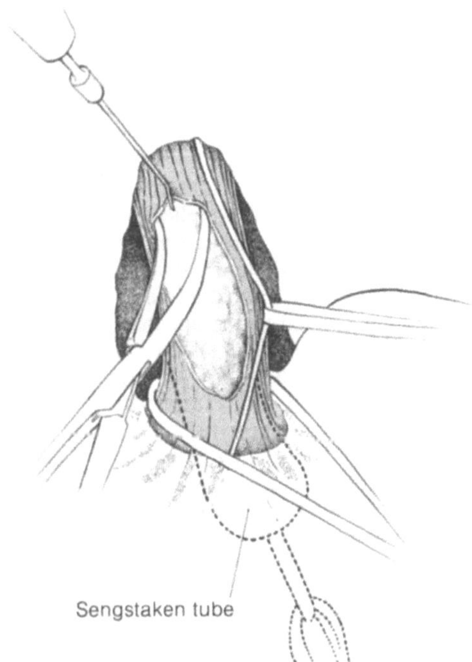

b

Fig. 117 a–c. Transabdominal myotomy of the lower esophageal sphincter. **a** The muscle bundles are spread apart to develop the plane between the muscularis and submucosa. **b** The muscle bundles of the lower esophageal sphincter are divided longitudinally with the electrocautery. The submucosa balloons outward under the pressure of the indwelling Sengstaken tube. **c** A semifundoplication is performed to cover the exposed mucosa and prevent reflux. The two most proximal sutures pierce the esophageal wall and the hiatal crura

nerve trunk is spared by identifying the nerve, encircling it with a tape, and retracted it toward the greater curvature side. The connective tissue overlying the esophagus is reflected upward by patty dissection, exposing the anterior circumference of the muscular tube. The esophagus is encircled with the thumb and forefinger, and both fingertips are brought together behind the esophagus while bluntly dissecting the connective tissue. The dissection is guided posteriorly by the aorta and spine, rather than the posterior wall of the esophagus, to avoid perforation. When the esophagus has been cleared sufficiently to encircle it with the index finger, a Guyon clamp is passed behind the esophagus, using the fingertip as a guide. The esophagus is then snared by grasping a rubber tape or drain with the clamp and pulling it through. The snare is pulled downward to bring the abdominal and lower thoracic portion of the esophagus into view. Residual overlying peritoneum and connective tissue are displaced laterally and superiorly, sparing the branches of the left gastric and inferior phrenic arteries that are distributed to the esophagus. It is unnecessary to expose the esophagus circumferentially far into the hiatus, because the myotomy will be performed only on the anterior side of the esophagus; the concomitant posterior myotomy described by Heller [13] is omitted. The disordered portion of the lower esophageal sphincter rarely extends more than 4 cm proximal to the esophagogastric junction. If the esophagus is not significantly dilated, the myotomy need not extend more than 1 cm beyond this zone to ensure an adequate operation. If the esophagus is dilated, we pull it downward until the lower portion of the distended body presents in the hiatus; we then divide the musculature into the dilated area. A schematized approach prescribing a myotomy length of 6 cm, 8 cm, or 10 cm lacks a physiologic rationale. The myotomy is extended distally only a few millimeters onto the stomach, i.e., to the point where transverse gastric veins are visible. We see no reason to extend the incision 2 cm or more onto the stomach, as some have advocated [5, 7]. The gastric musculature is not hypertrophied and shows no evidence of neuromuscular abnormality.

The muscle bundles are spread apart with an Overholt clamp until the submucosa appears (Fig. 117 a). The plane between the muscularis and submucosa is made easier to define by passing a Sengstaken tube into the lower esophagus and inflating it slightly. As the clamp is advanced along the submucosa, the muscle bundles are picked up on the tips of the opened blades and divided with an electrocautery, proceeding first in the proximal direction and then distally. When the last muscle fibers have been severed, the mucosa will pout through the incision under the pressure of the inflated Sengstaken tube (Fig. 117 b). Transverse fissures signify the presence of intact muscle fibers that still must be divided. When the myotomy is completed, the Sengstaken tube is replaced by a small-caliber stomach tube. Because small leaks may be overlooked during the myotomy, we recommend methylene blue injection to test the integrity of the esophageal wall.

The myotomy largely destroys the function of the lower esophageal sphincter, rendering it unable to close. Gastroesophageal reflux in this situation is avoided by adding an antireflux procedure. Another benefit of this procedure is that it covers the exposed part of the mucosa and so largely eliminates the effects of an overlooked or incipient wall injury. The semifundoplication (Fig. 117 c) in one of its various modifications (see 11.6) is superior to the Nissen fundoplication (see 11.5) in achalasia because it does not block the passage of food into the stomach, and there is no need to fear the dysphagia that can result from a complete fundic wrap around the terminal esophagus.

9.4.6 Transthoracic Myotomy of the Lower Esophageal Sphincter

Preoperative preparation: See Chap. C and 9.4.3.

Instruments: Basic set, extra thoracic set; Sengstaken tube (optional).

Position and approach: Left posterolateral thoracotomy in the seventh interspace.

Operative technique: The technique is similar to that of thoracic myotomy for diffuse ideopathic esophageal spasm (see 9.3); only the extent of the myotomy is different. The esophagus is exposed, mobilized, and snared. Its abdominal portion is delivered into the chest as far as the esophagogastric junction. The hiatal structures are carefully preserved so as not to provoke reflux. The myotomy is performed in standard fashion, extending proximally into the dilated portion of the esophagus and distally to the stomach. If an antireflux procedure is not desired, the hiatal ring is checked for competence, and if necessary its margins are approximated with sutures. The mediastinal pleura is closed over the myotomy by continuous suture, a chest tube is inserted, the lung is reexpanded, and the thoracotomy is closed in layers. If an antireflux procedure is elected, one should consider avoiding a fundoplication for the reasons stated above (see 9.4.5). The technique is described in 11.5.1.2. A semifundoplication, like fundoplication, requires that the fundus be mobilized through a thoracic approach. With the esophagogastric junction and part of the fundus transposed into the thorax, a fold of fundus is created, and its apex is fixed to the upper angle of the myotomy incision. The cut edges of the muscle are tacked to the sides of the fundic fold with interrupted sutures. One or two additional sutures are placed through the esophageal musculature near the tip of the upper angle of the myotomy, through the apex of the fundus, and through a corresponding site on the hiatal rim. These sutures are not tied; they will be used for a fundopexy after the esophagus has been returned to the abdomen. When a semicircular wrap of fundus has been secured around the esophagus, the latter is returned to the abdomen, and the hiatus is narrowed with 2 or 3 sutures placed through its margins. Then the fundopexy sutures are tightened and tied.

9.5 Surgical Treatment of Stage 3 Achalasia

In Stage 3 achalasia, characterized by a sigmoid dilatation of the lower thoracic esophagus, a simple myotomy is not sufficient to drain the "esophageal stump" adequately. It is necessary to rely on procedures like the esophagogastrostomy (see 4.3.6) or fundic patch graft (see 4.3.5) that create a broad communication between the dilated esophagus and stomach, or to augment myotomy with a vagotomy, pyloroplasty, gastropexy, semifundoplication and gastrostomy [24], or to combine myotomy with a procedure that reduces the caliber of the dilated esophagus [14, 21]. We believe that partial esophagectomy with reconstruction by interposed colon or jejunum is an adequate procedure in these cases, as it provides good function while avoiding the precancerous condition of a chronically inflamed esophagus [12].

The operation described by Thorbjarnarson [24], in which myotomy is combined with vagotomy, pyloroplasty, gastropexy, semifundoplication, and temporary gastrostomy, is done with the object of straightening the esophagus, eliminating its dependent pouch, and increasing the length of its intraabdominal segment. This procedure is technically complex, however, and produces the undesired sequelae of truncal vagotomy. An advantage of this procedure over simple abdominal advancement of the dilated esophagus with myotomy [20], which has shown little success in Stage 3 achalasia, apparently relates to the acid-reducing effect of the vagotomy with concurrent drainage of the stomach.

9.5.1 Treatment of Stage 3 Achalasia by Myoplication and by Strip Myectomy with Plication of the Mucosa

Both methods [14, 21] combine division of the lower esophageal sphincter with a reduction in the caliber of the dilated esophageal body. Unlike longitudinal strip resection of the esophageal wall, esophagogastrostomy or segmental resection, the lumen of the esophagus is not entered, and an anastomosis is not required. Consequently, both methods significantly reduce the operative risk compared with the two procedures described above.

9.5.1.1 Technique of Myoplication

Preoperative preparation: See Chap. C and 9.4.3.

Instruments: Basic set, extra thoracic set; Sengstaken tube (optional).

Position and approach: Right posterolateral thoracotomy in the sixth or seventh interspace (see Chap. B).

Steps in procedure:

(1) Exposure and snaring of the thoracic esophagus (see 2.1.1)
(2) Delivery of the cardia and fundus into the chest
(3) Myotomy of the lower esophageal sphincter
(4) Extension of the myotomy over the entire dilated esophagus
(5) Semifundoplication to cover the myotomy in the area of the lower sphincter
(6) Semicircular dissection of the muscular coat of the dilated esophagus from the mucosa
(7) Fixation of the muscle flaps in trapdoor fashion over the mucosa, which is splinted by an intraluminal Sengstaken tube
(8) Replacement of the semifundoplication in the abdomen, and narrowing of the hiatal ring
(9) Drainage and closure of the chest

Operative technique: The esophagus is exposed and snared just above the diaphragm (see 2.1.2). The lower esophageal sphincter is divided by an extramucosal myotomy that extends 1 cm past the sphincter proximally and distally. The gastric fundus is pulled through the hiatus into the thorax and sutured into the myotomy defect so that the gastric serosa covers the exposed mucosa of the esophagus while also preventing reapproximation of the divided muscle and gastroesophageal reflux. The myotomy is extended proximally, and the esophageal musculature is dissected back from the mucosa, exposing about half the circumference of the mucosal tube (Fig. 118 a). The medial and lateral muscle flaps thus formed are laid back over the mucosa in overlapping fashion so that the wall of the esophagus apposes snugly to the indwelling Sengstaken tube, inflated to a diameter of about 2.5 cm. The muscle wall is held in place with interrupted sutures (Fig. 118 b). Following the myotomy and antireflux procedure, the lower esophagus is returned to the abdominal cavity, and the hiatus is narrowed and fixed to the esophagus on the right side. Then the mediastinal pleura is closed by continuous suture, a chest tube is inserted, the lung is inflated, and the thoracic incision is closed in layers.

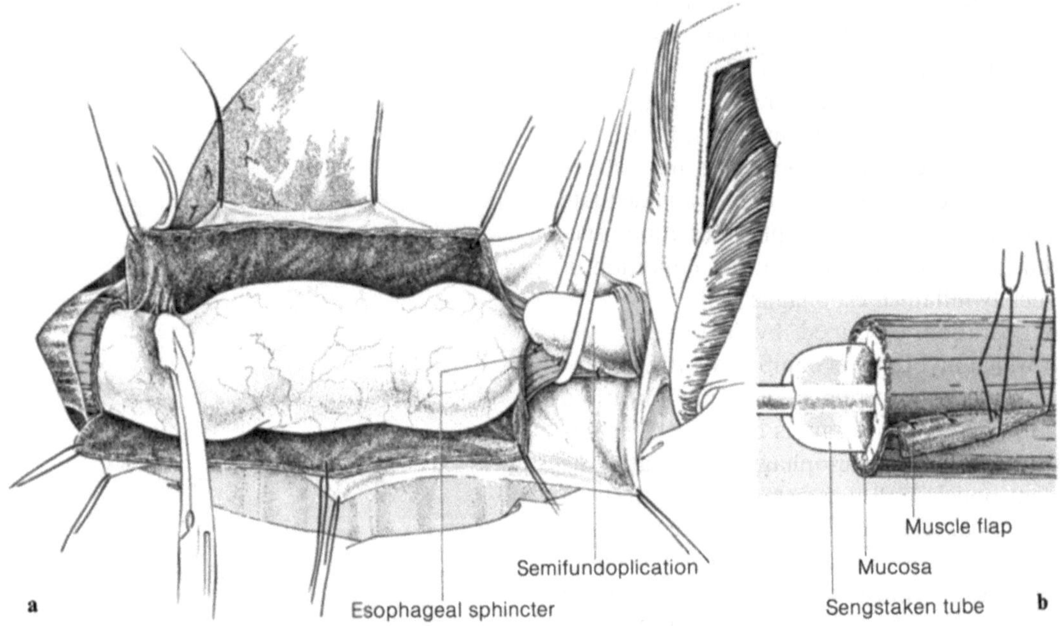

Fig. 118 a,b. Myoplication for the treatment of Stage 3 achalasia. **a** Part of the circumference of the muscle wall is dissected from the dilated esophageal body. The lower sphincter has been divided, and the mucosa has been covered with a semifundoplication. **b** The muscle flaps on the dilated esophageal body are fixed in trapdoor fashion around the mucosa, which is splinted by the indwelling Sengstaken tube

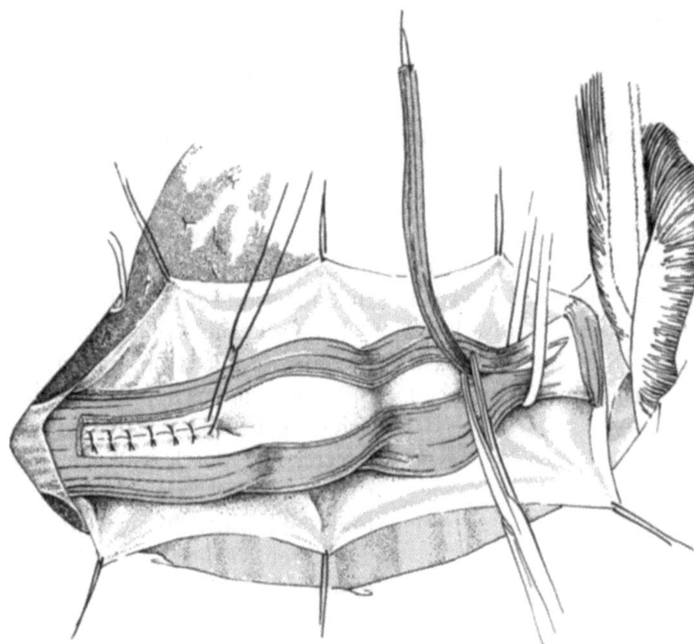

Fig. 119. Treatment of Stage 3 achalasia by strip myectomy and mucosal plication. A longitudinal muscle strip of sufficient width is resected, and the mucosal tube is plicated to narrow the dilated esophageal body. The muscle wall is reapproximated over the mucosa with interrupted sutures

9.5.1.2 Technique of Strip Myectomy and Mucosal Plication

This procedure is similar to the myoplication described above. The esophagus is exposed, and the lower sphincter is myotomized. A sufficiently wide longitudinal strip of muscle is dissected from the dilated body of the esophagus to reduce the caliber of the esophagus when the cut edges of the muscle wall are approximated. Before this is done, a series of inverting sutures are placed in the exposed submucosa to plicate and narrow the mucosal tube (Fig. 119). The muscle edges are approximated over that with interrupted sutures, and a fundoplication is performed through the thoracic incision (see 11.5).

References

1. Arvantakis C (1975) Achalasia of the esophagus: a reapraisal of esophagomyotomy vs. forceful pneumatic dilatation. Dig Dis 20:841
2. Belsey RH (1966) Functional disease of the esophagus. J Thorac Cardiovasc Surg 52:164
3. Bennett JR, Hendrix TR (1970) Treatment of achalasia with pneumatic dilatation. Mod Treat 7:1217
4. Bennett JR (1980) Treatment of achalasia: a review. J R Soc Med 73:649
5. Black J, Vosbach An, Collis JL (1976) Results of Heller's operation for achalasia of the esophagus. Br J Surg 63:949
6. Blakely WR, Gorety EJ, Smith DE (1968) Section of the cricopharyngeus muscle for dysphagia. Arch Surg 96:745
7. Bünte H (1977) Chirurgie des Ösophagus. Klinikarzt 6:128
8. Csendes A, Velaseo N, Braghetto J, Henriques A (1981) A prospective randomized study comparing forceful dilatation and esophagomyotomy in patients with achalasia of the esophagus. Gastroenterology 80:789
9. Ellis FH jr (1980) Surgical management of esophageal motility disturbances. Am J Sur 139:752
10. Ellis FH, Crozier RE (1981) Cervical esophageal dysphagia. Ann Surg 194:279
11. Gottstein G (1908) Über Pathologie und Therapie des Cardiospasmus. All med Centr Ztg 77:563
12. Hankins J, McLaughthin J (1975) The association of carcinoma of the esophagus with achalasia. J Thorac Cardiovasc Surg 69:355
13. Heller E (1914) Extramuköse Kardiaplastik beim chronischen Kardiospasmus mit Dilatation des Ösophagus. Mitt Grenzgeb Med Chir 27:141
14. Herfahrth C, Matthes P, Heil T (1979) Die Ösophagus-Myoplicatur in der Behandlung der dekompensierten Achalasie. Chirurg 50:681
15. Hollender LF, Meges C, Jamart J, Calderoli H (1977) L'operation de Heller dans the traitement du mégaesophage idiopathique. Med Chir Dig 6:89–94
16. Mills CP (1973) Dysphagia in pharyngeal paralysis treated by cricopharyngeal myotomy. Lancet 1:455
17. Okike N, Payne WS, Neufeld DM, Bernatz PE, Pairolero PC, Sanderson DR (1979) Esophagomyotomy versus forcefull dilation for achalasia of the esophagus: results in 899 patients. Ann Thorac Surg 28:119
18. Olsen AM, Harrington SW, Moersch HJ (1951) The treatment of cardiospasm: analysis of a twelve-year experience. J Thorac Card Surg 22:164
19. Payne WS, Olsen AM (1974) The esophagus. Lea and Febiger, Philadelphia
20. Rapant V, Kralik J (1970) Die Problematik der Therapie der Achalasie der Speiseröhre. Bruns Beitr Klin Chir 1:12
21. Reding R (1981) Die Streifenmyektomie und Raphie der Schleimhaut des Ösophagus zur Behandlung der dekompensierten Achalasia cardiae (Stadiu III). Zbl Chirurgie 106:335
22. Spitzer G, Hessler C, Sailer FX (1973) Therapie des Kardiospasmus. Med Welt 24:1256
23. Sutherland HD (1962) Cricopharyngeal achalasia. J Thorac Cardiovasc Surg 43:114
24. Thorbjarnarson B (1975) An operation for advanced achalasia. Am J Surg 129:111
25. Vantrappen G, Hellemans J (1980) Treatment of achalasia and related motor disorders. Gastroenterology 79:144
26. Yon J, Christensen J (1975) An uncontrolled comparison of treatment for achalasia. Ann Surg 182:672

10 Treatment of Stage 1 and 2 Achalasia by Dilatation of the Lower Esophageal Sphincter

In collaboration with G. BUESS

CONTENTS

The dilatation therapy of achalasia was introduced by Starck [1], who used a mechanical dilator. Since then, mechanical dilation has been largely replaced by pneumatic dilation using a bougie-shaped instrument that is advanced through the stenosed cardia under endoscopic or radiologic guidance with the aid of a guidewire system. The balloon portion of the instrument is then inflated, dilating the cardia to a specified caliber. A preference is emerging in favor of hollow balloon dilators [2, 3] designed for insertion on an endoscope ("piggy-back system"). The pros and cons of nonoperative dilation versus myotomy of the lower esophageal sphincter for Stage 1 and 2 achalasia were discussed previously (see 9.4.2).

Fig. 120. The Witzel dilator system [3]. *1* Tubing with dilating balloon. *2* Rings for attaching the dilator to the endoscope. *3* Bulb with manometer

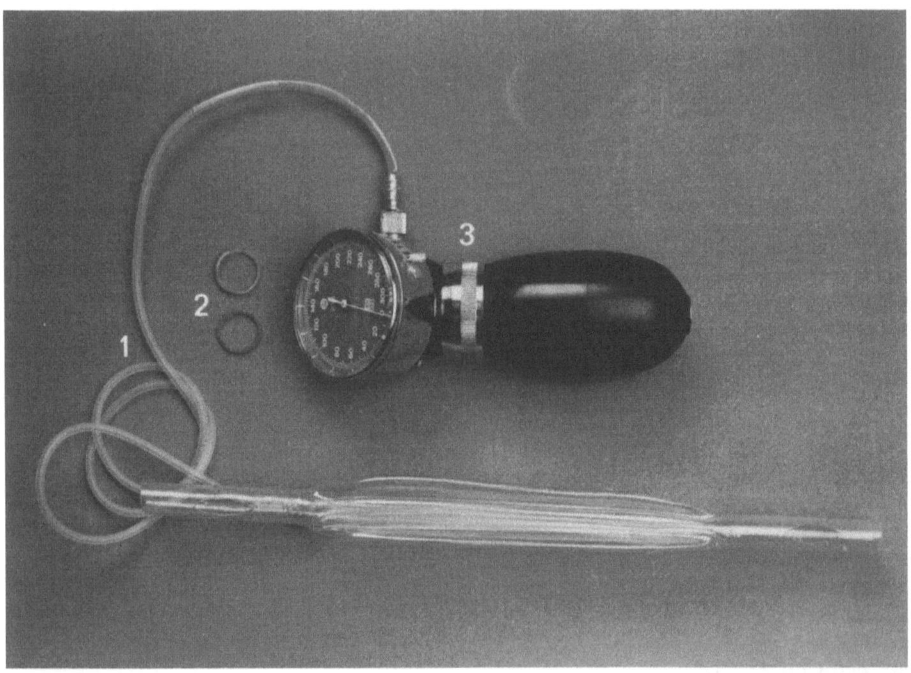

10.1 Balloon Systems with Endoscopic Guidance

10.1.1 The Witzel Dilator System [3]

The dilator consists of a short polyvinyl tube enclosed within a polyurethane balloon (Fig. 120). The balloon expands to a maximum external diameter of 40 mm when inflated under manometric control. For insertion, the dilator is fitted over a small-caliber fiberoptic endoscope so that the dilatation can be monitored by deflecting the tip of the scope 180° (Fig. 121). The use of rubber bands for attaching the dilator to the endoscope is less than optimum.

10.1.2 The Kaphingst Dilator

This model was introduced by Troidl et al. [2] (Fig. 122). It attaches directly to the endoscope via a tube. The latex balloon is enclosed within a nylon sheath that limits the inflation to a specified diameter.

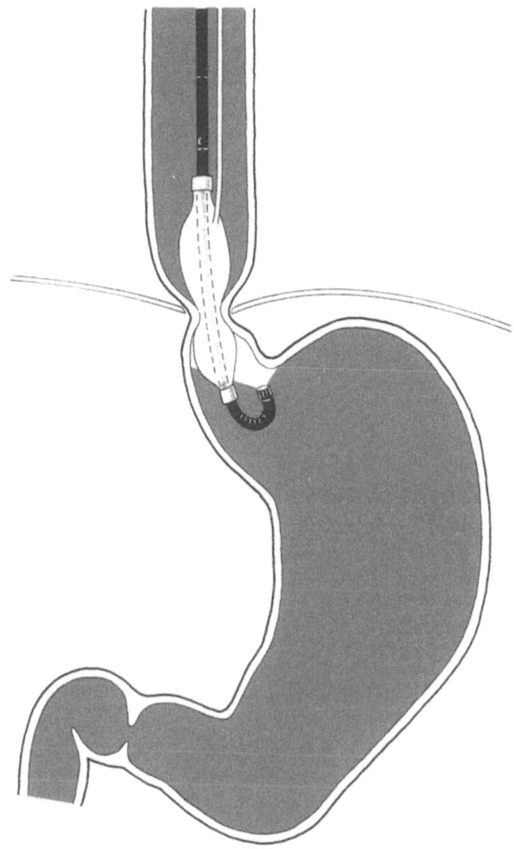

Fig. 121. The position of the dilator is checked by deflecting the tip of the endoscope 180°

Fig. 122. The Kaphingst dilator: tube with latex balloon, flexible endoscope tip, pump with manometer

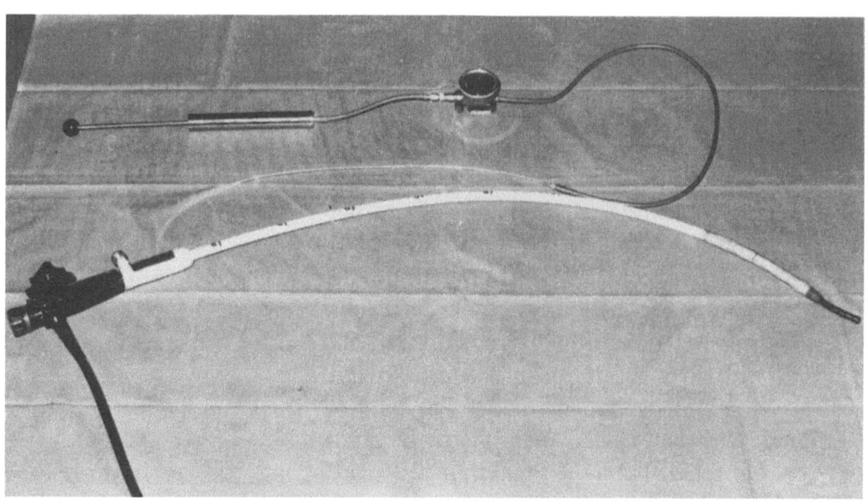

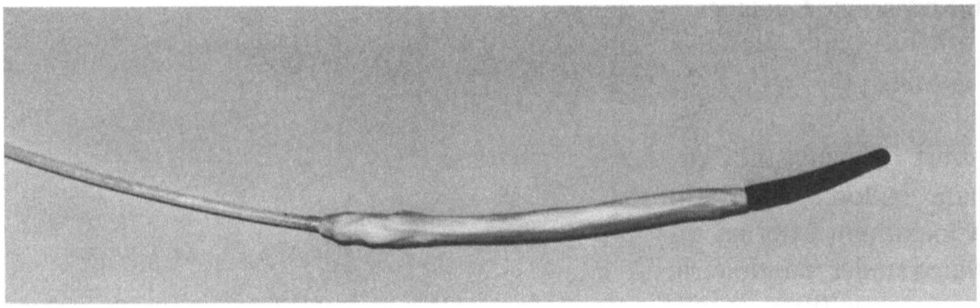

Fig. 123. A simple balloon dilator

10.2 Balloon Systems without Endoscopic Guidance

In these systems a balloon is mounted on a bougie with a soft rubber tip that helps guide the instrument through the cardia (Fig. 123). The latex balloon has the same design as the Kaphingst system (see 10.1.2).

10.3 Technique of Dilatation

10.3.1 Dilatation with Endoscopically Guided Balloon Systems

Preparation: The patient is fasted in preparation for the procedure. If the esophagus is markedly distended, it should first be irrigated to remove accumulated food and secretions. The patient is sedated with up to 10 mg diazepam i.v., and the pharynx is sprayed with a topical anesthetic.

Instruments: See 10.1.1 and 10.1.2.

Position: Left lateral decubitus.

Technique: The pneumatic dilator is fitted over the endoscope, and the assembly is inserted into the esophagus. Once the flexible tip of the endoscope has traversed the cardia, the advance of the balloon and its position prior to the dilation are monitored by retroversion of the endoscope tip (Fig. 121). Since the balloon may become displaced during the dilatation, its position should be monitored throughout the procedure so that necessary adjustments can be made. The balloon is inflated with air under manometric control. Pressures of 100–350 mm Hg, maintained for 1–5 min, are recommended.

We apply a dilating pressure of 200 mm Hg for 2 min in the first session and 250 mm Hg for 3 min in a second session, which is mandatory. When the dilatation is completed, the balloon is deflated, the endoscope is withdrawn, and the dilated area is inspected. After every treatment we opacify the esophagus and cardia with a water-soluble contrast medium and obtain a radiograph to exclude perforation.

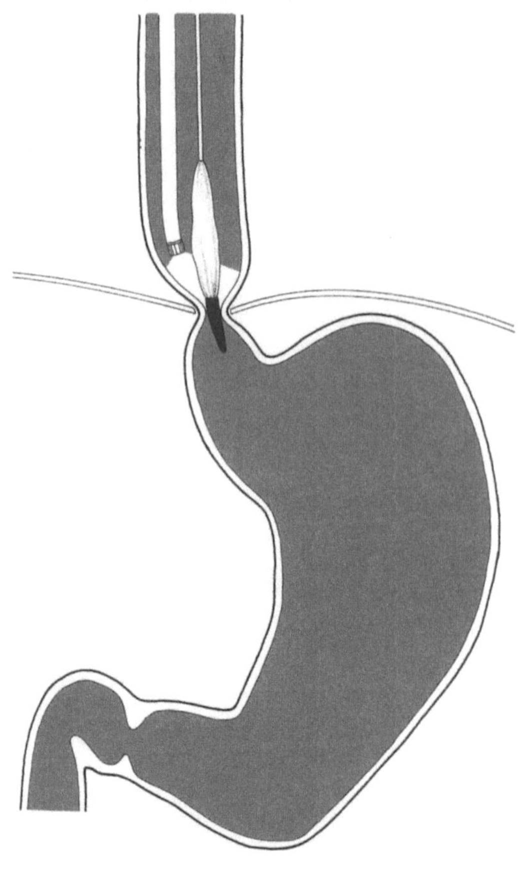

Fig. 124. The passage of the dilating balloon into the cardia can be monitored with a parallel endoscope

10.3.2 Dilatation with Non-Endoscopically Guided Balloon Systems

Preparation: See 10.3.1.

Instruments: See 10.2; facilities for fluoroscopy and/or endoscopy.

Position: Supine on a tiltable X-ray table; sitting or left lateral (for endoscopic control).

Technique: The dilator is introduced into the esophagus. There is a danger that the flexible tip will become misdirected at the angulation of the cardia, so the dilator should be advanced with great caution when resistance is felt. The instrument can be passed with greater accuracy under radiographic control by having the patient swallow a water-soluble contrast material. Before we began using the "piggyback system," we monitored difficult insertions by introducing an endoscope parallel to the dilating instrument and then negotiating the cardia under visual guidance (Fig. 124).

Once the instrument has been properly placed, the dilatation is performed as described in Sect. 10.3.1

References

1. Starck H (1952) Die Krankheiten der Speiseröhre. Med Praxis, Bd 36. Steinkopff, Darmstadt
2. Troidl H, Vestweber KH, Somma H (1980) Neues Verfahren zur pneumatischen Dehnung bei der Achalasie mit dem flexiblen Endoskop. Abstracts of the IVth European Congress of gastrointestinal endoscopy. Thieme, Stuttgart, 24, E 7:1
3. Witzel L (1981) Treatment of achalasia with a pneumatic dilatator attached to a gastroscope. Endoscopy 13:176

11 Surgical Treatment of Esophageal Diverticula

CONTENTS

11.1 Classification and Indications

Esophageal diverticula may be classified by their location as cervical or intrathoracic. While this simple classification disregards the formal pathogenesis of the lesion (pulsion/traction, acquired/congenital, epiphrenic/parabronchial) and its anatomy (true/false diverticulum), it simplifies considerations of patient selection and operating technique. Surgery is always indicated for a cervical diverticulum, because these lesions tend to enlarge and produce dysphagia, there is no proximal barrier against the aspiration of material spilled from the pouch, and the operation is well tolerated.

Surgery for intrathoracic diverticulum is associated with a disproportionately higher risk and so is indicated only if the lesion is causing significant clinical symptoms such as regurgitation with danger of aspiration or in the presence of a mass effect, diverticulitis, or tracheoesophageal fistula.

11.2 Choice of Operation

The surgical treatment of the diverticulum should be directed toward relieving the underlying cause. If the treatment leaves behind a blind sac that is isolated from the self-cleansing mechanisms of the esophagus, the sac must be removed or else invaginated or sutured in a way that will prevent food retention in the pouch and spillover. Inversion of the pouch is no longer practiced, but diverticulopexy is still occasionally used in addition to the standard procedure of diverticulectomy [2]. The latter is associated with a higher rate of postoperative complications than diverticulopexy due to the potential for suture line leak (1%–3%) and its sequelae, which depend on the location of the diverticulum. However, we are reluctant to leave behind a dead space that is not accessible to diagnostic evaluation, so we always make an attempt to excise the diverticular sac.

11.3 Treatment of Cervical Diverticulum by Myotomy, Excision, or Diverticulopexy

The importance of upper esophageal sphincter dysfunction in the pathogenesis of diverticula was previously noted (see 9.2). Cricopharyngeal myotomy is the first and probably the most important step in treatment. Gastroesophageal reflux also can increase the cricopharyngeal muscle tone [2, 6] and thus incite the formation of a cervical diverticulum. This observation demonstrates the necessity of total esophageal function testing, even if only its cervical portion appears to be affected. A procedure that simply weakens the cricopharyngeal muscle in the presence of gastroesophageal reflux would destroy the last barrier against the reflux of gastric contents into the oral cavity, and the danger of aspiration would be significant.

Preoperative preparation: See Chap. C; perioperative antibiotics as required.

Instruments: Basic set; Sengstaken tube or large-caliber stomach tube (Ch 32).

Position and approach: Unilateral Kocher collar incision or incision along the anterior border of the sternocleidomastoid muscle on the side toward which the diverticulum projects (see 2.1.1).

Operative technique: The esophagus and hypopharynx are exposed (see 2.1.1), and the parapharyngeal space is entered by blunt patty dissection. If identification of the diverticulum proves difficult because the lesion is embedded in connective tissue or fused to the muscle wall, it can be located by using the cricopharyngeal muscle as a guide. The neck of the diverticulum will always be cranial to the horizontal fibers of the muscle. The diverticu-

Steps in procedure:

(1) Exposure of the cervical esophagus (see 2.1.1)
(2) Circumferential exposure of the diverticulum
(3) Exposure of the cricopharyngeal muscle
(4) Development of the plane between the muscularis and submucosa with an Overholt clamp
(5) Division of the cricopharyngeal muscle between the blades of the Overholt clamp with an electrocautery
(6) Inspection of the myotomy incision for mucosal defects and undivided muscle fibers
(7) Progressive division of the neck of the diverticulum with simultaneous closure of the resulting defect by continuous or interrupted sutures
(8) Test of suture line integrity
(9) Insertion of a soft rubber drain and closure of the cervical incision

lum is grasped with a small Babcock clamp and carefully dissected free on all sides. The neck of the diverticulum is freed from all muscular structures so that its junction with the esophageal submucosa is clearly defined (Fig. 125 a). Cricopharyngeal myotomy follows (see 9.2.1). The rest of the procedure depends on the extent of the diverticulum and the shape of its neck. If the base of the diverticular sac is higher than the inferior margin of the neck after the myotomy, the myotomy will be an adequate procedure. If the diverticular neck is narrow and the base of the diverticulum remains below the level of the neck after the myotomy, excision or diverticulopexy must be added. We amputate the diverticulum by an open technique and generally close the defect obliquely. A Sengstaken tube or large-gauge stomach tube is passed into the esophagus to keep it from constricting during the closure. The initial suture serves as a traction suture. It is tied, grasped with a clamp, and held in slight tension. The closure can be completed with inverting interrupted sutures or with a continuous suture. The neck of the diverticulum is transected with a scissors in stepwise fashion, and the luminal opening is repaired at once with sutures (Fig. 125 b). A single suture layer is sufficient to provide watertight closure [5].

Undivided cricopharyngeal muscle fibers will jeopardize the integrity of the manual or mechani-

Fig. 125 a, b. Excision of a cervical esophageal diverticulum. **a** The neck of the diverticulum is cleared circumferentially, and cricopharyngeal myotomy (broken line) is performed. **b** The diverticular neck is incised in steps, and the defect is closed transversely in one layer

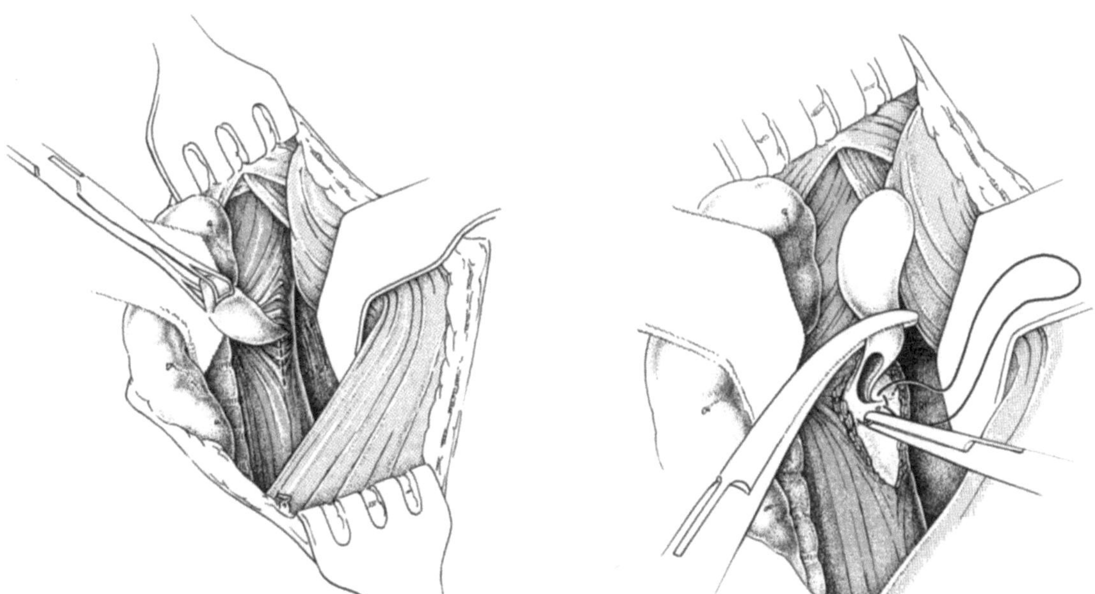

a b

cal closure by restoring a high pressure zone postoperatively that may blow out the suture line.

Diverticulopexy is recommended by Belsey [2] when the esophageal wall shows inflammatory changes about the neck of the diverticulum, making it hazardous to apply sutures in that area. In this situation the mobilized diverticular sac is up-ended and is fixed to the prevertebral fascia with 4 or 5 mattress sutures to provide dependent drainage of the pouch. The sutures pierce the full thickness of the diverticular wall to provide a secure fixation and partially obliterate the lumen of the sac.

Following diverticulectomy (but not diverticulopexy), a Penrose drain is placed next to the esophagus, and the wound is closed in layers.

11.4 Treatment of Thoracic Diverticulum by Myotomy, Excision, or Diverticulopexy

The surgical treatment of intrathoracic diverticula follows the same principles that apply to the treatment of cervical diverticula: elimination of the cause and, if necessary, direct attack on the diverticulum. With "pulsion" diverticula, a functional disorder of the esophagus can be demonstrated in two-thirds of cases [1]. A functional disorder is presumed to exist in the remaining third even if it cannot be demonstrated. Thus, in addition to eliminating a known cause (e.g., relieving gastroesophageal reflux by an antireflux procedure), we treat every pulsion diverticulum by incising the muscle wall from a point 1 cm above the diverticular neck to the esophagogastric junction.

Diverticulum-like outpouching of the entire esophageal wall in the direction of the tracheobronchial tree may result from the tension of an inflammatory process or may involve a gastroenteric cyst, incomplete separation of the trachea and esophagus, or incipient duplication [2, 3, 6]. It is extremely rare for this condition to require treatment. Surgery is indicated in the presence of a tracheobronchial-esophageal fistula or if an abscess has formed.

Special forms of intrathoracic diverticula are intramural diverticulosis [4] and postsurgery diverticula following an incomplete myotomy for achalasia or diffuse spasm of the esophagus. The treatment of intramural diverticulosis consists of systemic antibiotics to treat the possible infectious cause and also dilatation in patients with dysphagia and stenosis. An incomplete myotomy is either dilated or surgically revised.

Preoperative preparation: See Chap. C; perioperative antibiotics.

Instruments: Basic set, extra thoracic set; Sengstaken tube or large-caliber stomach tube (Ch 32).

Position and approach: Posterolateral thoracotomy according to the location of the diverticulum (see Chap. B).

Steps in procedure:

(1) Exposure of the thoracic esophagus (see 2.1.2)
(2) Circumferential dissection of the diverticulum
(3) Stepwise division of the diverticular neck and concomitant closure of the esophageal defect with continuous or interrupted sutures
(4) Approximation of the muscle wall over the mucosal repair with interrupted sutures
(5) Myotomy of the thoracic esophagus lateral to the closure site, extending to the esophagogastric junction
(6) Closure of the mediastinal pleura by continuous suture
(7) Insertion of a chest tube and closure of the chest

Operative technique: The esophagus is exposed and if necessary is encircled with a snare (see 2.1.2). A pulsion diverticulum is dissected free from surrounding connective tissue until its site of entry into the esophagus is clearly visualized. The size of the diverticulum and the shape of its neck will determine whether myotomy alone will suffice or whether excision should be added (see 11.3). A myotomy without diverticulectomy extends from a point 1 cm above the neck of the diverticulum to the esophagogastric junction (Fig. 126 a,b). If diverticulectomy is proposed, the myotomy may be placed lateral to the neck or below its site of transection. A lateral incision is advantageous as it permits the muscularis to be reapproximated over the mucosal suture following closure of the diverticular neck (Fig. 127 a,b). This reduces the danger of intrathoracic suture-line leakage, with its potentially grave consequences. The neck is closed using the same technique as for a cervical diverticulum (see 11.3). In the small percentage of cases where a parabronchial diverticulum is managed surgically, the diverticulum is exposed

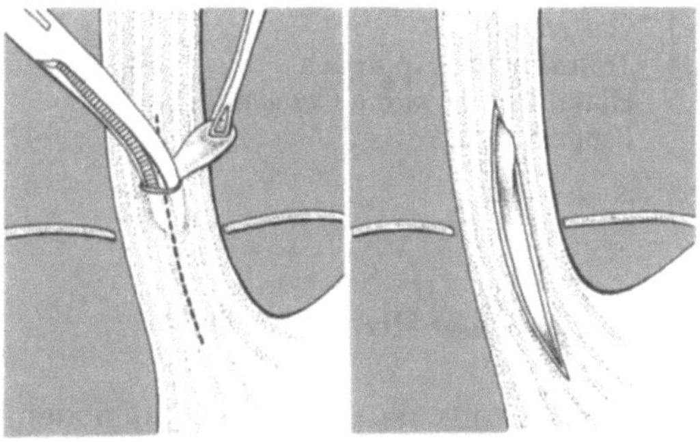

a b

Fig. 126a, b. Treatment of a small intrathoracic esophageal diverticulum by myotomy alone. **a** The intrathoracic diverticulum is circumferentially exposed, and the esophagus is myotomized above and below the neck of the lesion. **b** Status following the myotomy. There is only a small bulge of mucosa at the former site of the diverticulum. Since there is no dead space, it is unnecessary to excise the diverticulum

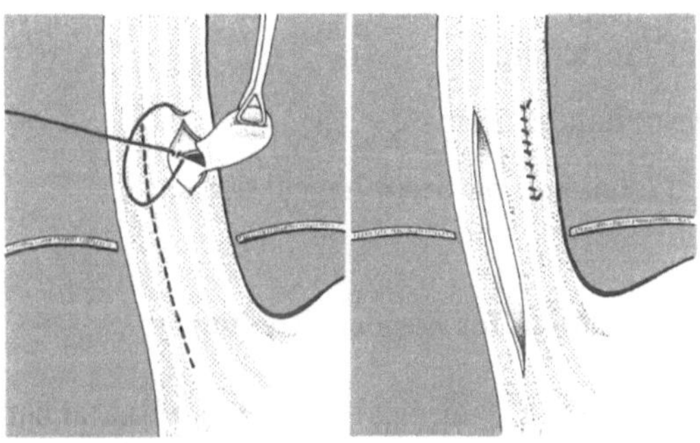

a b

Fig. 127a, b. Excision of an intrathoracic esophageal diverticulum. **a** The diverticulum is circumferentially cleared, progressively excised, and the defect closed transversely in one layer. The myotomy (broken line) is separate from the diverticulectomy. **b** Coapting muscle sutures cover the mucosa over the excised diverticulum. The myotomy is separate from the closure site

and is either divided between transfixion ligatures or closed using the technique described in 11.3. Generally a myotomy is unnecessary. If there is a coexisting peridiverticular abscess, it may be prudent to drain the abscess first and then repair the diverticulum in a second operation.

References

1. Allen TH, Clagett OT (1965) Changing concepts in the surgical treatment of pulsion diverticula of the lower esophagus. J Thorac Cardiovasc Surg 50:455
2. Belsey RH (1966) Functional disease of the esophagus. J Thorac Cardiovasc Surg 52:164
3. Borrie J, Wilson RLK (1980) Esophageal diverticula: principles of management and appraisal of classification. Thorax 35:759
4. Creely JJ, Trail ML (1970) Intramural diverticulosis of the esophagus. South Med J 63:1258
5. Hoehn JG, Payne WS (1969) Resection of pharyngoesophageal diverticulum using stapling device. Mayo Clin Proc 44:738
6. Ribbert H (1906) Die Traktionsdivertikel des Ösophagus. Virchows Arch 184:403
7. Smiley TB, Caves PH, Porter DC (1970) Relationship between posterior pharyngeal pouch and hiatal hernia. Thorax 25:725

12 Surgical Treatment of Hiatal Hernias

CONTENTS

12.1 Classification of Hiatal Hernias

Hiatal hernias involve the displacement of abdominal viscera, usually a portion or all of the stomach, into the thorax through the esophageal hiatus along with a sac of peritoneum. The following forms are recognized [39]:

Axial or sliding hernias:
- reversible or facultative form, usually without pathologic significance;
- axial hernia associated with reflux disease and possibly with a columnar-lined esophagus;
- fixed hernias associated with secondary esophageal shortening.

Paraesophageal hernias.

Mixed axial and paraesophageal hernias.

12.2 Indications for Surgical Treatment

Indications for the surgical treatment of hiatal hernia are based not on the anatomic defect itself but on the conditions that may precipitate, accompany, or follow the defect. Thus, the main criterion for the operative treatment of hiatal hernia is reflux disease [48]; in the columnar-lined esophagus it is the potential for malignant transformation, and in paraesophageal hernias it is the potential for strangulation or incarceration of the stomach wall or the presence of an intrathoracic mass. In mixed forms the principal component of the hernia will determine the need for operative treatment.

12.3 Choice of Operation for Esophageal Reflux Disease

12.3.1 Operative Method

Of the various surgical procedures available for the treatment of reflux disease, such as fundoplication [38, 44], semifundoplication [3, 4, 13, 17, 23, 25, 47], anatomic repair [1, 7, 19, 28, 34, 35], and procedures using ligament flaps [9, 27, 36, 42], more than 10 years' follow-up experience indicates that only fundoplication and the various types of semifundoplication have been able to provide objective relief of pathologic gastroesophageal reflux and associated complaints in 80% to 90% of patients [18, 22, 25, 25, 46, 49, 52]. We regard them, therefore, as the procedures of choice for the surgical treatment of reflux esophagitis. The possible superiority of a fundoplication over the various types of semifundoplication can be judged only on the basis of comparative prospective studies that take into account long-term efficacy as well as postoperative complications and late sequelae. To date, such studies have not been conducted or have taken insufficient account of the factors stated above [11]. Consequently we shall present the facts below as we know them, and we shall leave it to the operator to evaluate their significance.

1. The postoperative hospital mortality and complication rates of fundoplication and semifundoplication are almost identical. 2. Measurements of spontaneous and provoked acid reflux and of pressures in the lower esophageal sphincter indicate superior results with fundoplication. In the comparative prospective study of Demeester et al. [11], fundoplication was more effective than semifundoplication in the prevention of reflux. Also, the fundoplication increased the lower sphincter pressure more than the semifundoplication in comparison with preoperative levels. This finding is confirmed by experimental and clinical studies [2, 12, 32]. 3. If we take symptomatic recurrent reflux as the criterion for a successful outcome, we find no difference between the procedures due to variations in follow-up times and therapeutic goals. Generally the recurrence rate increases with the length of follow-up. 4. One cause of early and late recurrence of reflux is suture disruption in the fundic wrap. This seems to be a greater problem in semifundoplications due to the lower tear-out strength of the esophageal wall. 5. Postoperative dysphagia is more common after fundoplication than semifundoplication, although dilatation is rarely warranted. The ability of patients to belch and vomit decreases with the degree of the fundic wrap around the esophagus and so is most impaired after the fundoplication. Gas bloat syndrome, characterized by a feeling of fullness, abdominal distention, and inability to belch or vomit, is a significant complaint of many patients undergoing fundoplication and constitutes a major objection to that procedure. It may be preventable by employing a looser wrap [39].

12.3.2 Suture Material

We use absorbable suture material for all surgical procedures on the esophagus (see 1.3.2.1). A number of surgeons [4, 23, 38, 44, 50, 52] prefer nonabsorbable material for hiatal hernia repairs, claiming that it is necessary for a permanent reposition, i.e., for maintaining an intraabdominal segment of esophagus. Even if we allow that the structures to be united (e.g. the abdominal esophagus and fundus) should be broadly adherent to one another by the time the absorbable suture material loses its stability, we have seen instances where disruption occurred more than six weeks after a semifundoplication; hence we cannot entirely dismiss the foregoing argument. Our current recommendation would be to perform hiatal hernia repairs with a nonabsorbable suture material or at least to use an absorbable acid material that retains its stability for a relatively long period of time.

12.4 Approach

Once there was controversy as to the best approach for hiatal hernia repairs, but today it is generally acknowledged that the trauma of thoracotomy does not relate favorably to the benignity of the underlying disorder. Laparotomy is better tolerated by the great majority of patients, and it permits evaluation of the entire intestinal tract. It has become the standard approach for antireflux procedures. Only Belsey [4, 5] continues to advocate the transthoracic approach for his Mark IV operation. Modifications for all methods have been devised that enable surgeons to choose between a transabdominal or transthoracic approach.

The transthoracic approach is advantageous in obese patients, in patients with a short esophagus requiring extensive mobilization, and for repeat antireflux operations following a previous transabdominal procedure.

12.5 Fundoplication

The Rossetti modification [44], in which the wrap is formed from the anterior wall of the fundus, has become the standard technique of fundoplication, largely replacing the original technique of Nissen [38]. The advantage of confining the fundoplication to the anterior wall is that the lesser omentum and the retroperitoneal attachments of the proximal stomach remain intact. This preserves the hepatic branches of the vagus nerve, and the intact retroperitoneal attachments ensure that portions of the stomach will not herniate through the fundic wrap. The original technique is used in cases where the lesser omentum is already divided and the stomach has been previously mobilized (e.g., for a selective proximal vagotomy).

12.5.1 Original Technique

12.5.1.1 Transabdominal Approach

Preoperative preparation: See Chap. C.

Instruments: Basic set, stomach tube (Ch 32).

Position and approach: Upper midline laparotomy, which may be extended around the left side of the umbilicus.

Steps in procedure:

(1) Detachment of the left lobe of the liver from the diaphragm
(2) Transverse division of the peritoneum over the esophagogastric junction
(3) Extension of the incision into the gastrosplenic ligament on the left side and the gastrohepatic ligament on the right
(4) Dissection of 4–6 cm of the abdominal esophagus
(5) Snaring of the esophagus
(6) Creation of a wrap using folds from the anterior and posterior walls of the gastric fundus
(7) Fixation of the wrap with 4 interrupted sutures (1 piercing the anterior muscle wall of the esophagus)
(8) Confirmation of a loose wrap
(9) If necessary, stabilization of the wrap with 2 or 3 sutures uniting the lower margin of the wrap to the anterior stomach wall

Operative technique: The abdomen is entered, and the table is tilted slightly toward the foot end so that the viscera can sag distally. The condition of the hiatus is assessed by palpation, and the extent of the hernia is determined. A nasogastric tube inserted preoperatively is useful for orientation. The left lobe of the liver is retracted medially with a broad, curved retractor. If this does not give adequate exposure of the esophagogastric junctional area, the triangular ligament of the liver is divided prior to medial retraction of the left lobe. The nasogastric tube is positioned along the greater curvature. With its help, an assistant grasps the stomach and pulls it downward, placing tension on the peritoneal reflection and gastrophrenic ligament. The peritoneum is incised transversely over the gastroesophageal junction. On the left side the incision is extended through the gastrophrenic ligament to its junction with the gastrosplenic ligament. The short gastric arteries in this area are ligated and divided. On the right side the omental bursa is opened by dividing the superior portion of the gastrohepatic ligament (Fig. 128 a). Usually one cannot help dividing the hepatic branch of the vagus nerve at this time. The anterior vagus nerve trunk is left on the esophagus and is carefully preserved. Close to the nerve trunk are the ascending esophageal branches from the left gastric artery with their accompanying veins. They are ligated, since injury to these vessels during subsequent dissection can produce troublesome bleeding. Posterolateral branches from the inferior phrenic artery also are vulnerable when the esophagus is snared, and they may be divided without compromising the esophageal blood supply. The peritoneum, connective tissue, and the esophagophrenic membrane are mobilized 4–6 cm upward from the esophagus with a dissecting patty, carefully avoiding injury to the vagus nerve (Fig. 128 b). At this time the nasogastric tube is replaced by a large-gauge stomach tube (Ch 32). Then the esophagus is encircled with a snare. This maneuver is not without its hazards, for the posterior wall of the esophagus and the surrounding tissues are fragile, adherent, and easily injured as a result of the reflux disease. One should not be misled if the inflammatory changes in the anterior wall appear minor, for it is the posterior wall that is exposed most consistently to the effects of peptic reflux during recumbency. With the index finger of the right hand, the surgeon feels his way toward the pulsating aorta on the left side of the esophagus while carefully dissecting down through the connective tissue. When the finger reaches the aorta, it turns mediad along the anterior aspect of the vertebral column. The finger should now be able to palpate the thumb, which is inserted in similar fashion from the right side. The tips of the finger and thumb are moved together until they touch. Using the aorta and spinal column as guides, it should be possible to avoid esophageal wall injury even when a very high grade of esophagitis is present (Fig. 128 c). With the index finger encircling the esophagus, the tip of a Guyon clamp is placed against the fingertip for safe passage be-

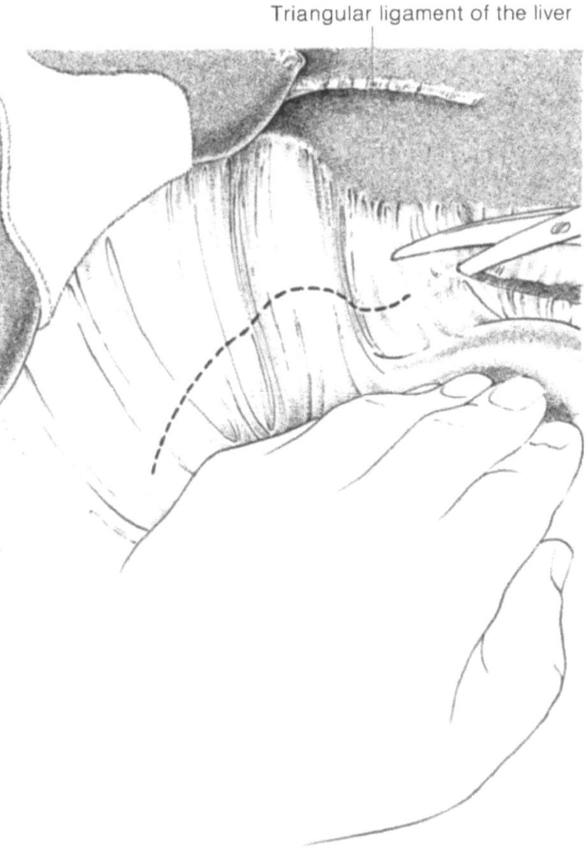

a

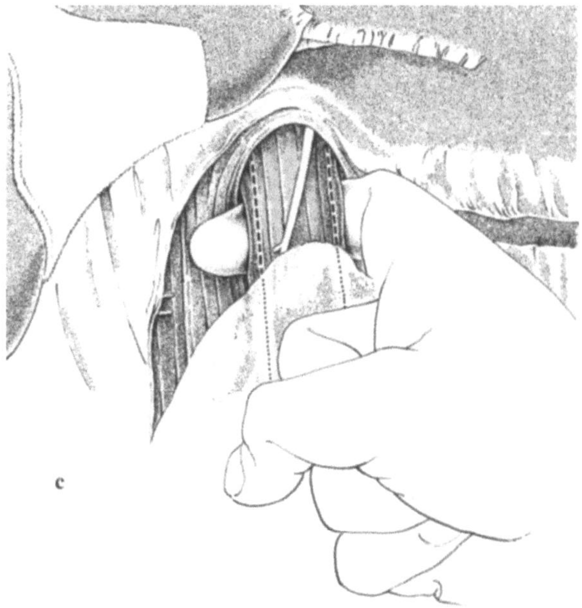

c

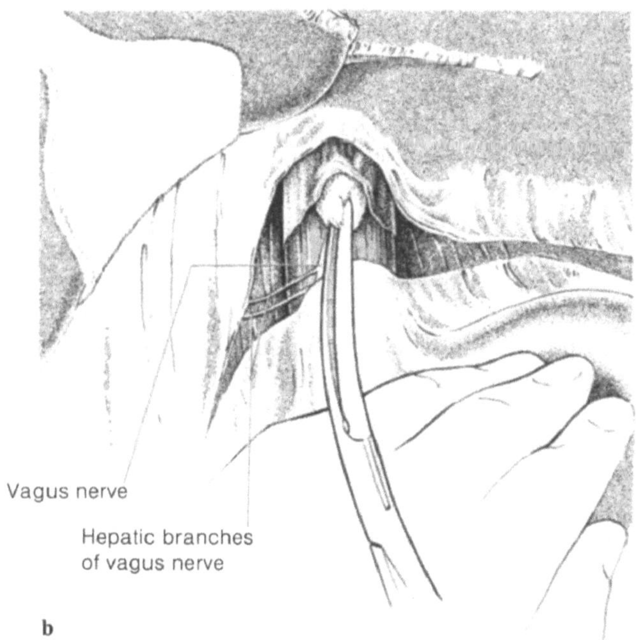

b

Fig. 128a–f. The original technique of fundoplication. **a** Transverse division of the gastrophrenic ligament, the peritoneal covering of the esophagus, and the upper portion of the gastrohepatic ligament. The left lobe of the liver is detached from the diaphragm. **b** The peritoneum and esophagophrenic membrane are dissected from the abdominal esophagus. **c** The esophagus is encircled with the finger. **d–f** see p. 410

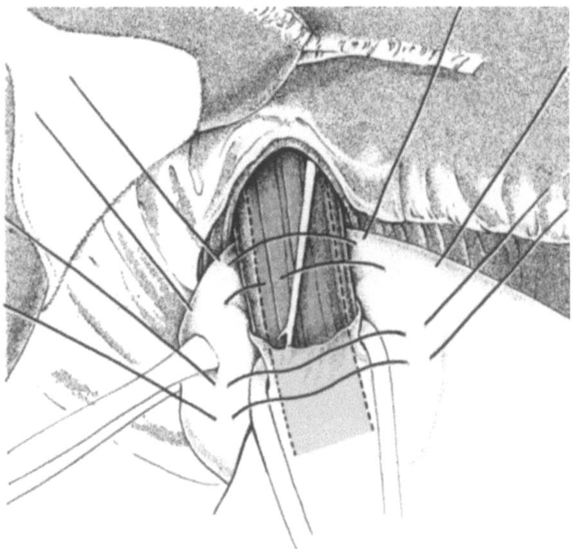

d

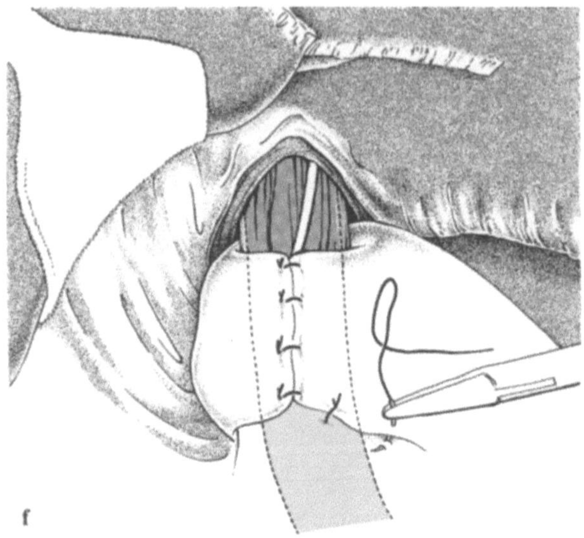

f

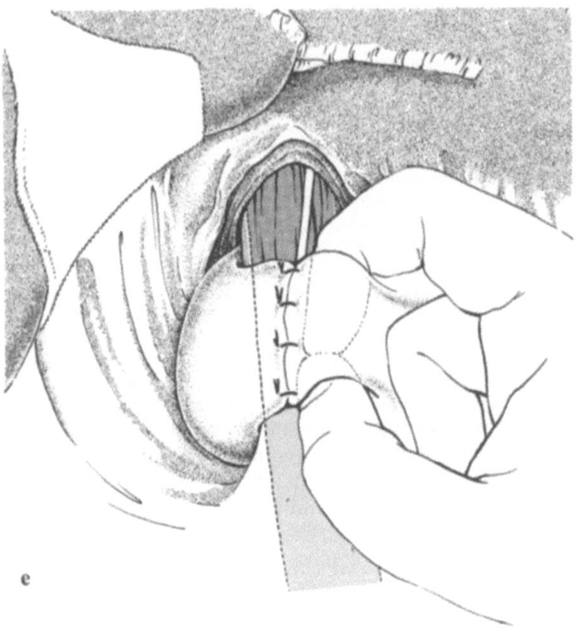

e

Fig. 128. d Sutures for creating the fundic wrap. The central suture is placed first and is the only suture that pierces the esophagus. **e** A loose wrap is confirmed. **f** The wrap is sutured to the anterior stomach wall to prevent telescoping

hind the esophagus. The clamp is then used to grasp and pull through a soft rubber drain, which is looped around the esophagus. With this technique the posterior vagus nerve trunk remains on the esophagus. In the absence of significant periesophageal inflammation, the nerve trunk can be dissected off the esophagus and snared. Later it will be routed outside the fundic wrap. The rubber drain encircling the esophagus is pulled laterally forward in preparation for mobilizing the stomach. The connective-tissue attachments joining the cardia and fundus with the retroperitoneum are divided. Then the posterior wall of the fundus is grasped with a Babcock clamp and passed behind the esophagus from left to right. Downward traction is applied to the esophageal snare to make sure the wrap is positioned over the esophagus and not over the proximal stomach. The first suture pierces the anterior wall of the fundus, the muscularis and submucosa of the esophagus, and the posterior wall of the fundus (Fig. 128 d). It is tightened at once to determine whether there is room to insert a finger easily between the fundic wrap and the esophagus, which is splinted internally by the stomach tube. If the wrap is sufficiently loose, the suture may be tied. One more suture is placed above it and two more below it. These sutures incorporate the anterior and posterior fundic walls but not the esophagus. The wrap is checked again to make sure it is not too tight (Fig. 128 e).

Some surgeons [29, 41, 52] recommend that all the fundoplication sutures pierce the esophageal wall to give added protection against telescoping, or slippage of the stomach through the fundic wrap. An alternative is to fix the lower margin of the wrap to the anterior stomach wall with two or three sutures (Fig. 128 f) close to the lesser curvature [50]. Then the rubber drain is removed, the large stomach tube is replaced with a nasogastric tube, and the abdomen is closed without drainage. Narrowing of the hiatus is not part of the original technique described by Nissen et al. [39].

12.5.1.2 Transthoracic Approach

Preoperative preparation: See Chap. C.

Instruments: Basic set, extra thoracic set; stomach tube (Ch 32).

Position and approach: Left posterolateral thoracotomy in the 6th interspace (see Chap. B).

Steps in procedure:

(1) Exposure and snaring of the thoracic esophagus (see 2.1.2)
(2) Dissection of the esophagus in the hiatus
(3) Mobilization of the fundus
(4) Exposure of the hiatal crura
(5) Placement of hiatal plication sutures
(6) Step 5 is omitted with a short esophagus, or the hiatus may have to be enlarged by incising into the central tendon of the diaphragm
(7) Construction of the fundic wrap (see 12.5.1.1)
(8) Replacement of the abdominal esophagus and fundoplication into the abdomen
(9) Narrowing of the hiatus with the preplaced sutures
(10) Steps 8 and 9 are omitted with a short esophagus, and instead the wrapped fundus is sutured to the hiatus or to the phrenotomy

Operative technique: The chest is entered, and the lower third of the esophagus is exposed and snared with a rubber tape (see 2.1.2). With cephalad traction on the tape, the pleura is divided over the hernial sac and the hiatus. The phrenoesophageal membrane under the pleura (linking the endoabdominal fascia with the endothoracic fascia) is incised anterolaterally, giving access to the retroperitoneal fat and peritoneal reflection. When these have been divided, the cardia can be freed circumferentially from its attachments with the diaphragm. The branch of the left inferior phrenic artery that ascends lateral to the vagus nerve is ligated. The cardia is now pulled into the thorax, bringing into view the hepatogastric ligament and the branch of the left gastric artery that ascends within the ligament. The esophageal branches of the left gastric artery are divided. The pars densa of the lesser omentum is divided, carefully avoiding injury to the vagus nerve trunks. The hepatic branches of the vagus nerve often are severed at this time. Now the esophagus is pulled anteriorly with the tape, and the fundus is mobilized by severing its connective-tissue attachments with the diaphragm (Fig. 129 a). If this does not free the stomach sufficiently for the fundoplication, mobility can gained by dividing the proximal short gastric arteries. When the mobilization has been completed, it should be possible to pass a finger completely around the esophagus within the hiatus. The stomach is returned to the abdominal cavity, and the esophagus is pulled anteriorly. The pericardium is bluntly separated from the diaphragm so that the tendinous origin of the diaphragm can be identified. The first suture is placed through the posterior margins of the hiatal crura close to the aorta (Fig. 129 b). Generally two or three additional sutures will be needed to narrow the hiatus sufficiently. For the time being the sutures are held with a clamp but not tied. If the esophagogastric junction cannot be returned to the abdomen due to shortening of the esophagus, the hiatus should not be narrowed. In fact, it is usually necessary to enlarge the hiatus in these cases by incising toward the central tendon of the diaphragm. This is to ensure that the fundic wrap will not be constricted by the narrow hiatus. The wrapped fundus is then anchored to the hiatus or phrenotomy with a few interrupted sutures (Fig. 129 c). The technique for constructing the wrap is the same as in the transabdominal approach (see 12.5.1.1). The two folds of fundus are brought together on line with the lesser curvature, the sutures are placed, and the wrap is checked for looseness. The tape is removed from the esophagus, and the abdominal esophagus and the wrap covering it are reduced into the abdominal cavity. The sutures previously placed through the hiatal crura are then tied, making sure that the tip of the forefinger can be admitted alongside the esophagus, which is splinted by the stomach tube. Finally the pleura is closed over the esophagus by continuous suture, a chest tube is inserted, the lung is inflated, and the thoracotomy is closed in layers.

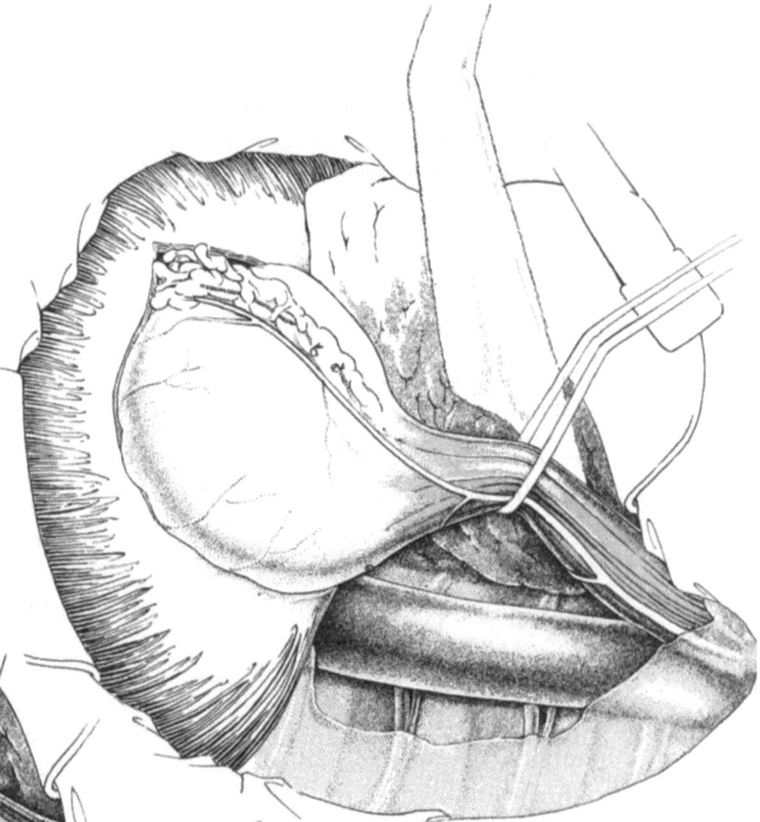

a

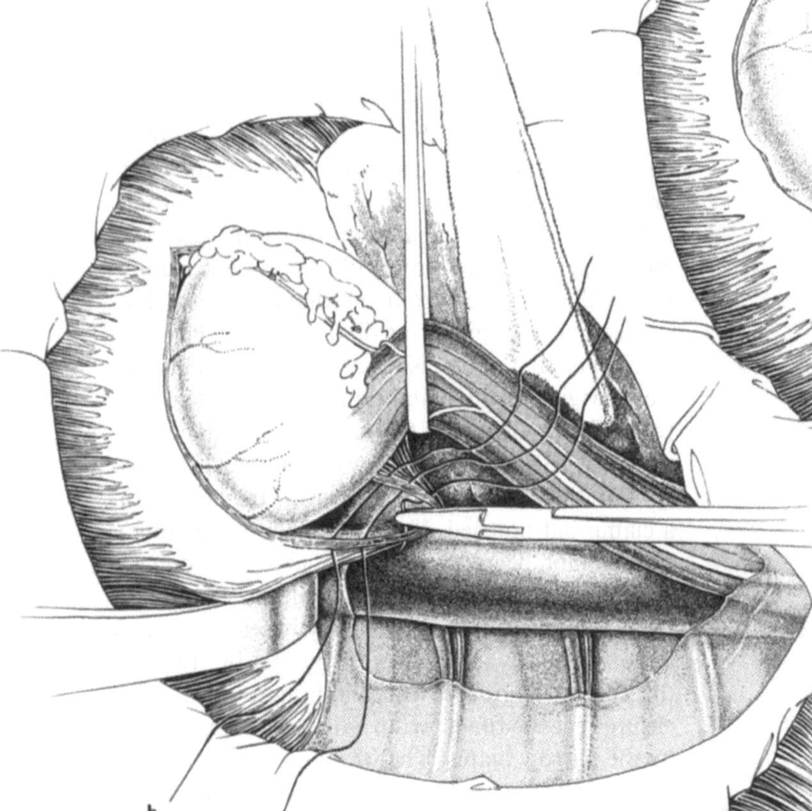

b

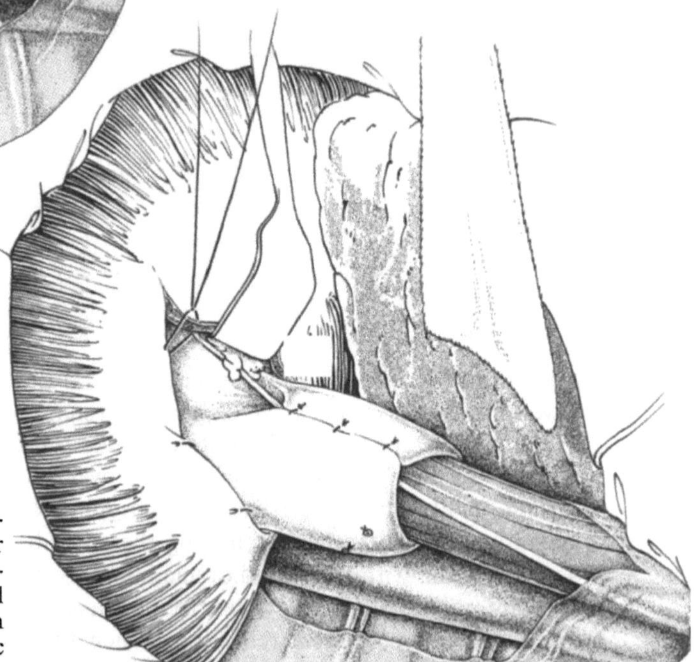

c

Fig. 129 a–c. Fundoplication through a transthoracic approach. **a** The fundus and proximal part of the lesser curvature are pulled into the thorax through the esophageal hiatus, which is enlarged by incising into the central tendon. **b** The crural margins are approximated with interrupted sutures to narrow the hiatus. **c** Intrathoracic fundoplication with a short esophagus. The hiatus is fixed to the fundic wrap with several sutures

12.5.2 Rossetti Modification [44]

Preoperative preparation, instruments, position and approach: See 11.5.1.

Steps in procedure:

(1) Transverse incision of the peritoneum over the esophagogastric junction
(2) Extension of the incision laterally to the gastrosplenic ligament
(3) Snaring of the esophagus
(4) Passage of a fold of anterior fundus behind the esophagus
(5) Creation of a counterfold from the greater curvature side of the anterior fundus
(6) Approximation of both folds with four seromuscular sutures, creating a 360° wrap around the abdominal esophagus
(7) Confirmation of a loose wrap
(8) Stabilization of the wrap by suturing its lower margin to the anterior stomach wall

Operative technique: The cardia and abdominal esophagus are exposed much as they are in the original Nissen technique (see 12.5.1.1). However, the peritoneal incision over the esophagus is carried only 1 cm into the uppermost portion of the hepatogastric ligament on the right side to ensure that the hepatic and hepatopyloric vagus nerve branches are spared. In addition, the posterior wall of the fundus is not freed from its peritoneal adhesions. The rubber tape on the esophagus is pulled forward and downward, and a loose fold of anterior fundic wall is passed behind the esophagus with one or two fingers of the right hand (Fig. 130 a). There it is grasped at its upper and lower edges with two small Bablock clamps and held in position. Usually only about a 1- to 2-cm length of fundus can be passed behind the esophagus in this fashion. The "counterfold" for making the wrap

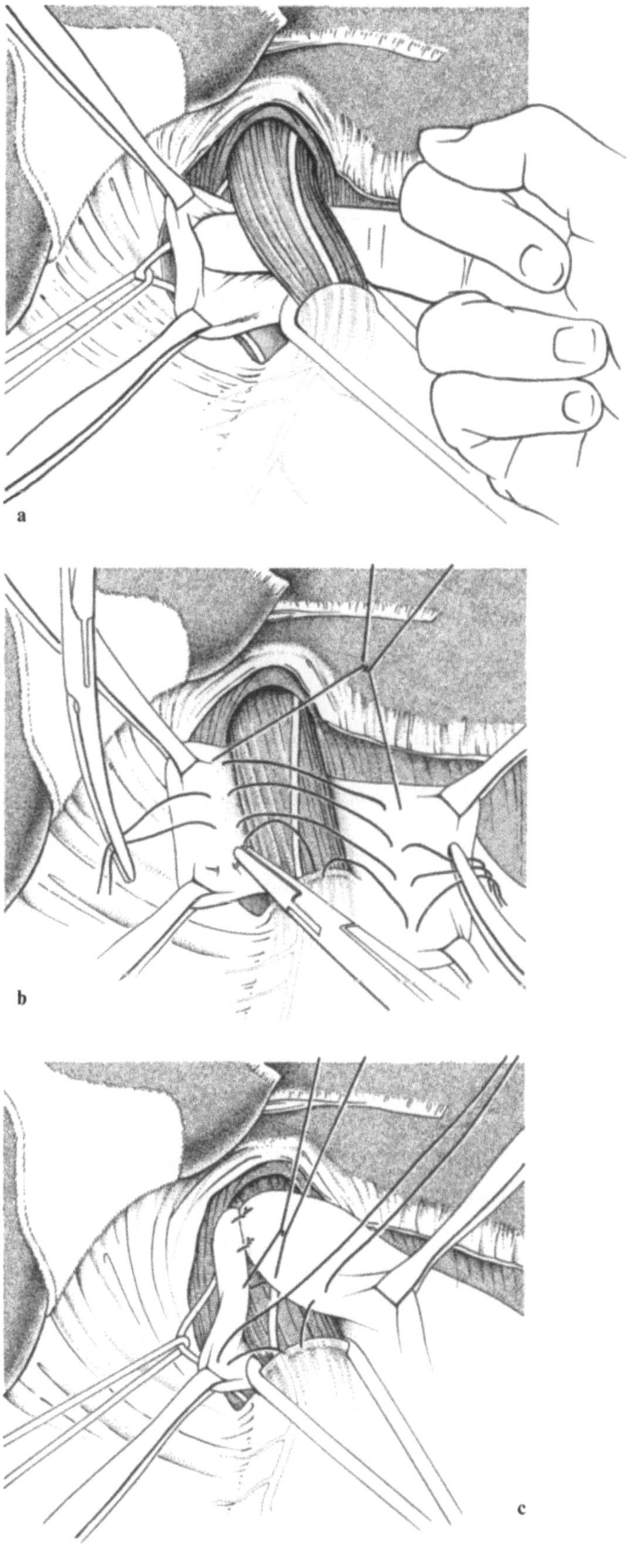

Fig. 130 a–c. Rosetti's modification of fundoplication [44]. **a** The wrap is initiated by passing a loose fold of the anterior wall of the fundus behind the mobilized esophagus with the finger. **b** A counterfold is developed from the greater curvature side of the anterior fundus. The lowermost suture is passed through the connective tissue of the esophagogastric junction to stabilize the wrap. **c** The folds of fundus are stitched together over the esophagus, which is splinted with an indwelling stomach tube is formed from the greater curvature side of the anterior fundus, at a slightly more distal level, and is marked with two clamps (Fig. 130 b). If there is not enough material for the fundoplication, it will be necessary to mobilize the greater curvature side of the fundus as far as the hilum of the spleen. The clamps are brought together to confirm that the wrap envelops the esophagus without tension.

The folds are stitched together with four seromuscular sutures that do not incorporate the esophagus. The most distal suture may pierce the connective tissue just below the junction of the esophageal muscularis with the serosa-covered stomach (Fig. 130 c). The looseness of the wrap is tested by inserting a finger or a blunt, slightly opened clamp. It is imperative that the wrap enclose the esophagus loosely and without tension. The position of the wrap can be secured by stitching its lower margin to the anterior stomach wall near the lesser curvature. Sutures are not placed to narrow the hiatal opening.

12.6 Semifundoplication

12.6.1 180° Semifundoplication

The various modifications of the 180° fundic wrap differ in whether the fundus is fixed to the anterior [13], posterior [17, 47], or lateral [23] aspect of the esophagus. In addition, a variety of measures may be used to narrow the hiatal sling and maintain an intraabdominal segment of esophagus.

12.6.1.1 Anterior or Posterior Semifundoplication

Preoperative preparation: See Chap. C.

Instruments: Basic set; stomach tube (Ch 32).

Position and approach: Upper midline laparotomy, which may be extended around the left side of the umbilicus.

Operative technique: The abdominal esophagus and cardia are exposed (see 12.5.1.1). The peritoneum over the gastroesophageal junction is incised transversely with a scissors. On the left side the incision is extended through the gastrophrenic ligament to the gastrosplenic ligament, which carries the short gastric vessels (Fig. 131 a). There is no need to extend the incision past the esophagus on the right side, so the hepatic branches of the vagus nerve are spared. The peritoneum and esophagophrenic membrane are bluntly dissected from the esophagus with a pledget, exposing slightly more than half its circumference (Fig. 131 b). The posterolateral branches of the left inferior phrenic artery are divided, as they are prone to bleed when the esophagus is snared. The anterior vagus nerve trunk is identified and left on the esophagus. At this point the nasogastric tube is replaced with

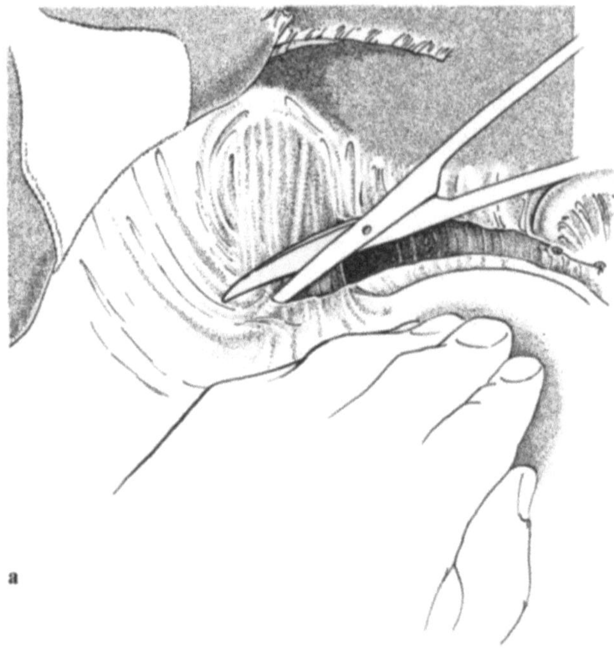

a

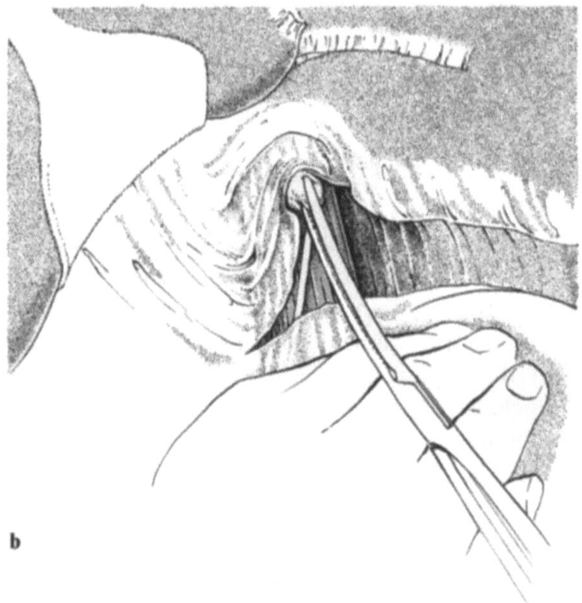

b

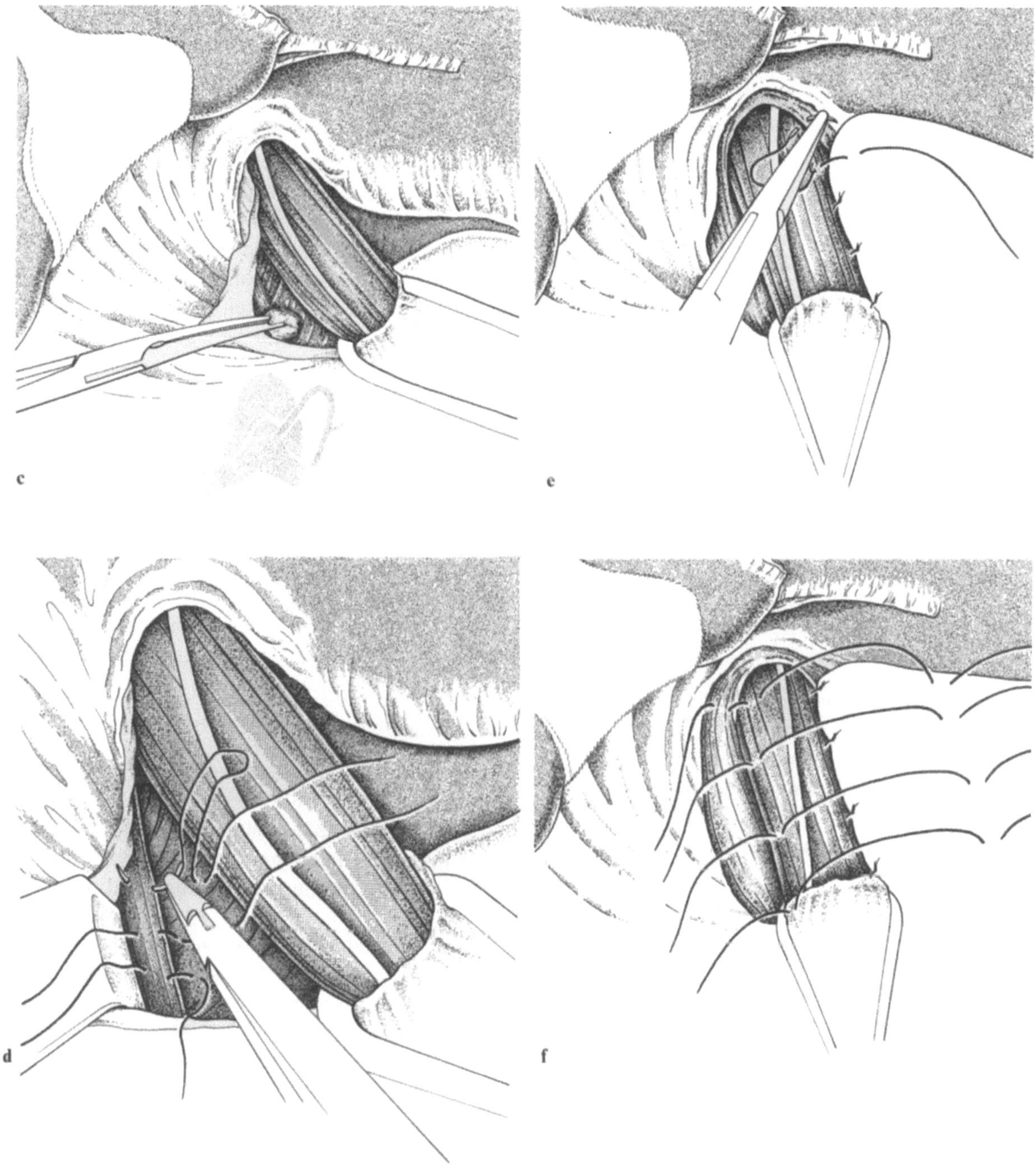

a large-caliber stomach tube, and the esophagus is encircled with a snare (see 12.5.1.1). This maneuver is not without its hazards due to the vulnerability of the posterior esophageal wall. We leave the posterior vagus nerve branch on the esophagus. This causes no problems in an anterior semifundoplication. For a posterior semifundoplication, Guarner et al. [17] try to keep the posterior vagus outside the wrap by dissecting it from the esophagus, unless this is prevented by inflammatory

Fig. 131 a–f. Anterior 180° semifundoplication. **a** The gastrophrenic ligament and the peritoneum covering the esophagus are divided. **b** The anterior esophageal body is dissected free. **c** The hiatal crura are exposed posterior to the esophagus. **d** A posterior hiatal repair is performed. **e** The gastric fundus is fixed to the left lateral esophageal wall. The most proximal suture pierces the rim of the esophageal hiatus. **f** The semifundoplication is performed by suturing the anterior wall of the fundus to the right lateral wall of the esophagus

Steps in procedure:

(1) Detachment of the left lobe of the liver from the diaphragm
(2) Incision of the peritoneum over the esophagogastric junction
(3) Extension of the incision to the gastrosplenic ligament
(4) Circumferential dissection of a 4- to 6-cm length of the abdominal esophagus
(5) Snaring of the esophagus
(6) Exposure of the hiatal crura
(7) Approximation of the crura with 2 or 3 sutures to narrow the hiatus
(8) Fixation of the fundus to the left lateral wall of the esophagus and to the hiatus with 3 or 4 sutures
(9) Anterior wall of the fundus is passed around the anterior side of the esophagus and fixed to its right lateral wall and hiatus with interrupted sutures

changes. The esophagus is pulled forward and downward with the snare, and a segment 4–6 cm long is cleared on all sides. The next step is to narrow the hiatal opening posterior to the esophagus. While Dor et al. [13] identify this step as part of the procedure, Guarner et al. [17] do not describe it explicitly. We personally use the anterior semifundoplication as our standard procedure and perform the hiatal repair routinely. The esophagus is pulled anterolaterally, and the hiatal crura are exposed by patty dissection (Fig. 131 c). Starting from the aorta and working toward the esophagus, the crural margins are approximated with heavy interrupted sutures, leaving enough space to accommodate a fingertip between the hiatal rim and the esophagus, which is splinted with the stomach tube. The two or three sutures that are used to narrow the hiatus pierce the crura at different depths to prevent fraying of the muscle fibers (Fig. 131 d). When all the sutures have been placed, they are tied right away.

Hermann [21] advises narrowing the hiatus anterior to the esophagus, stating that it is technically easier to perform the hiatal repair on that side than posteriorly. He points out that the hiatal crura are more strongly developed anterior to the esophagus near the central tendon of the diaphragm and will hold sutures more securely. He also notes that narrowing the hiatus anteriorly moves it to a more normal position near the spine and aorta and closes the hiatal defect at the site where it developed.

For an anterior semifundoplication the mobilized fundus is pulled medially, and a 4- to 6-cm length of its wall is fixed with 3 or 4 sutures to the left lateral wall of the esophagus (Fig. 131 e). The stitch pierces the serosa and muscularis of the fundus and incorporates the submucosa of the esophagus to ensure a solid hold. The lowermost suture is additionally reinforced by placing it level with the peritoneal reflection at the cardia. The uppermost suture incorporates a portion of the hiatal margin. Care is taken that none of the sutures catches the anterior vagus nerve trunk. The anterior wall of the fundus is passed around the anterior circumference of the esophagus and fixed to its right lateral wall with 3 or 4 sutures. Again, the lowermost suture is placed at the peritoneal reflection, and the uppermost suture incorporates the hiatus (Fig. 131 f). For a posterior semifundoplication [17] a fold is raised from the anterior wall of the fundus, passed behind the esophagus, and fixed to its left lateral wall with 3 or 4 sutures. At that time the large-gauge stomach tube is replaced with a nasogastric tube, and the abdomen is closed without drainage.

12.6.1.2 Lateral Semifundoplication

In the Hill repair [23], first described as a posterior gastropexy and later modified to a semifundoplication [22, 25, 56], intraabdominal fixation of the esophagus is accomplished by suturing the remaining phrenoesophageal tissue and the fundus to the arcuate ligament or, if the latter is poorly developed, to the tendinous origin of the right crus of the diaphragm. Attachment to these heavy structures is supposed to provide a more reliable fixation than attachment to the esophageal wall.

Preoperative preparation, instruments, position and approach: See 12.6.1.1.

Operative technique: The esophagus is exposed and encircled with a snare (see 1.5.1). The hiatus, the preaortic fascia, and the arcuate ligament above the celiac trunk are dissected free. The hiatus is narrowed posterior to the esophagus with several heavy sutures. The stomach is rotated posteriorly to expose the margins of the phrenoesophageal tissue in front of and behind the esophagus. This tissue is continuous with the hepatogastric ligament. The first suture is placed at the esophagocardiac junction and incorporates the posteror layer of the esophagophrenic tissue, the adjacent poste-

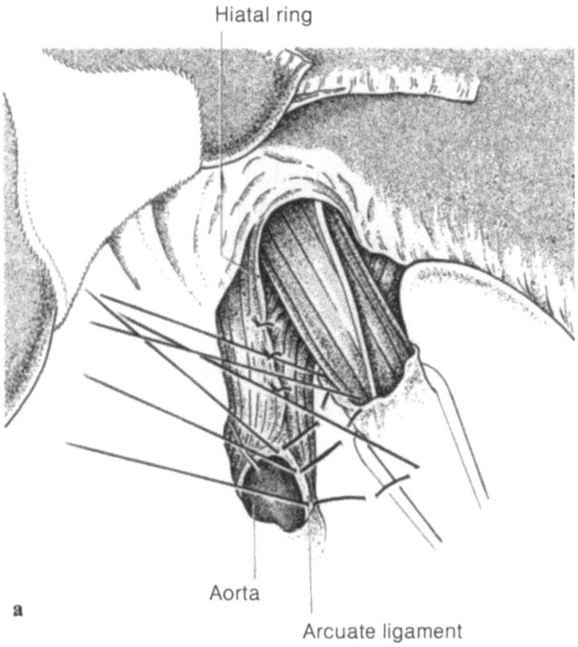

a

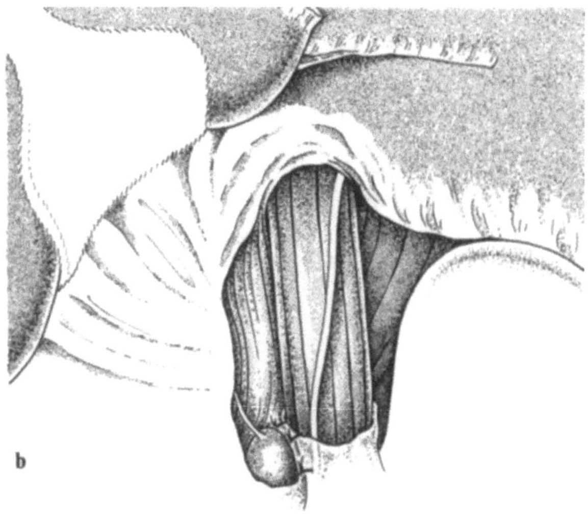

b

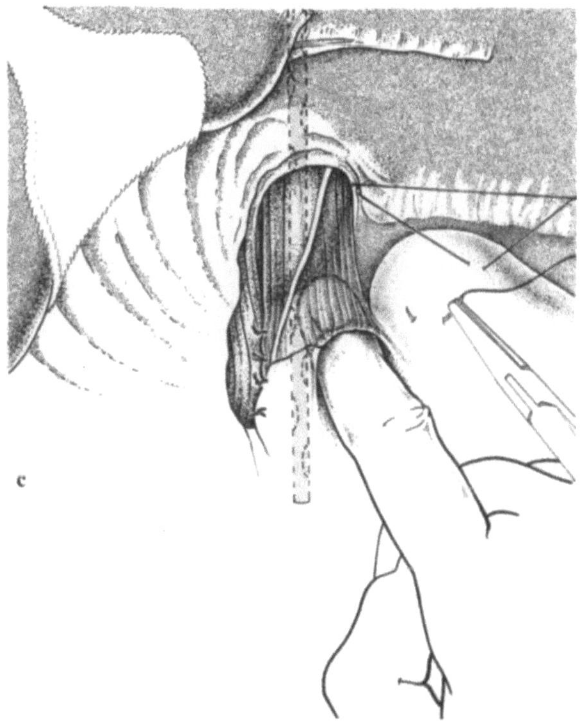

c

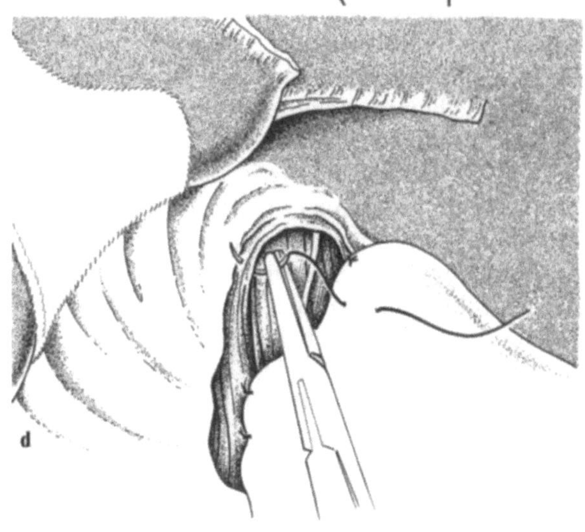

d

Fig. 132 a–d. Lateral 180° semifundoplication. **a** The esophagophrenic tissue is sutured to the arcuate ligament. The hiatal ring has been narrowed posteriorly with interrupted sutures. **b** The gastropexy sutures are tied, and the esophagogastric angle is restored. **c** The lumen of the esophagus is tested after completion of the gastropexy. **d** The anterior wall of the fundus is fixed to the anterior and posterior walls of the esophagus in two layers with interrupted sutures

rior wall of the fundus, and the center of the arcuate ligament of the aortic hiatus (Fig. 132 a). One or two additional sutures are placed proximal and distal to the first, incorporating both phrenoesophageal layers, the anterior and posterior walls of the stomach, and the arcuate ligament (Fig. 132 b). These sutures effectively prevent upward migration of the esophagus, restore tension to the cardial muscle sling, restore the esophagogastric angle, and create a type of valve mechanism. After each suture is tied, the surgeon invaginates the index finger into the lower esophagus to confirm an adequate lumen (Fig. 132 c). The competence of the antireflux barrier is tested by measuring the lower esophageal sphincter pressure intraoperatively [26]. The repair is completed by plicating part of the anterior fundic wall over the abdominal segment of the esophagus and suturing it to the esophagus or arcuate ligament and to the hiatus (Fig. 132 d).

12.6.2 270° Semifundoplication

The repair described by Belsey [4, 5] is performed exclusively through a thoracic approach.

Preoperative preparation, instruments, position and approach: See 12.5.1.2.

Steps in procedure:

(1) Exposure and snaring of the thoracic esophagus (see 2.1.2)
(2) Circumferential mobilization of the esophagus in the hiatus
(3) Dissection of the fundus
(4) Exposure of the hiatal crura
(5) Placement of 2 or 3 crural sutures
(6) Placement of the first row of 3 mattress sutures, creating a 3/4 wrap of fundus around the esophagus
(7) Placement of the second row of 3 mattress sutures, which incorporate the hiatal musculature
(8) Reduction of the abdominal esophagus into the abdomen
(9) Second row of mattress is tied
(10) Crural sutures are tied

Operative technique: The chest is entered as in a transthoracic fundoplication (see 11.5.1.2). The esophagus is exposed to the aortic arch, and the proximal part of the stomach is mobilized circumferentially through the hiatus. The esophagus is carefully cleared of all remaining fat and connective tissue so that the semifundoplication will appose the serosa of the stomach directly to the esophageal musculature, enabling the necessary cohesion to take place. The pleura between the diaphragm and pericardium is incised, and the pericardium is bluntly mobilized from the diaphragm so that its tendinous portion can be clearly identified. The diaphragm anterior to the hiatus is grasped with a clamp and pulled forward, exposing the tendinous portion of the right crus. Two or three heavy sutures are used to narrow the hiatus, depending on the extent of the herniation. The sutures are passed through the tendinous part of the right crus near its origin. On the left side they catch only a portion of the muscular cuff and the overlying pleura so that the muscle will not become strangulated when the sutures are tied. After the sutures have been placed, they are held with a clamp. They are not tied until the fundoplication is completed.

At this time it is determined whether the esophagogastric junction can be displaced about 4–6 cm distally into the abdominal cavity. If it cannot, the surgeon should abandon the semifundoplication and change to a fundoplication that leaves part of the wrapped fundus above the diaphragm (see 12.5.1.2). The semifundoplication is started by placing an initial row of three mattress sutures. The first is placed laterally, directly adjacent to the anterior vagus nerve; it pierces the seromuscular layer of the fundus and then the muscular and submucosal layers of the esophagus about 2 cm above the esophagogastric junction. The suture is reversed and passed back through the esophagus and gastric fundus, taking an oblique bite in the esophagus to obtain maximum anchorage in the muscle wall. The suture is tightened and tied at once to fix the fundus to the esophagus. Two additional mattress sutures are placed in similar fashion, one on the anterior aspect of the esophagus and one directly adjacent to the right vagus nerve. This creates a fundic wrap involving about 3/4 the circumference of the esophagus. In preparation for placing the second row of sutures, which incorporate the diaphragm, a spoon retractor is inserted through the hiatus to protect the underlying organs while the diaphragm is sutured. Again starting on the lateral side, the needle is passed through the tendinous part of the diaphragm about 1–2 cm from the hiatal margin into the bowl of the spoon and out through the hiatus (Fig. 133 a). The suture then pierces the seromuscularis of the fundus and the esophageal musculature and submucosa at sites 2 cm from the first row. The suture is reversed, as before, taking an oblique bite of the esophageal wall and passing back through the fundus, hiatus, and out through the diaphragm. Two more mattress sutures are placed parallel to the first row, imbricating an additional 2 cm of stomach over the first suture line (Fig. 133 b). The semifundoplication is placed below the diaphragm and held there until the sutures in the second row are tied. These sutures should not be tied too tightly lest they cut through the muscle wall of the esophagus. Finally the preplaced crural sutures are tightened behind the esophagus and tied. A chest tube is inserted, the lung is reexpanded, and the thoracotomy is closed in layers.

In the transabdominal modification of the 270° semifundoplication [33], the esophagus and fundus are mobilized through an abdominal incision as in the Nissen

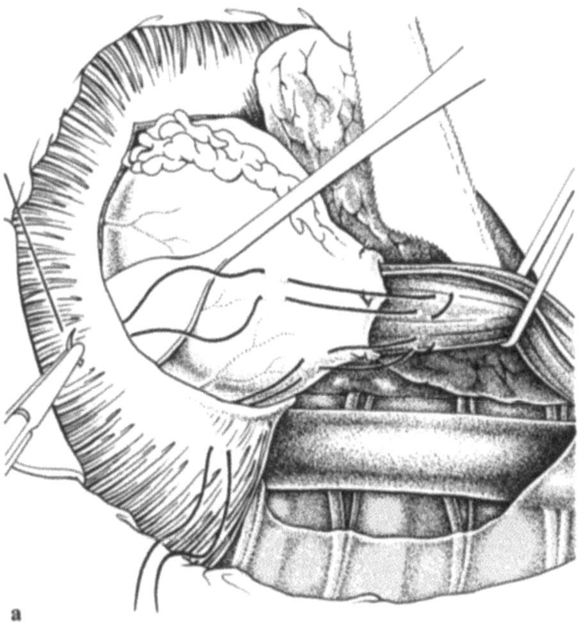

a

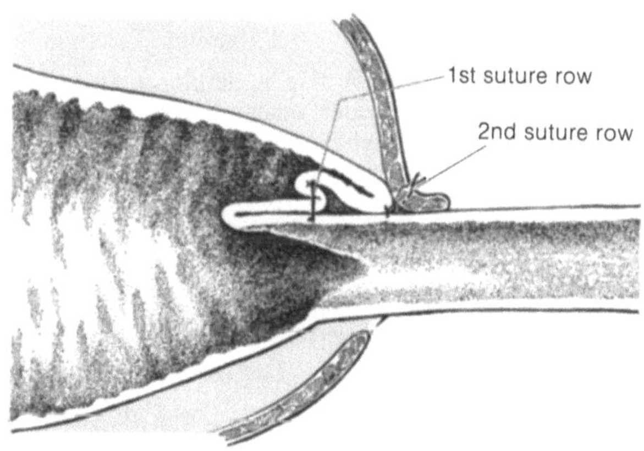

b

Fig. 133 a,b. The Belsey Mark IV semifundoplication [4, 5]. **a** The second row of mattress sutures is being applied. The initial row of 3 sutures has been placed and tied, imbricating the fundus over 3/4 of the circumference of the terminal esophagus. The second row of mattress sutures incorporates the hiatal musculature. The spoon passed into the hiatus protects the underlying viscera while the diaphragm is sutured. **b** Longitudinal section through the esophagus and stomach after completion of the semifundoplication

repair (see 12.5.1.1). The gastric fundus is fixed with interrupted sutures around the abdominal esophagus to create a two-thirds wrap. The fundus is not sutured to the diaphragm.

12.7 Anatomic Repairs

Anatomic repairs such as hiatal reconstruction [1, 19, 35], gastropexy [7, 37], and esophagofundopexy with posterior narrowing of the hiatus [34] are done for the purpose of eliminating a sliding hiatal hernia rather than preventing gastroesophageal reflux. Except for the procedure of Lortat-Jacob [34] and certain modifications [28], these repairs have been abandoned because they were unable to correct the underlying disorder.

12.7.1 Narrowing of the Hiatus Posterior to the Esophagus and Esophagofundophrenicopexy

The goal of this procedure is overcorrection of the Hiss angle, although the associated intraabdominal displacement of the esophagus provides a reflux-preventing factor.

Preoperative preparation: See Chap. C.

Instruments: Basic set; stomach tube (Ch 32).

Position and approach: Upper midline laparotomy.

Technique: The abdomen is entered, and the esophagus is exposed and snared (see 12.5.1.1). The esophagus is pulled anterolaterally, and the hiatal crura are exposed by patty dissection. Heavy crural sutures are placed and tied behind the esophagus to narrow the hiatus. Then the esophagus is pulled distally and, starting from the esophagogastric junction, the fundus is fixed with interrupted sutures to the esophagus, the hiatal crura, and the diaphragm.

12.7.2 Narrowing of the Hiatus Anterior to the Esophagus and Fundophrenicopexy

The advantage of this operation is its technical simplicity. There is no need to mobilize the esophagus circumferentially, so a major risk factor, perforation, is eliminated. The disadvantage is the high rate of recurrence.

Preoperative preparation, instruments, position and approach: See 12.7.1.

Technique: The abdomen is entered, and the region of the cardia is exposed. It is rarely necessary to divide the triangular ligament of the liver. The hiatal hernia is reduced by downward traction on the stomach. There is no need to open the hernial sac or to mobilize the cardia or abdominal esophagus. The margins of the enlarged hiatus are easily identified with the palpating finger. Without further dissection, the hiatus is narrowed anterior to the esophagus with several heavy sutures, leaving just enough room to accommodate the tip of the index finger. The gastric fundus is fixed to the diaphragm with a curved suture line that begins next to the cardia.

12.8 Use of Ligamentous Flaps

The snaring or fixation of the lower esophagus under tension with endogenous or foreign material to maintain the reduction of an hiatal hernia [27, 42] was initially abandoned in favor of the methods described above but recently has found new application [11, 36].

12.8.1 Omental Cuff

Preoperative preparation, instruments, position and approach: See 12.5.1.1.

Technique: After the abdomen is entered, the greater omentum is cleared of adhesions and exteriorized. Starting from its left margin, a well-perfused flap of omentum about 8 cm wide is mobilized as far as the transverse colon. Then the stomach is pulled distally, the peritoneum is incised directly over the cardia for a length of 3 cm, and the esophagus is encircled with a rubber tape. The distal end of the omental tag is attached to the tape, pulled through behind the esophagus, and brought laterally downward until its ascending and descending portions touch at the level of the anterior stomach wall. The flap should be slightly tense, but not to the point of displacing the transverse colon from its normal position. The ascending and descending parts of the omental cuff are stitched together with 3 or 4 interrupted sutures in front of the anterior gastric wall (Fig. 134). Additionally the right margin of the descending limb and the left margin of the ascending limb are fixed to the anterior stomach wall with several interrupted sutures.

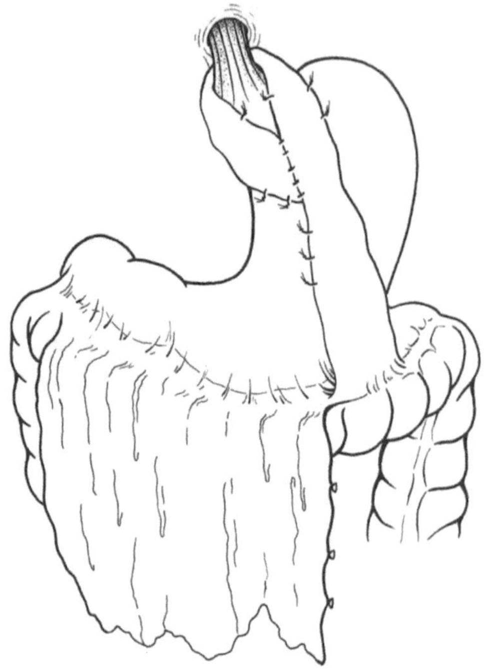

Fig. 134. Omental cuff. A flap is developed from the left portion of the greater omentum and is looped around the terminal esophagus to keep it reduced below the diaphragm

12.8.2 Ligamentum Teres Flap

Preoperative preparation, instruments, position and approach: See 12.5.1.1.

Operative technique: The skin, subcutaneous tissue, and fascia are divided. The peritoneum is bluntly dissected from the underside of the fascia until about a palm-sized sheet of peritoneum is exposed. This area is sharply circumscribed and mobilized upward from the umbilicus to the level of the xyphoid, leaving about a 3-cm wide pedicle superiorly. The space between the xyphoid and peritoneum is developed to allow the insertion of

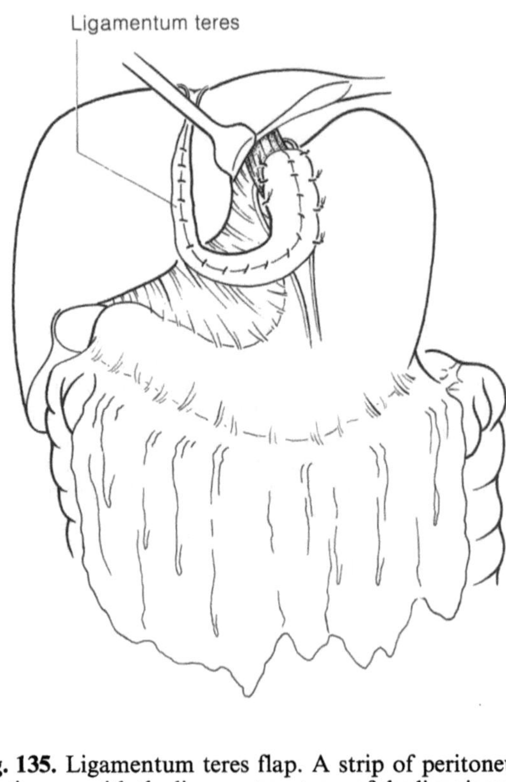

Fig. 135. Ligamentum teres flap. A strip of peritoneum continuous with the ligamentum teres of the liver is sutured across the fundus and distal esophagus

a Rochard retractor. Now the peritoneal margins of the mobilized sheet are sutured together from below upward, creating a strong, tubular flap that is enclosed by peritoneum and is continuous with the ligamentum teres of the liver and the falciform ligament. The distal esophagus is exposed and its peritoneal covering incised longitudinally on both sides for a length of 2 cm. The exposed portion of the esophagus is then encircled with the finger and snared. After reduction of the hernia, the free distal end of the ligamentum teres flap is laid across the fundus and terminal esophagus and stitched in place with 3 or 4 heavy sutures (Fig. 135). The sutures pass from the fundus to the esophagus and thence through the posterior side of the free end of the ligamentum teres. Since the esophagus was not skeletonized, the sutures can incorporate enough periesophageal tissue anteriorly to avoid esophageal injury. The hiatus is narrowed only in the presence of a large hernial opening.

12.9 Treatment of Peptic Strictures with or without a Short or Columnar-Lined Esophagus

The surgical treatment of peptic strictures with or without a short or columnar-lined esophagus is guided by the severity of inflammatory changes in the esophagus, the level of the stricture, and the underlying cause.

Peptic strictures at the esophagogastric junction are usually associated with secondary reflux disease brought on by impaired gastric emptying and coexisting incompetence of the lower esophageal sphincter. Strictures at higher levels may be caused by primary reflux disease or by local acid production in the esophagus in the presence of an intact lower sphincter (Barrett's syndrome).

The treatment of peptic stricture consists of pre- or intraoperative esophageal dilatation followed by an antireflux procedure. This is combined with vagotomy and pyloroplasty or with a gastric resection if gastric emptying is impaired. Stelzner [55] considers dilatation followed by a two-thirds gastric resection and Y anastomosis to be adequate treatment for peptic esophageal strictures. In the rare cases where the esophagus is shortened to the degree that an intraabdominal esophageal segment cannot be established even with extensive mobilization, it is necessary either to perform a fundoplication above the diaphragm or to perform a Collis-type gastric tube extension of the esophagus [10] so that the fundoplication or semifundoplication can be placed within the abdomen [14, 40]. If the stricture is not dilatable, several plastic procedures are available for enlarging the esophagus (see Sect. 4), but we prefer to manage these cases by segmental resection with interposition of colon or jejunum (see 7.4 and 7.5), which we also use for Barrett's esophagus and cases where the esophagus has been irreversibly damaged by secretions or prior surgery.

12.9.1 Treatment of Low Strictures

The primary concern in the treatment of low strictures is the elimination of secondary reflux. Pre- or intraoperative dilatation of the stricture is indicated. We prefer intraoperative dilation, either blind or endoscopically controlled (see Sect. 5), performed without gastrotomy and assisted by the surgeon, who guides the dilator manually across the esophagogastric junction and supports the fragile, inflamed wall of the esophagus to avoid perforation.

The esophagus is dilated to 32 Ch if possible. In the rare cases where the guidewire for endoscopic dilatation or the smallest size rubber bougie cannot be passed perorally into the stomach, transgastric dilatation with Hegar dilators may be attempted via a small gastrostomy placed near the cardia. After dilatation is completed, the obstruction is relieved by resection or by vagotomy with pyloroplasty, and a semifundoplication is added. We avoid a 360° wrap in these cases due to the risk of supercontinence. If the stricture cannot be adequately dilated even by the transgastric route, a segmental esophageal resection is performed in the same sitting with reconstruction by colon or jejunum.

12.9.2 Treatment of High Strictures without Local Acid Production

These cases are managed initially by endoscopic dilatation and medical therapy. Then an antireflux procedure is performed by the transabdominal route. If this cannot be done, plastic repair of the stricture or single-stage resection and reconstruction may be appropriate, depending on the level of the stricture. At present it is unclear whether a selective proximal vagotomy should be added in these cases to control the peptic component of the disease. The markedly poorer late results of dilatation and antireflux surgery in the treatment of high strictures compared with antireflux procedures in patients with reflux disease but no strictures may justify this additional measure.

12.9.3 Treatment of High Strictures with Local Acid Production

Because the strictures in these cases are not caused by gastroesophaeal reflux but by local acid production within the esophagus, and the lower esophageal sphincter is intact, there is no rationale for performing an antireflux procedure. Treatment consists of dilatation and measures to reduce acid production in the body of the esophagus. If medical control is unsuccessful, an intrathoracic vagotomy may be beneficial, making certain that the vagus nerve branches proximal to the stricture are divided to destroy the fibers supplying the gastric mucosa in the tubular esophagus. If response to this treatment is also poor, segmental esophageal resection with reconstruction in the same sitting remains an alternative.

12.9.4 Treatment of Strictures in the Columnar-Lined Esophagus

The same concept of dilatation followed by an antireflux procedure applies to the management of peptic strictures in the columnar-lined esophagus. Because the cardia in these cases tends to lie below the strictured area and slightly above the diaphragm, it is usually possible to mobilize the esophagus through an abdominal approach sufficiently so that a segment can be reduced below the diaphragm and an antireflux procedure performed. If the esophagus is too short for this, the fundus and lower esophagus are mobilized for a fundoplication (see 12.5.1.1) through a laparotomy. The abdomen is closed, and the patient is repositioned for a left posterolateral thoracotomy, through which the actual fundoplication is carried out (see 12.5.1.2). All or part of the fundic wrap is left within the thorax. A possible alternative is gastroplasty [10]. Although Collis [10] considered this procedure inferior to interposition, he recommended it for high-risk patients and for surgeons with little experience in the technique of interposition.

12.9.4.1 Gastroplasty

Preoperative preparation: Perioperative antibiotics; see Chap. C.

Instruments: Basic set, extra thoracic set; GIA; stomach tube (Ch 32).

Position and approach: Left thoracoabdominal incision in the bed of the seventh or eighth rib or posterolateral thoracotomy in the seventh intercostal space (see Chap. B).

Steps in procedure:

(1) Exposure and snaring of the thoracic esophagus
(2) Circumferential mobilization of the cardioesophageal junction and adjacent stomach in the esophageal hiatus
(3) Passage of a large-caliber stomach tube along the lesser curvature
(4) Creation of a gastroplasty tube with the GIA stapler applied adjacent to the stomach tube
(5) Reduction of the severed portion of the fundus into the abdomen
(6) Placement of crural sutures to narrow the hiatus
(7) Fundoplication (see 12.5.1.1)

Operative technique: The esophagus is dissected free as far as the aortic arch and encircled with a snare (see 2.1.2). Then the gastric sac is freed from its hiatal attachments. If it is found that sufficient material is present to reduce the stomach into the abdomen, a Belsey (see 12.6.2.1) or Nissen (see 12.5.1.2) antireflux repair is carried out, and the opertion is concluded. If the stomach cannot be reduced, a large-gauge stomach tube is passed through the esophagus into the stomach. The construction of a gastroplasty tube from the lesser curvature is accomplished most easily with the GIA stapling instrument. It is applied adjacent to the preplaced stomach tube so that its tip points toward the lesser curvature (Fig. 136 a). After the stapler has been fired and the tissue severed, the cut edge is examined for mucosal bleeding points, which are cauterized or suture-ligated as required. The staple line is tested for watertightness by the injection of methylene blue dye. Then the projecting portion of the fundus is reduced into the abdomen. The crura of the diaphragm and arcuate liga-

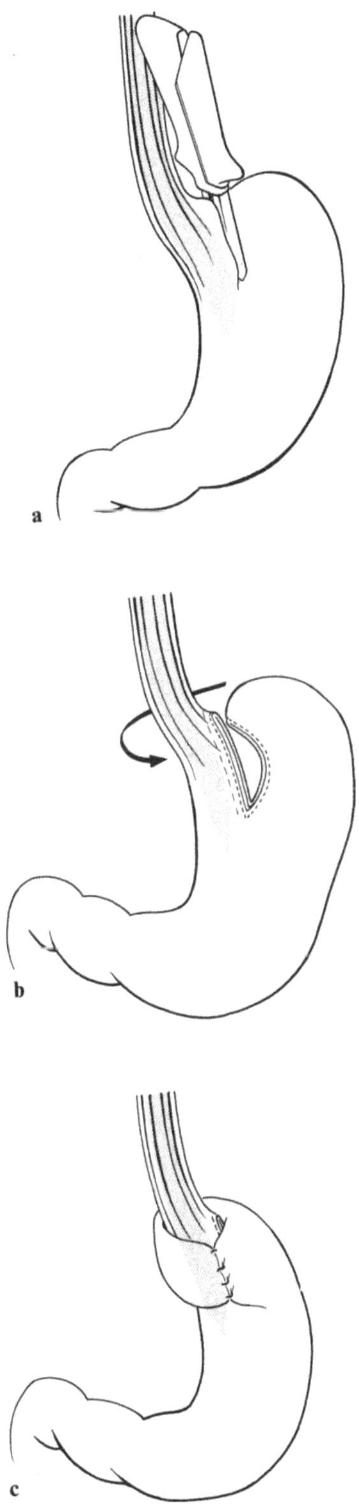

Fig. 136 a–c. Collis gastroplasty [10] (schematic). **a** A tubular extension of the lower esophagus is formed from the proximal part of the lesser curvature using the GIA instrument. **b** The fundus is passed behind the new terminal esophagus. **c** The completed fundoplication

ment are exposed. The lesser curvature is fixed to the arcuate ligament with several heavy sutures at the level of the newly created Hiss angle. The hiatus is narrowed anterior to the esophagus with sutures passed through the crura. The stomach is additionally sutured to the diaphragm through an abdominal incision. Better reflux control is obtained, however, by wrapping the fundus around the newly created distal esophageal tube (Fig. 136 b,c).

12.10 Treatment of Paraesophageal Hernia

12.10.1 Choice of Operation

The surgical repair of paraesophageal hernias follows the same principles that apply to hernia surgery in general: reduction of the stomach below the diaphragm, where it is secured by fixation to the abdominal wall, diaphragm, or both; narrowing of the hernial opening at the hiatus; and removal of the hernial sac if required. However, because the viscera do not tend to remain in the hiatus as they would, say, in the inguinal ring, it is sufficient to reduce the size of the hernial opening [1, 24, 35] or effect a permanent reduction [7, 37]. The hernial sac is removed if this can be done without excessive risk due to the presence of extensive adhesions [15, 54]. Mixed axial and paraesophageal hernias are by definition sliding hernias. Their treatment corresponds to that for paraesophageal hernia, and an antireflux procedure is added only if reflux is positively diagnosed. While paraesophageal hernias can be approached either transthoracically or transabdominally, the transabdominal approach has come to be preferred. The esophagus, its lower sphincter, and the structures of the posterior mediastinum are normal, so they are not disturbed. The abdominal approach gives better exposure than the thoracic for reducing the herniated viscera, securing them in place, and narrowing the widened hiatus. There is no question that a very large sac that is fused to adjacent structures can be removed more readily through a thoracic incision. However, since we do not excise the hernial sac in these cases, this advantage is not a factor.

12.10.2 Reduction and Hiatal Repair

Preoperative preparation: See Chap. C.

Instruments: Basic set; stomach tube (Ch 32).

Position and approach: Upper midline laparotomy.

Steps in procedure:

(1) Detachment of the left lobe of the liver from the diaphragm
(2) Reduction of the hernia
(3) If possible, excision of the hernial sac and closure of the defect by continuous suture
(4) Narrowing of the hiatus lateral, posterior, or anterior to the esophagus
(5) With hiatus communis, fixation of the superior edge of the fundus to the hiatus and diaphragm in two layers

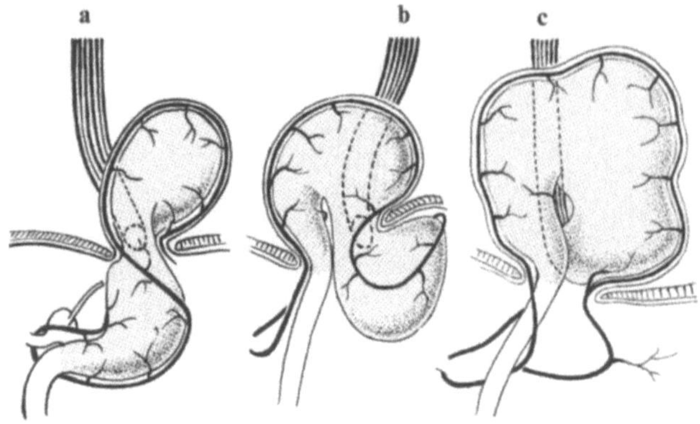

Fig. 137 a–c. Paraesophageal hernias. **a** Organoaxial rotation of the stomach with displacement of its proximal portion into the thorax. **b** Mesoaxial rotation of the stomach with displacement of its distal portion into the thorax. **c** "Intrathoracic stomach"

Operative technique: The abdomen is entered, the left lobe of the liver is retracted anteromedially, and the triangular ligament is divided. Then the lobe is turned downward and held mediad with a broad, curved retractor to get an unobstructed view of the cardia and hiatus. Anatomic relationships in this condition can be somewhat confusing, depending on the extent of the herniation of the stomach, its type of rotation (organoaxial or mesoaxial), and whether its proximal or distal portions have ascended into the thorax (Fig. 137). Occasionally, portions of other viscera such as the colon, spleen, or greater omentum may also be displaced into the chest. Reduction of the stomach usually presents no difficulties. Adhesions with the hernial sac are rare and, if present, usually occur at the neck of the sac and result from local circulatory deficits or ulcerations caused by transient incarceration or strangulation of the herniated stomach. After its return to the abdomen, the stomach is carefully examined visually and by palpation. If an ulcer is found and there is no past history of ulcer disease, it is reasonable to assume that the ulcer developed under the conditions of the hernia. Even so, the nature of the lesion should be established by intraoperative gastroscopy with multiple excisional biopsies or by open excision of the ulcer. We prefer intraoperative endoscopic biopsy, as it avoids the risks of gastrotomy. We continue to use endoscopy postoperatively to monitor the progress of ulcer healing. If an ulcer is found in a patient who has a positive history of gastric ulceration, the repair should be combined with a two-thirds gastrectomy and continuity restored by a Roux-en-Y anastomosis.

If the hernial sac is to be excised, it is grasped with a clamp at its highest point, and an attempt is made to pull it into the abdomen. If this cannot be done right away, the sac is incised at the anterior rim of the hiatus and is carefully dissected from the thorax, avoiding injury to the structures adherent to it. If the entire sac can then be displaced into the abdomen, it is fixed close to the diaphragm with a clamp at its lateral end. Starting from that point the sac is excised in piecemeal fashion while the defect is concurrently repaired by continuous suture (Fig. 138 a,b).

A large-caliber stomach tube is passed into the esophagus to aid evaluation of the hiatus. The hernial opening at the hiatus may be closed from the lateral, posterior, or anterior side. The stomach is pulled distally, and the hiatal crura are exposed with a dissecting patty. They are grasped with long Ellis clamps and pulled forward. The hiatal margins are approximated with several heavy, interrupted sutures that pierce the muscle bundle of each crus at different depths to avoid fraying. The hiatus is narrowed until it can just accommodate a fingertip inserted alongside the esophagus, which is splinted internally with the stomach tube (Fig. 138 c).

If an hiatus communis exists, i.e., if the descending aorta apposes directly to the posterior side of the esophagus with no intervening muscu-

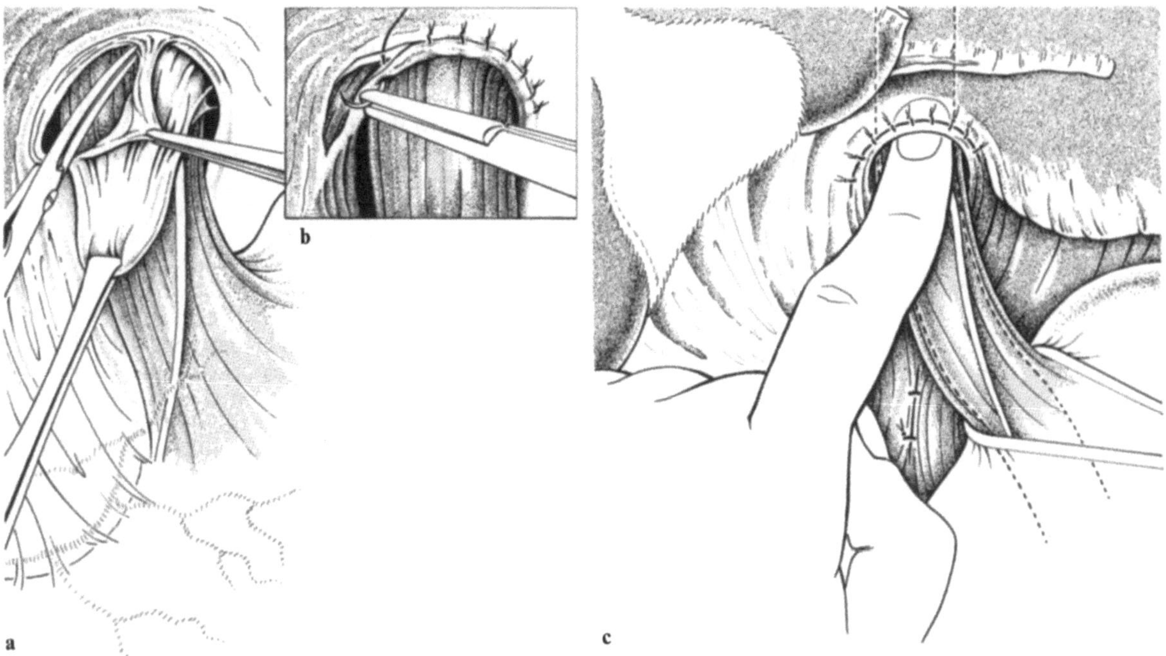

Fig. 138 a–c. Repair of a paraesophageal hernia. **a** Excision of the hernial sac after reduction of the hernia. **b** Closure of the peritoneum after excision of the hernial sac. **c** The width of the hiatus is checked after plication of the crura

lar crura, it may not be possible to narrow the hiatus effectively. These cases can be managed by suturing the superior margin of the mobilized fundus to the anterior rim of the hiatus. To maximize the area of attachment and further limit access to the hiatus, a second suture line is placed to imbricate additional fundus onto the diaphragm (Fig. 139).

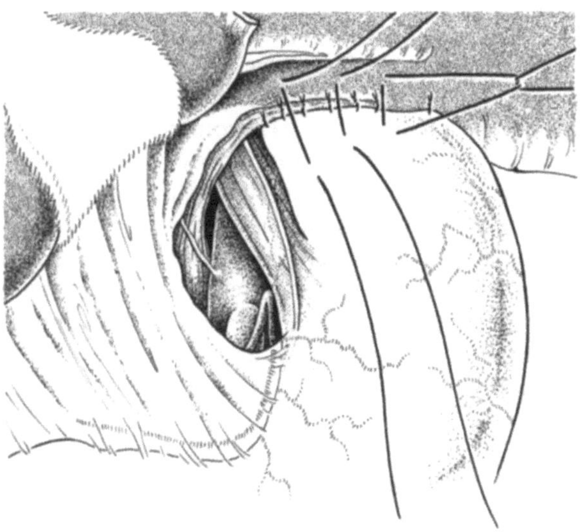

Fig. 139. Phrenicopexy in hiatus communis. The fundus is fixed to the anterior hiatal margin with an initial row of sutures and to the diaphragm with a second row to prevent recurrence of the herniation

12.10.3 Gastropexy

This term may be broadly applied to all operations described for the treatment of reflux disease, since all involve the intraabdominal fixation of the stomach.

In the absence of reflux, however, it is sufficient to suture the lesser curvature [7, 24], the fundus [19, 35], the body, or the body and fundus of the stomach [37, 39, 45] to the peritoneum of the anterior abdominal wall or to the diaphragm. The gastropexy sutures are spaced about 1.5 cm apart. Nissen et al. [39] anchor the fundus to the diaphragm just anterior to the laterally narrowed hiatus with 4 or 5 sutures. This creates an effective barrier to the hiatus while preserving a physiologic esophagogastric angle (Fig. 140 a). A second suture line along the esophageal axis fixes the body of the stomach to the peritoneum of the anterior abdominal wall. These sutures, placed under slight

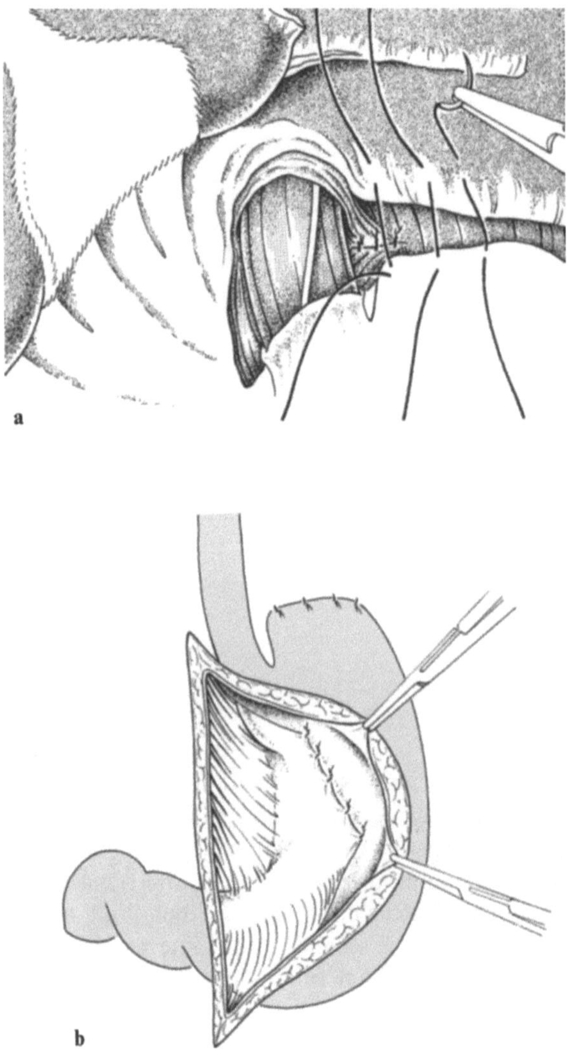
a

b

Fig. 140 a,b. Nissen gastropexy [37]. **a** A fundophrenicopexy is performed at the level of the hiatus. The hiatal crura have been approximated laterally. **b** The anterior stomach wall is fixed to the peritoneum of the anterior abdominal wall

tension, retain the stomach in an anatomic position, eliminate gliding in the area of the cardia, and prevent rotation (Fig. 140 b).

Preoperative preparation, instruments, position and approach: See 12.10.2.

Operative technique: For gastropexy of the body or lesser curvature of the stomach, the peritoneum and the fascia at the left margin of the laparotomy are grasped with Mikulicz clamps and pulled forward. The suture is passed through the seromuscular layer of the stomach wall at the proposed gastropexy site, directing the needle toward the greater curvature. The suture is partially pulled through. Tension on the Mikulicz clamps is released to allow the abdominal wall to sag to its natural position, and the level of the fixation site on the abdominal wall is determined by placing slight tension on the preplaced suture in the stomach wall. The needle is passed through the peritoneum at the designated site and also through the posterior rectus sheath, which is engaged for a width of about 3 cm. The suture may be tightened at tied at this point if there is doubt that it will exert adequate tension on the esophagus, although it is simpler and less traumatizing to the gastric wall if the remaining 3 or 4 fixation sutures are placed in the same fashion before any are tied. Finally the abdominal wall is allowed to sag back to its normal position, and the threads are tied. Since no hollow viscus has been entered, it is unnecessary to insert a drain before closing.

12.11 Hiatal Hernias in Children

The indications for the surgical repair of congenital or acquired axial or paraesophageal hiatal hernias in children are largely identical to those in adults. Operative repair is always indicated for paraesophageal hernias. With an axial hiatal hernia, surgery is indicated for Grade I or Grade II reflux esophagitis that has not responded promptly to medical treatment, and also in small children who are failing to thrive. Hecker [20] advocates surgical repair for large hiatal hernias even when they are not associated with reflux.

12.11.1 Choice of Operation

Anatomic repair by hiatal reconstruction or gastropexy is preferred by a number of pediatric surgeons [2, 20, 26, 43] over fundoplication [6, 31], as it does not permanently alter anatomic relations in the area of the cardia and fundus. This is believed to be desirable in children. The authors state that, in contrast to adults, the results of anatomic repairs in children are just as good as the results of fundoplication.

12.11.2 Approach

The standard approach is by laparotomy. The transthoracic approach is preferred for the shortened esophagus, as it permits the esophagus to be mobilized past the aortic arch.

12.11.3 Transabdominal Approach

12.11.3.1 Hiatal Repair

Preoperative preparation: See Chap. C.

Instruments: Basic set; Ch 20 stomach tube.

Position and approach: Upper midline laparotomy.

Steps in procedure:

(1) Division of the ligamentum teres of the liver and detachment of the left lobe from the diaphragm
(2) Transverse incision of the peritoneum over the esophagogastric junction
(3) Extension of the incision to the gastrosplenic ligament and far into the gastrohepatic ligament
(4) Circumferential dissection and snaring of the abdominal esophagus
(5) Mobilization of the cardia and fundus
(6) Exposure of the hiatal crura
(7) Narrowing of the posterior angle of the hiatus
(8) Fixation of the esophagus in the hiatus with interrupted sutures
(9) Fixation of the fundus to the intraabdominal esophagus and along the diaphragm if desired [16]

Operative technique: The abdomen is entered, and the portions of the fundus and cardia displaced into the thorax are reduced by traction on the stomach. The ligamentum teres of the liver is divided close to the umbilicus and the surface of the liver. Tension is placed on the left hepatic lobe, and the triangular ligament is transected. The liver is retracted mediad. The uppermost part of the gastrohepatic ligament or the entire ligament is divided. The esophagus is circumferentially cleared and snared with a soft rubber tape. Then the peritoneum and the remaining tissue layers that fix the cardia and lower esophagus in the hiatus are divided. The gastric fundus is separated from the hiatal opening, the left hemidiaphragm, and the spleen. The cardia and fundus should be completely mobile at this stage. Next the crura of the hiatus are exposed with a dissecting patty. Rehbein [43] recommends snaring the crura with three traction sutures placed to the right, front, and left of the esophagus. He places another traction suture in the angle formed by the intersecting crura anterior to the aorta (Fig. 141 a). This is done to avoid

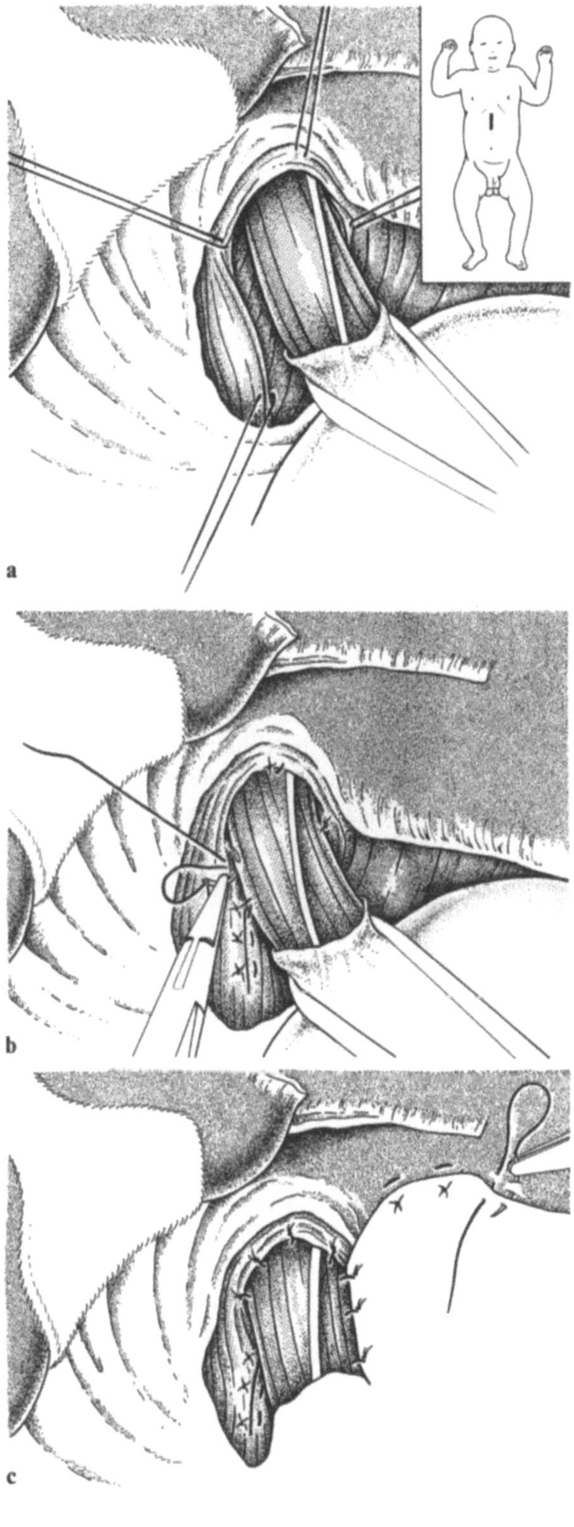

Fig. 141 a–c. Hiatal repair in a pediatric diaphragmatic hernia. **a** Traction sutures are placed in the hiatus. **b** The crura are plicated, and the esophagus is fixed within the hiatus. **c** The fundus is fixed to the intraabdominal esophagus and to the diaphragm using the Gross technique [16]

damage to the muscle fibers by forceps or retractor pressure. The hiatus is held open by traction on the sutures or by holding back the crura with a closed forceps, enabling the surgeon to dissect the esophagus free in the posterior inferior mediastinum. The vagus nerve trunks are carefully preserved. The hernial sac is left in place.

The esophagus is pulled anterolaterally by traction on the rubber tape, and the hiatal opening is narrowed with interrupted crural sutures placed forward from the aorta, the last suture taking a bite of the esophageal muscle wall. If traction sutures have been placed as described above, they are used at this time to anchor the right and left sides of the esophagus to the hiatal rim (Fig. 141 b). The sutures should not catch the vagus nerve trunks or pierce the esophageal mucosa. Neither should they be placed too tightly, or they may cut through the soft hiatal crura and esophageal musculature. If traction sutures have not been used, multiple interrupted sutures are placed around the circumference of the esophagus to anchor it within the narrowed hiatus. Gross [16] additionally fixes the fundus to the intraabdominal esophagus and also along the diaphragm using a curved suture line (Fig. 141 c). Hecker [20] considers it unnecessary to suture the esophagus to the hiatus.

12.11.3.2 Gastropexy

Gastropexy may be performed alone or in conjunction with an hiatal repair.

Preoperative preparation, instruments, position and approach: See 12.11.3.1.

Operative technique: The abdomen is entered, and the hernia is reduced (see 12.11.3.1). Two or three interrupted seromuscular sutures are placed in the proximal part of the lesser curvature. Then the stomach is made slightly tense, and the lesser curvature is sutured to the anterior abdominal wall to the right of the abdominal incision using the preplaced threads. Rehbein [43] incorporates these sutures into the laparotomy closure. Starting inferiorly, the fascia and peritoneum are closed in one layer. When the upper abdomen is reached, temporary traction is placed on the gastropexy threads to determine the site for incorporating them into the fascia and the peritoneal suture. The cardia and esophagus should be under considerable tension after the threads are tied. When the sutures have been tied, the rest of the abdomen is closed.

12.11.4 Transthoracic Approach

Preoperative preparation: See Chap. C.

Instruments: Basic set, extra thoracic set.

Position and approach: Left thoracotomy.

Operative technique: The lung is retracted anteriorly with a broad spatula, and the mediastinal pleura is opened over the esophagus. The esophagus is freed by blunt dissection and snared with a soft rubber tape. With gentle traction on the tape cephalad, the hernial sac and stomach are displaced into the thorax, and the distal esophagus and stomach are freed from their attachments with the sac. Next the esophagus is mobilized proximally to gain the length needed for reducing the stomach back into the abdomen. When this has been done, a paracostal incision is made in the diaphragm, and the ends of the tape around the esophagus are passed through the hiatus and out of the phrenotomy. Traction is then placed on the tape to reduce the cardia and terminal esophagus below the diaphragm (Fig. 142). The hiatus is narrowed

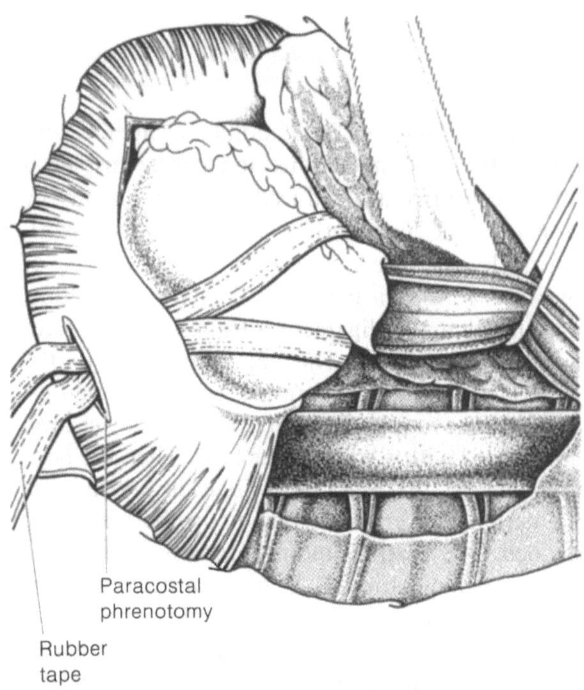

Fig. 142. Hiatal repair for pediatric hiatal hernia through a thoracic approach. The hernia is reduced. While the hiatus is repaired, the reduction is maintained with a rubber tape brought out through a paracostal phrenotomy

posterior to the esophagus without constricting it, and the crura are additionally fixed to the circumference of the esophagus with interrupted sutures. Finally the rubber tape holding the esophagus within the abdomen is brought out through the separate incision, and the phrenotomy is closed. The mediastinal pleura is closed by continuous suture, a chest tube is inserted, the lung is inflated, and the thoracotomy is closed.

12.11.5 Hiatal Hernia with a Congenital or Peptic Stricture

The primary treatment of pediatric hiatal hernia associated with a congenital or peptic esophageal stricture is gastrostomy with dilatation, which may be done using a continuous loop of thread. The hiatal hernia is repaired operatively in a second sitting. Generally this is sufficient to restore a normally functioning esophagus, and only a few children will require esophageal resection and reconstruction, Thal's operation (see Sect. 4), or an esophagogastric bypass [20].

References

1. Allison PR (1951) Refluxesophagitis, sliding hiatal hernia and the anatomy of repair. Surg Gyncc Obstet 92:419
2. Balison JR, Woodward ER (1973) Effect of hiatus hernia repair and truncal vagotomy on human lower esophageal sphincter. Press Res Ann Surg 177:554
3. Baue AE, Belsey RH (1967) The treatment of sliding hiatal hernia and reflux esophagitis by the Mark IV technique. Surg 62:396
4. Belsey RH (1966) Functional disease of the esophagus. J Thorac Cardiovasc Surg 52:164
5. Belsey RH (1977) Mark IV repair of hiatal hernia by the transthoracic approach. World J Surg 1:475
6. Bettex M, Kuffer F (1977) Fundoplication in hiatal hernia. Results after 10 years. Prog Pediat Surg 10:25
7. Boerema I, Germis R (1955) Gastropexia anterior geniculata wegen Hiatusbruch des Zwerchfells. Zbl Chir 80:1585
8. Cahill JL, Aberdeen E, Waterston DJ (1969) Results of surgical treatment of hiatal hernia in infancy and childhood. Surg 66:597
9. Cesnik H (1980) Operative Behandlung der Hiatushernie durch Umschlingung mit einer Netzmanschette. Chir 51:115
10. Collis JL (1957) An operation for hiatal hernia with short esophagus. J Thorac Cardiovasc 34:768
11. Demeester TR, Johnson LW, Kent AH (1974) Evaluation of current operations for the prevention of gastroesophageal reflux. Ann Surg 180:511
12. Dilling EW, Peyton MD, Cannon JQ, Kanaly PJ, Elkins RC (1977) Comparsion of Nissen Fundoplicatio and Belsey Mark IV in the management of gastroesophageal reflux. Am J Surg 134:733
13. Dor J, Humbert P, Dor V (1962) L'intériet de la technique de Nissen du reflux après cardio-myotomie extramuqueuse de Heller. Mém Acad Chir 88:877
14. Ellis FH, Leonardi HK, Dabuzhsky L, Crozier RE (1978) Surgery short esophagus with stricture: An experimental and clinical manometric study. Ann Surg 188:341
15. Ellis FH (1978) Para-esophageal hiatus hernia. In: Nyleus LM, Condors RE (eds) Hernia, 2nd edn. Lippincott, Philadelphia
16. Gross RE (1970) An atlas of children's surgery. Saunders, Philadelphia
17. Guarner V, Degooade JR, Nelson TM (1975) A new antireflux procedure at the esophagogastric junction. Arch Surg 110:101
18. Guarner V, Martinez M, Gavino JF (1980) Ten years evaluation of posterior fundoplasty in the treatment of gastroesophageal reflux. Am J Surg 139:200
19. Harrington SW (1955) Esophageal hiatal hernia. Surg Gynecol Obstet 100:277
20. Hecker WCH (1975) Die Eingriffe in der Bauchhöhle im Neugeborenen Säuglings- und Kindesalter. In: Zenker R, Berchtold R, Hamelmann H (Hrsg) Die Eingriffe in der Bauchhöhle. Springer, Berlin Heidelberg New York (Allgemeine und spezielle chirurgische Operationslehre, 3. neubearb. Aufl, Bd VII/1)
21. Hermann RE (1968) Transabdominal repair of esophageal hiatal hernia anterior to the esophagus. Surg Gynecol Obstet 126:844
22. Hermeck AS, Coates NR (1980) Results of the Hill antireflux operation. Am J Surg 140:764
23. Hill LD (1967) An effective operation for hiatal hernia: An eight year appraisal. Ann Surg 166:681
24. Hill LD, Tobias JA (1968) Paraesophageal hernia. Arch Surg 96:735
25. Hill LD (1977) Progress in the surgical management of hiatal hernia. World J Surg 1:425
26. Hill LD (1978) Intraoperative measurement of lower esophageal sphincter pressure. J Thoracic Cardiovasc 75:378
27. Hoffmann TH (1968) Zur Frage der Rezidive operierter Hiatushernien. Langenbecks Arch Klin Chir 322:424
28. Höhnle KO, Kümmerle F (1972) Eine neue Methode zur Behandlung von Hiatushernien durch Fundopexie und Hiatusschlitzeinengung. Langenbecks Arch for Chir Suppl, p 255
29. Keen G (1981) Operative surgery and management. Wright, PSG, Bristol London Boston
30. Larrain A (1971) Technical considerations in posterior gastropexy. Surg Cynecol Obstet 299:300
31. Leape LL, Ramenofsky ML (1980) Surgical treatment of gastroesophageal reflux in children. Am J Dis 134:935

32. Leonardi HK, Lee MF, El-Kurd MF (1977) An experimental study of the effectiveness of various antireflux operations. Ann Thorac Surg 24:215
33. Lind JF, Burris CM, McDougall JT (1965) "Physiological" repair for hiatus hernia – A manometric study. Arch Surg 91:239
34. Lortat-Jacob JL (1957) Le traitment chirurgical des maladies de reflux gastro-esophagies. Presse méd 65:455
35. Madden JL (1956) Anatomic and technical consideratony in the treatment of esophageal hiatal hernia. Surg Gynecol Obstet 102:187
36. Mahmud H, Ulrich B, Kremer K (1979) Die Teresplastik. Chirurg 50:322
37. Nissen R (1956) Gastropexie als alleiniger Eingriff bei Hiatushernien. DMW 81:185
38. Nissen R (1956) Eine einfache Operation zur Beeinflussung der Refluxösophagitis. Schweiz Med Wschr 86:590
39. Nissen R, Rossetti M, Siewert R (1981) Fundoplicatio und Gastropexie bei Refluxkrankheit und Hiatushernie. Thieme, Stuttgart New York
40. Pearson FG, Cooper JD, Nelems JM (1978) Gastroplasty and fundoplication in the management of complex reflux problems. J Thoracic Cardiovasc 76:665
41. Polk HC, Zeppa R (1971) Hiatal hernia and esophagitis. Ann Surg 173:775
42. Rampal M, Perrilat P, Frigatelle J, Julien R, Bounet J (1967) Traitement des hernies hiatales et du reflux esophagies par la cardio-pexie avec le ligament rond du foie. Presse Med 75:617
43. Rehbein F (1976) Kinderchirurgische Operationen. Hippokrates, Stuttgart
44. Rossetti M (1968) Zur Technik der Fundoplicatio. Aktuelle Chir 3:229
45. Rossetti M, Geering P (1976) Paraoesophagealer Magenvolvolus. Helv Chir Acta 43:543
46. Rossetti M, Hell K (1977) Fundoplication for the treatment of gastroesophageal reflux in hiatal hernia. World J Surg 1:439
47. Rudler JC (1960) Pour l'opération de Heller. Helv Chir Acta 27:411
48. Salvary M, Miller G (1977) Der Ösophagus. Glassmann, Solothurn
49. Siewert R, Wallet M, Kotsch M, Peiper MJ (1975) Klinische Ergebnisse der Fundoplicatio. Langenbecks Arch Chir 338:9
50. Siewert R, Lespien G, Weisen MF, Schattenmann G, Peiper MJ (1977) Das Teleskop-Phänomen. Chirurg 48:640
51. Skinner DB, Booth DJ (1970) Assessment of distal esophageal function in patients with hiatal hernia and gastroesophageal reflux. Ann Surg 172:627
52. Skinner DB, DeMeester TH (1976) Gastroesophageal reflux. Curr Probl Surg 13:52
53. Skinner DB (1977) Complications of surgery for gastroesophageal reflux. World J Surg 1:485
54. Skinner DB (1981) Hiatal hernia. In: Keen G (ed) Operative surgery and management Wright, PSG, Bristol Boston London
55. Stelzner F (1982) Ergebnisse der Behandlung der peptischen Ösophagusstriktur mittels einer Magenresektion. Chirurg 53:778
56. Vasant JH, Baker JW, Ross DG (1976) Modification of the Hill technique for repair of hiatal hernia. Surg Gynecol Obstet 143:637

13 Surgical Treatment of Esophageal Injuries

CONTENTS

13.1 Treatment of Esophageal Perforations and Ruptures

13.1.1 Indications for Surgical Treatment

Operative treatment is indicated for virtually all perforations and ruptures of the esophagus, whether they are spontaneous or caused by internal or external violence. Exceptions to this rule should be made only in selected cases following a careful assessment of the clinical situation. An expectant approach may be taken if the perforation is not diagnosed until several days after the traumatic episode, and there is no clincal evidence of local or generalized infection [2, 17]. A few authors [4, 10, 21] claim that with a confined perforation like that following the dilatation of a peptic stricture or achalasia, a wait-and-see approach may be taken during which time oral intake is suspended and the patient is managed conservatively with large antibiotic doses, nasogastric suctioning, and total parenteral nutrition. We do not subscribe to this view. It cannot be predicted how the confined perforation will progress, and if a free perforation develops later on, it would place the patient in far greater jeopardy than an operative procedure. Moreover, the surgical treatment of a confined perforation can be performed electively under favorable conditions.

13.1.2 Choice of Procedure

The surgical management of esophageal perforations and ruptures is guided by the location of the defect and the length of time that has elapsed between the injury and its diagnosis or treatment.

Adjunctive measures such as nasogastric suctioning, pharmacologic acid reduction, large antibiotic doses, and total parenteral nutrition are integral parts of the surgical treatment concept and should be applied diligently until healing of the defect is confirmed radiographically.

In the absence of an abscess, which is simply drained, a defect in the cervical esophagus is managed by direct suture repair, and the area is drained. The extra dissection required is slight compared with simple drainage and adds minimal risk or discomfort to the procedure. If the repair is unsuccessful and a fistula ultimately develops, the situation will correspond to that occurring with simple drainage. If the superior mediastinum is already involved by infection, a cervical mediastinotomy must be added and copious drainage established (see Chap. G).

A perforation or rupture of the abdominal esophagus is repaired by direct suture of the debrided wound and then covered with a fundoplication (see 12.5), regardless of how much time has passed between the formation of the defect and its diagnosis. If the esophageal wound margins will not retain a direct suture, the wound may be repaired with a fundic patch using Thal's technique (see 4.3.5). The operative area is copiously irrigated with antiseptic solution and then drained. The additional need to defunctionalize the esophagus by constructing a cervical stoma (see 2.2) must be considered on a case-by-case basis. Often, however, the primary closure is so secure that it obviates the need for an esophagostomy.

Injuries of the thoracic esophagus pose the greatest therapeutic challenge. It is widely agreed that perforating injuries of the intrathoracic esophagus presenting for surgical care within 12 to 24 h after the traumatic episode should be managed by opening the injured side of the thorax, oversewing the defect, irrigating the pleural cavity with antiseptic solution, and establishing drainage [2, 5, 12, 13, 19]. Additional coverage of the defect with gastric fundus (see 12.5) or with a pedicled flap of diaphragm, pleura, or omentum (see 1.6), depending on the level of the injury, can be beneficial and will depend on the specific situation. The same applies to concomitant defunctioning of the esophagus by cervical esophagostomy (see 2.2).

An extensive laceration of the esophagus secondary to major thoracic trauma or a perforation secondary to a fresh corrosive injury, a long high-grade stricture, or esophageal carcinoma is managed (in good surgical candidates) by resecting the thoracic esophagus and constructing a cervical esophagostomy and Witzel fistula [19]. We feel that most of these patients are too ill to tolerate concomitant reconstruction of the esophagus in the same sitting. An alternative to open surgery, especially in carcinoma patients, is occlusion of the defect by endoesophageal intubation [3, 11]. If pleural effusion or empyema exists, a chest tube is inserted.

If the perforation or rupture is more than 24 h old, the patient's general condition will dictate further management. If the patient can tolerate thoracotomy, direct suture repair should be attempted. If it appears at operation that a direct repair will not be feasible, we would advocate resection as the best way of preventing permanent infection of the pleural cavity by gastric juice or saliva. Temporary ligation of the esophagus below the defect [16, 20] combined with the construction of a cervical or thoracic T-tube esophagostomy [1, 15, 18] is reserved for exceptional cases.

If the patient cannot tolerate thoracotomy, other options include drainage alone, drainage with esophageal intubation (see Chap. 5), drainage with complete defunctionalization of the esophagus through a cervical or abdominal approach, and blunt dissection (see 6.7). We question the value of esophageal exclusion by balloon catheters placed proximal and distal to the perforation through a cervicostomy and gastrostomy [6, 9], because we doubt the ability of these devices to keep saliva and gastric fluids from entering the pleural cavity. In cases where the perforation has led to abscess formation in the posterior mediastinum without involvement of the pleural cavity, the abscess can be drained through a posterior extrapleural mediastinotomy (see Chap. G).

13.1.3 Primary Repair and Drainage of the Intrathoracic Esophagus

Preoperative preparation: Antibiotic therapy; see Chap. C.

Instruments: Basic set, extra thoracic set.

Position and approach: Posterolateral thoracotomy placed according to the site of the perforation (see Chap. B).

Steps in procedure:

(1) Thoracotomy
(2) Copious irrigation of the pleural cavity
(3) Incision of the mediastinal pleura over the perforation site
(4) Determination of the extent of the defect in the esophageal muscularis and mucosa (circumferential mobilization of the esophagus is performed only if needed for better exposure)
(5) Closure of the defect in two layers (the pleural cavity is not closed)
(6) Irrigation of the pleural cavity
(7) Chest tube drainage, closure of the thoracotomy

Operative technique: The chest is entered, and the pleural cavity is cleaned and irrigated with several liters of antiseptic solution. The site of the injury is determined. This is not difficult if the mediastinal pleura over the perforation has been breached. Otherwise the mediastinal pleura is incised vertically over the esophagus at the level of the defect. Localization of the injury can be aided by instilling methylene blue dye into the esophagus. If the perforation cannot be visualized, it will be necessary to encircle and snare the esophagus and mobilize it past the upper and lower limits of the perforation (see 2.1.2) so that the extent of the injury can be accurately assessed. If an open defect is found after incision of the pleura, the site should not be mobilized, since this may cause excessive soilage of the mediastinum. The muscularis of the esophagus is bluntly dissected from the mucosa in the area of the perforation so that the mucosal defect, which is usually larger than the muscular defect, can be seen in its entirety. The mucosa is repaired by continuous suture. The muscularis is loosely approximated over the first suture line with simple interrupted sutures. The mediastinal pleura is left open so that any material leaking from the suture line can be aspirated through the chest tube. Leakage below a closed mediastinal pleura can incite mediastinitis that is difficult to control. After the pleural cavity is again irrigated copiously with antiseptic solution, a chest tube is placed at the site of the repair, a second tube may be placed at the most dependent point in the chest, the lung is inflated, and the thoracotomy is closed in layers.

13.1.4 Exclusion of the Thoracic Esophagus by Cervical Esophagostomy and by Temporary Ligation of the Esophagus below the Defect

Urschel et al. [20] and Schwarz and McQuarrie [16] recommend the following treatment for very extensive injuries of the thoracic esophagus or for injuries that are more than 12–24 h old when diagnosed: If the patient can tolerate thoracotomy, the perforation site is identified and the defect repaired. To keep gastric juice out of the injured esophagus, the latter may be occluded proximal to the hiatus with a small Teflon band 1 cm wide [20]. A gastrostomy is constructed in the same sitting for gastric decompression and for later feeding. When complete healing of the defect is confirmed radiographically, the band is removed through the same approach.

Schwartz and McQuarrie [16] modified the technique by placing a Silastic band around the infradiaphragmatic portion of the esophagus (Fig. 143). They chose Silastic because it incites fewer adhesions, and they placed it below the diaphragm to keep foreign material out of the infected pleural cavity.

Closure of the esophagus distal to the perforation site with the TA stapler should be considered only in cases where the patient is not in immediate danger, and resection of the esophagus is planned. Once occluded, the esophagus cannot be reopened by removal of the staples.

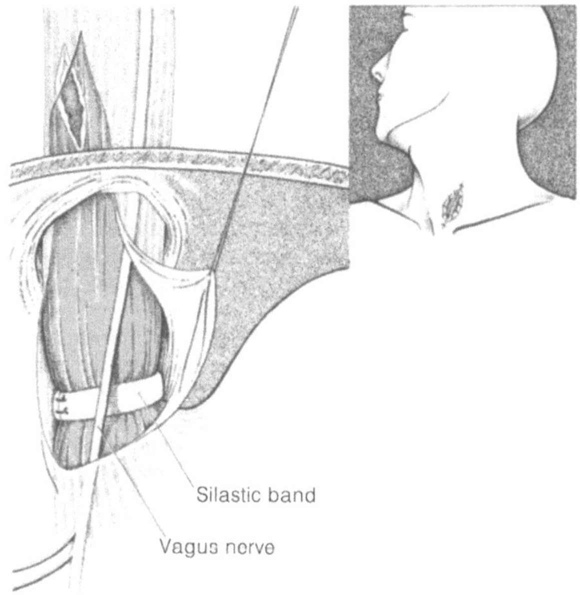

Fig. 143. Temporary infradiaphragmatic occlusion of the esophagus with a Silastic band. A cervical esophagostomy is established in the same operation

13.1.5 Treatment of Intrathoracic Esophageal Perforation by Thoracic Esophagostomy

The T-tube thoracic esophagostomy was introduced by Thorek [18] for the treatment of high-grade inflammatory esophageal strictures but was later abandoned due to the potential for leakage around the exteriorized limb of the T tube. In recent years various surgeons [1, 15] have successfully used the technique to treat perforations that are more than 24 h old and are not amenable to direct repair because of the fragility of the tissue, or in cases of leakage following an unsuccessful primary repair.

Through a thoracotomy on the injured side, the defect is identified, and a large-caliber T tube is inserted

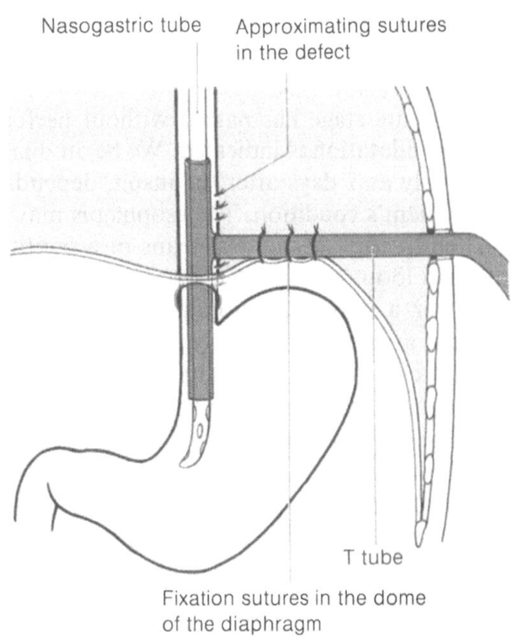

Fig. 144. Thoracic esophagostomy for drainage of the perforated thoracic esophagus

through it into the esophagus. The aboral limb of the tube must be long enough to extend into the stomach to ensure drainage of saliva and keep it from collecting above the lower esophageal sphincter. A nasogastric tube is passed through the lumen of the T tube into the stomach to retain the position of the tube and allow for continuous suctioning of gastric contents (Fig. 144). The margins of the defect are approximated over the limbs of the T tube with interrupted sutures. Then the exterior limb of the tube is sutured to the dome of the diaphragm with surgical gut and brought out through a stab incision separate from the thoracotomy wound. A chest tube is additionally placed at the inferior border of the esophagus. Within a few weeks, when the patient is out of danger, the T tube will be walled off by a fistulous tract and may be removed, leaving an esophagostomy opening that may close spontaneously. If it does not, the defect can be repaired by direct suture or covered with prosthetic material, since the scarred rim of the defect will now provide good purchase for sutures.

13.2 Treatment of Corrosive Injuries

The primary management of a fresh corrosive injury is conservative and consists in treatment for shock, the administration of steroids and antibiotics, pain relief, the passage of a soft nasogastric tube, and parenteral nutrition with total suspension of oral feeding. The administration of neutralizing agents is not essential. If perforation or necrosis of the esophagus occurs in the acute stage, it is pointless to attempt to close the defect [14]. In these cases the esophagus is bluntly resected, and a cervical stoma and gastrostomy are constructed.

If the acute stage has passed without perforation, early dilatation is indicated. We begin dilatation as early as 7 days after the insult, depending on the patient's condition. The esophagus may be dilated endoscopically or by means of a continuous thread loop (see Sect. 3). The response is followed over a period of months, and additional dilatations are performed as required (see Sect. 3). If a total caustic stricture cannot be dilated, or if an adequate esophageal lumen cannot be established despite repeated dilations, reconstruction should be undertaken. We feel that the question of bypass versus resection and replacement in these cases has been adequately resolved. If the patient's current status permits, and his life expectancy is not seriously limited by advanced age or coexisting disease, the burned esophagus should be removed. Left in place, it may create a nidus for ulcer formation with perforation or hemorrhage [8] since the scarred lower sphincter is an incompetent reflux barrier, and the self-cleaning mechanism of the esophagus is abolished by the failure of peristalsis. The bypassed esophagus is poorly accessible to radiologic evaluation and is wholly inaccessible to endoscopy. This removes the possibility of early carcinoma detection in a group that has a 1000 times greater risk of developing carcinoma than the population at large [7]. Blunt dissection without thoracotomy (see 6.5) is a particularly appropriate technique in these cases, provided the esophagus is not fused to posterior mediastinal structures due to previous periesophagitis. Otherwise the resection must be performed through a right thoracic incision. We prefer colon over stomach or jejunum for the reconstruction of these cases (see Sect. 7), as we do whenever the underlying disease is benign.

References

1. Abbott OA, Mansour KA, Logan WD (1970) Atraumatic socalled "spontaneous rupture of the esophagus". J Thorac Cardiovasc Surg 59:67
2. Bergdahl L, Henze A (1978) The treatment of oesophageal perforations. Scand J Cardiovasc Surg 12:137
3. Berger RL, Donato AT (1972) Treatment of esophageal disruption by intubation: A new method of management. Ann Thorac Surg 13:27
4. Cameron JL, Kieffer RF, Hendrix TR, Mehigan DG, Baker RR (1979) Selective nonoperative management of contaminated intrathoracic esophageal disruptions. Ann Thorac Surg 27:404
5. Finley RJ, Pearson FG, Weisel RD, Todd TRJ, Ilves R, Cooper J (1980) The management of nonmalignant intrathoracic esophageal perforations. Ann Thorac Surg 30:575
6. Hinder RA, Baskind AF, Le Grange F (1981) A tube system for the management of ruptured oesophagus. Br J Surg 68:182
7. Höllwarth M, Sauer H (1975) Speiseröhrenverätzungen im Kindesalter. Z Kinderchir 16:1
8. Imre J, Wooler G (1969) Peptic ulceration of the esophagus following corrosive burns. Thorax 24:762
9. Lebsien G, Siewert JR (1981) Traumatische Perforationen und Fisteln im Bereich von Ösophagus und Magen. In: Allgöwer M, Harder F, Hollender LF, Peiper H-J, Siewert JR (Hrsg) Chirurgische Gastroenterologie 1, Springer, Berlin Heidelberg New York, S 374
10. Lyons WS, Seremetis MG, deGuzman VC, Peobody JW (1978) Ruptures and perforations of the esophagus: The case for conservative supportive management. Ann Thorac Surg 25:346
11. Messner K (1977) Der „Verschluß" instrumenteller Perforationen des stenosierten Ösophagus durch Endoprothese. Langenbecks Arch Chir 344:93–99

12. Michel L, Grillo HC, Malt RA (1981) Operative and nonoperative management of esophageal perforations. Ann Surg 194:57
13. Pague WS, Brown PW, Fontana (1974) Esophageal perforation, Mallory-Weiss Syndrome, and acquired esophageal fistulas. In: Payne WS, Olsen AM (eds) The Esophagus. Lea and Febiger, Philadelphia, p 171
14. Ritter FN, Gago O, Kirsch MM (1971) The rationale of emergency esophago-gastrectomy in the treatment of liquid caustic burns of the esophagus and stomach. Am Otol Rhinol Laryngol 80:513–520
15. Schroeder L, Bock JU (1978) Zur chirurgischen Problematik iatrogener Ösophagusperforationen. Langenbecks Arch Chir 346:201–208
16. Schwartz ML, McQuarrie DG (1980) Surgical management of esophageal perforation. Surg Gynecol Obstet 151:669
17. Skinner DB, Little AG, DeMeester TR (1980) Management of esophageal perforation. Am Journ Surg 139:760–764
18. Thorek P (1951) Surgical treatment of stenosis due to esophagitis: Formation of temporary external fistula over T-tube. JAMA 147:640–642
19. Triggiani E, Belsey R (1977) Oesophageal trauma: Incidence, diagnosis and management. Thorax 32:241–249
20. Urschel HC, Razzuk MA, Wood RE, Galbraith N, Pockey M, Paulson DL (1974) Improved management of esophageal perforation: Exclusion and diversion in continuity. Ann Surg 179:587
21. Van Trappen G, Helleman J (1980) Treatment of achalasia and related motor disoders. Gastroenterology 79:144–154

14 Operations for Congenital Malformations of the Esophagus

CONTENTS

14.1 Esophageal Atresia

14.1.1 Classification of Atresias

The most common type of atresia (Fig. 145) in the original Vogt classification [31] is Type IIIb, followed by Type II. Type I, esophageal agenesis, is generally associated with major coexisting anomalies that are incompatible with survival.

14.1.2 Special Diagnostic Studies

When a presumptive diagnosis of esophageal atresia is made clinically, a radiopaque rubber catheter (14–18 Ch) is passed into the esophagus under radiologic control. The roentgenogram must cover the thorax and abdomen to give information on the pulmonary status and the presence of air in the abdomen. If the abdomen is devoid of air, a Type II atresia may be diagnosed. The only initial treatment to be considered is gastrostomy. An air-filled abdomen establishes the presence of a fistulous communication between the distal esophageal segment and the trachea. Marked distention of the gastric bubble, possibly accompanied by distended loops of bowel, signifies duodenal atresia or some other stenosing malformation of the intestinal tract. The surgeon should not insist upon contrast visualization of the proximal esophageal segment. The almost inevitable spillover of contrast medium into the trachea would inflict additional harm. The information to be gained on the length of the proximal segment, the existence of a tracheoesophageal fistula, and the presence or absence of a stricture

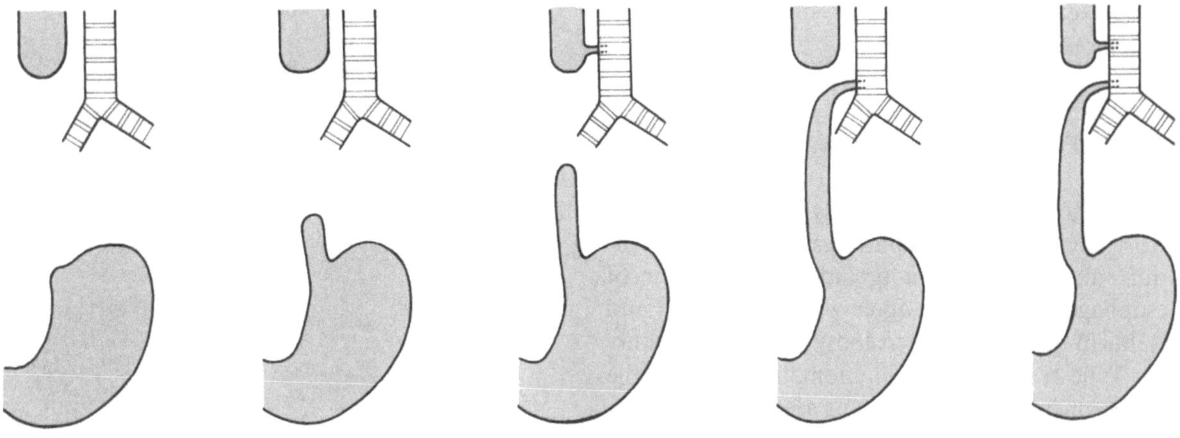

Fig. 145. The Vogt classification of esophageal atresia [31]

are either irrelevant for operative treatment or are so rare that they do not justify the risk of the examination.

14.1.3 Preoperative Preparation

Prior to operation a double-lumen Reploge tube is introduced into the proximal esophageal segment, and the contents of the pouch are evacuated at 20- to 30-min intervals with an intermittent suction pump or, preferably, by manual technique. The catheter is flushed at regular intervals with 1–2 ml saline, to which a mucolytic agent may be added. If a fistula exists between the distal esophagus and trachea, the infant is placed in a head-up posture to prevent reflux of gastric juice into the trachea. Moving the infant frequently from one side to the other and regular tracheobronchial suctioning are indicated to decrease the risk of pneumonia. Antibiotic treatment is optional and will depend on the pulmonary findings. Meanwhile measures are taken to establish a normal water-electrolyte-acid-base balance via a peripheral or central venous line based on the results of blood studies.

14.1.4 Plan of Surgical Treatment

The plan for surgical repair depends chiefly on the status of the infant and the presence or absence of esophagotracheal fistula. Anastomosis of the esophageal segments is not a primary therapeutic concern. The risk categories developed by Waterston et al. [32], based on survival rates of newborns with esophageal atresia, are useful for devising a treatment strategy:

Category A: Mature newborns (birthweight over 2500 g) with minimal signs of pneumonia and no other congenital anomalies.

Category B: Newborns with a birthweight of 1800 to 2500 g and no signs of pneumonia or coexisting anomalies, and mature newborns with moderate pneumonia or minor coexisting anomalies.

Category C: Newborns with a birthweight under 1800 g or higher-birthweight newborns with either severe pneumonia or a severe coexisting anomaly.

Category C babies are poor candidates for a major operation, especially thoracotomy. Surgical repair is undertaken using a staged approach [14] that conforms to the status of the infant. A gastrostomy is performed as soon as the baby is hospitalized. If a type IIIb anomaly exists, measures are taken through the same approach to eliminate the regurgitation of gastric contents into the trachea (see 14.1.9). Closure of the fistula and anastomosis of the esophagus are undertaken in one or two subsequent stages. A more flexible policy is applied to the treatment of Category A and B patients. Surgical repair is urgent but is not conducted on an emergency basis. The infant is examined every 4 h to determine whether an existing esophagotracheal fistula should be closed and esophageal continuity established primarily, or whether the patient should be maintained on intensive care until the risk of surgery is reduced to a more acceptable level.

14.1.5 Preliminary Gastrostomy

While Holder [17, 18] routinely recommends gastrostomy for gastric decompression, reflux prevention, and feeding as a prelude to the repair of esophageal atresia, we agree with Haight [11] and Rehbein [27] that gastrostomy is necessary only for Type II and Type IIIa anomalies. Usually the two segments of the esophagus are so widely separated in these cases that an anastomosis cannot be performed without first elongating the segments. In Type IIIb atresia, on the other hand, a primary anastomosis can be accomplished in the majority of patients. If reflux is minimal, the stomach can be satisfactorily decompressed through a small-caliber tube. Gastric secretions will be slight in any case when the infant is on parenteral nutrition, which we prefer over tube feeding and maintain until X-rays confirm a watertight anastomosis. If it is found at operation that the esophageal segments cannot be united primarily, a Kader gastrostomy [9, 27] is performed after the thoracic part of the operation is completed.

14.1.5.1 Rehbein Modification of the Gastrostomy [27] (Fig. 146)

Preoperative preparation: See 14.1.3 and Chap. C.

Instruments: Basic set.

Position and approach: Upper midline laparotomy (3–4 cm).

Steps in procedure:

(1) Placement of two parallel sutures in the anterior stomach wall, spaced apart by the diameter of the gastrostomy tube
(2) Placement of preliminary ties
(3) Incision of the stomach between the sutures
(4) Insertion of the gastrostomy tube
(5) Fixation of the tube with the preplaced sutures
(6) Single-layer closure of the peritoneum and fascia with extraperitonealization of the gastrostomy

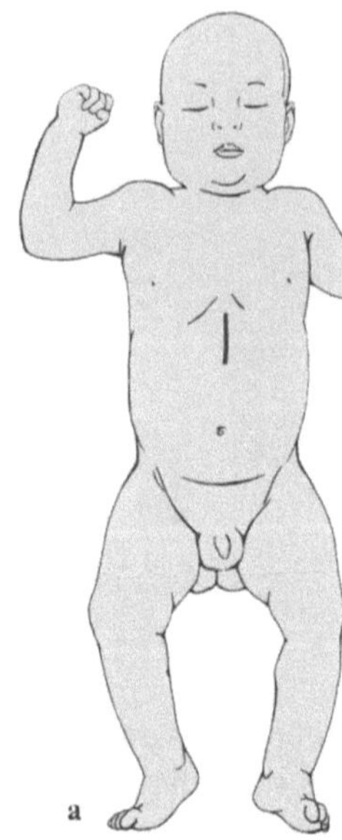

Fig. 146 a–e. Rehbein gastrostomy [27]. **a** Upper midline laparotomy (3–4 cm). **b** The anterior stomach wall is opened between parallel sutures. Two knots are tied 0.5 cm apart in the threads on the left side. **c** The gastrostomy tube is marked 2 cm from its tip to aid insertion. **d** The gastrostomy tube is secured with the preplaced threads. **e** The abdominal wall is closed, extraperitonealizing the gastrostomy. The sutures for closing the abdominal wall around the gastrostomy incorporate the anterior stomach wall

Operative technique: The abdomen is entered, and the lower portion of the body of the stomach is grasped with small Babcock clamps and pulled forward. The site for the gastrostomy is defined by placing two parallel sutures in the anterior stomach wall. Each suture pierces the stomach wall twice, the distance between them equaling the diameter of the gastrostomy tube. The left ends of the threads are tied together. A second knot is tied 0.5 cm above the first and will be used for subsequent fixation of the tube. The right ends of the threads are prepared for tying. The full thickness of the stomach is incised between the two sutures (Fig. 146 b), and a rubber catheter (2–12 Ch) with a terminal opening is inserted. A mark is placed 2–2.5 cm from the end of the tube (Fig. 146 c) to indicate the desired depth of insertion and ensure that the tube does not impinge on the opposite wall. The right ends of the sutures

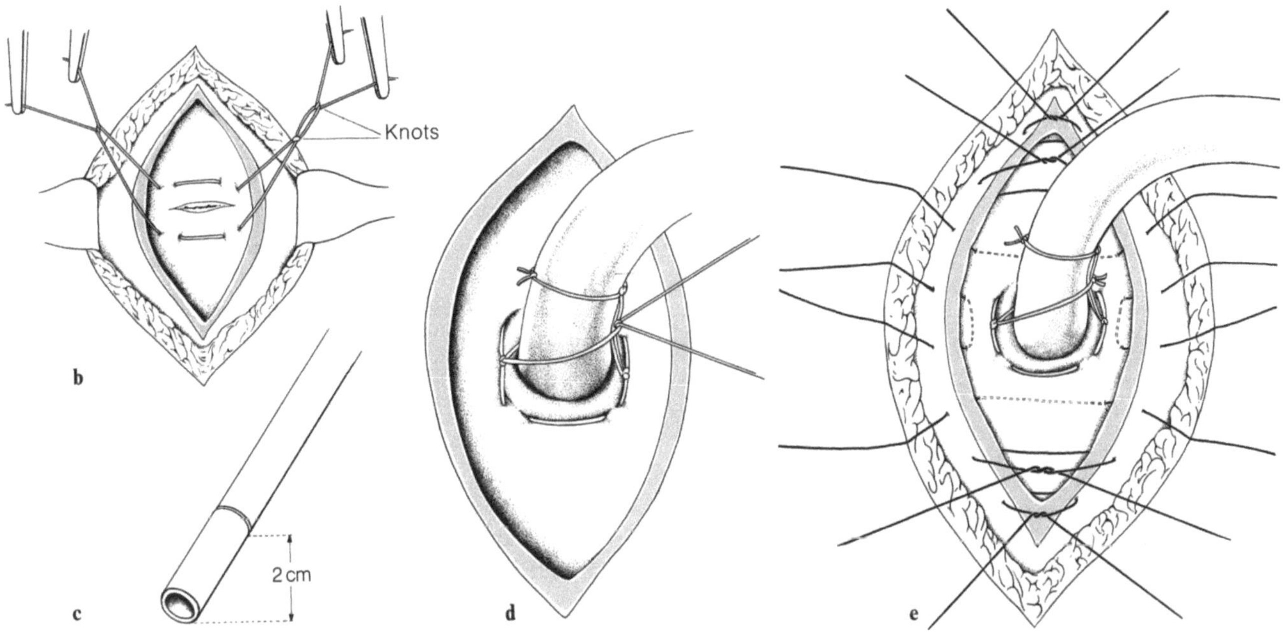

are now tied so that the gastrostomy margins appose snugly to the tube. The tube is additionally secured by tying the free ends of the sutures around it (Fig. 146 d). At this point air is injected into the stomach with a syringe, and the appearance of air in the jejunum is confirmed. Absence of jejunal air implies duodenal atresia, which is corrected in the same operation. The peritoneum and fascia are closed in a single layer. The stomach wall above and below the gastrostomy is incorporated into the abdominal wall closure (Fig. 146 e) so that the gastrostomy is extraperitonealized. The skin is closed, and the gastrostomy tube is additionally secured with a skin suture placed just below its site of emergence.

14.1.5.2 Gross Modification of the Gastrostomy [10]

Preoperative preparation and instruments: See 14.1.5.1.
Position and approach: Upper transrectus laparotomy (3–4 cm) on the left side.
Operative technique: The procedure is basically the same as that used in adults (see 2.5.3.1), except that the de Pezzer catheter is brought out through the laparotomy incision, and the uppermost pursestring suture is incorporated into the peritoneal closure.

14.1.6 Surgical Treatment of Type IIIb Atresia

14.1.6.1 Transpleural or Extrapleural Approach

The advantage of the transpleural approach is that it provides better exposure and shortens operating time, since it takes more time to dissect and retract the pleura than to incise it [10]. Disadvantages are the inevitable traumatization of the delicate infant lung, which can occur with even the most careful handling. If a postoperative anastomotic leak develops, the inflammation will spread rapidly and incite a potentially devastating pleural empyema.

The extrapleural approach gives somewhat poorer exposure than the transpleural, especially in patients with a short proximal segment or a low fistula. The major advantage of this approach is that the lung is protected throughout the operation by its pleural envelope. Thus an anastomotic leak will not communicate with the pleural cavity, and an associated purulent infection can be controlled by drainage of the extrapleural space. While there are no comparative prospective studies demonstrating the superiority of one approach over the other, a number of retrospective studies [9, 13, 14, 27, 32, 34] indicate that the extrapleural approach is the more favorable.

14.1.6.2 Extrapleural Approach

Preoperative preparation: See 14.1.3 and Chap. C.

Instruments: Basic set, extra thoracic set; set VI if required.

Position and approach: Posterolateral thoracotomy through the third or fourth interspace (see Chap. B).

Steps in procedure:

(1) Progressive dissection of the parietal pleura from the endothoracic fascia
(2) Exposure of the proximal esophageal segment
(3) If necessary, ligation of the azygos vein
(4) Identification of the distal esophageal segment
(5) Placement of traction sutures in both segments
(6) Dissection of the fistulous connection between the lower esophagus and trachea
(7) Placement of a traction suture at the upper border of the fistula
(8) Division of the fistula
(9) Closure of the tracheal defect with interrupted or continuous sutures
(10) Confirmation of airtight closure of the trachea

Operative technique: For approach through the fourth intercostal space, an assistant spreads the fourth and fifth ribs apart with a small periosteal elevator or forceps point to make the intercostal muscle tense. The muscle is divided with a scalpel for a length of 5–6 cm along the superior border of the fifth rib in the midaxillary area until the pleura appears. Fibers in contact with the pleura are pushed aside bluntly with a moist dissecting patty, or they may slip off the pleura spontaneously as the fourth and fifth ribs are spread apart. The exposed parietal pleura is progressively separated from the endothoracic fascia by patty dissection, carrying the dissection proximally and distally until there is sufficient room to insert a rib spreader. As the spreader is carefully opened, the pleura becomes tense and is further mobilized along the fourth intercostal space so that the division of the intercostal muscles can be continued anteromedially to the nipple line and posterolaterally almost to the spine. If access is obstructed by the inferior angle of the scapula, it may be held out of the way by an assistant or fixed to the blade of the spreader with a suture. The extrapleural space is further developed toward the posterior mediastinum, proceeding very carefully and in small steps to avoid tearing the pleura. If a pleural tear occurs, it is immediately repaired with sutures. Special care is taken at the costovertebral junction, where the pleura tends to be in intimate contact with the heads of the ribs and the sympathetic trunk (Fig. 147 a). When the pleura has been separated from the superior part of the posterior mediastinum, the distal pouch of the esophagus will become visible. A traction suture is placed in the segment to mark it and to serve as a handle for manipulations. The azygos vein may be freed from its pleural sheath, ligated and divided, or it may be left on the pleura after division of the intercostal veins and retracted anteriorly. The posterior pleural reflection is mobilized as far as the right pulmonary hilum, where the distal esophageal segment is usually encountered. If the lower segment is not found there, it will be necessary to mobilize the pleura farther distally. If necessary the segment can be located by tracing the vagus nerve downward. The pleura and lung are retracted medially with a broad, padded retractor. The side of the distal esophageal segment opposite the aorta is exposed with a dissecting patty, carefully avoiding injury to the vagus nerve. The upper part of the segment is encircled with a small, curved clamp, and a thin rubber tape is passed around it (Fig. 147 b). Further mobilization of the lower segment distally and toward the aorta should be minimized due to the risk of devascularization. The site of entry of the lower esophageal segment into the trachea is carefully dissected free. Before division of the fistula, a traction suture is placed at the superior border of the tracheal fistula and is tied. The distal esophagus is divided close to the trachea and engaged with two all-coats traction sutures placed in inside-to-outside fashion. A smear is taken from the open tracheal fistula to serve as a guide for postoperative antibiotic therapy. The previously placed traction suture may now serve either as the first suture of a double continuous row or as an initial interrupted suture for closure of the tracheal fistula. The sutures should not incorporate too much of the tracheal wall to avoid stenosis. The closure is best performed with the aid of a magnifying loupe (Fig. 148). One should avoid leaving too much of the fistula on the trachea, as the resulting pocket may become a source

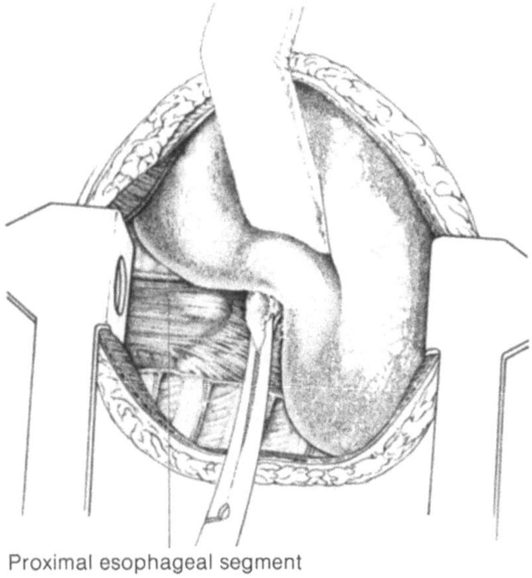

a

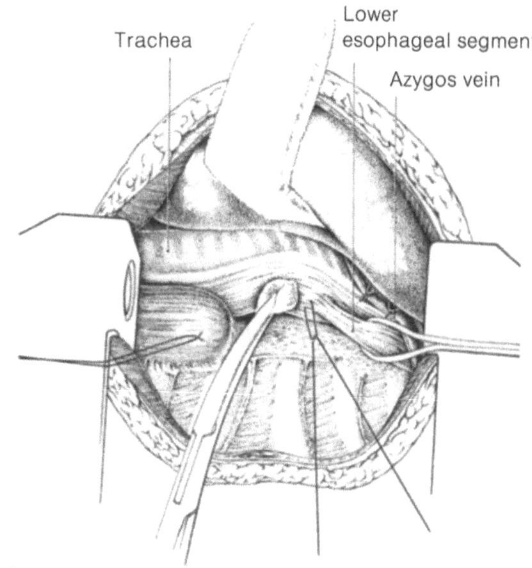

b

Fig. 147 a,b. Exposure of the proximal and distal esophageal segments through an extrapleural approach. **a** The pleura is dissected from the proximal esophageal segment. **b** The fistulous junction of the lower esophagus with the trachea is dissected free. The ends of both segments are held with traction sutures

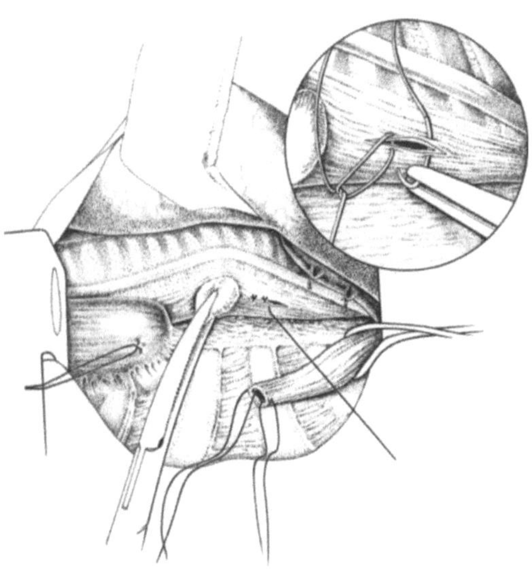

Fig. 148. Closure of the tracheoesophageal fistula

of infection. Airtight closure of the fistula is tested by immersing it in water while positive-pressure ventilation is briefly applied. Bubbling indicates an air leak, which usually is from a needle track but is occasionally due to inadequate closure of the fistula. In the latter case additional sutures are placed, bearing in mind the danger of tracheal stenosis. Generally the needle tracks will close spontaneously. Fibrin glue may be placed in the suture line to ensure aerostasis. The open lumen of the lower esophageal segment is cleaned with dissecting patties soaked in antiseptic to reduce the bacterial count. If a preliminary gastrostomy was not performed, a catheter is passed into the stomach, and accumulated air and secretions are removed by suction. After removal of the catheter, the stump is covered with an antiseptic-soaked compress.

14.1.6.3 Transpleural Approach

Preoperative preparation and instruments: See 14.1.6.2.

Position and approach: Posterolateral thoracotomy in the third or fourth interspace on the right side (see Chap. B).

Operative technique: The pleural cavity is entered, and the lung is retracted downward and medially with a padded retractor. The pleura is incised about 0.5 cm posterior to the palpable vagus nerve from the apex of the chest to the azygos vein, and the proximal esophageal segment is identified. If necessary, the azygos vein is ligated and divided. Then the pleural incision is continued downward to a point just above the hiatus. The rest of the procedure, especially closure of the esophagotracheal fistula, is like that in the extrapleural approach.

14.1.6.4 Mobilization of Both Esophageal Segments

A catheter previously passed down into the upper esophageal segment is advanced until the pouch becomes tense and its intrathoracic extent can be appreciated. Tracheal injury must be avoided during isolation of the pouch. The blind end of the segment is elevated away from the trachea with a traction suture, and the tissue between the pouch and trachea is spread apart with a small scissors. The tissue is divided only when it is certain that the blades are not entering the membranous part of the trachea or the esophagus (Fig. 149 a). If the gap between the esophageal segments is small, further mobilization is unnecessary. But if a larger gap exists, the proximal segment may be mobilized past the thoracic inlet without risk of devascularization. The segments are brought together with the traction sutures so that the remaining distance between them can be estimated (Fig. 149 b). It is reported that the proximal segment can be elongated by about 1–1.5 cm by performing one or more circumferential myotomies in its wall [23, 24] (Fig. 149 c). It is possible to lengthen the distal segment by dissecting the side adjacent to the aorta, but this may jeopardize the blood supply to the segment. The rest of the procedure depends on the distance that remains between the two segments. A good rule of thumb is that a primary anastomosis is too hazardous if a gap of more than 5 mm remains between the segments after maximum prudent mobilization. Neither should an anastomosis be forced if one of the two segments appears discolored.

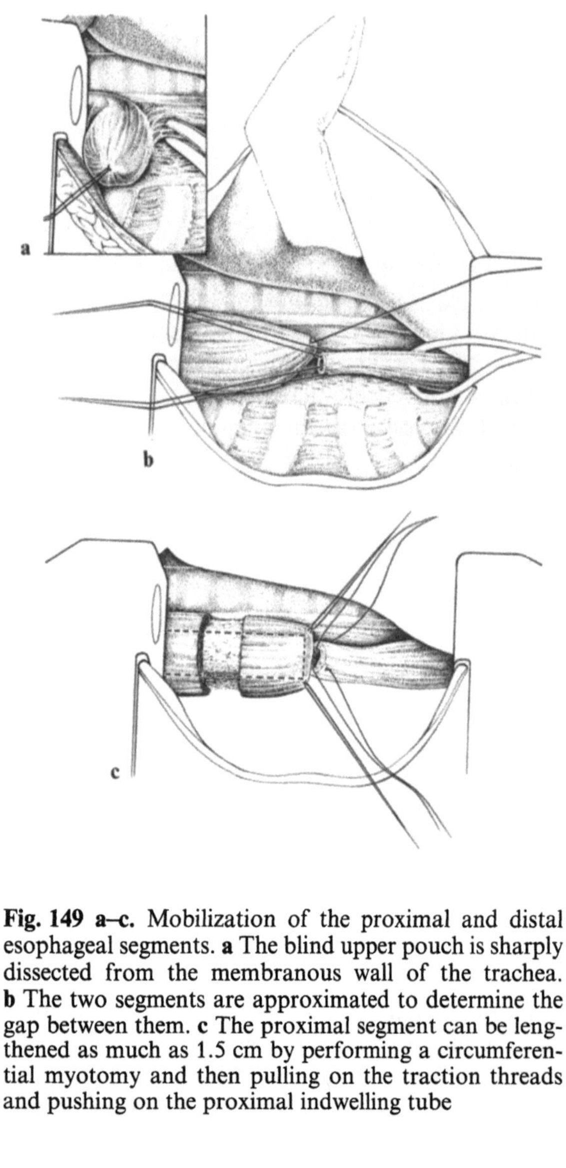

Fig. 149 a–c. Mobilization of the proximal and distal esophageal segments. **a** The blind upper pouch is sharply dissected from the membranous wall of the trachea. **b** The two segments are approximated to determine the gap between them. **c** The proximal segment can be lengthened as much as 1.5 cm by performing a circumferential myotomy and then pulling on the traction threads and pushing on the proximal indwelling tube

14.1.6.5 Anastomosis of the Esophageal Segments

Steps in procedure:

(1) The upper esophageal segment is opened at its lowest point
(2) Two all-layer corner sutures are placed in the upper and lower esophageal segments
(3) The segments are held open with the corner sutures, and 2 or 3 all-coats sutures are placed posteriorly
(4) The segments are approximated by traction on the corner threads, and the posterior sutures are tied
(5) Anterior all-coats sutures are placed

The upper esophageal pouch is elevated with the traction suture, and its blind tip is opened with a small scissors. The opening should be no larger than the lumen of the lower segment, which tends to have a smaller diameter than the upper segment.

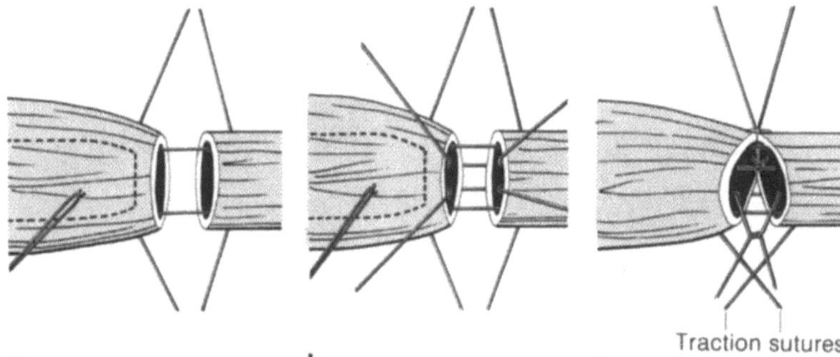

Fig. 150 a–c. Anastomosis of the esophageal segments. a The lumina are stretched to their full size between the corner sutures. b Interrupted sutures are placed through the full thickness of the posterior walls. c The posterior sutures are tied from onc corner thread to the other. The corner sutures are drawn up simultaneously and with equal tension to distribute the strain when approximating the esophageal segments

If the opening in the upper segment appears too large, or if the lumen of the lower segment is unusually narrow, the end of the lower segment may either be beveled or opened longitudinally with a 1- to 2-mm incision. The traction sutures previously placed in the lower segment will form the corner sutures for the anastomosis. They are passed through the full thickness of the upper segment at corresponding sites about 3 mm from the cut edge (Fig. 150 a) and initially are left untied. The sutures are carefully retracted apart to stretch the stoma of each segment to its full diameter, and 2 or 3 all-coats sutures are placed between them to begin the posterior part of the anastomosis (Fig. 150 b). The segments are apposed, and the threads are sequentially tied starting from one corner suture and proceeding around the posterior wall to the other corner suture (Fig. 150 c). Before the anterior sutures are applied, a nasogastric tube is passed through the anastomosis and into the stomach under vision. Then the anterior wall sutures are placed and sequentially tied using the same technique as before. Tension can be removed from the anastomosis by anchoring the proximal segment to the prevertebral fascia with several sutures [18]. Rehbein [27] interposes small pieces of muscle between the trachea and esophagus to prevent recurrence of the fistula.

If the two segments overlap, they can be united by a two-layer anastomosis (see 1.3.2) or by the Haight telescopic anastomosis [11] (Fig. 151).

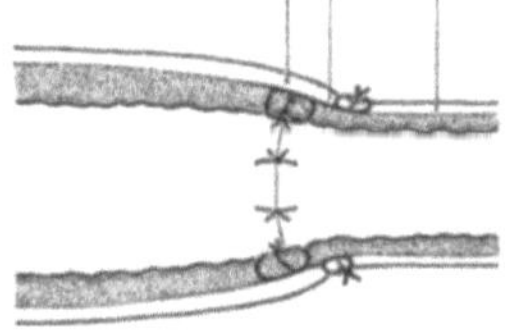

Fig. 151. Haight telescopic anastomosis [11]. This is a two-layer technique in which the muscularis of the proximal segment is drawn over the initial mucosal suture and sutured to the muscularis of the distal segment

14.1.6.6 Closure of the Thoracotomy

After the anastomosis is completed, an attempt should be made to approximate the pleura over it if the transpleural approach has been used. Generally, however, there is not enough material for the margins of the pleura to be sutured together. A chest tube is inserted, and the lung is reexpanded. When the extrapleural approach has been used, a Penrose drain may be placed in the area of the anastomosis, or drainage may be omitted. In either case the chest wall is closed with six or seven pericostal stitches, over which the divided muscle layers are approximated with interrupted sutures.

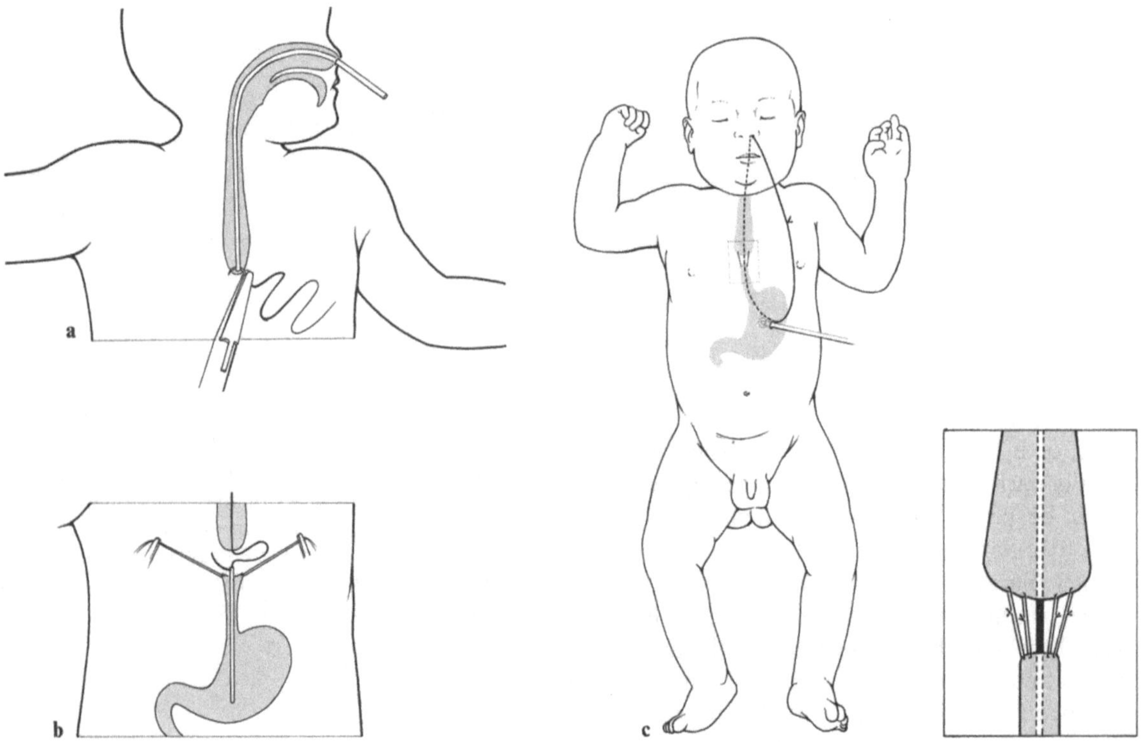

Fig. 152 a–e. Thread technique of Rehbein [27]. **a** A Perlon thread on a needle is passed through the upper pouch and through a rubber catheter inserted transnasally. **b** The Perlon thread is passed through the lower esophageal segment into the stomach. **c** The thread is brought out through the gastrostomy. It passes freely through the posterior mediastinum. The upper and lower esophageal segments are held in approximation by interrupted sutures (insert). **d** Instrumentation: *a* filiform dilator with swaged-on plastic thread and screw connector. *b* Screw connector of the filiform dilator and tip of the esophageal dilator with thread. *c* Various sizes of esophageal dilator (available range is from No. 16 to 48). **e** Insertion of the esophageal dilator. The Perlon thread is brought out through the mouth and fastened to the filiform dilator, to which the esophageal dilator is connected

14.1.6.7 Postoperative care following a Primary Anastomosis

Postoperatively the infant is fed parenterally. If contrast roentgenograms taken on the seventh to tenth postoperative day show no evidence of anastomotic leak, oral liquids may be started with a stomach tube in place. If the child has no difficulty swallowing, the tube may be removed within a few days. If dysphagia is noted, bougienage may be initiated as early as the fourth postoperative week. Because every anastomosis tends to undergo constriction, Rehbein [27] advises routine bougienage before discharging any child who has undergone an atresia repair.

14.1.6.8 Atresia Repair with a Major Gap between the Esophageal Segments

We feel that every means should be exhausted for securing anastomosis of the esophageal segments with available material before resorting to a reconstructive procedure using other portions of the alimentary tract.

14.1.6.8.1 Thread and Olive Technique of Rehbein [27]. If a primary anastomosis cannot be accomplished after maximum mobilization of the esophageal segments, a heavy Perlon thread is passed through the base of the upper segment and through the tip of an indwelling rubber catheter (Fig. 152 a). As the catheter is withdrawn, the Perlon thread is pulled out through the nose and grasped with a clamp. The end of the thread still

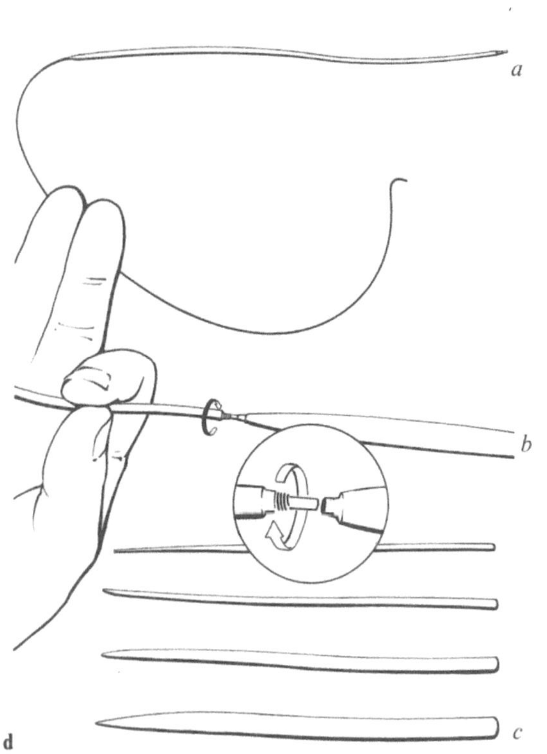

d

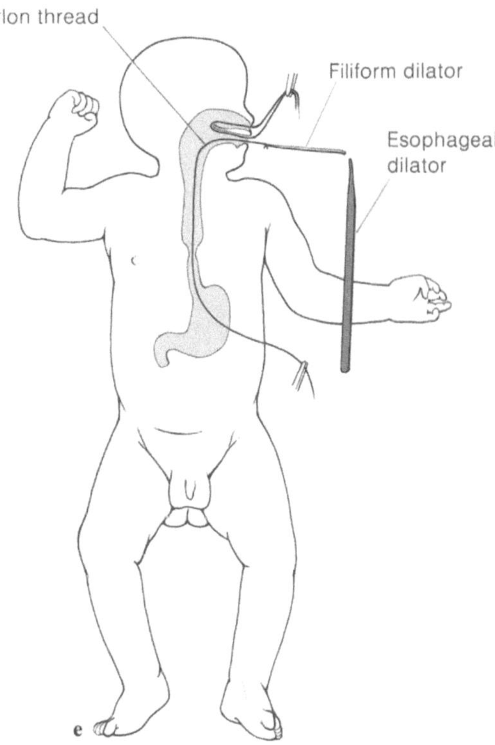

e

in the chest is attached to a feeding catheter about 15 cm long, which is passed into the stomach through the open distal esophageal segment (Fig. 152 b). The distal segment is closed around the Perlon thread. Then three or four approximating sutures of nonabsorbable material are placed between the esophageal segments with minimal tension (Fig. 152 c), the Perlon thread passing freely through the mediastinum across the gap that is to be bridged. The thoracotomy is closed, and the patient is repositioned for gastrostomy (see 14.1.5). The Perlon thread is brought out adjacent to the gastrostomy tube, and the abdominal wall is closed. The ends of the Perlon thread are tied together.

Following surgery the infant will require three to four weeks of intensive care that includes regular, frequent suctioning of the upper pouch. During this time a fibrous tract will form around the Perlon thread, establishing a communication between the upper and lower segments. Initially the tract is composed of connective tissue, but with passage of time its inner surface will become lined with esophageal mucosa. When decreased salivary flow and the presence of gastric contents in the mouth indicate that a serviceable canal has formed, bougienage may be initiated if the gap between the segments was smaller than 15 mm. For longer gaps, the olive technique may be used.

The bougienage is performed under general anesthesia. The gastrostomy tube is removed and the Perlon thread cut. The ends of the thread are held with clamps. The upper part of the Perlon thread is identified in the posterior pharynx with the laryngoscope, pulled forward with a small, blunt hook, and cut again. The transnasal part of the thread is held with a clamp, while a filiform dilator is attached to the transesophageal part. A plastic thread is swaged onto the end of the dilator, and the opposite end carries a screw connector (Fig. 152 d) to which the smallest-size esophageal dilator is attached (Fig. 152 e). By pulling carefully on the part of the Perlon thread protruding from the gastrostomy, both dilators are successively drawn through the site of the stenosis. The esophageal dilator is left in place for a short time, then withdrawn perorally and replaced with a larger size. If the dilator does not pass easily or is blood-streaked when withdrawn, the bougienage is discontinued. The Perlon thread protruding from the mouth is cut off at the dilator and tied to the lower end of the transnasal thread. A new Perlon

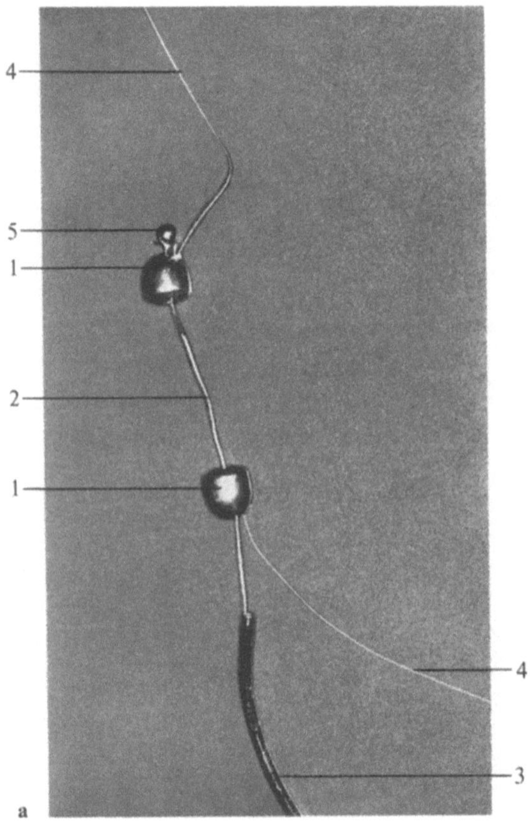

a

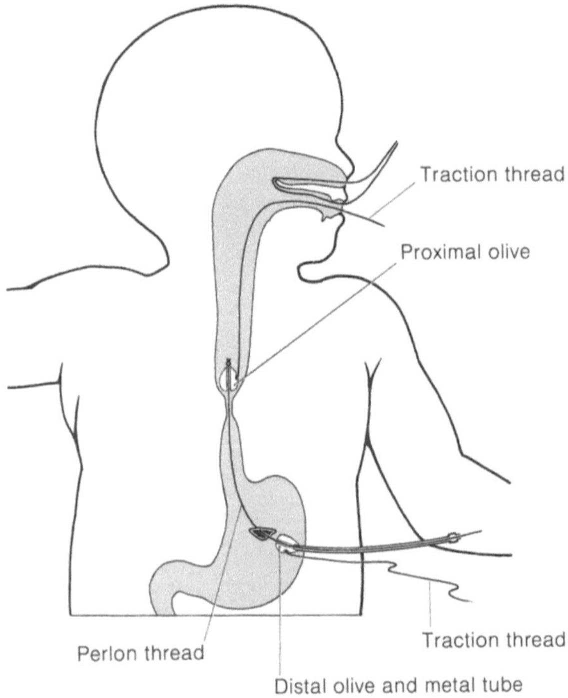

b

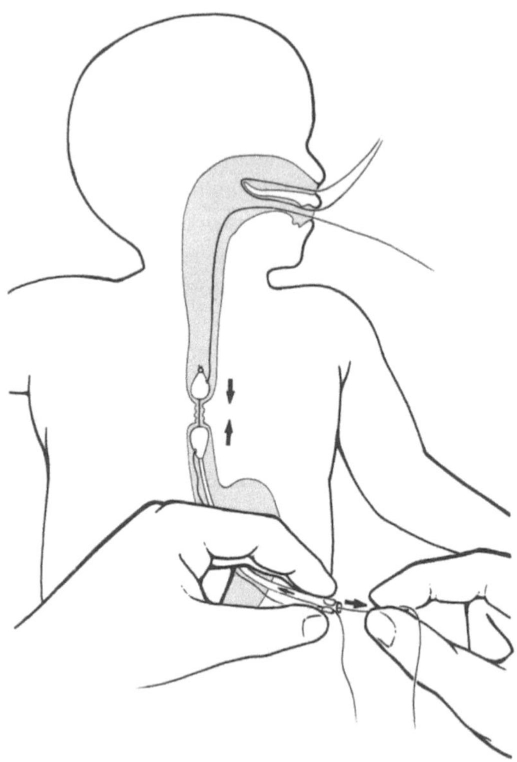
c

Fig. 153 a–c. Olive technique of Rehbein [27]. **a** Instrumentation: *1* silver olives, *2* Perlon thread, *3* thin metal tube, *4* pullout thread tied to an eye on the olive, *5* metal ball with central perforation for attachment of the Perlon thread. **b** Insertion of the olives into the esophagus. **c** The esophageal segments are approximated by traction on the Perlon thread and pressure on the metal tube

thread is tied to the upper end of the transnasal thread and is pulled through the stenosis and out the gastrostomy. The ends of the new thread are tied together.

The bougienage is performed once or twice weekly. In infants less than 10 weeks of age, we dilate to a maximum of 17 Ch. The thread is not removed at that time, but is left in place for several months so that necessary dilatations can be performed quickly and safely. The thread is removed when the patient is swallowing normally and two to three months have passed since the last dilation. Generally the gastrostomy will close spontaneously after the tube is withdrawn.

The olive technique is used when the esophageal segments are widely separated. When a satisfactory fibrous tract has formed around the Perlon thread, the thread is pulled out through the mouth, divided, and secured as described above. The transoral part of the thread is passed through the central bore of a flat-based silver olive dilator and fastened to a small metal ball at the top of the olive (Fig. 153 a). A separate pullout thread is fastened to an eye loop on the side of the silver olive. When the Perlon thread is pulled through the gastrostomy, the olive is drawn down through the esophagus, where it engages against the base of the upper segment (Fig. 153 b). An olive of similar design is threaded over the end of the Perlon thread protruding from the gastrostomy, and a thin, curved metal tube is threaded on behind it. The Perlon thread is pulled taut, and the second olive is pushed into the lower esophageal segment by pressure on the metal tube. Resistance will be felt as the base of the olive seats against the roof of the lower segment. The distance between the two olives is checked with an image intensifier. By pulling on the transoral thread and simultaneously pushing on the metal tube, the two segments are approximated (Fig. 153 c). With the system under slight tension, the Perlon thread is tied off to an eye loop at the end of the metal tube. The system is left in place for about 1–2 h. With a regimen of one or two of these sessions per week, the distance between the esophageal segments will gradually diminish. Finally all that remains is a thin intervening septum, which is crushed. If a stricture remains, it is either dilated by bougienage over the Perlon thread or is resected.

14.1.6.9 Reconstruction of the Pediatric Esophagus

Reconstruction of the atretic esophagus is appropriate only in the relatively few cases where the gap between the segments is so large, even after elongating measures, that a primary anastomosis is not possible or an attempted primary anastomosis has failed, leaving a large residual defect. The functional result of esophageal reconstruction is satisfactory in the great majority of patients, especially when colon is used. Most children swallow well after the procedure and go on to develop normally without special dietary measures. Colon makes the most suitable esophageal substitute, followed by jejunum and stomach. The preparation of the transplant, routes for transplantation, and construction of the anastomosis are basically the same as in adults (see Sect. 7). Here we shall focus on aspects that apply specifically to esophageal replacement in small children.

Waterston [33] states that the most favorable time for operation is the 6th month of life. Gross [9] advises that the procedure be undertaken when the child attains a body weight of 10 kg. In our opinion and that of Rehbein [27], 12 months is the optimum age for the reconstruction.

14.1.6.9.1 Final Intrathoracic Measures in Preparation for the Esophagoplasty. If the esophagotracheal fistula has been closed and the segments mobilized, and it is found that the gap between the segments is large enough to justify segmental esophageal replacement with an intrathoracic transplant, the lumen of the lower esophagus is closed with inverting interrupted sutures. Both segments are fixed to the prevertebral fascia. Continuous suctioning of the upper pouch should be maintained until the definitive reconstruction is undertaken. If the proximal segment is very short, or if a retrosternal route of transplantation or cervical anastomosis is preferred on general principles, the upper pouch is mobilized past the thoracic inlet before the thoracotomy is closed. After closure an end-cervical esophagostomy (see 2.2.2) is constructed.

14.1.6.9.2 Reconstruction Using Colon. Colon esophagoplasty in children is most often performed with a left colon isoperistaltic transplant based on the left colic artery or proximal sigmoid artery. The transplant may consist only of the left transverse colon or may include the descending colon, depending on the length of the defect (see 7.5.2.1). If the right colon is to be used, the ileocecal valve should be left in situ [1, 28] to avoid bacterial contamination of the small intestine and malabsorption.

Within the abdomen, the mobilized segment is always brought up posterior to the stomach and reanastomosed colon (see 7.2.1). For the thoracic phase, either a retrosternal or transpleural route may be employed (see 7.2.2).

Waterston [33], who always prepares the colon segment through a thoracic approach after detaching the diaphragm from the costal margin, recommends bringing the transplant up through a phrenotomy made about 3 cm from the esophageal hiatus. He notes that this route preserves the integrity

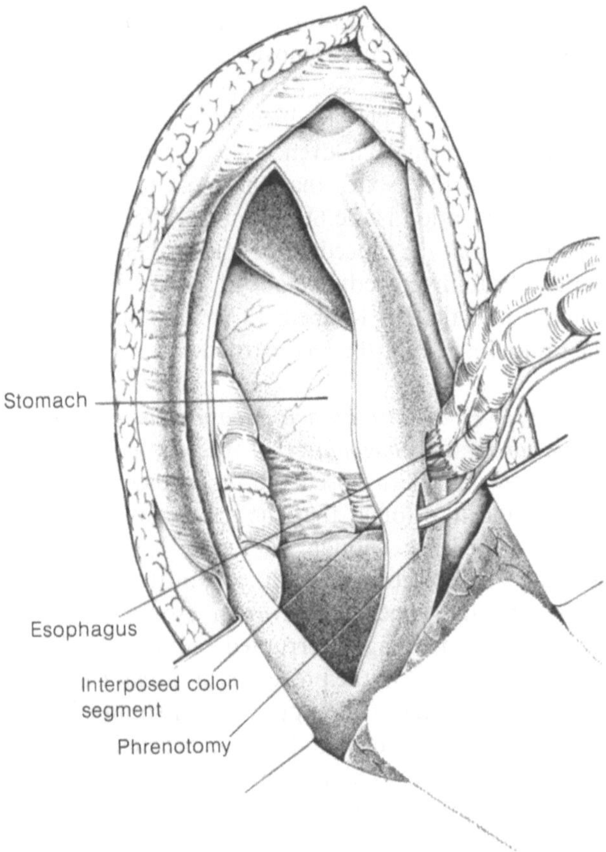

Fig. 154. Bringing the isolated colon segment up through a phrenotomy incision separate from the hiatus

of the cardia and hiatus as barriers against reflux. After widening the incision, he passes a blunt, curved forceps under digital guidance down behind the splenic vessels and pancreas and plunges the forceps through the retroperitoneum distal to the inferior border of the pancreas. By repeatedly opening the forceps blades, he creates a tunnel through which the prepared colon segment can be pulled up into the thorax (Fig. 154). Because the colon transplant has very little peristaltic activity, there is a potential for severe dilatation of the segment when the lower esophageal sphincter is intact. Rehbein [27], who observed this situation repeatedly, recommended that the intrathoracic colon segment be ensheathed within a mesh of absorbable material.

Pyloroplasty is not essential if the vagus nerves are intact. A Perlon thread can be passed through the interposed colon segment and subsequently brought out perorally and through the gastrostomy. This provides a safe means of dilating the reconstructed esophagus if anastomotic stricture ensues. Before the transplant is anastomosed to the lower esophageal segment, the luminal disparity is corrected either by making a wedge excision from the antimesenteric colon wall or by longitudinal incision of the esophagus. The colon segment should take a straight course within the thorax but should be free of tension. The proximal anastomosis may be performed in the thorax or the neck, depending on the length of the upper esophageal segment. Space limitations in the cervical area may make it necessary to resect part of the manubrium sterni or the head of the clavicle and incise the sternocleidomastoid muscle to make room for the esophageal substitute [28].

14.1.6.9.3 Reconstruction Using Jejunum. The delicate vascular system of small children greatly limits the use of small intestine for reconstructing the atretic esophagus. Segmental jejunum interposition (see 7.4.3) and the Roux-en-Y anastomosis (see 7.4.4) have been successfully utilized in older children with severe strictures secondary to gastroesophageal reflux [5, 10].

14.1.6.9.4 Reconstruction Using Stomach. In children, bringing the stomach into the chest for anastomosis to the esophagus is fraught with complications such as reflux esophagitis and peptic stricture, and we do not recommend this procedure. Reconstruction with a reverse gastric tube (see 7.3.5) has been successfully accomplished in several children from 12 to 18 months of age [4, 8]. This method may be considered when the esophageal atresia is accompanied by an anal malformation, and it is desirable to preserve the colon for a possible pull-through operation. The spleen should be preserved whenever possible due to the risk of infection that follows splenectomy.

14.1.7 Surgical Treatment of Type II Atresia

Type II atresia is the second most common form, accounting for 5%–10% of cases. There is no associated fistula, and a major gap can exist between the upper and lower esophageal segments. The initial step is to perform a gastrostomy once the diagnosis is confirmed (see 14.1.5). Esophagostomy should definitely be avoided, as it will necessitate an esophageal replacement procedure. The blind

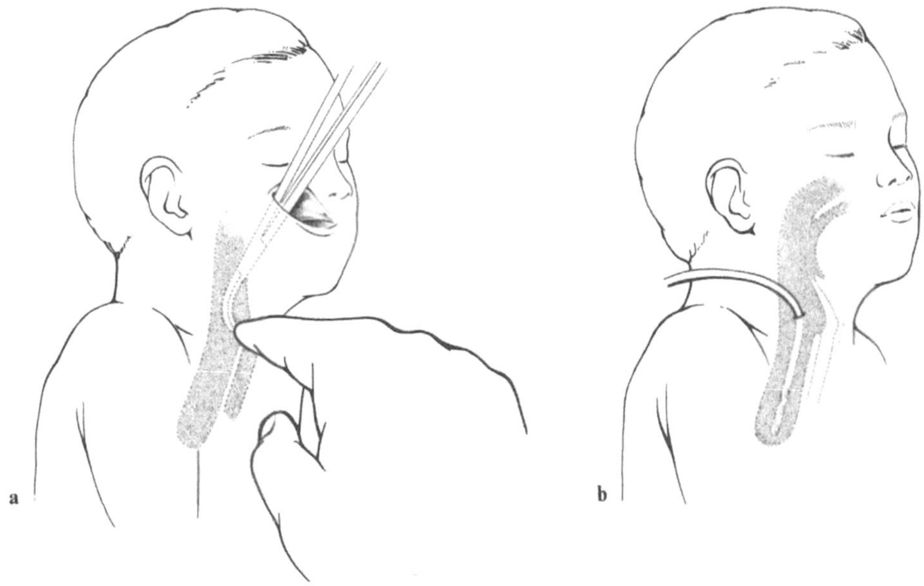

Fig. 155 a,b. Temporary tube pharyngostomy. **a** A curved clamp is passed into the pharynx. The end of the clamp is palpated with the fingertip, and the overlying skin is incised. **b** Position of the tube in the blind upper pouch

upper pouch is suctioned frequently through a double-lumen Reploge tube until the definitive repair is undertaken. However, the frequent catheter changes are not without risk, and the transnasal position of the catheter hampers nasal respiration, upon which the child must rely. An alternative is the temporary tube pharyngostomy [29]. Its main advantage over the transnasal catheter is that a considerably larger-caliber tube can be used without causing appreciable injury or irritation of the pharynx or esophagus. The nasal mucosa is not disturbed, and the tube does not interfere with respiration. The fistulous tract heals rapidly after the tube is removed. In addition, the pharyngostomy leaves open the option for elongation and anastomosis of the esophageal segments.

Preoperative preparation: See 14.1.3.

Instruments: Pediatric basic set.

Position: Supine.

Operative technique: A curved clamp is introduced through the mouth until its tip can be palpated through the anterolateral pharyngeal wall at the level of the hyoid bone. The skin over the palpable tip is incised, and the clamp is gently pushed through the soft tissues of the neck toward the finger in the skin wound, avoiding injury to the neurovascular bundle (Fig. 155 a). When the tip of the clamp is visible, the channel is enlarged by carefully opening the blades of the clamp. A catheter of appropriate size is grasped with the clamp and pulled into the pharynx. The catheter tip is then advanced to the floor of the upper pouch under laryngoscopic guidance (Fig. 155 b). The catheter is fixed to the skin with a suture. Within 48 h a satisfactory tract is established, making it easy to insert a fresh tube.

14.1.7.1 Methods of Elongating the Esophageal Segments

The distance between the segments is determined fluoroscopically. A rubber catheter containing a flexible metal tube is passed transorally into the blind upper pouch, and a similar catheter is inserted into the blind lower pouch via the gastrostomy. The esophageal segments are carefully approximated, and the residual gap is documented by X-ray. If the ends are too widely separated for a direct anastomosis, the upper pouch is stretched and lengthened by daily dilatations until radiographs show that maximum elongation has been obtained [19]. If a significant gap persists, an attempt may be made to lengthen the proximal pouch further by mobilizing it through a cervical approach [4].

Hendren and Hale [13] developed the technique of electromagnetic bougienage for lengthening the esophageal segments in congenital atresia. A steel "bullet" attached to a metal wire is introduced into each of the two segments (Fig. 156). The infant's upper body is placed into an electromagnetic field ("atresia coil"), which pulls the bullets toward each other. The field is intermittent, on for 40 s and off for 60 s for a total of 4 h, 3 times per day [6]. The infant is accessible to nursing care while in the coil. Through repeated sessions the two segments can be lengthened sufficiently to enable a primary anastomosis, or the tissue remaining between the segments is so thin that it is easily crushed or penetrated.

Okmian [26] devised an endoscopic technique for placing a Perlon thread through both esophageal segments and the mediastinum. A cystoscope is passed through the gastrostomy into the lower pouch, and an infant esophagoscope is passed into the upper pouch. Using continuous two-plane fluoroscopic guidance, a needle with Perlon thread attached is introduced through the cystoscope and is pushed through the upper end of the distal pouch and through the lower end of the proximal pouch. The esophagoscope is used to grasp the needle and attached thread and pull them out through the proximal pouch. The operator can then proceed with Rehbein's silver olive dilatation procedure (see 14.1.6.8.1).

If the two segments cannot be adequately approximated using the methods described above, thoracotomy is performed. The rest of the procedure then corresponds to that for a Type IIIb atresia after closure of the tracheoesophageal fistula (see 14.1.6).

14.1.8 Surgical Treatment of Type IIIa and Type IIIc Atresia (Atresia with a Proximal Fistula)

Atresia with a fistula between the upper esophageal pouch and trachea is less a problem of treatment than of diagnosis. The prevalence of this anomaly, at 1%, is low. A fistula involving the cervical part of the esophagus is closed via a cervical approach. The repair of an intrathoracic fistula follows the technique described for Type IIIb atresia (see 14.1.6).

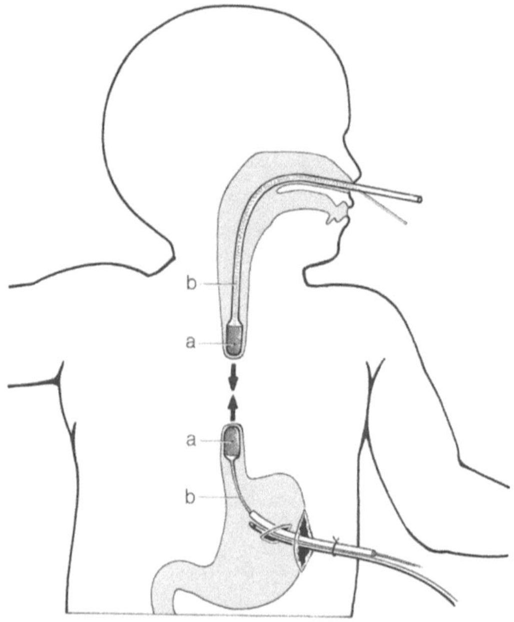

Fig. 156. Electromagnetic bougienage of Hendren and Hale [13]. *a* Steel "bullets," *b* metal wires for inserting the bullets into the esophageal segments

14.1.8.1 Closure of the Fistula through a Cervical Approach

Preoperative Preparation See 14.1.3 and Chap. C.

Instruments: Pediatric basic set.

Position and approach: See 2.1.1.

Steps in procedure:

(1) Exposure of the esophagus in the neck (see 2.1.1)
(2) Localization of the fistula
(3) Circumferential dissection of the fistulous junction
(4) Snaring of the fistula
(5) Placement of traction sutures on the esophagus and trachea above and below the fistula
(6) Division of the fistula
(7) Closure of the tracheal opening with continuous or interrupted sutures
(8) Closure of the defect in the upper esophageal segment with a transfixion ligature
(9) Drainage of the operative area

Operative technique: The esophagus is exposed (see 2.1.1). Usually the fistula can be identified by an audible and palpable bruit that is synchronous with respirations. Distal to the presumed site of the fistula, the esophagus is separated from the trachea using small dissectors or small dissecting patties. Extreme care is taken not to injure the membranous part of the trachea or the esophageal wall. When a portion of the esophagus has been freed from the trachea, it is encircled with a small, curved clamp and snared with a thin rubber tape. If the bruit persists when the tape around the esophagus is tightened, the fistula is assumed to be located above the tape. The area above the fistula is dissected in a similar fashion, and a second tape is passed around the esophagus at that level. Both tapes are pulled laterally. The site of entry of the fistula into the trachea is exposed, cleared, and encircled with a tape. A pair of traction sutures are placed in the trachea, one above the fistulous junction and one below, and the trachea is pulled toward the medial side of the field (Fig. 157). A traction suture is also placed on the esophageal side of the fistula, about 3 mm from the trachea, to keep the esophagus from retracting after division of the fistula. The fistula is divided with a scalpel, and the tracheal defect is repaired with continuous or interrupted sutures (see 14.1.6.2). The proximal stump of esophagus is closed with a transfixion ligature. The operative area is drained with a small-caliber Penrose drain.

14.1.8.2 Measures after Closure of the Proximal Tracheoesophageal Fistula

Closure of the proximal tracheoesophageal fistula converts a Type IIIa anomaly into a Type II configuration. A gastrostomy is performed during the primary operation. Further measures are like those described for the treatment of Type II atresia (see 14.1.7).

Closure of the proximal fistula in Type IIIc atresia leaves a Type IIIb configuration, which is managed as described in 14.1.6.

14.1.9 Staged Repair for Infants with Serious Accompanying Illness, Prematurity, or Coexisting Anomalies

In Category C babies, who are considered poor candidates for a primary anastomosis, the treatment regimen is adapted to the patient's current status and stage of development. Initial surgery should be minimal in its extent.

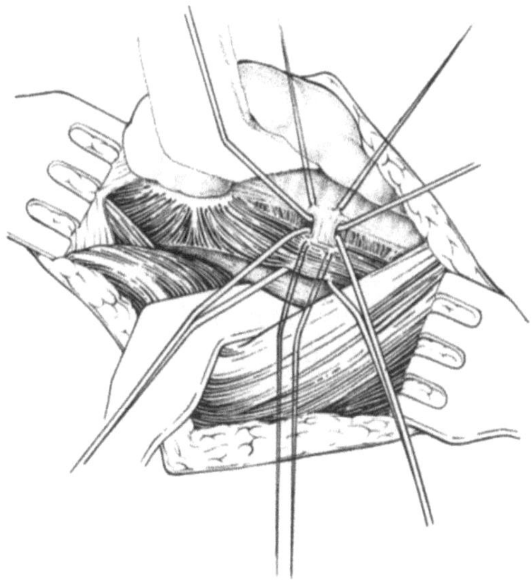

Fig. 157. Closure of a tracheoesophageal fistula through a cervical approach. Snares have been placed around the esophagus and fistula. Traction sutures on the esophageal side of the fistula prevent retraction of the esophagus when the fistula is divided

14.1.9.1 First Stage of Treatment

For Type II atresia, a gastrostomy is performed under local anesthesia. Pooled secretions are suctioned from the blind upper pouch through a Reploge tube or temporary tube pharyngostomy (see 14.1.7). If a fistula exists between the upper esophageal segment and trachea (Type IIIa/c), it is closed through a cervical approach in the same operation (see 14.1.8.1).

Gastrostomy alone is inadequate for Type IIIb atresia. It cannot eliminate the reflux of gastric juice into the trachea, especially if the gastrostomy is additionally used for feeding. This led Firor [7] to advise that gastrostomy be combined with a feeding jejunostomy in these infants. Holder and Ashcraft [17] insert a small-caliber feeding catheter alongside the gastrostomy tube and advance it through the pylorus into the duodenum or jejunum. While both methods are superior to simple gastrostomy, neither is completely effective in eliminating gastric reflux into the trachea. This underscores the need for additional measures such as temporary ligation of the esophagus [21], division of the stomach or esophagus [25, 30], or sealing of the fistula with Histacryl [8] to prevent the aspiration of gastric fluids. We cannot recommend temporary ligation of the esophagus [21] due to the danger of ischemic necrosis.

14.1.9.1.1 Gastric Division. Gastric division with double gastrostomy continues to be the most effective method of preventing gastric reflux into the trachea in infants with esophageal atresia. Disadvantages are that the procedure may be poorly tolerated by critically ill babies, and a second operation is needed to repair the stomach once esophageal continuity is established.

Preoperative preparation, instruments, position and approach: See 14.1.5.

Operative technique: The abdomen is entered, and the stomach is pulled downward. The transverse line of the gastric division separates the proximal third of the stomach from the distal two-thirds. The greater omentum is detached at the proposed site of the transection, and the left gastric artery is palpated and mobilized. The lesser omentum is divided between the ascending and descending branches of the artery to ensures that both parts of the stomach will have an adequate blood supply. The stomach is divided with the GIA instrument, and a gastrostomy is constructed in each pouch (see 14.1.5). The gastrostomy tubes are brought out through separate incisions to the right and left of the laparotomy wound (Fig. 158). The anterior wall of each gastric pouch is fixed to the peritoneum. The distal tube provides a route for feeding, and the proximal tube is for decompression.

Touloukian and Stinson [30] devised a procedure in which the stomach is temporarily partitioned by a full-thickness plication technique. The gastrocolic ligament is divided at the junction of the fundus and body of the stomach. A finger or dissecting patty is passed into the lesser sac and advanced to the lesser curvature. A gastrostomy is performed in the proximal third of the stomach for drainage, and the tube is brought out through a separate stab incision to the left of the laparotomy. A suture of nonabsorbable monofilament is passed into the peritoneal cavity over a plastic button. The stomach is partitioned by plicating the full thickness of its anterior and posterior walls, starting on the greater curvature and proceeding toward the lesser curvature. At the lesser curvature the suture is brought outside the abdominal wall, passed through a second plastic button, and returned to the abdominal cavity. The suture is brought back across the stomach, making a second

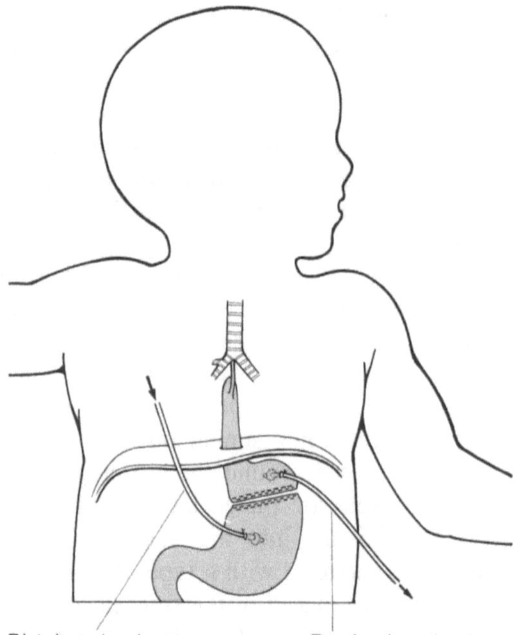

Fig. 158. Gastric division. The stomach is divided transversely between its proximal third and distal two-thirds with the GIA instrument. The proximal gastrostomy provides for gastric drainage; the distal gastrostomy is for tube feeding

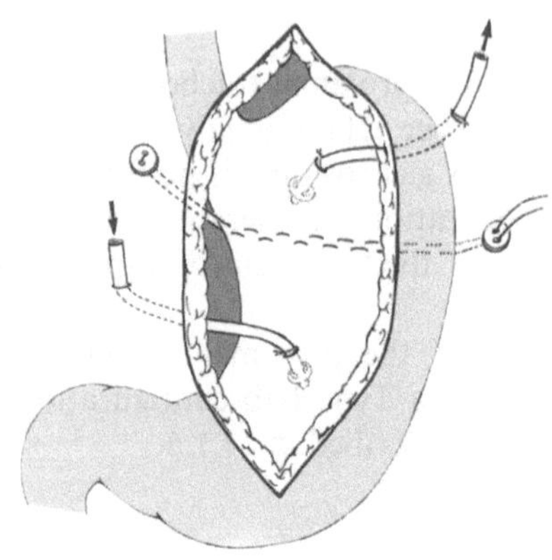

Fig. 159. Temporary gastric partition of Touloukian and Stinson [30]. A pullout plication suture divides the stomach into a proximal and distal pouch. Separate gastrostomies provide for drainage of gastric juice and for tube feeding

suture line parallel to the first, and is tied to the first button. This partitions the stomach into a proximal and a distal pouch (Fig. 159). A second gastrostomy is performed in the distal gastric pouch, and the tube is brought out through a separate incision to the right of the laparotomy. After closure of the laparotomy, the plication suture is tightened sufficiently to fix the anterior stomach wall to the abdominal wall and secure the gastric partition. Once the tracheoesophageal fistula has been closed and esophageal continuity established, it is unnecessary to perform a second operation to reanastomose the stomach. The partition is removed by cutting and withdrawing the sutures.

14.1.9.1.2 Supragastric Division of the Esophagus. Supragastric division of the esophagus with closure of both ends and fixation of the esophagus to the anterior wall of the fundus has several disadvantages. Reanastomosis is more difficult than after a gastric division, and the functional integrity of the cardia and hiatus is destroyed. Postoperative reflux is common following reanastomosis.

14.1.9.1.3 Sealing Off the Tracheoesophageal Fistula. The regurgitation of gastric juice into the trachea can be prevented by sealing off the tracheoesophageal fistula with Histacryl [8]. The fistulous opening is identified with a tracheoscope, and the plastic material is injected into the neck of the fistula through a thin tube. It is unclear how effective this technique is in occluding the fistula, and long-term efficacy is untested. To date the procedure has been used successfully in two infants.

14.1.9.2 Subsequent Treatment Stages

If the child shows satisfactory recovery in the ensuing weeks or months, the operator may proceed with division and closure of the tracheoesophageal fistula. The fistula repair may be combined with a primary anastomosis or with one of the foregoing methods of lengthening the esophageal segments. Gastric continuity is restored in a third stage. The gastrostomy is maintained until it is certain that dysphagia is relieved. Usually the wound will close spontaneously after the tube is removed.

14.1.10 Treatment of Esophageal Atresia with Associated Intestinal Anomalies

From twenty to thirty percent of infants with esophageal atresia have coexisting intestinal malformations. In the absence of other complicating circumstances such as cardiac anomalies, respiratory distress or prematurity, the thoracic part of the operation may be combined with the abdominal part.

14.1.10.1 Esophageal Atresia Combined with Duodenal Atresia

In otherwise healthy infants, duodenoduodenostomy is performed at the time the gastrostomy is established. This is followed immediately by the thoracic phase. If the infant is too sick to tolerate a primary repair of both anomalies, the duodenal atresia is corrected, and the stomach is transversely divided. The timing of the esophageal atresia repair depends on how well the infant does after the initial surgery.

14.1.10.2 Esophageal Atresia Combined with Anal Atresia

In girls with an anovestibular or rectovaginal fistula, there will be little impairment of defecation. Enemas can be given to evacuate the bowel, and the surgeon may proceed with thoracotomy. In boys with an infralevator or membranous obstruction, a perineal anoplasty is performed and the bowel evacuated before thoracotomy is undertaken. With supralevator anal atresia, an abdominoperineal pull-through procedure will be necessary in newborn males. Under no circumstances should this be combined with the thoracic procedure. A temporary colostomy is performed first, then esophageal continuity is established, and finally the anal atresia is corrected and the definitive colostomy is constructed.

14.2 Isolated Tracheoesophageal Fistula

Tracheoesophageal fistula is extremely rare as an isolated anomaly. The fistulous tract runs obliquely upward from the esophagus to the trachea. The technique of operative repair depends on the exact location of the fistula. However, approximately 80% of these fistulas involve the cervical part of the esophagus, entering at the level of the thoracic inlet. Diagnostic localization relies on esophagoscopy while positive-pressure ventilation is applied. A characteristic bruit will be heard during ventilation of the intubated infant. The fistula can be visualized with the esophagoscope, and small blebs may be seen about the fistulous opening. Localizing the fistula to the cervical or thoracic part of the esophagus dictates the surgical approach. Fistulas in the thoracic inlet pose special problems, and the operation should be planned so that either a thoracic or cervical approach may be taken. The cervical approach should be made first, as it is the lesser procedure [29]. If no pathology is found there, the chest is opened in the same operation. Repair of the fistula through a cervical approach follows the technique described for Type IIIa esophageal atresia (see 14.1.8.1). Repair of thoracic fistulas follows the procedure recommended for Type IIIb anomalies (see 14.1.6).

References

1. Azar H, Crispin AR, Waterston DJ (1971) Esophageal replacement with transverse colon in infants and children. J Pediatr Surg 6:3
2. Burrington JD, Stephens CA (1968) Esophageal replacement with a gastric tube in infants and children. J Pediatr Surg 3:2
3. Cohen DH, Middleton AW, Fletcher J (1974) Gastric tube esophagoplasty. J Pediatr Surg 9:451
4. Daum R, Hecker W, Heiss W (1970) Der Wert der aufgeschobenen End-zu-End Anastomose nach Elongation des kurzen proximalen Segmentes bei Ösophagusatresie. Z Kinderheilkunde 8:359
5. Ferer JM, Bruch HM (1968) Jejunal and colonic interposition for non-malignant disease of the esophagus. Ann Surg 169:533
6. Filler D, Effenhauser P (1982) Magnetische Bougierung bei primär nicht rekonstruierbarer Ösophagusatresie. Diagnostik und Intensivtherapie 7:405
7. Firor HV (1970) New techniques in the management of esophageal atresia. S Afr J Surg 8:59
8. Gdanietz K, Krause I (1975) Plastic adhesives for closing oesophago-tracheal fistula in children. International Symposium on oesophageal atresia, Bremen
9. Gross RF (1953) The surgery of infancy and childhood. Saunders, Philadelphia
10. Gross RF (1970) An atlas of childrens surgery. Saunders, Philadelphia
11. Haight C (1969) Congenital atresia and tracheo-esophageal fistula. In: Mustard WT, Ravitch MM, Snyder WH, Welch KJ, Benson CD (eds) Pediatric Surgery, 2nd edn. Year Book Medical Publishers, Chicago
12. Heimburger IL, Alford WC, Wooler GH (1965) Hiatal hernia and reflux esophagitis in children. J Thorac Cardiovasc Surg 50:467
13. Hendren WH, Hale JR (1975) Electromagnetic bougienage to lengthen esophageal segments in congenital esophageal atresia. N Engl J Med 293:428
14. Holder TM, McDonald DB, Wooley MM (1962) The premature or critically ill infant with esophageal atresia: Increased success with a staged approach. J Thorac Cardiovasc Surg 44:344
15. Holder TM, Cloud DT, Lewis JE, Pilling GP (1964) Esophageal atresia and tracheo-esophageal fistula. A survey of its members by the surgical section of the American Academy of Pediatrics. Pediatrics 34:542
16. Holder TM (1964) Transpleural versus retropleural approach for repair of tracheo-esophageal fistula. Surg Clin North Am 44:1433
17. Holder TM, Ashcraft KW (1966) Esophageal atresia and tracheo-esophageal fistula. Curr Probl Surg 1:1
18. Holder TM (1978) Current trends in the management of esophageal atresia and tracheo-esophageal fistula. The Am Surg 31:12
19. Howard R, Myers NA (1965) Esophageal atresia. A technique for elongating the upper pouch. Surgery 58:725
20. Hrabovsky E, Boles ET (1978) Long term results following esophageal anastomosis in the neonate. Surg Gynecol Obstet 147:30
21. Koop CE, Schnaufer L, Broennie AM (1974) Esophageal atresia and tracheo-esophageal fistula: Supportive measures that affect survival. Pediatrics 54:558
22. Leininger BJ (1972) Silastic banding of esophagus with subsequent repair of esophageal atresia and tracheo-esophageal fistula. J Pediat Surg 7:404
23. Livaditis A, Björk G, Fängström LG (1969) Esophageal myectomy. Scand J Thorac Cardiovasc Surg 3:181
24. Livaditis A (1973) Esophageal atresia: A method of overbridge large segmental gaps. Z Kinderchirurgie 13:298
25. Meeker IA, Hags DM, Woolley MM, Snyder WH (1962) Changing techniques in the management of esophageal atresia. Arch Surg 92:611
26. Okmian L, Booss D, Ekelund L (1975) An endoskopic technique for REHBEIN's silver olive method. Z Kinderchir 16:212
27. Rehbein F (1976) Kinderchirurgische Operationen. Hippokrates, Stuttgart
28. Rodgers BM, Talbert JL, Moazam F, Felman AH (1978) Functional and metabolic evaluation of colon replacement of the esophagus in children. Journ Ped Surg 13:35
29. Talbert JL, Haller JA (1965) Temporary tube pharyngostomy in the staged repair of congenital tracheo-esophageal fistula. Ped Surg 58:737
30. Touloukian RJ, Stinson KK (1970) Temporary gastric partition: A model for staged repair of esophageal atresia with fistula. Ann Surg 171:184
31. Vogt EC (1929) Congenital esophageal atresia. Am J Roentgenol 22:463
32. Waterston DJ, Bonham-Carter RE, Aberdeen E (1962) Esophageal atresia: Tracheo-esophageal fistula. A study of survival in 218 infants. Lancet 1:819
33. Waterston DJ (1964) Colonic replacement of esophagus (intrathoracic). Surg Clin N Amer 44:1441
34. Woolley MM (1980) Esophageal atresia and tracheo-esophageal fistula: 1939 to 1979. Am Journ Surg 139:771

Subject Index

K. Topography of Surgically Important Regions
15 Anatomic Plates

K. Zilles and U. Demmel

This section presents 15 anatomic plates demonstrating the topography of surgically important regions in the neck, thorax, and upper abdomen. Special emphasis is placed on portraying the aspects from which these regions are most commonly viewed by the operating surgeon. Each plate is accompanied by a brief explanation of the principal structures of interest. Thus, the present section is concerned less with depicting topographic anatomy in the conventional sense than with providing a practical guide to understanding problems of surgical anatomy. More comprehensive presentations may be found in the pertinent literature.

References

Braus H, Elze C (1956) Anatomie des Menschen, Bd II. Springer, Berlin Göttingen Heidelberg

Corning HK (1939) Lehrbuch der topographischen Anatomie. Bergmann, München

Hafferl A (1969) Lehrbuch der topographischen Anatomie. Springer, Berlin Heidelberg New York

Pernkopf E (1979/80) Atlas der topographischen und angewandten Anatomie des Menschen. Band 1+2

Rohen JW (1977) Topographische Anatomie. Schattauer, Stuttgart New York

Rohen JW, Yokochi CH (1982, 1983) Anatomie des Menschen. Band 1+2. Schattauer, Stuttgart New York

Töndury G (1981) Angewandte und topographische Anatomie. Thieme, Stuttgart

Lanz T von, Wachsmuth W (1955) Praktische Anatomie. 1. Band/Teil 2: Hals. Springer, Berlin Heidelberg New York

Plate I: The Arteries, Veins, and Nerves of the Anterior and Lateral Chest Wall

The cutaneous and perforating branches of the intercostal arteries, the internal thoracic artery, the lateral thoracic artery, and the thoracodorsal artery supply the skin of the anterior and lateral chest wall. The perforating intercostal arterial branch emerging from the corresponding intercostal space is usually of large caliber. All the cutaneous arteries anastomose with one another. Venous drainage is accomplished by the lateral thoracic vein, the thoracoepigastric vein, and the median xiphoid vein, which likewise interanastomose. The thoracoepigastric vein forms an anastomotic chain with the superficial epigastric vein, which empties into the femoral vein via the saphenous vein; this system establishes a communication between the inferior and superior venae cavae. Impairment of portal venous drainage can cause the damming back of blood into the paraumbilical veins ("Medusa's head") and into the superior vena cava by way of the median xiphoid, thoracoepigastric, and lateral thoracic veins. The skin is innervated by the lateral and anterior branches of the intercostal nerves and by the supraclavicular nerves.

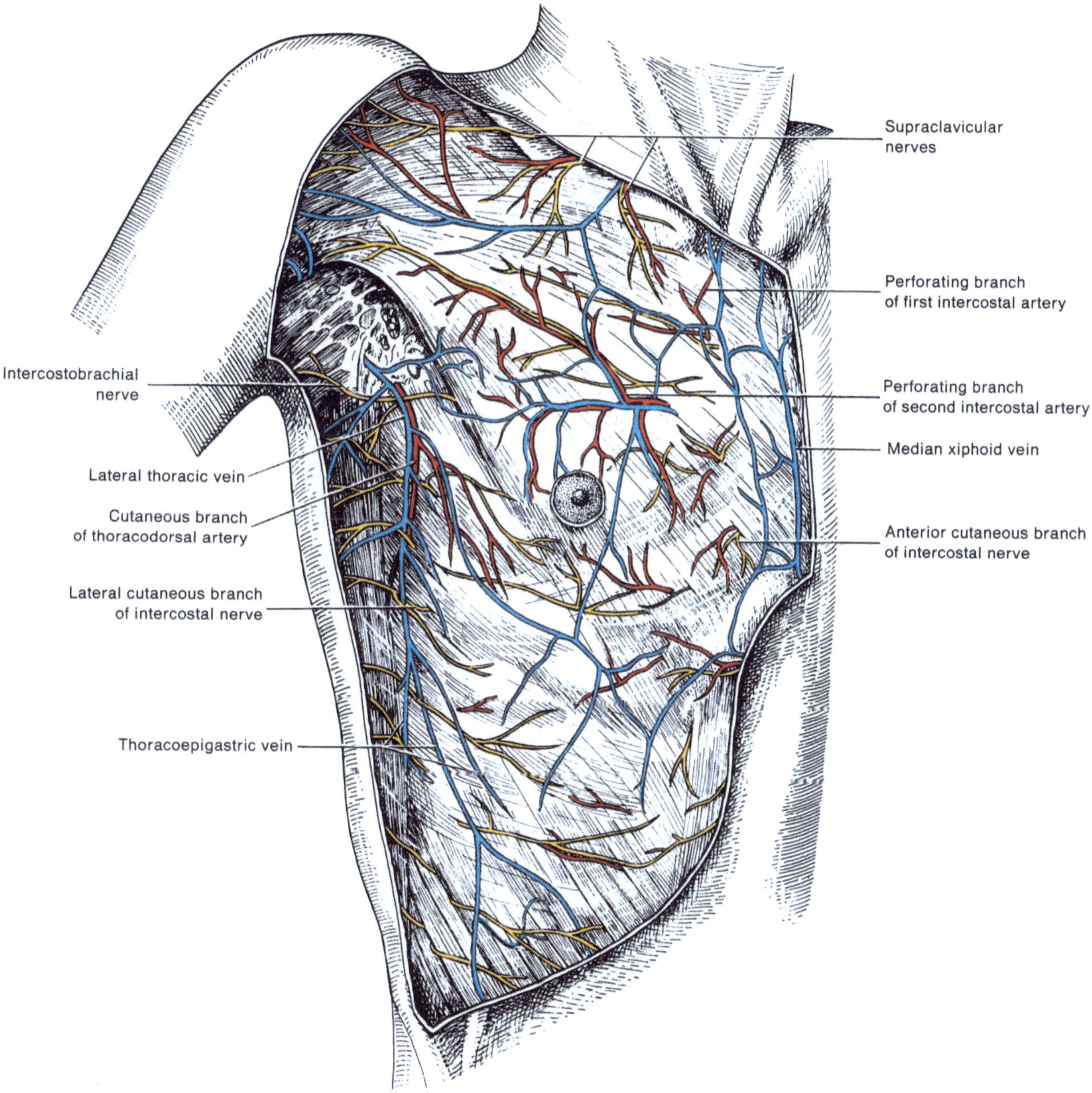
Supraclavicular nerves
Perforating branch of first intercostal artery
Intercostobrachial nerve
Perforating branch of second intercostal artery
Median xiphoid vein
Lateral thoracic vein
Cutaneous branch of thoracodorsal artery
Anterior cutaneous branch of intercostal nerve
Lateral cutaneous branch of intercostal nerve
Thoracoepigastric vein

Plate II: Posterior View of the Neck, Shoulder, and Chest Wall

The trapezius muscle has been severed from its origins a few centimeters lateral to the spinous processes. This muscle is innervated from its inferior surface by the accessory nerve and cervical plexus. Removal of the trapezius exposes arteries that also enter the undersurface of the muscle: the superficial cervical and transverse cervical arteries. A twig from the deep branch of the transverse cervical artery passes through the connective-tissue interval between the rhomboideus major and minor muscles.

The latissimus dorsi muscle has been divided in its upper portion with a curved incision and reflected medially downward. Branches of the intercostal arteries and veins as well as the intercostal nerves of the lower thoracic segments pierce the muscle and supply the overlying skin. The serratus anterior and serratus posterior inferior muscles are visible below the reflected latissimus dorsi muscle.

The suprascapular artery, vein, and nerve disappear beneath the supraspinatus muscle. Their inferior continuation can be seen by stripping the infraspinatus muscle from the scapular spine and from the upper part of the infraspinous fossa. The suprascapular artery anastomoses in the infraspinous fossa with the circumflex scapular artery, which passes through the medial triangular space.

The deltoid muscle has been divided and reflected upward to expose the lateral quadrangular space, which is traversed by the axillary nerve and posterior circumflex humeral artery.

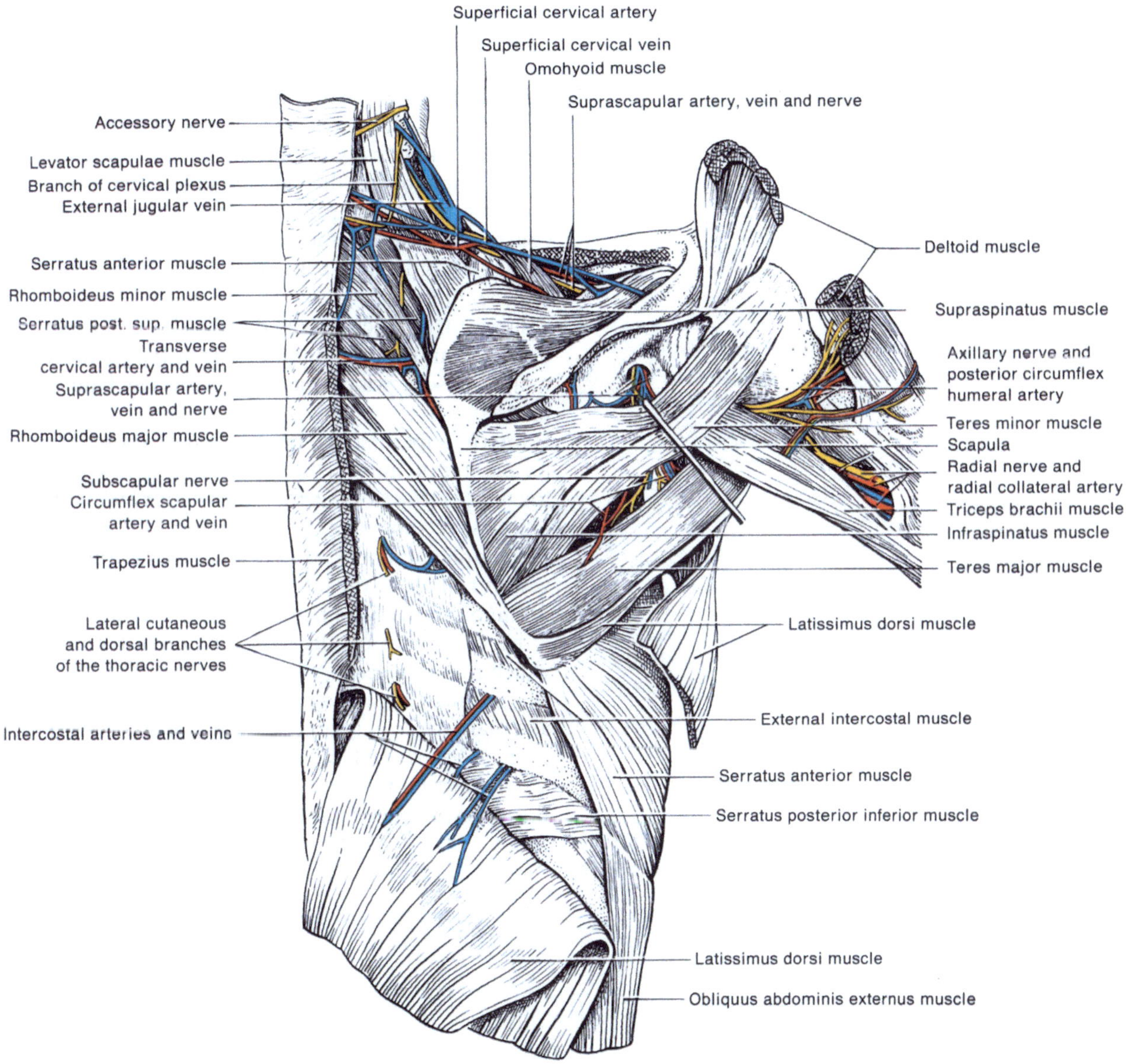

Superficial cervical artery
Superficial cervical vein
Omohyoid muscle
Suprascapular artery, vein and nerve
Accessory nerve
Levator scapulae muscle
Branch of cervical plexus
External jugular vein
Deltoid muscle
Serratus anterior muscle
Rhomboideus minor muscle
Serratus post. sup. muscle
Supraspinatus muscle
Transverse cervical artery and vein
Axillary nerve and posterior circumflex humeral artery
Suprascapular artery, vein and nerve
Rhomboideus major muscle
Teres minor muscle
Scapula
Subscapular nerve
Radial nerve and radial collateral artery
Circumflex scapular artery and vein
Triceps brachii muscle
Infraspinatus muscle
Trapezius muscle
Teres major muscle
Lateral cutaneous and dorsal branches of the thoracic nerves
Latissimus dorsi muscle
External intercostal muscle
Intercostal arteries and veins
Serratus anterior muscle
Serratus posterior inferior muscle
Latissimus dorsi muscle
Obliquus abdominis externus muscle

Plate III: Anterior View of the Inferolateral Cervical Region and Right Chest Wall

The sternocleidomastoid muscle has been divided at its sternal and clavicular origins and removed, exposing the infrahyoid muscle group. The intermediate tendon of the omohyoid muscle crosses the internal jugular vein. The phrenic nerve courses on the scalenus anterior muscle, and behind it the brachial plexus emerges in the posterior scalene interval.

A large curved incision divides the clavicular, sternocostal, and abdominal portions of the pectoralis major muscle, which has been reflected laterally upward.

From the superomedial border of the exposed pectoralis minor muscle, the pectoral nerves pass to the undersurface of the pectoralis major and minor muscles, accompanied by the pectoral branches of the thoracoacromial artery. The lateral thoracic vessels run along the lateral border of the pectoralis minor muscle, and behind them the long thoracic nerve courses on the serratus anterior muscle, which it innervates.

The intercartilaginous muscles, covered in the parasternal intercostal spaces by the external intercostal membrane, and the overlying pectoralis major are pierced by the anterior cutaneous branches of the anterior intercostal nerves.

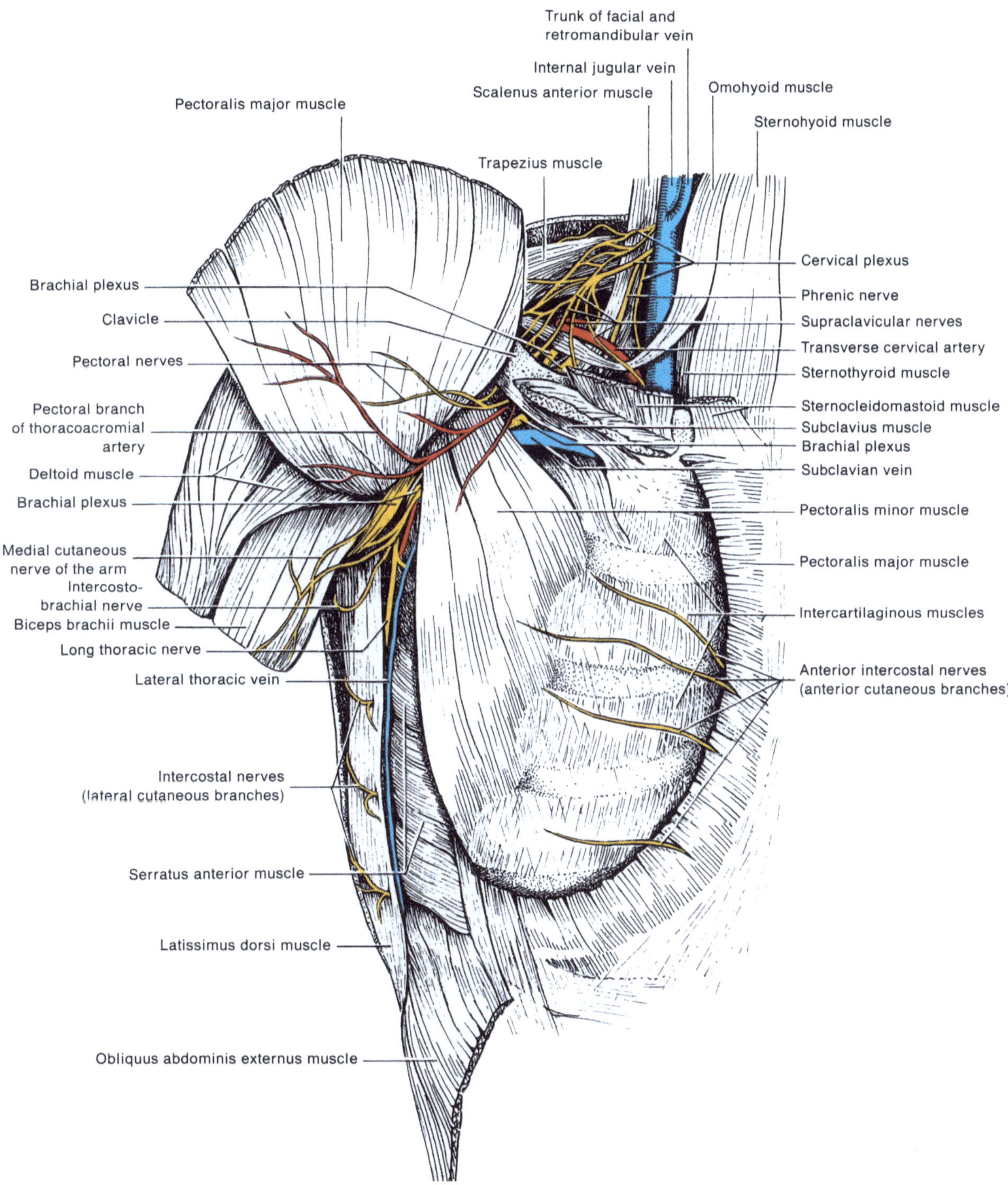

Trunk of facial and retromandibular vein
Internal jugular vein
Scalenus anterior muscle
Omohyoid muscle
Pectoralis major muscle
Sternohyoid muscle
Trapezius muscle
Cervical plexus
Brachial plexus
Phrenic nerve
Clavicle
Supraclavicular nerves
Transverse cervical artery
Pectoral nerves
Sternothyroid muscle
Pectoral branch of thoracoacromial artery
Sternocleidomastoid muscle
Subclavius muscle
Brachial plexus
Deltoid muscle
Subclavian vein
Brachial plexus
Pectoralis minor muscle
Medial cutaneous nerve of the arm
Pectoralis major muscle
Intercosto-brachial nerve
Intercartilaginous muscles
Biceps brachii muscle
Long thoracic nerve
Anterior intercostal nerves (anterior cutaneous branches)
Lateral thoracic vein
Intercostal nerves (lateral cutaneous branches)
Serratus anterior muscle
Latissimus dorsi muscle
Obliquus abdominis externus muscle

Plate IV: Right Axilla and Lateral Chest Wall

The sternal and abdominal portions of the pectoralis major muscle have been divided several centimeters from their origin with a curved incision, and the whole muscle has been reflected superiorly. The underlying pectoralis minor muscle has been detached from its three-part origin and reflected superomedially. The pectoral branches of the thoracoacromial vessels and the pectoral nerves that supply the pectoralis major and minor muscles are visible on the undersurface of the muscles.

In most cases the intercostobrachial nerve arises from the second thoracic segment (less frequently from Th3) and pierces the upper digitations of the serratus anterior muscle at the lateral border of the pectoralis minor muscle. Looping through the axilla, the nerve anastomoses with the medial cutaneous nerve of the arm from the medial cord of the brachial plexus.

The latissimus dorsi muscle has been divided and its lower portion reflected laterally to expose the thoracodorsal nerve and thoracodorsal vessels on its inferior surface.

The broken line indicates the path of the incision through the deeper tissue layers in the anterior and posterior thoracotomy. The incision passes through the superior or transverse part of the serratus anterior muscle twice and cuts the diverging and converging fibers almost at right angles to their course. It also divides the lateral thoracic artery and the lateral thoracic vein, which anastomoses inferiorly with the thoracoepigastric vein. Both vessels course on the serratus anterior muscle, which they supply. The incision spares the main trunk of the long thoracic nerve. From the depths of the axilla this nerve emerges from behind the brachial plexus and courses downward on the muscle, deep to the accompanying vessels. The nerve, unlike the vessels, is covered by the muscular fascia.

Plate IV

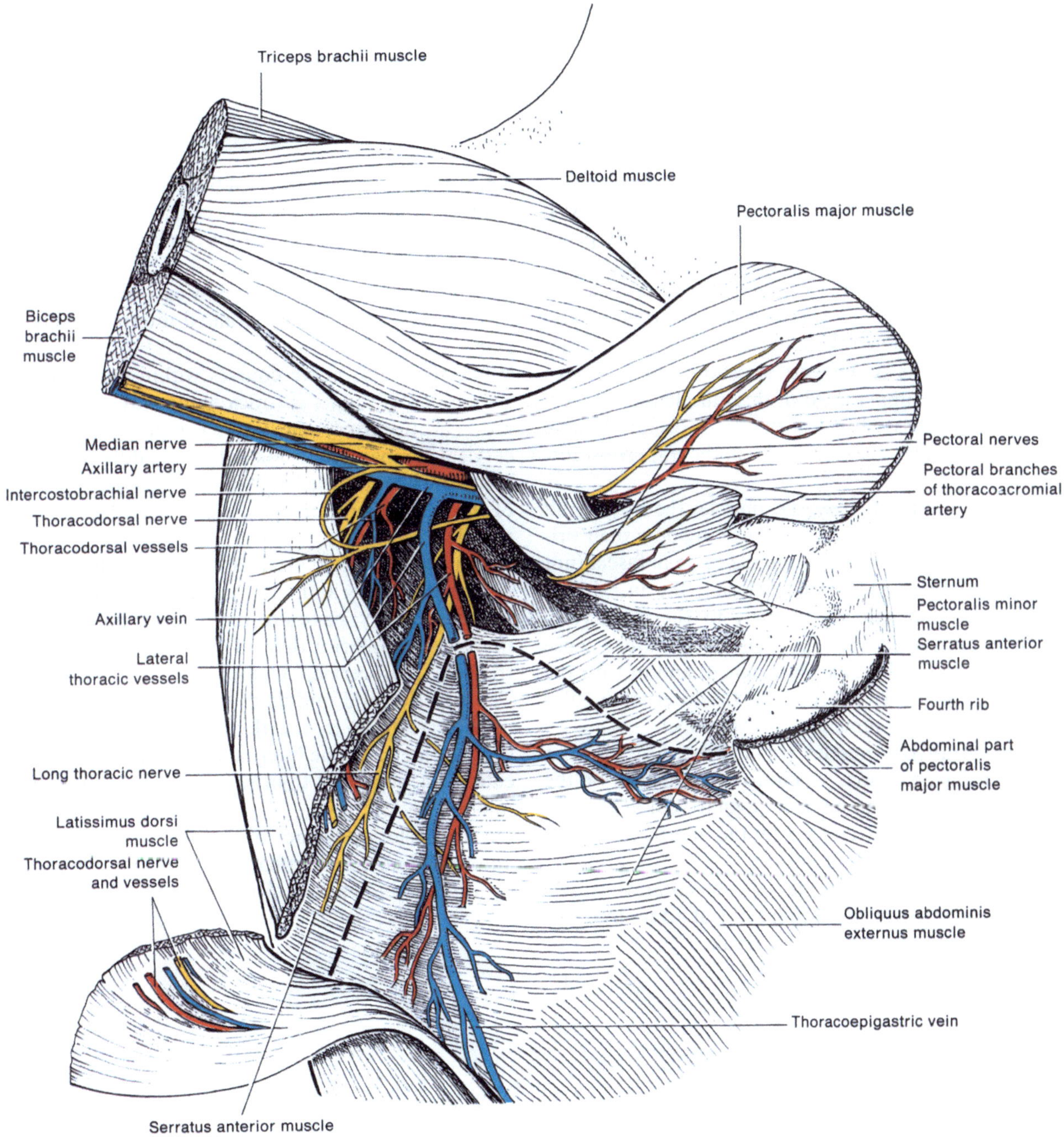

Triceps brachii muscle
Deltoid muscle
Pectoralis major muscle
Biceps brachii muscle
Median nerve
Axillary artery
Intercostobrachial nerve
Thoracodorsal nerve
Thoracodorsal vessels
Axillary vein
Lateral thoracic vessels
Long thoracic nerve
Latissimus dorsi muscle
Thoracodorsal nerve and vessels
Pectoral nerves
Pectoral branches of thoracoacromial artery
Sternum
Pectoralis minor muscle
Serratus anterior muscle
Fourth rib
Abdominal part of pectoralis major muscle
Obliquus abdominis externus muscle
Thoracoepigastric vein
Serratus anterior muscle

Plate V: Deep Lateral Cervical Region

The plastysma has been removed, and the underlying cutaneous branches of the cervical plexus, which have an almost common site of emergence at the level of the third cervical vertebra (Erb's point) just above the center of the sternocleidomastoid muscle, are reflected and individually shown. The sternocleidomastoid muscle has been divided at its origin and insertion and removed. Deep to the upper third of this muscle the accessory nerve crosses beneath the lesser occipital nerve at right angles and terminates in the trapezius muscle.

Except for the thyrohyoid muscle, the infrahyoid muscles have been removed, leaving only their origins and insertions. The middle cervical fascia (not shown) forms a sheath enclosing the infrahyoid muscles and extends laterally to the omohyoid. The omohyoid muscles make this fascia tense when the head is sharply inclined, and in turn the fascia, which is adherent to the internal jugular vein, keeps the lumen of this vein open.

The infrahyoid muscles are innervated by the ansa cervicalis profunda, which usually is placed on the lateral wall of the internal jugular vein at the site where the vein is crossed by the intermediate tendon of the omohyoid muscle.

The phrenic nerve on the scalenus anterior muscle accompanies the ascending cervical artery as it origins from the thyrocervical trunk.

The posterior scalene interval between the scalenus anterior and medius muscles is traversed by the brachial plexus and, at a more inferior level, by the subclavian artery.

The bifurcation of the common carotid artery is obscured by the laterally situated internal jugular vein.

While the vagus nerve courses within the fibrous sheath of the vagina carotica along with the common carotid artery and internal jugular vein, the cervical sympathetic trunk with its middle cervical ganglion is embedded in the deep cervical fascia of the prevertebral muscles, where it is almost immobile.

The superior thyroid artery springs from the external carotid artery and, after giving off the superior laryngeal artery, passes to the superior pole of the thyroid. The inferior thyroid artery takes its origin from the thyrocervical trunk.

The superior and middle thyroid veins are shown in their relation to the thyroid gland, and their sites of entry into the internal jugular vein are indicated. The unpaired thyroid plexus opens into the inferior thyroid vein.

On the posterior surface of the pharynx, retracted anteromedially, is the pharyngeal plexus, supplied by afferent and efferent fibers from the glossopharyngeal nerve, vagus nerve, and sympathetic trunk.

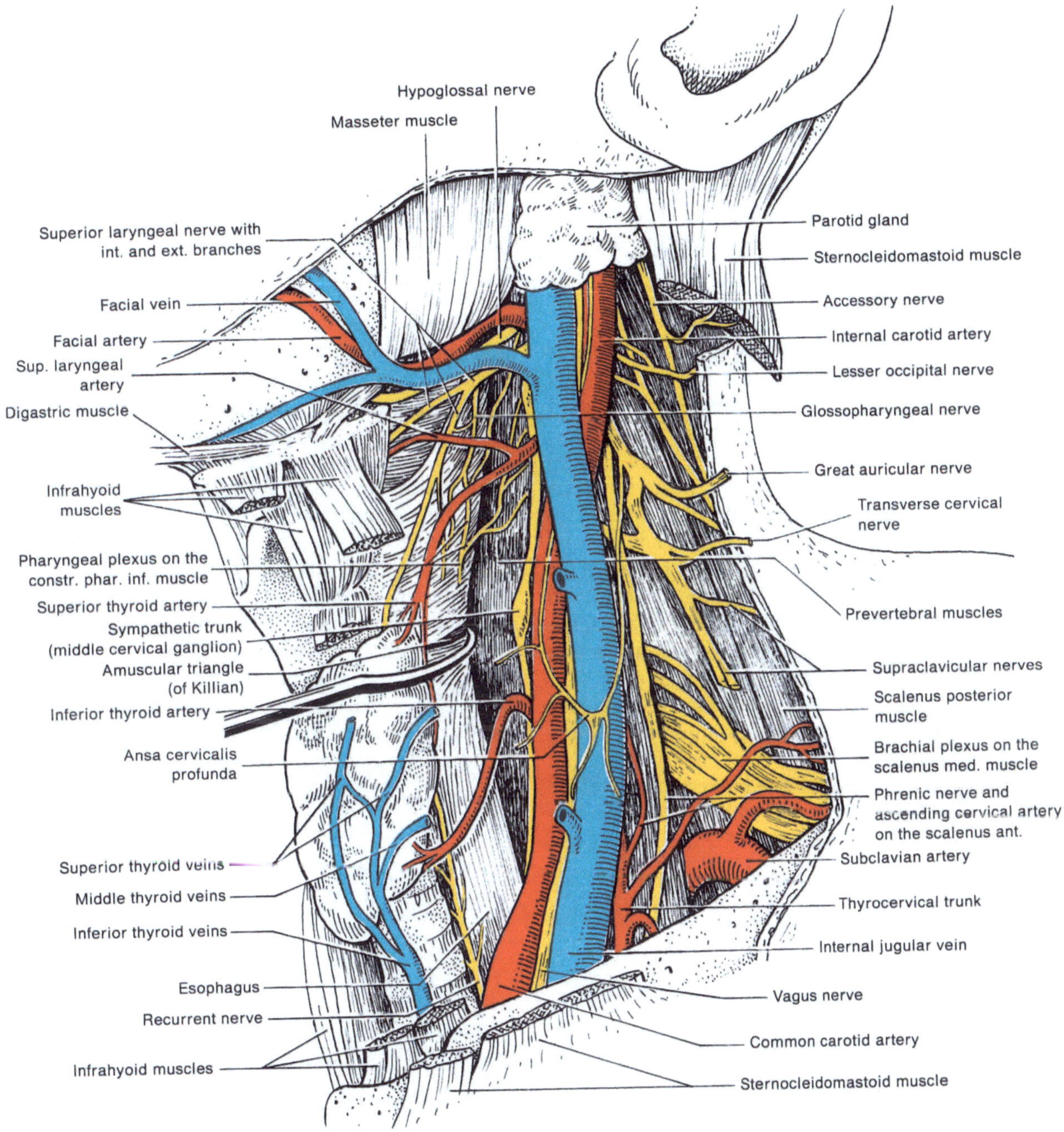
Hypoglossal nerve
Masseter muscle
Superior laryngeal nerve with int. and ext. branches
Facial vein
Facial artery
Sup. laryngeal artery
Digastric muscle
Infrahyoid muscles
Pharyngeal plexus on the constr. phar. inf. muscle
Superior thyroid artery
Sympathetic trunk (middle cervical ganglion)
Amuscular triangle (of Killian)
Inferior thyroid artery
Ansa cervicalis profunda
Superior thyroid veins
Middle thyroid veins
Inferior thyroid veins
Esophagus
Recurrent nerve
Infrahyoid muscles
Parotid gland
Sternocleidomastoid muscle
Accessory nerve
Internal carotid artery
Lesser occipital nerve
Glossopharyngeal nerve
Great auricular nerve
Transverse cervical nerve
Prevertebral muscles
Supraclavicular nerves
Scalenus posterior muscle
Brachial plexus on the scalenus med. muscle
Phrenic nerve and ascending cervical artery on the scalenus ant.
Subclavian artery
Thyrocervical trunk
Internal jugular vein
Vagus nerve
Common carotid artery
Sternocleidomastoid muscle

Plate VI. View into the Right Thoracic Cavity from Below

The transverse section through this part of the thorax is placed so that it cuts the second rib at its sternal attachment anteriorly and the body of the T 5 vertebra posteriorly.

The parietal pleura and endothoracic fascia have been removed. The internal intercostal muscles extend anteriorly to the sternum (intercartilaginous muscles) and terminate posteriorly at the costal angle. The external intercostal muscles are exposed by removal of the internal intercostal membrane.

The arteries of the intercostal space form anastomoses between the thoracic aorta (posterior intercostal artery) and the internal thoracic artery (anterior intercostal branch). The first and second posterior intercostal arteries usually arise from the supreme intercostal artery (from the costocervical trunk). The remaining right intercostal arteries spring from the posterior wall of the aorta and pass behind the esophagus and azygos vein. The posterior intercostal veins open into the right side of the azygos vein. The posterior intercostal artery and vein undercross the sympathetic trunk in front of the heads of the ribs. The intercostal nerve and posterior intercostal vessels disappear at the costal angle between the internal and external intercostal muscles.

Behind the insertion of the scalenus anterior muscle on the first rib, the subclavian artery and brachial plexus cross the first rib through the "scalene interval," while the subclavian vein enters the thorax in front of the scalenus anterior muscle, passing through the "anterior scalene interval." There it is joined by the vertebral vein, which enters it from behind and above.

The vagus nerve crosses the subclavian artery (origin of the recurrent nerve). The sympathetic trunk is visible behind the artery and forms the stellate ganglion on the head of the first rib.

The internal thoracic vessels pass below the first rib to the parasternal chest wall and are directly apposed in the upper intercostal spaces to the endothoracic fascia and parietal pleura.

The reflection at the junction of the epicardium and pericardium is clearly visible behind the retrosternal fat pad on the ascending aorta.

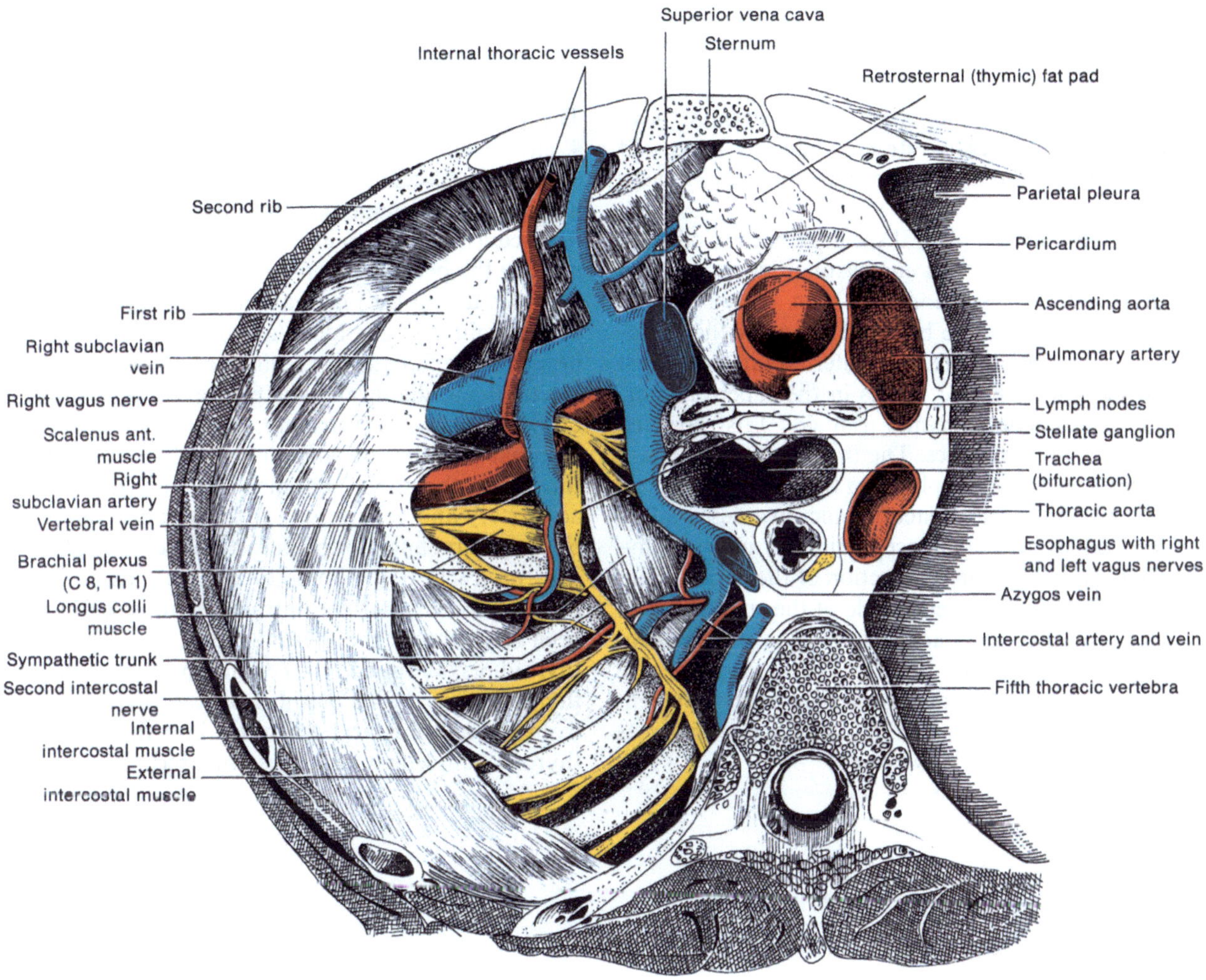
Superior vena cava
Sternum
Internal thoracic vessels
Retrosternal (thymic) fat pad
Second rib
Parietal pleura
Pericardium
First rib
Ascending aorta
Right subclavian vein
Pulmonary artery
Right vagus nerve
Lymph nodes
Stellate ganglion
Scalenus ant. muscle
Trachea (bifurcation)
Right subclavian artery
Thoracic aorta
Vertebral vein
Esophagus with right and left vagus nerves
Brachial plexus (C 8, Th 1)
Azygos vein
Longus colli muscle
Intercostal artery and vein
Sympathetic trunk
Fifth thoracic vertebra
Second intercostal nerve
Internal intercostal muscle
External intercostal muscle

Plate VII. Lower Cervical Organs and View into the Superior and Anterior Mediastinum (Sternum Split and Retracted)

The manubrium and body of the sternum have been split and widely retracted laterally to so that the superior and anterior mediastinum can be visualized.

The right and left pleural sac have been windowed in their anterior and mediastinal portions, and slight lateral retraction has been placed on the lungs to disclose the bilateral extent of the costomediastinal recess. The retrosternal fat pad, a rest of the paired thymic bodies in the superior interpleural triangle ("thymic triangle"), is retracted laterally on both sides. The thymus or its remnant derives its blood supply from the internal thoracic artery and pericardiacophrenic arteries and is drained by the brachiocephalic and inferior thyroid veins. The upper reflection of the pericardium is applied to the anterior side of the superior vena cava and ascending aorta. Lateral to the ligamentum arteriosum (of Botalli), the recurrent nerve winds around the aortic arch. The right recurrent nerve loops below the right subclavian artery as it leaves the vagus nerve trunk.

The phrenic nerve, which arises mainly from C 4, enters the chest cavity through the thoracic aperture and descends in front of the pulmonary hilum, passing through the connective tissue between the mediastinal pleura and pericardium. Accompanied by the pericardiacophrenic vessels, this nerve provides the motor innervation for the diaphragm on the right and left sides. Additionally, its pleural branches provide sensory innervation to the mediastinal and diaphragmatic pleura, its pericardial branches to the pericardium, and its phrenicoabdominal branches to portions of the parietal peritoneum in the upper abdomen. The internal thoracic artery and vein pass over the anterior surface of the pleural apex to the parasternal chest wall.

The pretracheal (or middle) cervical fascia has been removed, and the infrahyoid muscles have been divided over the thyroid gland. The unpaired thyroid plexus applied to the inferior poles of both thyroid lobes drains blood from the thyroid and from the inferior laryngeal veins into the inferior thyroid vein, which usually is unpaired.

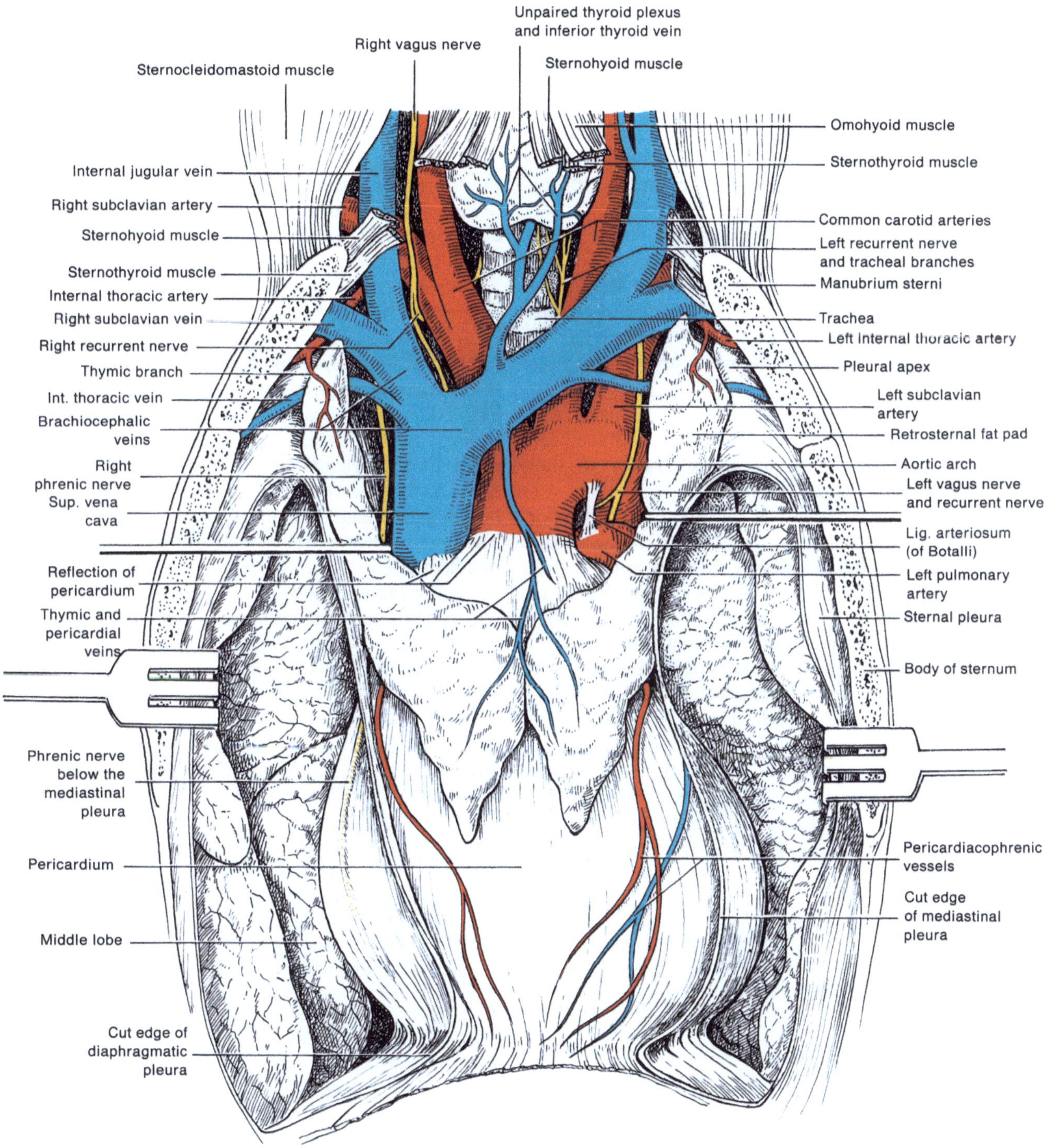
Unpaired thyroid plexus and inferior thyroid vein
Right vagus nerve
Sternohyoid muscle
Sternocleidomastoid muscle
Omohyoid muscle
Internal jugular vein
Sternothyroid muscle
Right subclavian artery
Common carotid arteries
Sternohyoid muscle
Left recurrent nerve and tracheal branches
Sternothyroid muscle
Manubrium sterni
Internal thoracic artery
Right subclavian vein
Trachea
Left internal thoracic artery
Right recurrent nerve
Thymic branch
Pleural apex
Int. thoracic vein
Left subclavian artery
Brachiocephalic veins
Retrosternal fat pad
Right phrenic nerve
Aortic arch
Left vagus nerve and recurrent nerve
Sup. vena cava
Lig. arteriosum (of Botalli)
Reflection of pericardium
Left pulmonary artery
Thymic and pericardial veins
Sternal pleura
Body of sternum
Phrenic nerve below the mediastinal pleura
Pericardiacophrenic vessels
Pericardium
Cut edge of mediastinal pleura
Middle lobe
Cut edge of diaphragmatic pleura

Plate VIII. Brachial Plexus and Vessels of the Neck and Axilla; Neurovascular Bundle in the Upper Arm

The clavicle and pectoralis minor muscle have been partially resected. With the right shoulder pulled slightly laterally, the pectoralis major muscle has been divided at its origins on the thorax and reflected laterally and superiorly. The pectoral nerves that innervate the muscle are visible on its undersurface; like the pectoral branches for the pectoralis minor muscle, these nerves arise from the supraclavicular portion of the brachial plexus. The pectoral branches of the thoracoacromial artery supply the pectoralis major and minor muscles.

The pretracheal layer of the cervical fascia and its junction with the clavipectoral fascia have been removed along with the axillary fascia so that deeper layers can be visualized.

A "scalenus interval" is formed by the anterior scalenus muscle, on which the phrenic nerve descends, and by the medial scalenus muscle. The brachial plexus courses through the upper part of this interval. The subclavian artery emerges through the lower part of the "scalenus interval" passing directly over the first rib. Arising from the C 5 segment, the long thoracic nerve passes through the scalenus medius and descends on the serratus anterior, covered by its fascia. There it is accompanied by the lateral thoracic artery, which arises from the axillary artery in its midaxillary portion (behind the pectoralis minor muscle). Farther distally the thoracodorsal artery arises from the axillary artery via the subscapular artery. The thoracodorsal artery descends laterally with the thoracodorsal nerve (from the posterior cord of the plexus), and they both disappear below the anterior border of the latissimus dorsi muscle, which both supply.

The cephalic vein courses between the clavicular part of the pectoralis major muscle and the clavicular part of the deltoid muscle in Mohrenheim's fossa. It passes deeply and pierces the clavipectoral fascia to unite with the subclavian vein.

The axillary vein has been resected to expose the axillary artery, around which are grouped the cords of the brachial plexus (the key landmark is the median nerve, which arises directly from the lateral and medial cords).

The axillary nerve arises from the posterior cord behind the subclavian artery and passes through the quadrangular space in company with the posterior circumflex humeral artery. The musculocutaneous nerve leaves the lateral cord and passes to the coracobrachialis muscle, which it pierces and innervates. The lateral cutaneous branch of the second intercostal nerve passes as the intercostobrachial nerve to the upper arm and anastomoses with the medial cutaneous nerve of the arm from the medial cord of the brachial plexus.

Plate VIII

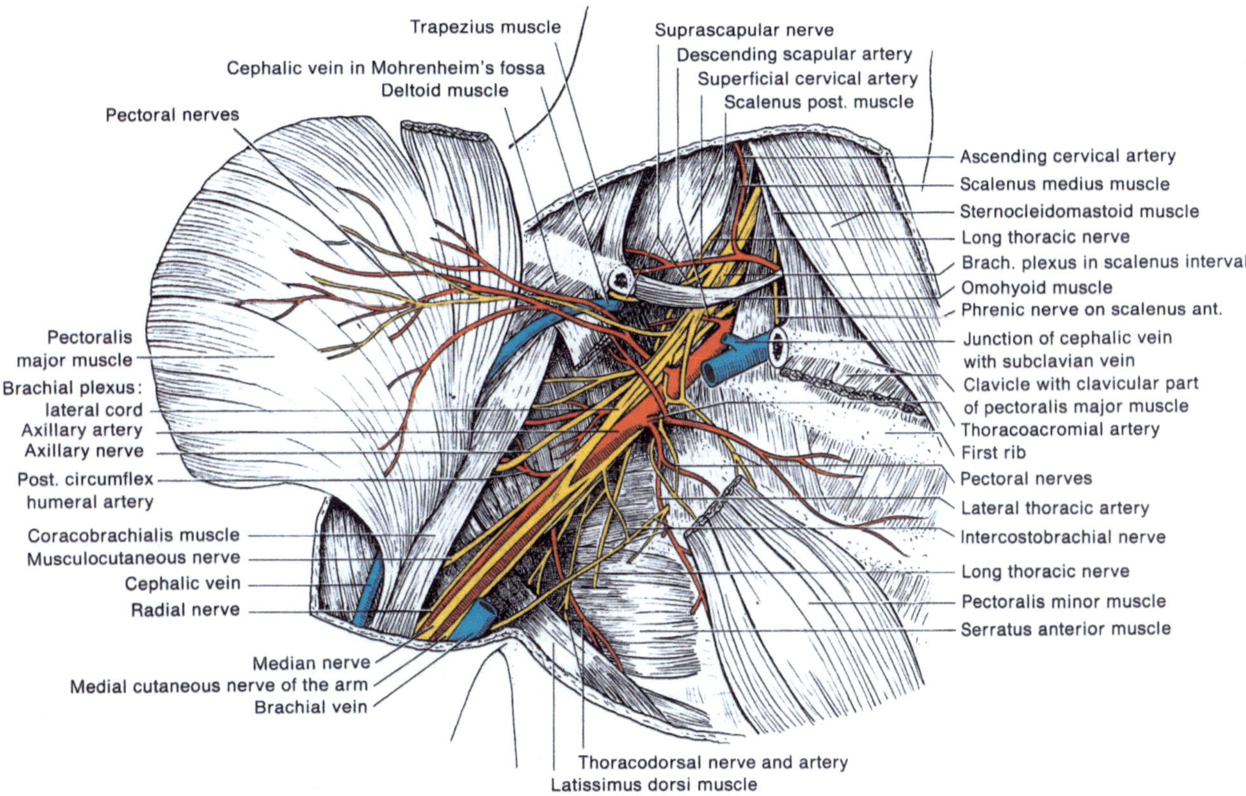
Trapezius muscle
Cephalic vein in Mohrenheim's fossa
Deltoid muscle
Pectoral nerves
Suprascapular nerve
Descending scapular artery
Superficial cervical artery
Scalenus post. muscle
Ascending cervical artery
Scalenus medius muscle
Sternocleidomastoid muscle
Long thoracic nerve
Brach. plexus in scalenus interval
Omohyoid muscle
Phrenic nerve on scalenus ant.
Junction of cephalic vein with subclavian vein
Clavicle with clavicular part of pectoralis major muscle
Thoracoacromial artery
First rib
Pectoral nerves
Lateral thoracic artery
Intercostobrachial nerve
Long thoracic nerve
Pectoralis minor muscle
Serratus anterior muscle
Pectoralis major muscle
Brachial plexus: lateral cord
Axillary artery
Axillary nerve
Post. circumflex humeral artery
Coracobrachialis muscle
Musculocutaneous nerve
Cephalic vein
Radial nerve
Median nerve
Medial cutaneous nerve of the arm
Brachial vein
Thoracodorsal nerve and artery
Latissimus dorsi muscle

Plate IX. Right Pulmonary Hilum and Organs of the Superior and Anterior Mediastinum

The right chest wall has been widely resected, and the upper and middle lobes of the right lung are retracted laterally to expose the right hilum. The mediastinal pleura and pulmonary pleura are not shown.

The superior vena cava is located ventrally to the hilar structures of the right side. Just before its entry into the pericardium, the superior vena cava is joined by the azygos vein, which arches over the right main bronchus. This bronchus is the most posterior and superior of the hilar structures; caudal to it are the pulmonary artery and vein. The right upper lobe bronchus is eparterial to the pulmonary artery, which gives off a large branch to the upper lobe (the "anterior trunk") while still outside the hilum.

The right superior pulmonary vein is the most anterior of the hilar structures and largely obscures the right inferior pulmonary vein. The right vagus nerve descends on the lateral tracheal wall, passing behind the hilum to the esophagus in the posterior mediastinum.

The right phrenic nerve, in company with the pericardiacophrenic vessels, courses somewhat more posteriorly than on the left side. It descends along the superior vena cava and then passes between the mediastinal pleura and pericardium, providing both with sensory fibers, before proceeding to the diaphragm. The internal thoracic vessels pass over the retrosternal fat pad to the anterior chest wall, upon which they descend in a parasternal position.

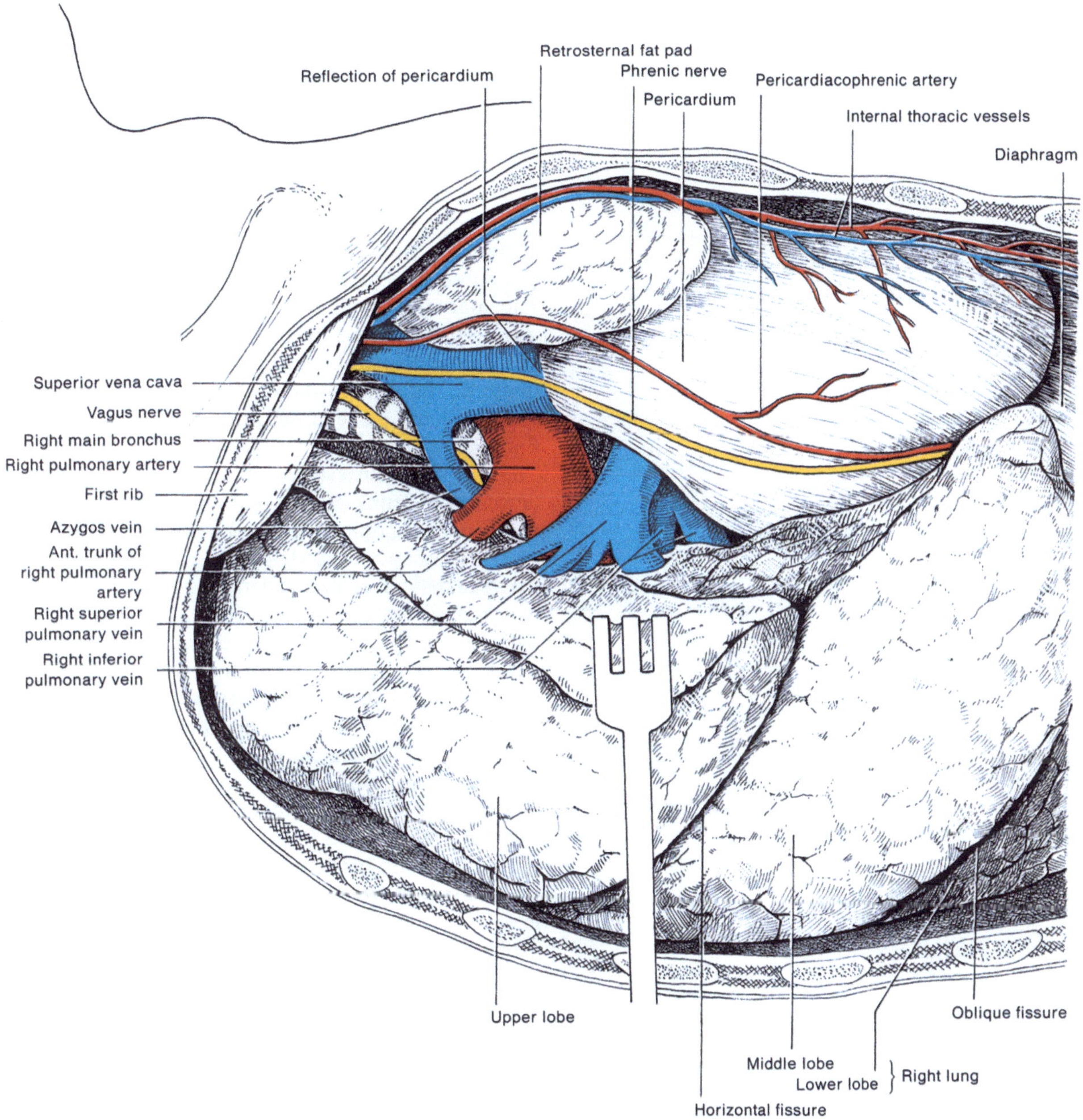

Retrosternal fat pad
Reflection of pericardium
Phrenic nerve
Pericardium
Pericardiacophrenic artery
Internal thoracic vessels
Diaphragm
Superior vena cava
Vagus nerve
Right main bronchus
Right pulmonary artery
First rib
Azygos vein
Ant. trunk of right pulmonary artery
Right superior pulmonary vein
Right inferior pulmonary vein
Upper lobe
Oblique fissure
Middle lobe
Lower lobe
Right lung
Horizontal fissure

Plate X. Left Pulmonary Hilum and Organs of the Superior and Anterior Mediastinum

The left chest wall has been widely resected and the upper lobe of the left lung retracted postero-laterally to expose the left hilum. The mediastinal and pulmonary pleurae are not shown.

The internal thoracic artery arises from the subclavian and, accompanied by the internal thoracic vein, courses laterally and anteriorly over the retrosternal fat pad. Both vessels reach the anterior chest wall and descend on it in a parasternal position.

The left phrenic nerve crosses the aortic arch and descends in front of the pulmonary hilum with the pericardiacophrenic vessels, somewhat more anteriorly than on the right side, passing between the mediastinal pleura and pericardium, both of which receive sensory fibers from the nerve. The trunk of the phrenic nerve provides motor innervation to the diaphragm, while its phrenicoabdominal branches pierce the diaphragm and send sensory fibers to portions of the parietal peritoneum in the left upper abdomen.

The cardiac plexus, formed from branches of the vagus nerve and sympathetic trunk, presents on the anterior side of the aortic arch, which "rides" on the left main bronchus. Lateral to the ligamentum arteriosum (of Botalli) the left recurrent nerve leaves the vagus trunk and winds posteriorly around the aortic arch. The vagus nerve descends behind the left hilum into the posterior mediastinum.

The left superior pulmonary vein is the most anterior of the left hilar structures. The left pulmonary artery presents superior to the vein, coursing between it and the arch of the aorta. The left inferior pulmonary vein is largely obscured by the left superior pulmonary vein, and a portion of it is just visible in the lower hilar region. The left main bronchus is deep to these structures and, like the right bronchus, cannot be seen from the anterior aspect. The accessory hemiazygos vein, representing a superior continuation of the hemiazygos, terminates at the left brachiocephalic vein.

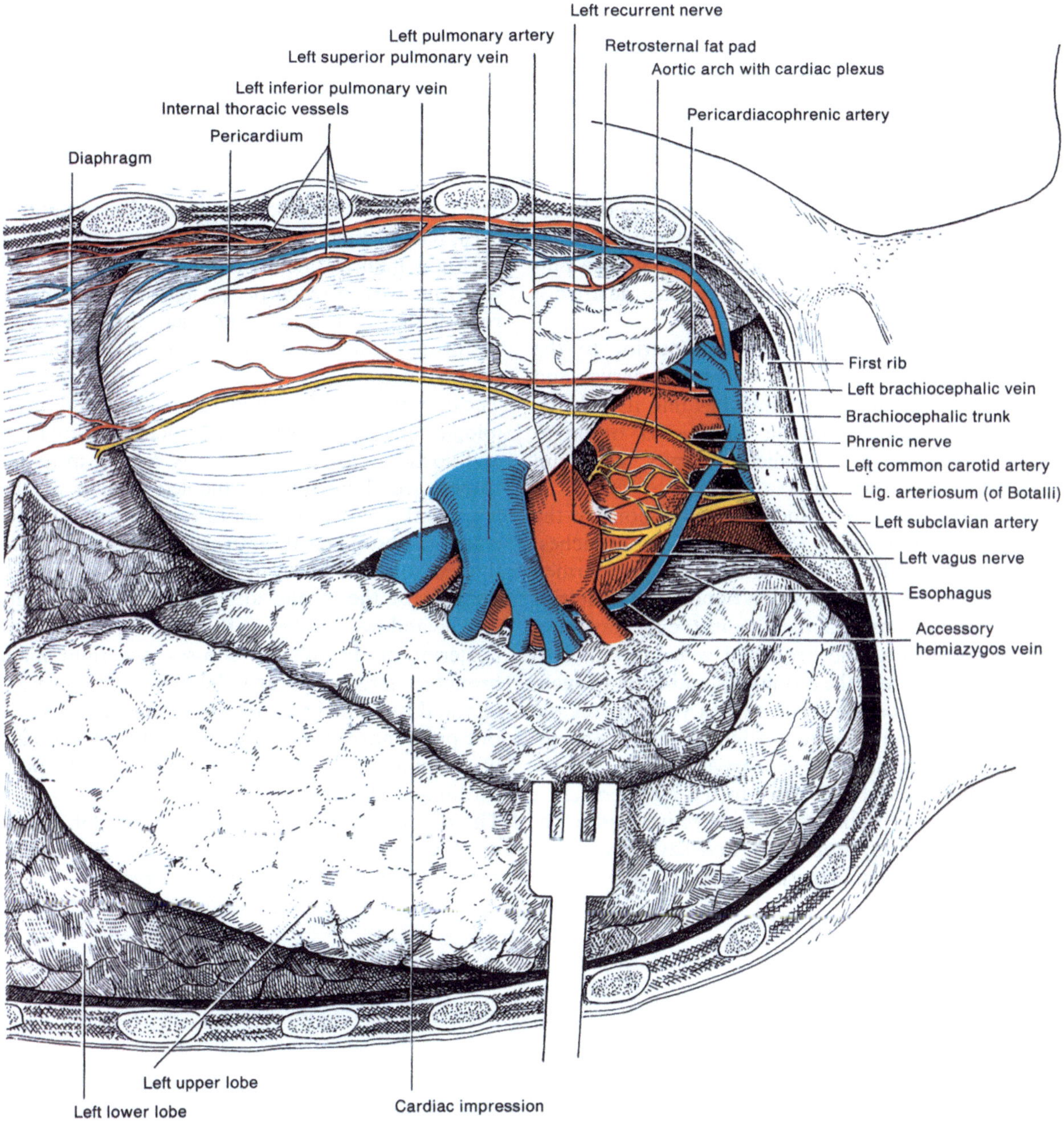

Left recurrent nerve
Left pulmonary artery
Retrosternal fat pad
Left superior pulmonary vein
Aortic arch with cardiac plexus
Left inferior pulmonary vein
Internal thoracic vessels
Pericardiacophrenic artery
Pericardium
Diaphragm
First rib
Left brachiocephalic vein
Brachiocephalic trunk
Phrenic nerve
Left common carotid artery
Lig. arteriosum (of Botalli)
Left subclavian artery
Left vagus nerve
Esophagus
Accessory hemiazygos vein
Left upper lobe
Left lower lobe
Cardiac impression

Plate XI. Right Pulmonary Hilum and Organs of the Posterior Mediastinum

The right lateral chest wall has been widely resected, and the middle and lower lobes of the right lung are retracted upward and forward. The pulmonary, mediastinal, and vertebral pleurae are not pictured.

The sympathetic trunk courses anterior to the heads of the ribs and the intercostal nerves and vessels. Communicating branches link it with the intercostal nerves, and the trunk gives origin to the greater and lesser splanchnic nerves, which run forward and downward.

The azygos vein is joined in this region by the segmental intercostal veins (posterior branches) and by the right superior intercostal vein (formed from the union of the second and third posterior intercostal veins). Small veins in the mediastinum (the esophageal and bronchial veins, not shown) drain blood from the esophagus and main bronchi into the azygos vein. The azygos vein crosses the right main bronchus from behind and opens posteriorly into the superior vena cava.

The thoracic duct is visible in the right posterior mediastinum in the loose connective tissue between the aorta, esophagus, and azygos vein before ascending and crossing to the left side.

The right vagus nerve descends parallel to the trachea, passing medial to the azygos vein and behind the right main bronchus (which here is retracted well forward) to reach the posterior aspect of the root of the right lung. From there it descends on the posterior aspect of the esophagus and pierces the diaphragm.

The esophagus, having undergone its second physiologic constriction behind the tracheal bifurcation and aortic arch, becomes closely related in its retropericardial portion to the left atrium of the heart and then, tending more toward the left side, enters the esophageal hiatus in the diaphragm (at the level of the 10th–11th thoracic vertebra).

Because of the strong anterior retraction of the middle and lower lobes of the right lung, the most posterior of the hilar structures, the right main bronchus, largely obscures the right pulmonary artery and its branches. The right inferior and superior pulmonary veins are visible in the inferior part of the hilum, and their site of entry into the pericardium is apparent.

The phrenic nerve takes a more posterior course on the right side and reaches the diaphragm anterolateral to the inferior vena cava.

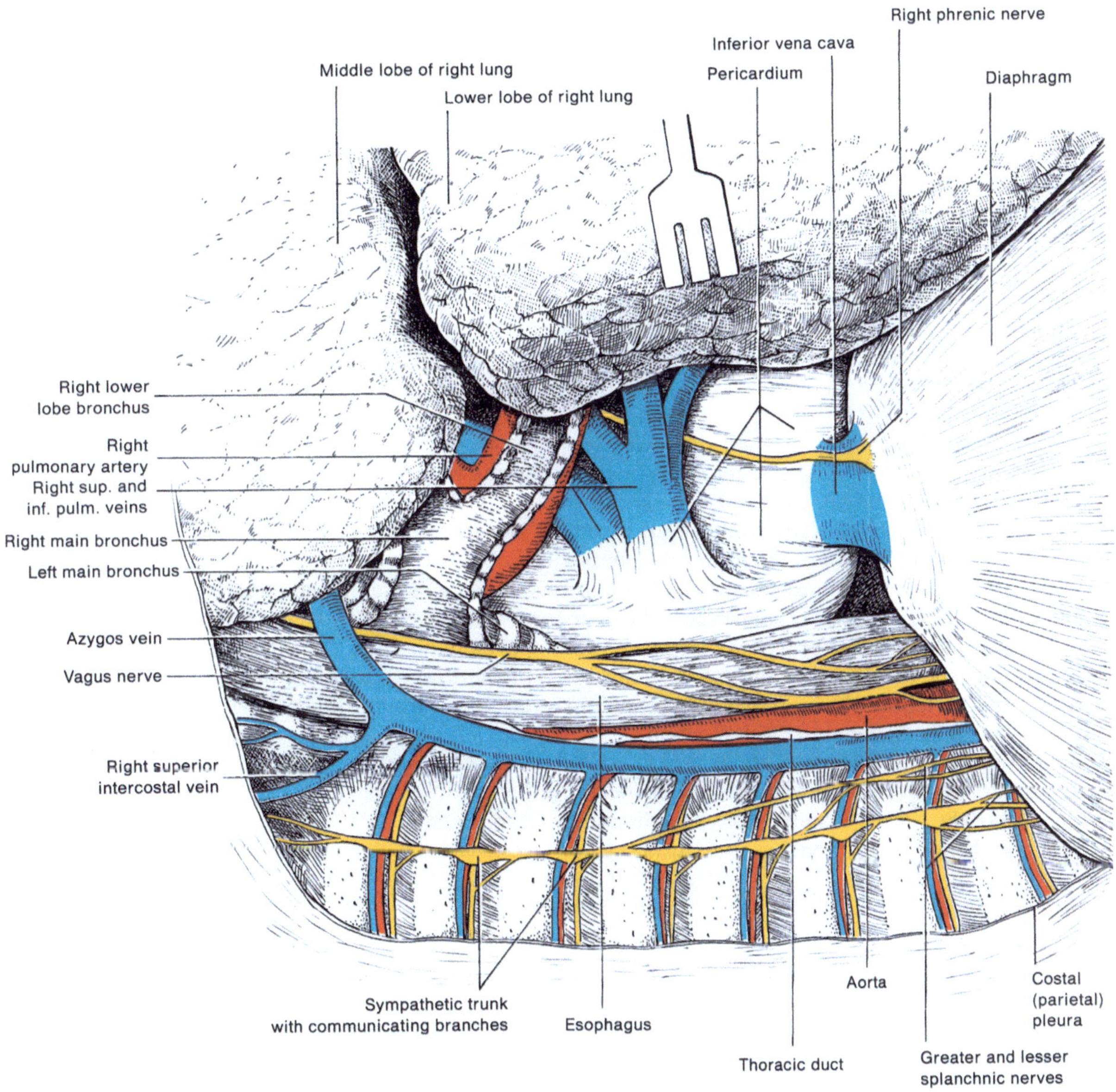
Right phrenic nerve
Inferior vena cava
Middle lobe of right lung
Pericardium
Diaphragm
Lower lobe of right lung
Right lower lobe bronchus
Right pulmonary artery
Right sup. and inf. pulm. veins
Right main bronchus
Left main bronchus
Azygos vein
Vagus nerve
Right superior intercostal vein
Sympathetic trunk with communicating branches
Esophagus
Aorta
Costal (parietal) pleura
Thoracic duct
Greater and lesser splanchnic nerves

Plate XII: Left Pulmonary Hilum and Organs of the Posterior Mediastinum

The left lateral chest wall has been widely resected. The upper and lower lobes of the left lung are retracted anteriorly and superiorly. The pulmonary, mediastinal, and vertebral pleurae are not shown.

The sympathetic trunk, covered by parietal pleura, courses anterior to the heads of the ribs and the intercostal nerves and vessels and is linked by communicating branches with the intercostal nerves. The greater and lesser splanchnic nerves arise from the 6th–9th and 10th–11th thoracic ganglia.

The hemiazygos vein is joined by the lower segmental intercostal veins (posterior branches). It has a superior continuation in the accessory hemiazygos vein which, after receiving the left superior intercostal vein (union of the posterior superior intercostal veins), usually establishes a communication with the left brachiocephalic vein. The intercostal arteries (posterior branches) arise as paired branches of the thoracic aorta, which descends between the vertebral pleura (not shown) and the esophagus. The aortic arch "rides" upon the left main bronchus. There the left recurrent nerve leaves the vagus trunk and loops upward behind the aorta. The left vegus nerve, often dividing into branches between the bronchus and aorta, passes behind the root of the left lung and descends on the lateral and especially the anterior side of the esophagus, accompanying it as it pierces the diaphragm.

The esophagus has its second physiologic constriction between the tracheal bifurcation and aortic arch. It passes behind the left atrium of the heart (retropericardiac part), usually slightly to the right of the midline, then turns back toward the left side to enter the esophageal hiatus (its third physiologic constriction). The posterior inferior "weak spot" of the mediastinum occurs between the posterior wall of the esophagus, the anterior wall of the aorta, and the diaphragm.

The left pulmonary artery and its branches are visible between the aortic arch and the left main bronchus, which is retracted far anteriorly. Inferior to the bronchus the left inferior pulmonary vein partially obscures the left superior pulmonary vein in the lower part of the hilum. The site of entry of both veins into the pericardium is visible.

The left phrenic nerve, which courses more anteriorly than on the right side, passes between the pericardium and mediastinal pleura to reach the diaphragm.

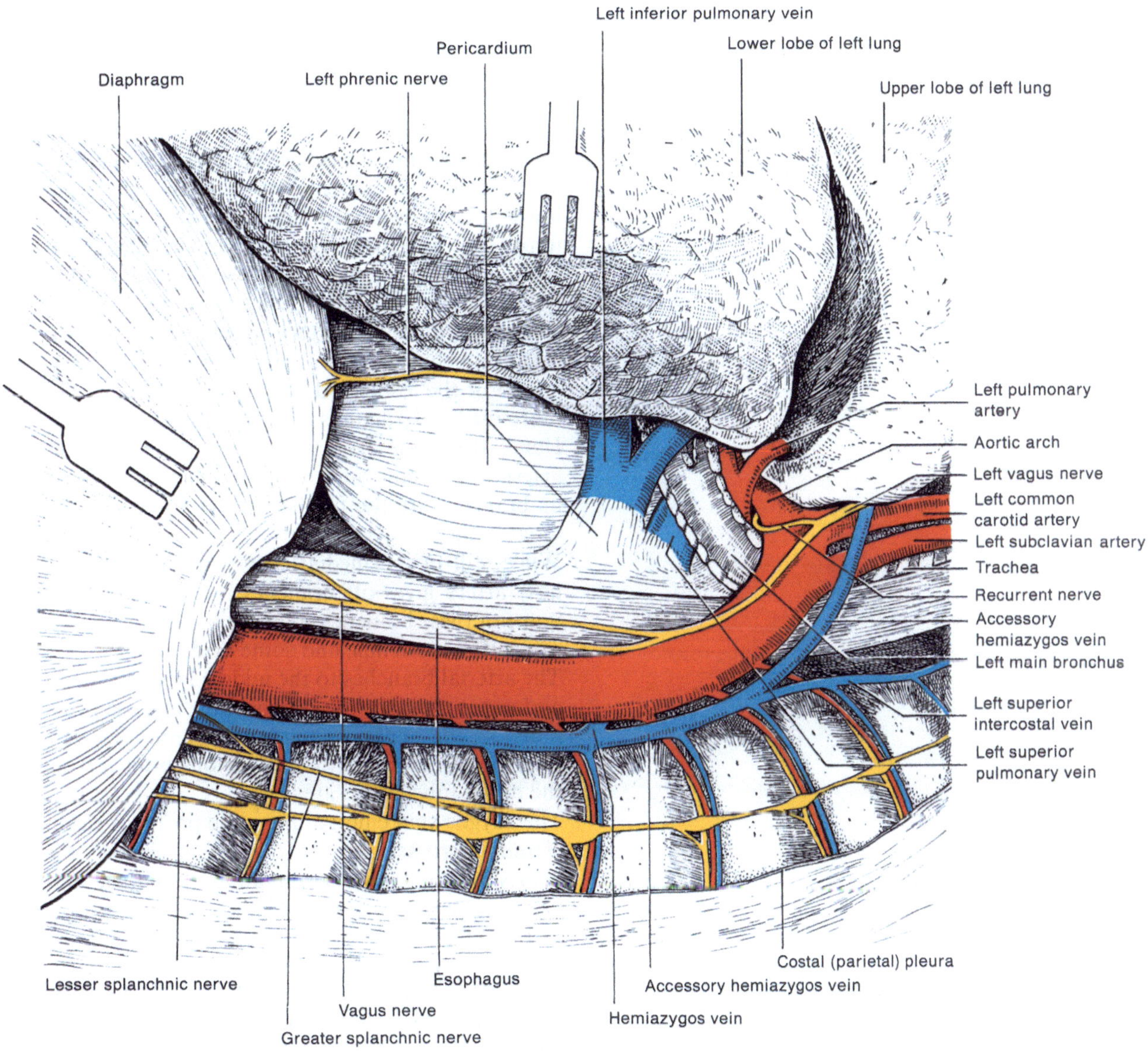
Left inferior pulmonary vein
Pericardium
Lower lobe of left lung
Diaphragm
Left phrenic nerve
Upper lobe of left lung
Left pulmonary artery
Aortic arch
Left vagus nerve
Left common carotid artery
Left subclavian artery
Trachea
Recurrent nerve
Accessory hemiazygos vein
Left main bronchus
Left superior intercostal vein
Left superior pulmonary vein
Costal (parietal) pleura
Lesser splanchnic nerve
Esophagus
Accessory hemiazygos vein
Vagus nerve
Hemiazygos vein
Greater splanchnic nerve

Plate XIII. View into the Oblique Fissure of the Right Lung

The right chest wall has been removed; the parietal and visceral pleurae are not shown. The right lower lobe is retracted far posteriorly, the right upper lobe anterosuperiorly, and the right middle lobe anteroinferiorly to expose the interlobar fissure, oblique fissure, of the right lung.

The right pulmonary artery crosses anterior to the main bronchus and, ramifying, passes to the lateral side of the lower and middle lobe bronchi. The most medial structures are the pulmonary veins. Hence the lobar bronchi are placed between the arteries and veins, and the pulmonary artery and its branches are the first structures to be encountered in the oblique fissure.

While still in the mediastinum, the right pulmonary artery gives off branches to the upper lobe. Some of these branches enter the upper lobe posterior to the bronchus, and some medial to it.

The arterial branches to the middle lobe are lateral and superior to the lobar bronchus, in close proximity to the superior pulmonary vein. The vein receives a posterior tributary venous branch from the upper lobe in this area.

The azygos vein emerges from the posterior mediastinum, crosses the right main bronchus, and "rides" on it before terminating at the superior vena cava.

In the inferior part of the posterior mediastinum, the lower portion of the esophagus is visible between the middle and lower pulmonary lobes. The right vagus nerve becomes the posterior vagal trunk on the right and posterior wall of the esophagus.

The bronchial arteries and veins are not shown, nor are the pulmonary plexus or the lymph vessels and nodes.

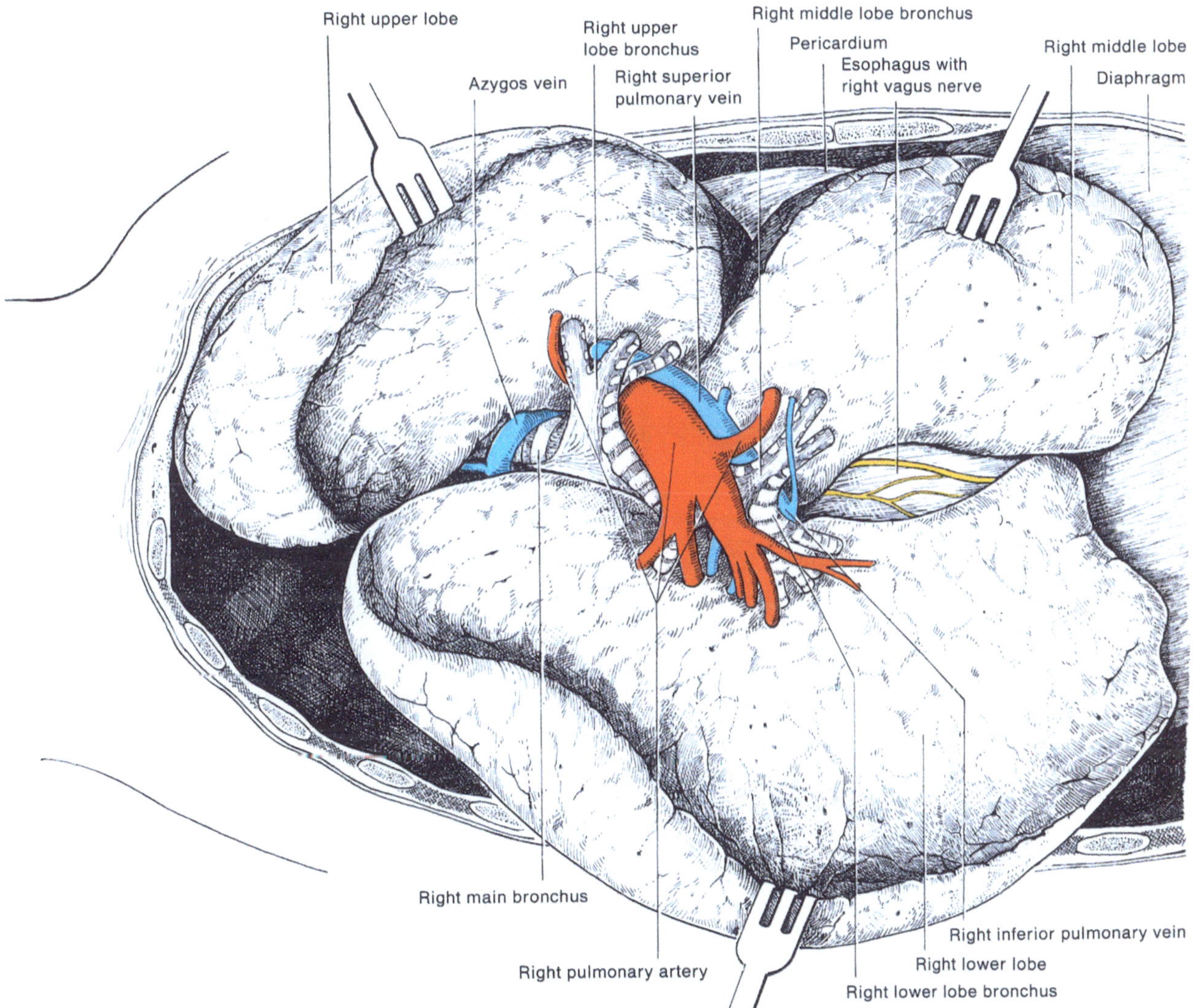

Right upper lobe
Right upper lobe bronchus
Right middle lobe bronchus
Pericardium
Right middle lobe
Azygos vein
Right superior pulmonary vein
Esophagus with right vagus nerve
Diaphragm
Right main bronchus
Right inferior pulmonary vein
Right lower lobe
Right pulmonary artery
Right lower lobe bronchus

Plate XIV. View into the Oblique Fissure of the Left Lung

The left hemithorax has been opened and most of the chest wall removed. The parietal and visceral pleurae are not shown. The left upper lobe is retracted anteriorly and superiorly, while the lower lobe is retracted posteriorly to give an unobstructed view into the interlobar fissure, the oblique fissure of the left lung.

The trunk of the left pulmonary artery crosses the left main bronchus, "riding" on its posterior surface. On the lateral side of the lobar bronchi the pulmonary artery ramifies, usually into four branches, that are distributed to the upper lobe and lingula and to the lower lobe, paralleling the bronchial divisions.

As on the right side, the left pulmonary veins are the most medial of the hilar structures. Only a few branches of the pulmonary veins are visible through the left oblique fissure. The pulmonary artery and its branches are encountered first, followed by the lobar bronchi, which occupy an intermediate position between the arteries and veins.

The thoracic aorta is posterior and medial to the vessels and bronchi of the left hilum. It is visible in the upper part of the interlobar fissure at its junction with the aortic arch. The left vagus nerve crosses the aortic arch, giving off the left recurrent laryngeal nerve superiorly, and disappears behind the pulmonary hilum, which it supplies with bronchial branches. The left phrenic nerve and pericardiacophrenic vessels course on the pericardium, which is covered by mediastinal pleura (not shown). The phrenic nerve supplies the pericardium and pleura with sensory fibers, and its trunk descends to the diaphragm, which it provides with motor and sensory innervation.

The bronchial arteries and veins, the pulmonary plexus, and the lymph nodes and vessels are not shown.

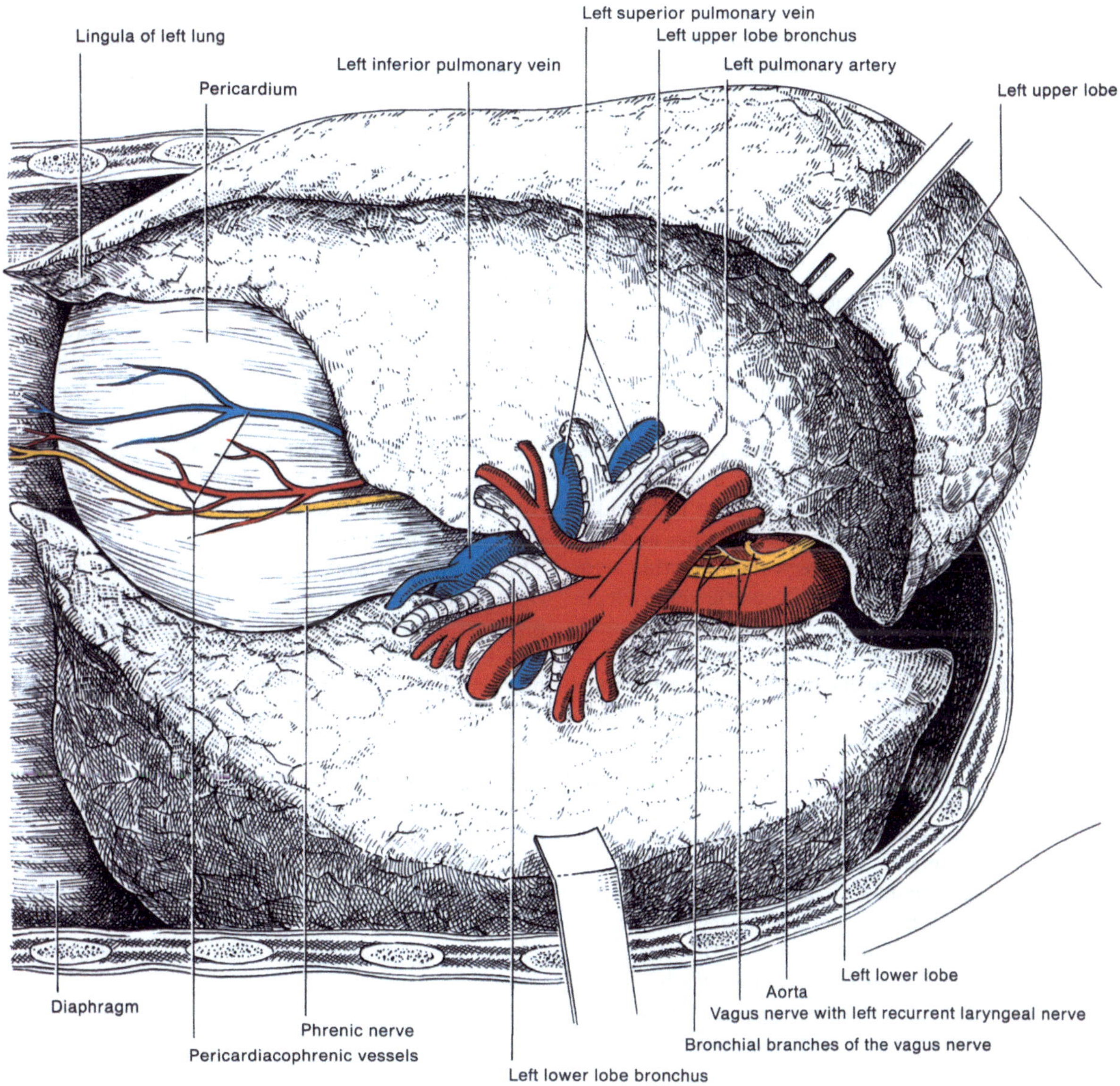
Left superior pulmonary vein
Left upper lobe bronchus
Lingula of left lung
Left inferior pulmonary vein
Left pulmonary artery
Pericardium
Left upper lobe
Left lower lobe
Aorta
Diaphragm
Vagus nerve with left recurrent laryngeal nerve
Phrenic nerve
Bronchial branches of the vagus nerve
Pericardiacophrenic vessels
Left lower lobe bronchus

Plate XV. Upper Abdomen about the Esophageal Hiatus and Lesser Curvature of the Stomach

The attachment of the falciform ligament on the superior surface of the liver marks the line of demarcation between the right and left hepatic lobes. (This division does not correspond to the lobation defined by the vascular structure of the liver.) In the drawing the right lobe is elevated slightly with a retractor while most of the left lobe has been resected, exposing the caudate lobe, the abdominal part of the esophagus, the gastric cardia, and structures in the lesser omentum.

The parietal and visceral peritoneum are not shown, nor are peritoneal folds such as the lesser omentum and its parts (hepatogastric and hepatoduodenal ligaments). All the biliary and vascular channels leading to or from the porta hepatis course within the hepatoduodenal ligament (not shown): the common bile duct on the right side, the hepatic artery proper on the left side, and the portal vein behind and between them. In this area the portal vein receives the left gastric vein, which drains the lesser curvature of the stomach and forms anastomoses with the inferior esophageal veins at the gastric cardia (portocaval anastomoses).

The common hepatic artery arises from the celiac trunk and, after giving off the gastroduodenal artery, reaches the porta hepatis as the hepatic artery proper. The cystic artery originates from the right branch of the hepatic artery proper to supply the wall of the gallbladder. The right gastric artery arises from the common hepatic artery (or the hepatic artery proper) and passes to the stomach, where it enters the arterial arcade of the lesser curvature. This arcade also receives blood from the left gastric artery, the smallest branch of the celiac trunk.

Behind the lesser curvature of the stomach, the omental tuberosity of the pancreas bulges into the omental bursa. The splenic artery, the third branch of the celiac trunk, disappears behind the stomach, which it supplies with short gastric arteries.

The celiac plexus with the celiac ganglia surrounds the origin of the celiac trunk from the aorta. It contains parasympathetic fibers mainly from the posterior vagal trunk, which traverses the diaphragm on the posterior wall of the esophagus. The splanchnic nerves (not visible), which arise from the 5th–11th thoracic ganglia of the sympathetic chain, transmit sympathetic fibers for the celiac plexus. The greater splanchnic nerve pierces the diaphragm together with the azygos or hemiazygos vein. The lesser splanchnic nerve accompanies it or pierces separately the lumbar attachment of the diaphragm.

The esophageal hiatus is bounded chiefly by the right medial crus of the lumbar part of the diaphragm, for a large fiber bundle of the right medial crus crosses to the left side, forming also the left margin of the hiatal opening.

The caudate lobe of the liver, separated from the left lobe by the fissure for the ligamentum venosum, largely obscures the inferior vena cava, which ascends in the sulcus venae cavae on the posterior surface of the liver. Three to five hepatic veins open into the inferior vena cava just before it traverses the diaphragm.

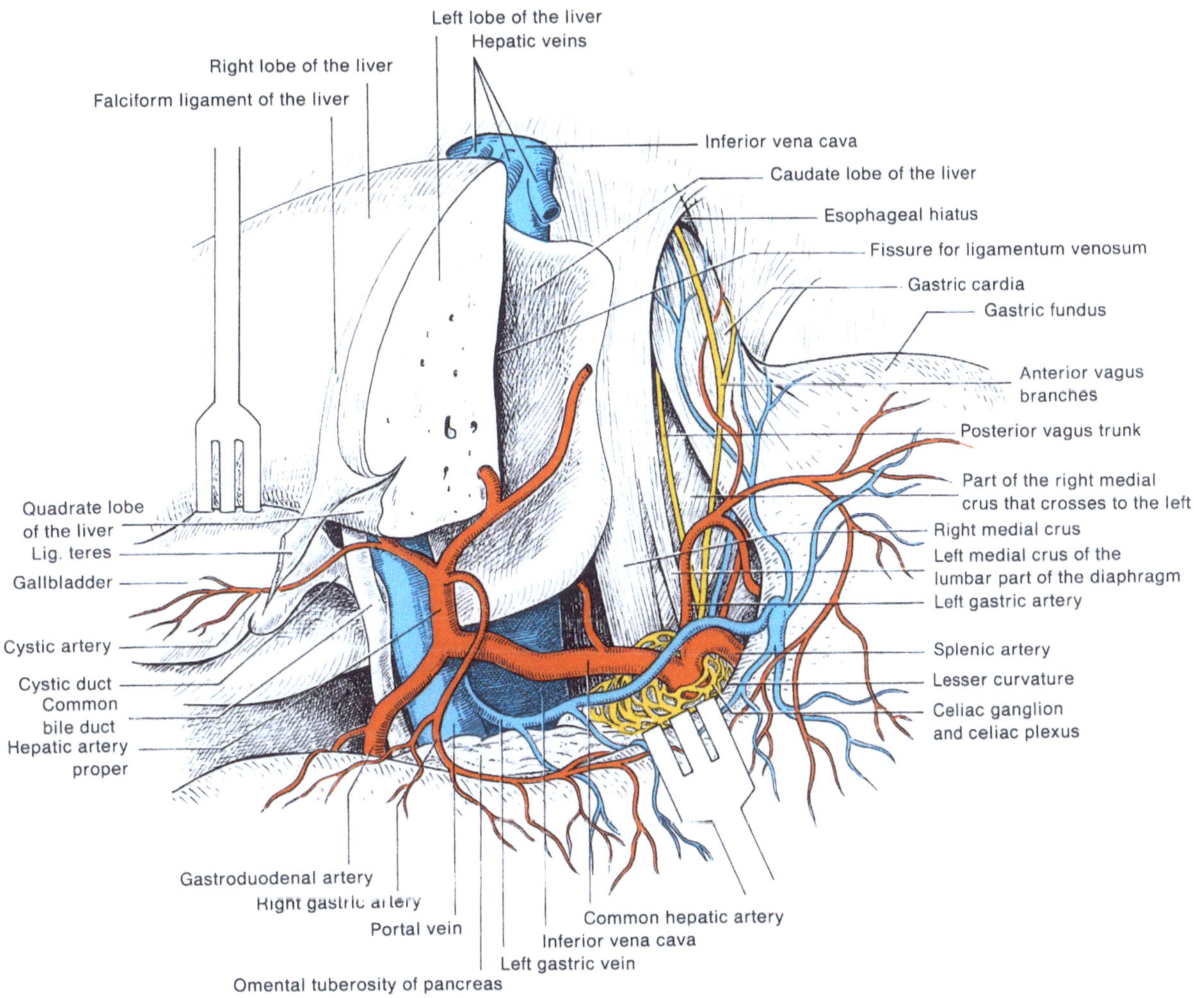
Left lobe of the liver
Hepatic veins
Right lobe of the liver
Falciform ligament of the liver
Inferior vena cava
Caudate lobe of the liver
Esophageal hiatus
Fissure for ligamentum venosum
Gastric cardia
Gastric fundus
Anterior vagus branches
Posterior vagus trunk
Part of the right medial crus that crosses to the left
Right medial crus
Left medial crus of the lumbar part of the diaphragm
Left gastric artery
Splenic artery
Lesser curvature
Celiac ganglion and celiac plexus
Quadrate lobe of the liver
Lig. teres
Gallbladder
Cystic artery
Cystic duct
Common bile duct
Hepatic artery proper
Gastroduodenal artery
Right gastric artery
Portal vein
Common hepatic artery
Inferior vena cava
Left gastric vein
Omental tuberosity of pancreas

K. Topography of Surgically Important Regions

15 Anatomic Plates

K. Zilles and U. Demmel

MIX
Papier aus verantwortungsvollen Quellen
Paper from responsible sources
FSC® C105338

If you have any concerns about our products,
you can contact us on
ProductSafety@springernature.com

In case Publisher is established outside the EU,
the EU authorized representative is:
Springer Nature Customer Service Center GmbH
Europaplatz 3, 69115 Heidelberg, Germany

Printed by Libri Plureos GmbH
in Hamburg, Germany